Dedication

To C.A.F.

Essentials of
Environmental Health

Second Edition

Robert H. Friis, PhD

Professor and Chair
Department of Health Science
California State University, Long Beach
Long Beach, California

JONES & BARTLETT
LEARNING

Jones & Bartlett Learning
40 Tall Pine Drive
Sudbury, MA 01776
978-443-5000
info@jblearning.com
www.jblearning.com

Jones & Bartlett Learning
Canada
6339 Ormindale Way
Mississauga, Ontario L5V 1J2
Canada

Jones & Bartlett Learning
International
Barb House, Barb Mews
London W6 7PA
United Kingdom

Jones & Bartlett Learning books and products are available through most bookstores and online booksellers. To contact Jones & Bartlett Learning directly, call 800-832-0034, fax 978-443-8000, or visit our website, www.jblearning.com.

Substantial discounts on bulk quantities of Jones & Bartlett Learning publications are available to corporations, professional associations, and other qualified organizations. For details and specific discount information, contact the special sales department at Jones & Bartlett Learning via the above contact information or send an email to specialsales@jblearning.com.

This publication is designed to provide accurate and authoritative information in regard to the Subject Matter covered. It is sold with the understanding that the publisher is not engaged in rendering legal, accounting, or other professional service. If legal advice or other expert assistance is required, the service of a competent professional person should be sought.

Production Credits
Publisher: Michael Brown
Associate Editor: Catie Heverling
Editorial Assistant: Teresa Reilly
Associate Production Editor: Kate Stein
Senior Marketing Manager: Sophie Fleck
Manufacturing and Inventory Control Supervisor: Amy Bacus
Composition: Publishers' Design and Production Services, Inc.
Art: diacriTech
Assistant Photo Researcher: Rebecca Ritter
Cover Design: Scott Moden
Cover, Section Opener, Chapter Opener, and Study Questions Image: © Szabo Photography/ShutterStock, Inc.
Background Images: Petri dish © Olivier Le Queinec/ShutterStock, Inc.; Crowd of people © Veer; Biohazard symbol © Richard C. Bennett/ShutterStock, Inc.; Poison symbol © Yobidaba/ShutterStock, Inc.; Radioactive symbol © WilleeCole/ShutterStock, Inc.
Printing and Binding: Malloy, Inc.
Cover Printing: John Pow Company

Library of Congress Cataloging-in-Publication Data
Friis, Robert H.
    Essentials of environmental health / Robert H. Friis. — 2nd ed.
            p. ; cm.
    Includes bibliographical references and index.
    ISBN-13: 978-0-7637-7890-3 (pbk.)
    ISBN-10: 0-7637-7890-7 (pbk.)
    1. Environmental health.   I. Title.
    [DNLM: 1. Environmental Health. 2.   Environmental Pollution.   WA 30.5]
    RA565.F75 2012
    616.9'8—dc22
                                                    2010027788
6048

Printed in the United States of America
14   13   12   11   10 9 8 7 6 5 4

Contents

The *Essential Public Health* Series

Essentials of Public Health Communication—Claudia Parvanta, PhD; David E. Nelson, MD, MPH; Sarah A. Parvanta, MPH; & Richard N. Harner, MD

Essentials of Public Health Ethics—Ruth Gaare Bernheim, JD, MPH & James F. Childress, PhD

Essentials of Management and Leadership in Public Health—Robert Burke, PhD & Leonard Friedman, PhD, MPH

Essentials of Public Health Preparedness—Rebecca Katz, PhD, MPH

ABOUT THE EDITOR:

Richard K. Riegelman, MD, MPH, PhD, is Professor of Epidemiology-Biostatistics, Medicine, and Health Policy, and Founding Dean of The George Washington University School of Public Health and Health Services in Washington, DC. He has taken a lead role in developing the Educated Citizen and Public Health initiative which has brought together arts and sciences and public health education associations to implement the Institute of Medicine of the National Academies' recommendation that "…all undergraduates should have access to education in public health." Dr. Riegelman also led the development of George Washington's undergraduate major and minor and currently teaches "Public Health 101" and "Epidemiology 101" to undergraduates.

Prologue

Dr. Robert Friis' *Essentials of Environmental Health* was the first book in the *Essential Public Health* Series. In the 4 years since the first edition was published, the importance of environmental health has been brought to the world's attention by crises and challenges ranging from oil spills to climate change, lead in toys, and pandemic influenza.

The second edition of *Essentials of Environmental Health* builds upon the first edition. It keeps up with the changes in environmental health to produce a state-of-the-art introductory text. The second edition provides a wide range of additions and updates including a new chapter on injuries, updates on pandemic flu, and coverage of recent environmental controversies, such as use of bisphenol A in plastics.

Dr. Friis also has produced a comprehensive website to accompany the text. The website provides the most recent information to broaden students' knowledge of environmental health. It also provides faculty with resources to challenge students and deepen their understanding of environmental health.

The *Essential Public Health* Series will soon include over 20 books, readers, and workbooks covering the full range of introductory texts. Dr. Friis has also authored *Epidemiology 101* as part of the series. *Epidemiology 101* is a core undergraduate public health text and a key component of the "101" approach to undergraduate public health education that also includes *Public Health 101* and *Global Health 101*. *Essentials of Environmental Health* has rapidly become a core text as well, key to a comprehensive curriculum in public health.

Dr. Friis brings to all his writing in environmental health and epidemiology a lifetime commitment to teaching, a personal connection to students as they begin their study of public health, and an impressive ability to clearly present complex subjects. I know that you will enjoy and benefit from this book.

Richard Riegelman, MD, MPH, PhD
Series Editor—*Essential Public Health*

Preface

When you follow the media, dramatic pictures and accounts of chemical spills, industrial fires, and other environmental disasters are not unusual. If you read the newspaper, surf the Internet, watch television, or merely observe what is happening around you, you will become aware of the environmental threats that are occurring on a worldwide scale. Within the past decade, public debate about global warming—a controversial topic—has escalated. Some worldwide climate changes such as extreme weather events have been attributed to global warming. The devastation caused by the August 2005 Hurricane Katrina in New Orleans was particularly moving. Other examples of extreme climate variations are increases in desertification in some parts of the world, while at the same time, other areas have experienced periodic massive flooding, such as Pakistan and China during summer 2010. As a consequence of the warming of the Earth's temperature, mountain glaciers, masses of ice in Greenland, and glaciers and sea ice in the Arctic region have been melting. Everyone should be concerned about the potential impact of these dramatic trends and incidents on the global physical environment and the health and survival of the world's population. At the same time, a hopeful attitude is warranted because of the progress that has been made in protecting environmental quality.

I have always been interested in the environment, especially the impact of rapid growth in California, my home state. During my lifetime, I have witnessed the conversion of pastoral northern California farmlands and orchards into densely populated urban zones with consequential environmental degradation. Although destruction of Brazilian rainforests is a focus of environmental advocates, wide swaths of the redwood forests of northern California and the wooded areas of the Pacific Northwest also are impacted by deforestation and are in need of protection.

In addition to urbanization in my home state, rapid growth has also been a global phenomenon. In my travels over the past decades, I have observed this phenomenon in Mexico and some parts of Europe. One example is the transformation of small cities in Baja, California into booming metropolises. Another example is the residential and commercial development that now fills the open, snow-covered fields that I traipsed through as a student in western Germany on the way to language classes. Despite urban growth, German cities have adopted exemplary programs for urban planning and recycling solid wastes. Other northern European countries, such as Sweden, have implemented development policies that preserve open space and encourage citizens to use public transportation. Member states of the European Union have been leaders in the development of wind and solar power, alternative fuels such as biodiesel, and energy-saving technologies.

Increasing population and development pressures affect southern Europe as well. As a result of water overdraft, some European cities along the Mediterranean have had salt water intrude into their public water supplies. When I first traveled to Europe as a student, I was impressed with the fact that people used bottled water instead of tap water, and later I began to understand why—most of the time, the tap water simply was not as palatable as bottled water. Nowadays, however, it is also common for people in the United States to tote around bottles of "prestige water," perhaps because of their fear of contaminants and microbes that may be present in the tap water. (In most cases, this fear is unwarranted because the quality of municipal tap water is highly regulated.)

Back in California, we now know that because of the introduction of toxic chemicals and pesticides, sewage contamination, and overfishing, our once abundant fisheries are declining and fishing must be limited. For example, it was once possible to consume fresh abalone, but now this delicious crustacean is almost unavailable from the wild due to excessive human predation. Seafood lovers are advised not to consume certain species of fish, which may be contaminated with mercury and other harmful substances.

During the spring and summer of 2010, a catastrophe at the Deepwater Horizon oil rig off the Louisiana coast caused the largest marine oil spill up to that time—about 5 million barrels. Aside from the immediate impact on wildlife and the fishing and tourism industries, the long-term environmental effects will require years to be ascertained. This catastrophe has called into question the safety of offshore oil drilling operations and focused attention on the adverse environmental consequences of oil extraction in general.

Still another concern is the impact of environmental factors on the safety of the global food supply. During late summer 2010, millions of eggs produced in the midwestern United States and sold widely by supermarket chains were found to be contaminated with *Salmonella* bacteria. Inspection of the poultry farms revealed that chickens were raised in despicable environmental conditions, which could contribute to the proliferation of *Salmonella* contamination. Within the past decade, other foodborne disease outbreaks in the United States have been associated with tomatoes (*Salmonella*) as well as lettuce and ground beef (*E. coli*). Noteworthy is the increasing internationalization of the world's food supply—adulterated and unsafe foodstuffs produced in one country can be shipped globally and threaten all of humanity. An example is the melamine-contaminated baby formula manufactured in China.

The picture is not entirely bleak, however; much progress has been made in informing the public about environmental health hazards and introducing regulations and procedures for the control of these hazards. Notable are the use of unleaded fuels and catalytic converters in automobiles to control air pollution and lead contamination. Not only have important environmental protections such as these been implemented in the United States, they also have been adopted by European countries and elsewhere.

Another example of a successful environmental policy that is now enforced in many parts of the world is the regulation of smoking in alcohol-serving establishments. This policy originated as California's Smokefree Bars Law, which controls occupational exposure to environmental tobacco smoke and also protects bar and restaurant patrons. At national and international levels, regulatory agencies conduct research and develop and enforce laws that control environmental health hazards. Although these efforts hold much promise for maintaining environmental quality, it must be kept in mind that policy and regulation are strongly influenced by the political process. Often economic considerations such as the need to maintain jobs and the prospect of increased taxation must be balanced against environmental protections.

This textbook addresses the major topics and methodological approaches in the environmental health field in order to provide a diversity of learners (from the beginning student to the experienced health professional) with an overview of the field. I believe that knowledge of environmental health issues can lead to an appreciation of humankind's connection with the earth and the precarious balance between human activities and environmental resources.

Robert H. Friis, PhD

Acknowledgments

My colleagues and students were extremely helpful in providing comments and background information necessary to complete this project. For the first edition of the book, I wish to thank the following former students: Ibtisam Khoury, Lillian Camacho, Sheetal Monga, Manohar Sukumar, and Heidi Burkey from California State University, Long Beach; and Nada Hamade from the University of California, Irvine. Students helped with literature searches, reviewed written text materials, and provided feedback. I also acknowledge the contributions of Dr. Robert Phalen and Dr. Yee-lean Lee, University of California, Irvine; Dr. Jan Semenza, European Center for Disease Prevention and Control; Dr. Glenn Paulson, School of Public Health, University of Medicine and Dentistry of New Jersey; and Dr. Michelle Saint-Germain and Dr. Javier Lopez-Zetina, California State University, Long Beach. These professional colleagues carefully reviewed chapters that were relevant to their areas of expertise. For the second edition, I express my gratitude to the following students who helped with literature searches and review of the text: Sarah Long, Paula Griego, Jane Kil, and Dexter Dizon.

Also, I would like to thank anonymous reviewers whose insightful comments greatly enhanced the quality of this text. Mike Brown, publisher for Jones & Bartlett Learning, provided continued encouragement and motivation for completion of the project; Jones & Bartlett Learning staff offered much expertise. Finally, my wife, Carol Friis, was involved extensively with this project—she provided detailed editorial comments, typed final versions of the document, verified the accuracy of the references, and helped with many other aspects of the project. Without her support and assistance, completion of the text would not have been possible.

About the Author

Robert H. Friis, PhD, is a Professor of Health Science and Chair of the Department of Health Science at California State University, Long Beach (CSULB), and Director of the CSULB Veterans Affairs Medical Center, Long Beach, Joint Studies Institute. Previously, he was a faculty member in the Department of Medicine, Department of Neurology, Department of Community and Environmental Medicine, and School of Social Ecology, University of California, Irvine. He is past president and a member of the Governing Council of the Southern California Public Health Association. He serves on the advisory boards of several health-related organizations, including the California Health Interview Survey. He is an epidemiologist by training and profession.

As a health department epidemiologist, Dr. Friis led investigations in environmental health problems such as chemical spills and air pollution. He has taught courses on environmental health at universities in New York City and southern California. He has conducted research and published and presented numerous papers related to tobacco use, mental health, chronic disease, disability, minority health, and psychosocial epidemiology. Dr. Friis has been the principal investigator or a coinvestigator on grants and contracts from the University of California's Tobacco-Related Disease Research Program, the National Institutes of Health, the METRANS program, and other agencies. This funding has supported investigations into topics such as geriatric health, depression in Hispanic populations, and nursing home infections. His interests have led him to conduct research in Mexico City and European countries. He has been a visiting professor at the Center for Nutrition and Toxicology, Karolinska Institute, Stockholm, Sweden; the Max Planck Institute, Munich, Germany; and two times at the Technical University of Dresden, Germany. He reviews articles for scientific journals, including *Public Health*, *Health Education Research*, *International Migration Review*, and *Social Science and Medicine*.

Dr. Friis is a fellow of the Royal Society for Public Health and a member of the Society for Epidemiologic Research and the American Public Health Association. He was awarded a postdoctoral fellowship for study at the Institute for Social Research, University of Michigan, and the Achievement Award for Scholarly and Creative Activity from California State University, Long Beach. His biography is listed in *Who's Who in America*.

He is author of *Epidemiology 101* (Jones & Bartlett Learning), senior author of *Epidemiology for Public Health Practice, Fourth Edition* (Jones & Bartlett Learning), coauthor of *Introductory Biostatistics for the Health Sciences* (Wiley), and editor of the *Praeger Handbook of Environmental Health* (Praeger).

Introduction

The purpose of this text is to inform the reader about the key areas of environmental health and instill awareness about the crucial role of the environment in the health of the planet and all living creatures. The second edition has been updated extensively to reflect the rapidly changing context of the environmental health field. Organized according to three major domains—background, environmental disease agents, and applications—the text begins with background material and "tools of the trade" (environmental epidemiology, environmental toxicology, and environmental policy and regulation). The text then covers specific agents of environmental diseases (e.g., microbial agents, toxic metals, pesticides, and ionizing and nonionizing radiation). Finally, applications and domains of environmental health are addressed (water and air quality, food safety, waste disposal, occupational health, and injuries).

This work is intended for graduate and undergraduate students who take environmental health courses in a variety of settings. Often, these courses are offered by schools of public health and health science departments. The text can also be used in online courses and instruction in intensive courses offered in a nontraditional format. Taking a nontechnical approach, the book should be accessible and interesting to students who have not had a great deal of previous introductory background, especially in the sciences. Nevertheless, the text should appeal to more advanced students as well. In order to generate interest in the subject matter, the author has included many examples and illustrations of environmental health issues. Text boxes provide detailed information on selected topics. Other learning aids are a list of learning objectives at the beginning of each chapter and study questions and exercises at the end.

A summary of the content of each chapter follows. Part I: Background of the Field, includes Chapters 1 through 4. Chapter 1 illustrates the role of environmental health in contemporary society, presents examples from the history of environmental health, and delimits the scope of the environmental health field; in addition, career opportunities are featured. Chapter 2 covers environmental epidemiology, one of the fundamental disciplines used in the study of environmental health. The subject of Chapter 3 is environmental toxicology, which, along with environmental epidemiology, is one of the key disciplines of the environmental health field. Chapter 4 focuses on environmental policy and regulation. Sometimes this content is placed near the end of environmental health textbooks. The author has elected to move it closer to the beginning because an appreciation of policy issues is crucial to the understanding of specific domains of environmental health. In addition, Chapter 4 contains extensive coverage of major environmental regulatory agencies and major U.S. environmental health laws. It is important to cover these topics early in the book because references to agencies and laws are made in the chapters that follow. The reader may want to use this material for reference and consult it later while reading the remaining chapters.

The next group of chapters, Part II: Agents of Environmental Disease, Chapters 5 through 8, covers agents of environmental disease. The respective topics are zoonotic and vector-borne diseases, toxic metals and elements, pesticides and other organic chemicals, and ionizing and nonionizing radiation. Part III: Applications of Environmental Health, Chapters 9 through

14 (Chapter 14 is new to the second edition), deals with applications of environmental health: water quality, air quality, food safety, solid and liquid wastes, occupational health, and injuries.

Other components of the textbook are a glossary of key definitions and a list of abbreviations. For additional information and learning aids that reinforce the didactic content of the textbook, the author recommends that readers access http://go.jblearning.com/friisEH. Some instructors enhance the learning experience by conducting field visits to environmentally relevant sites in the community (e.g., the municipal water plant). Other means to support the course are the use of videos and online resources.

Abbreviations

Term	Definition
APHIS	Animal and Plant Health Inspection Service (of USDA)
AQI	air quality index
ATSDR	Agency for Toxic Substances and Disease Registry
BHA	butylated hydroxyl anisole
BHT	butylated hydroxytoluene
BLL	blood lead level
BLS	Bureau of Labor Statistics
BRI	building-related illness
BSE	bovine spongiform encephalopathy
CAA	Clean Air Act
CDC	Centers for Disease Control and Prevention
CERCLA	Comprehensive Environmental Response, Compensation, and Liability Act, 1980
CFR	case fatality rate
CFSAN	Center for Food Safety and Applied Nutrition
CHD	coronary heart disease
Ci	Curie
CNS	central nervous system
CO	carbon monoxide
COHb	carboxyhemoglobin
COPD	chronic obstructive pulmonary disease
Cr(VI)	hexavalent chromium
CTS	carpal tunnel syndrome
CWP	coal workers' pneumoconiosis
dB	decibel

Term	Definition
DBPs	disinfection byproducts (of water)
DDT	dichlorodiphenyltrichloroethane
DES	diethylstilbestrol
DHF/DSS	dengue hemorrhagic fever/dengue shock syndrome
DHHS	Department of Health and Human Services
DNA	deoxyribonucleic acid
EBCLIS	EMF and Breast Cancer on Long Island Study
EDTA	ethylenediaminetetraacetic acid
EEA	European Environment Agency
EIA	environmental impact assessment
ELF	extremely low frequency radiation
EMF	electromagnetic field
EPA	U.S. Environmental Protection Agency
ETS	environmental tobacco smoke
EU	European Union
FAO	Food and Agricultural Organization (of United Nations)
FDA	Food and Drug Administration
FEMA	Federal Emergency Management Agency
FIFRA	Federal Insecticide, Fungicide, and Rodenticide Act, 1996
FoodNet	Foodborne Diseases Active Surveillance Network (of CDC)
FSIS	Food Safety and Inspection Service (of USDA)
FWS	Fish and Wildlife Service
GM	genetically modified
GRAS	generally recognized as safe
HACCP	hazard analysis of critical control points
HAV	hepatitis A virus
HBV	hepatitis B virus
HCV	hepatitis C virus
HIA	health impact assessment
HIV/AIDS	human immunodeficiency virus/acquired immunodeficiency syndrome
HPS	hantavirus pulmonary syndrome
HSEES	Hazardous Substances Emergency Events Surveillance (of ATSDR)
HUS	hemolytic uremic syndrome
IARC	International Agency for Research on Cancer
LD_{50}	lethal dose 50
MIC	methyl isocyanate
MM	malignant melanoma
MSD	musculoskeletal disorder

Term	Definition
MSG	monosodium glutamate
MSHA	Mine Safety and Health Administration
MSW	municipal solid waste
NAAQS	National Ambient Air Quality Standards
NCHS	National Center for Health Statistics
NEPA	National Environmental Policy Act, 1969
NIEHS	National Institute of Environmental Health Sciences
NIH	National Institutes of Health
NIOSH	National Institute for Occupational Safety and Health
NMSC	non-melanoma skin cancer
NO_x	nitrogen oxides
NORA	National Occupational Research Agenda
NPL	National Priorities List
NRDC	Natural Resources Defense Council
NTOF	National Traumatic Occupational Fatalities Surveillance System
NTP	National Toxicology Program
O_3	ozone
OAQPS	Office of Air Quality Planning and Standards (of EPA)
OECD	European Organization for Economic Cooperation and Development
OPs	organophosphates
OR	odds ratio
OSCAR	Osteoporosis with Cadmium as a Risk Factor [study]
OSHA	Occupational Safety and Health Administration
PAHs	polycyclic aromatic hydrocarbons
PAYT	pay-as-you-throw
PCBs	polychlorinated biphenyls
PEP	post-exposure prophylaxis
PM	particulate matter
POPs	persistent organic pollutants
ppb	parts per billion
PPCPs	pharmaceutical and personal care products
PPE	personal protective equipment
ppm	parts per million
PSP	paralytic shellfish poison
RCRA	Resource Conservation and Recovery Act, 1976
RDD	radiological dispersal device
RF	radio frequency
RMSF	Rocky Mountain spotted fever

Term	Definition
RR	relative risk
RVF	Rift Valley fever
SARA	Superfund Amendments and Reauthorization Act
SBS	sick building syndrome
SCE	sister chromatid exchange
SDWD	Safe Drinking Water Act
SI	System International
SMR	standardized mortality ratio
SO$_2$	sulfur dioxide
SPL	sound pressure level
TCDD	2,3,7,8-tetrachlorodibenzo-p-dioxin
TCE	trichloroethylene
TFR	total fertility rate
TLV	threshold limit value
TSCA	Toxic Substances Control Act, 1976
UNEP	United Nations Environment Programme
USDA	U.S. Department of Agriculture
USGS	United States Geological Survey
USPHS	U.S. Public Health Service
UVR	ultraviolet radiation
vCJD	Creutzfeldt-Jakob disease, new variant
VHF	viral hemorrhagic fever
VOCs	volatile organic compounds
VSP	Vessel Sanitation Program (operated by CDC)
WHO	World Health Organization
WNV	West Nile virus

PART I

Background of the Field

Introduction: The Environment at Risk

INTRODUCTION

This chapter will illustrate how environmental health relates to our lives and delimit the scope of the environmental health field. The author will define key terms used in environmental health, present some of the distinguishing features of the field, and introduce several of the basic concepts, which are essential to students of this discipline. For example, one of these concepts is the relationship between world population growth and the environment. Another concept relates to historically significant environmental events and how they influenced the topics that are of current importance to the environmental health field. An additional topic involves employment classifications, career roles, and opportunities for environmental health workers. The chapter will conclude with an overview of the textbook: the roles of **environmental epidemiology** and **toxicology**, policy aspects of environmental health, examples of environmentally related agents and diseases, and specific content areas of environmental health such as air quality, water quality, food safety, and waste disposal.

Maintaining environmental quality is a pressing task for the 21st century. Improvement in environmental quality is an official goal of the US government, as articulated in *Healthy People 2010.* This goal (number 8, Environmental Health) is formatted as follows: "Promote health for all through a healthy environment."[1(p55)] A list of environmental objectives is shown in Table 1-1. Note that *Healthy People 2020*, which will provide updated objectives, was not available as of this writing.

According to *Healthy People 2010:*

> Physical and social environments play major roles in the health of individuals and communities. The physical environment includes the air, water, and soil through which exposure to chemical, biological, and physical agents may occur. The social environment includes housing, transportation, urban development, land use, industry, and agriculture and results in exposures such as work-related stress, injury, and violence.[1(p41)]

Protecting the environment means creating a world in which the air is safe to breathe, the water is safe to drink, the land is arable and free from toxins, wastes are managed effectively, infectious diseases are kept at bay, and natural areas are preserved. Figure 1-1 illustrates a beautifully maintained natural area in the United States.

The requirements of a growing world population need to be balanced against the demands for environmental preservation. Although developed countries such as the United

TABLE 1-1 Objectives for *Healthy People 2010*—Goal Number 8, Environmental Health: Promote Health for All through a Healthy Environment

Outdoor Air Quality
8-1 Harmful air pollutants
8-2 Alternative modes of transportation
8-3 Cleaner alternative fuels
8-4 Airborne toxins

Water Quality
8-5 Safe drinking water
8-6 Waterborne disease outbreaks
8-7 Water conservation
8-8 Surface water health risks
8-9 Beach closings
8-10 Fish contamination

Toxics and Waste
8-11 Elevated blood lead levels in children
8-12 Risks posed by hazardous sites
8-13 Pesticide exposures
8-14 Toxic pollutants
8-15 Recycled municipal solid waste

Healthy Homes and Healthy Communities
8-16 Indoor allergens
8-17 Office building air quality
8-18 Homes tested for radon

8-19 Radon-resistant new home construction
8-20 School policies to protect against environmental hazards
8-21 Disaster preparedness plans and protocols
8-22 Lead-based paint testing
8-23 Substandard housing

Infrastructure and Surveillance
8-24 Exposure to pesticides
8-25 Exposure to heavy metals and other toxic chemicals
8-26 Information systems used for environmental health
8-27 Monitoring environmentally related diseases
8-28 Local agencies using surveillance data for vector control

Global Environmental Health
8-29 Global burden of disease
8-30 Water quality in the US-Mexico border region

Source: Data from US Department of Health and Human Services. *Healthy People 2010: Understanding and Improving Health.* 2nd ed. Washington, DC: US Government Printing Office; November 2000:55.

States have made substantial progress in clearing the air and reducing air pollution, significant challenges to the environment and human health remain. For example, among the current and continuing threats to the environment in the United States are the following: trash that fouls our beaches, hazardous wastes (including radioactive wastes) leaching from disposal sites, continuing episodes of air pollution in some areas, exposures to toxic chemicals, and destruction of the land through deforestation.

The hallmarks of environmental degradation are not difficult to find: Warning signs posted on beaches advise bathers not to enter ocean water that is unsafe because of sewage contamination. In some areas of the United States, drinking water is threatened by toxic chemicals that are leaching from disposal sites. Factories in some areas continue to belch thick, black smoke. Avoidance of air pollution, which at best insults our aesthetic senses and at worst endangers our health, is often impossible. Society's appetite for lumber and new housing to satisfy the burgeoning population has resulted in clear-cutting of forests and destruction of wildlife habitats in order to accommodate new habitations for humans.

Pollution and population growth, often associated with adverse economic circumstances, are closely connected with environmental health. In his classic article, Professor Warren Winkelstein wrote that "the three P's—pollution, population, and poverty—are principal determinants of health worldwide. . . ."[2(p932)] The three P's are interrelated: Population growth is associated with poverty, and both poverty and population growth are associated with pollution.

An example of the first "P" is pollution from combustion of fossil fuels (e.g., petroleum and coal), which disperses greenhouse gases along with other pollutants into the atmosphere. This process is believed to be a cause of global warming that in turn may have wide-ranging effects. One such effect is to advance the range of disease-carrying insects, bringing them into new geographic areas; for example, mosquito-borne diseases such as the West Nile virus and dengue fever may appear in areas that previously were free from these conditions. (Refer to Chapter 5 for more information.) The second "P" is population, which is growing exponentially in many parts of the world, especially the less developed areas, and may result in a worldwide population of up to 10 to 12 billion people during the 21st century; the presence of so many people may exceed the carrying capacity (defined later in the chapter) of the earth by a factor of two. The third "P," poverty, is linked to population growth; poverty is one of the well-recognized determinants of adverse health outcomes.

A recent environmentally related adverse health outcome may be attributed, at least in part, to one of the three P's: population growth (which is associated with urban crowding). As a result of known and unknown environmental and other factors, threats to the human population periodically arise from infectious disease agents. (This topic is discussed in Chapter 5.) For example, influenza viruses threaten the world's population from time to time. Environmental fac-

FIGURE 1-1 A natural ecosystem in the United States. Maintaining environmental quality is a pressing task for the 21st century.

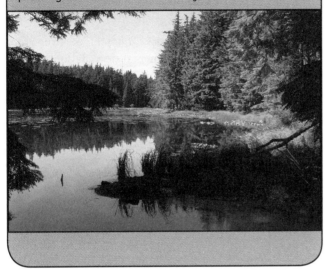

tors that are likely to advance the spread of influenza viruses include intensive animal husbandry practices needed to supply food to the world's growing population. These practices create extremely crowded conditions among food animals coupled with their close residential proximity to humans. Several years ago, public health officials became concerned about the possible occurrence of a human pandemic of avian influenza, caused by the avian influenza A (H5N1) virus. Large outbreaks of avian influenza occurred on poultry farms in Asia. Apparently, some transmission of the virus from birds to humans also occurred. The disease (called bird flu) produces a severe human illness that has a high fatality rate. Health officials were concerned that the virus might mutate, enabling human-to-human transmission; if human-to-human transmission of the virus erupted, a pandemic might result. In addition, contributing to the possible epidemic transmission of influenza (and other communicable diseases) is the ability of human beings to travel rapidly from one area of the globe to another. Exhibit 1-1 presents a case study of pandemic influenza (H1N1). In 2009, swine flu (H1N1 influenza) spread through North America to other parts of the globe. The World Health Organization (WHO) declared a pandemic.

SIGNIFICANCE OF THE ENVIRONMENT FOR HUMAN HEALTH

The environment is intimately connected with human health, illness, and mortality: Some estimates place the toll of the world's deaths caused by environmental factors at 40%.[3] Ex-

posures to potentially hazardous agents such as microbes, toxic chemicals and metals, pesticides, and ionizing radiation account for many of the forms of environmentally associated morbidity (acute and chronic conditions, allergic responses, and disability) and mortality that occur in today's world. These environmentally related determinants are believed to be important for the development of chronic diseases such as cancer, although most chronic diseases are thought to be the result of complex interactions between environmental and genetic factors.[4] All human beings are affected in some way by exposure to environmental hazards associated with lifestyle: at work, at home, during recreation, or while traveling on the expressway. Table 1-2 provides examples of the scope of disease burden associated with exposure to environmental hazards.

TABLE 1-2 The Scope of Environmental Health Problems in the World and the United States

Some estimates report that 25% to 33% of the global burden of disease is linked to environmental sources.

During the late 1900s, approximately 1.2 billion pounds of potentially neurotoxic chemicals were released into the air and waterways in the United States.

Elevated blood levels of lead continue to be an important problem in the United States with nearly 1 million children exceeding the threshold for acceptable blood lead levels.

The prevalence and mortality of asthma in the United States have increased since 1980 by 58% and 78%, respectively.

Exposure to toxic chemicals is thought to cause as many as 3% of developmental and neurological problems in children in the United States.

Using air quality standards established by the World Health Organization (WHO), experts have estimated that 1.3 billion of the world's urban inhabitants breathe air that exceeds these quality standards.

Environmental factors are thought to contribute significantly to many forms of cancer, including cervical cancer, prostate cancer, and breast cancer.

Definition of terms used in the table:

Burden of disease is defined as "The total significance of disease for society beyond the immediate cost of treatment. It is measured in years of life lost to ill health as the difference between total life expectancy and disability-adjusted life expectancy."[5]

Life expectancy refers to the expectation of the number of years of life at birth; **disability-adjusted life expectancy** refers to the number of years of healthy life expected in a particular population.[5]

Source: Data from PG Butterfield. Upstream reflections on environmental health: An abbreviated history and framework for action. *Advances in Nursing Science.* 2002;25:34.

Vulnerable Subgroups of the Population

The elderly, persons with disabilities and chronic diseases, pregnant women, and children are more likely to be affected by environmental hazards than are members of the general population. For example, children represent an especially vulnerable group with respect to exposure to hazardous materials, including pesticides and toxic chemicals. Their immune systems and detoxifying organs are still developing and are not fully capable of responding to environmental toxins.[6] Children may be exposed more often than adults to toxic chemicals in the ambient outdoor air and in the soil because they spend more time outside.[7,8]

Environmental Health and the Developing World

Residents of developing countries suffer far more from problems associated with environmental degradation than do those who live in developed countries; this observation holds true despite the fact that developed countries are highly industrialized and disseminate vast quantities of pollutants

---

Exhibit 1-1

CASE STUDY:
Pandemic Influenza (H1N1) 2009

On April 17, 2009, the CDC determined that two cases of febrile respiratory illness occurring in children who resided in adjacent counties in southern California were caused by infection with a swine influenza A (H1N1) virus. . . . Neither child had contact with pigs; the source of the infection is unknown. . . . Although this is not a new subtype of influenza A in humans, concern exists that this new strain of swine influenza A (H1N1) is substantially different from human influenza A (H1N1) viruses, that a large proportion of the population might be susceptible to infection, and that the seasonal influenza vaccine H1N1 strain might not provide protection. The lack of known exposure to pigs in the two cases increases the possibility that human-to-human transmission of this new influenza virus has occurred.

Since April 21, 2009, the CDC has reported cases of respiratory infection with a swine-origin influenza A (H1N1) virus (S-OIV) transmitted through human-to-human contact. . . . As of April 28, the total number of confirmed cases of S-OIV infection in the United States had increased to 64, with cases in California (10 cases), Kansas (two), New York (45), Ohio (one), and Texas (six).

Since mid-April 2009, the CDC, state and local health authorities in the United States, the World Health Organization (WHO), and health ministries in several countries have been responding to an outbreak of influenza caused by a novel influenza A (H1N1) virus. In March and early April 2009, Mexico experienced outbreaks of respiratory illness subsequently confirmed by the CDC and Canada to be caused by the novel virus. The influenza strain identified in US patients was genetically similar to viruses isolated from patients in Mexico. . . . On April 29, the WHO raised the level of pandemic alert from phase 4 to phase 5, indicating that human-to-human spread of the virus had occurred in at least two countries in one WHO region. The government of Mexico has instituted several measures to slow disease transmission and reduce mortality, including closure of all schools and avoidance of large public gatherings.

The emergence and spread of the 2009 pandemic influenza A (H1N1) virus (2009 H1N1) resulted in extraordinary influenza activity in the United States throughout the summer and fall months of 2009. . . . During this period, influenza activity reached its highest level in the week ending October 24, 2009, with 49 of 50 states reporting geographically widespread disease. As of January 9, 2010, overall influenza activity had declined substantially. Since April 2009, the dominant circulating influenza virus in the United States has been 2009 H1N1.

February 5, 2010—As of January 31, 2010, worldwide more than 209 countries and overseas territories or communities have reported laboratory confirmed cases of pandemic influenza H1N1 2009, including at least 15,174 deaths.

Source: Adapted and reprinted from the Centers for Disease Control and Prevention. Swine influenza A (H1N1) infection in two children—Southern California, March–April 2009. *MMWR.* 2009;58:400; the Centers for Disease Control and Prevention. Update: Infections with a swine-origin influenza A (H1N1) virus—United States and other countries, April 28, 2009. *MMWR.* 2009;58:431; the Centers for Disease Control and Prevention. Update: Novel influenza A (H1N1) virus infections—worldwide, May 6, 2009. *MMWR.* 58:453; the Centers for Disease Control and Prevention. Update: Influenza activity—United States, August 30, 2009–January 9, 2010. *MMWR.* 2010;59:38; and the World Health Organization. Pandemic (H1N1) 2009—update 86. Weekly update. Available at: http://www.who.int/csr/don/2010_02_5/en. Accessed February 7, 2010.

into the environment from industrial processes and motor vehicles. In comparison with developing countries, wealthy nations provide better access to medical care and are better able to finance pollution controls.

In the developing world, the pursuit of natural resources has caused widespread deforestation of tropical rain forests and destruction of wildlife habitat. Although these two issues have been the focus of much publicity, less widely publicized environmental hazards such as water contamination, air pollution, unsanitary food, and crowding take a steep toll in both morbidity and mortality in developing countries.[9]

One region of the world that at present confronts serious environmental threats is Asia. Many of the countries in this region are experiencing declines in the amount of forest land, unintentional conversion of arable land to desert, and rising levels of pollution. In order to meet the demands of the rapidly increasing populations of South Asia, rural farmers clear forests and cultivate land that erodes easily and eventually becomes useless for agriculture.[10] **Runoff** from the land contributes to water pollution. The world's most populous country, China, faces many challenging environmental problems including water shortages in the northwest; severe air pollution in major cities, such as Beijing; and increasing desertification.[11]

Environmental Risk Transition

The term **environmental risk transition** has been used to characterize changes in environmental risks that happen as a consequence of economic development in the less developed regions of the world. Environmental risk transition is characterized by the following circumstances:

> In the poorest societies, household risks caused by poor food, air, and water quality tend to dominate. The major risks existing in developing countries today are of this type—diarrhea is attributable to poor water/sanitation/hygiene, acute respiratory diseases to poor housing and indoor air pollution from poor quality household fuels, and malaria to poor housing quality, although all are of course influenced by other factors as well (malnutrition in particular). . . . As these problems are brought under control, a new set tends to be created at the regional and global level through long-term and long-range pollutants, such as acid rain precursors, ozone-depleting chemicals, and greenhouse gases.[12(p38)]

POPULATION AND THE ENVIRONMENT

Currently increasing at a geometric rate, the human population threatens to overwhelm available resources; some areas of the world face periodic food scarcity and famine. A number of factors have contributed to population growth, including increases in fertility and reductions in mortality. One of the consequences of population growth has been to encourage the conversion of large rural and forested areas of the earth into cities. Urbanization is linked to numerous adverse implications for the health of populations, including increasing rates of morbidity and mortality. Refer to the following text box, which discusses the consequences of continued population growth.

Population Growth Trends

The human population has grown exponentially over the past 200 years and reached the figure of 6 billion in June 1999.[13] The current trend is for world population growth to continue at a high rate, as noted in the following passage:

> Every day we share the earth and its resources with 250,000 more people than the day before. Every year there are another 90 million mouths to feed. That is the equivalent of adding a city the size of Philadelphia to the world population every week; a Los Angeles every two weeks; a Mexico every year; and a United States and Canada every three years.[14(p30)]

Homo Sapiens—A Suicidal Species?

Largely as a result of human action, profound changes are occurring in our environment. . . . The basic cause of almost all of these problems is the world's large and growing human population, which consumes so much energy and produces such large quantities of toxic wastes. . . . Environmental changes, if accompanied by economic and political instability, could lead to the collapse of organized health services. In an era of scarcities of food, water, and other resources, and of a threat to survival, priorities should be reassessed.[15(pp121,123)]

Figure 1-2 characterizes this burgeoning growth for a single year—2002. During that year the world population increased by 2⅓ persons per second, or 141 persons per minute. This annual growth rate would be equivalent to a Boeing 737 jetliner carrying a new group of 141 passengers each minute.

From the origin of the species *Homo sapiens* (assumed to be about 250,000 years ago) to AD 1800, the population of the world grew by 1 billion individuals.[16] From 1800 to 1922 (122 years), the population added another 1 billion persons. Since 1922, the population has increased at a phenomenal rate: another billion persons were added after 37 years, 15 years, and 13 years, respectively. Only 12 years elapsed before an additional billion persons were added between 1987 and 1999. See Figure 1-3.

Another perspective on population growth is the time that it takes for the population to double. From 1931 to 1974 (a 43-year interval), the earth's population doubled; it is projected to double again during approximately the same interval (1974 to 2018).[17] Estimates suggest that the world's population will reach 8 billion persons between the years 2018 and 2028.

In 1950, the world's five most populous countries were China, India, the United States, Russia, and Japan; at the turn of the 21st century, Russia and Japan were replaced by Indonesia and Brazil. In 2050, India will become the world's most populous country; China will fall to second place, the United States will remain in third place, Indonesia will be in fourth place, and Brazil will be replaced by Nigeria.

Around the 1960s, annual rates of population increase topped out at slightly more than 2% (an 81 million absolute increase annually since the 1980s).[18] Demographers project that the human population eventually may stabilize at a size—about 10 billion persons—that is about three quarters larger than it was around 2000.

Population Dynamics

The term **population dynamics** refers to the ever-changing interrelationships among the set of variables that influence the demographic makeup of populations as well as the variables that influence the growth and decline of population sizes. Among the factors that relate to the size as well as the age and sex composition of populations are fertility, death rates, and migration.

Fertility

One of the measures of fertility is the **total fertility rate (TFR)**, which "is a hypothetical estimate of completed fertility. It indicates how many births a woman would have by the end of her reproductive life. . . ."[19(p1)] (A definition of a statistical weighting procedure that is used to compute the TFR is beyond the scope of this text.) In the United States, the fertility rate fluctuates from around 2.0 to 2.1 births per woman; the natural population replacement rate is estimated to be 2.1.[19] During the baby boom era at the end of the 1950s, the US fertility rate exceeded 3.5 births per woman. Presently, Western European countries have low fertility rates; also, the rates are declining in most regions of the developing world.[20] The United States, Canada, Japan, South Korea, Thailand, China, and many countries in Europe are at or below the replacement rate for fertility. Despite the declines in fertility rates in some Asian countries to lev-

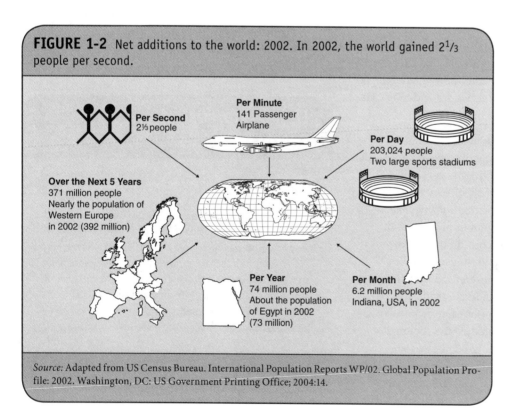

FIGURE 1-2 Net additions to the world: 2002. In 2002, the world gained 2⅓ people per second.

Per Second
2⅓ people

Per Minute
141 Passenger Airplane

Per Day
203,024 people
Two large sports stadiums

Over the Next 5 Years
371 million people
Nearly the population of Western Europe in 2002 (392 million)

Per Year
74 million people
About the population of Egypt in 2002 (73 million)

Per Month
6.2 million people
Indiana, USA, in 2002

Source: Adapted from US Census Bureau. International Population Reports WP/02. Global Population Profile: 2002. Washington, DC: US Government Printing Office; 2004:14.

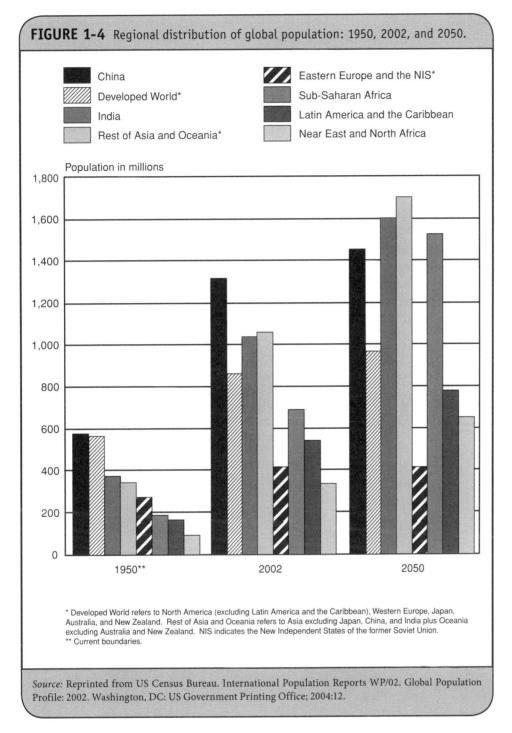

FIGURE 1-4 Regional distribution of global population: 1950, 2002, and 2050.

Legend:
- China
- Developed World*
- India
- Rest of Asia and Oceania*
- Eastern Europe and the NIS*
- Sub-Saharan Africa
- Latin America and the Caribbean
- Near East and North Africa

Population in millions

* Developed World refers to North America (excluding Latin America and the Caribbean), Western Europe, Japan, Australia, and New Zealand. Rest of Asia and Oceania refers to Asia excluding Japan, China, and India plus Oceania excluding Australia and New Zealand. NIS indicates the New Independent States of the former Soviet Union.
** Current boundaries.

Source: Reprinted from US Census Bureau. International Population Reports WP/02. Global Population Profile: 2002. Washington, DC: US Government Printing Office; 2004:12.

In comparison with the developed world, the fertility rates are considerably higher (at about 4.0 births per woman) in many Asian countries, Latin American countries, and African countries. In the future, their relatively higher fertility rates will enable these regions of the developing world to claim the largest population sizes. (See Figure 1-4.)

Mortality

Mortality has declined markedly over time in both industrialized and less developed countries. Adult mortality and infant and child mortality have demonstrated downward trends. Declining mortality in the developed world began approximately 200 years ago; in the developing world, substantial declines in mortality have occurred more recently during the past 50 years or so. The reduction in mortality has been accomplished through measures that have included public health improvements, famine control, and increased availability of drugs and vaccines.

Migration

Migration contributed to population growth in many areas of the world. However, migrants tend to cluster in a limited group of nations located in North America, Europe, and the former Soviet Union. In 2005, the three leading countries for receiving international migrants were the United States, Russia, and Germany.[21] Reasons for migration include the search for economic betterment, escape from persecution for religious and political reasons, and relief from unstable conditions in one's home country. Census estimates indicate that by the year 2050, the US population will grow by

els approaching replacement rates, the populations in these countries will continue to increase because of births among the large cohort of persons of childbearing age who were born when fertility rates were high. Those individuals form a substantial proportion of the population in China and other rapidly industrializing countries.

another 100 million and that about one-third of this growth will be from migration.

Demographic Transition

Demographic transition is the alteration over time in a population's fertility, mortality, and makeup.[13] (Note that demographic transition theory does not include the effects of migration upon the age and sex composition of a population.) According to the demographic transition theory, developed societies have progressed through three stages that have affected their age and sex distributions.

The three phases can be demonstrated by hypothetical population pyramids, which are graphs that show the distribution of a population according to age and sex. Examples of the population pyramids at stages 1 through 3 are shown in Figure 1-5. Stage 1 characterizes a population at the first stage of demographic transition when most of the population is young and fertility and mortality rates are high; overall,

the population remains small. Stage 2 shows a drop in mortality rates that occurs during the demographic transition; at this stage fertility rates remain high, and there is a rapid increase in population, particularly among the younger age groups. In comparison with the narrow triangular shape of the population distribution at Stage 1, this population pyramid also is triangular in shape but has a wider base. Stage 3 reflects dropping fertility rates that cause a more even distribution of the population according to age and sex.

Epidemiologic Transition

The term **epidemiologic transition** is used to describe a shift in the pattern of morbidity and mortality from causes related primarily to infectious and communicable diseases to causes associated with chronic, degenerative diseases. The epidemiologic transition accompanies the demographic transition. The epidemiologic transition already has taken place in the populations of most developed countries (a process that re-

FIGURE 1-5 The demographic transition in three stages of age and sex composition: stage 1 (left), stage 2 (middle), and stage 3 (right).

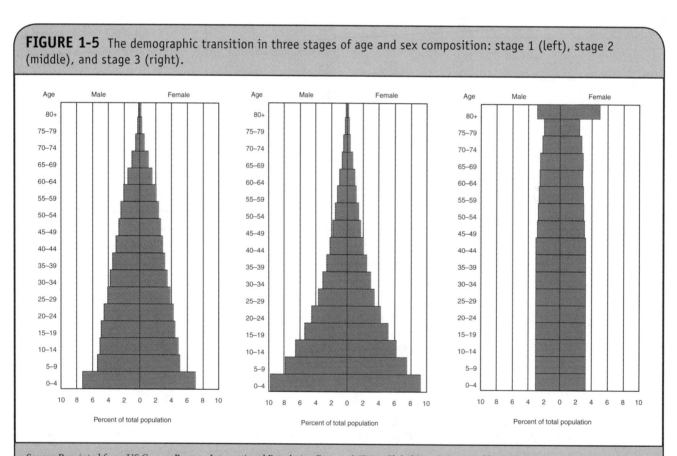

Source: Reprinted from US Census Bureau. International Population Reports WP/02. Global Population Profile: 2002. Washington, DC: US Government Printing Office; 2004:35.

quired approximately one century) but has not occurred yet in many developing countries.

One reflection of the epidemiologic transition is the growing burden of chronic, degenerative diseases, especially in developed countries and to a lesser extent in developing countries, as a consequence of population aging. Chronic, degenerative diseases include cardiovascular diseases, cancer, neuropsychiatric conditions, and injuries; these conditions are becoming the major causes of disability and premature death in many nations. Nevertheless, in developing countries communicable and infectious diseases remain the leading causes of morbidity and mortality.

Consequences of Population Increases

Rapid growth of the world's population contributes to the deterioration of the environment through widespread depletion of natural resources and by causing the levels of air, water, and other forms of pollution to increase. Also, the resources available per person decrease as the total number of individuals on the planet continues to increase geometrically. Consequently, population growth is a determinant of the number of persons who live in poverty. In already-crowded regions, an even larger population means that the size of most people's living spaces must decline and population density must increase. Population density and associated urban crowding are dimensions of environmental degradation associated with increases in the spread of infectious and communicable diseases.

Unless significant technological innovations can be introduced, merely feeding the world's hungry population will become problematic. Many developing countries, where population growth rates are among the highest in the world, are reaching the limit of their abilities to provide for the economic and social needs of their citizens. The United Nations Secretariat states that

> excessive population pressure in specific geographical areas can pose serious ecological hazards, including soil erosion, desertification, dwindling supplies of firewood, deforestation and the degradation of sources of fresh water. Often the link between population pressure and those types of environmental stress is the growth in the relative and absolute number of persons living in poverty. The result is marginalization of small-scale farmers and pressure on larger numbers to migrate from distressed areas. In many cases the result is also the prevalence of environmentally-related diseases.[22(p32)]

The effects of rapid growth of the world's population include:

- Urbanization
- Overtaxing carrying capacity (defined later in this chapter)
- Food insecurity
- Loss of biodiversity

Urbanization and the Environment

The past two centuries have seen a rapid increase in the number of cities over the entire globe.[23] The proportion of urban residents has increased from about 5% in 1800 to 50% in 2000 and is expected to reach about 66% by 2030. Figure 1-6 illustrates the growth of the world's urban population between 1974 and 2000 for developing and developed countries.[22] Although the proportion of urban residents has increased in both categories, a relatively larger growth in the number of urban residents is projected to occur among developing countries. This trend is apparent in the figure and is forecast to continue into the future.

The factors that lead to urbanization include industrialization, food availability, employment opportunities, lifestyle considerations, and escape from political conflict.[23] Tied to increases in urbanization are numerous adverse health impacts, particularly in developing countries. Among the most important causes of morbidity and early death in urban environments of developing countries are environmentally related diseases and accidents.[24] According to McMichael:

> Large cities in the least developed countries typically combine the traditional environmental health problems of poverty, particularly respiratory and enteric infections, with those of poor quality housing and unregulated industrialization. Residents therefore are often at **risk** from diseases and injuries associated with poor sanitation, unsafe drinking-water, dangerous roads, polluted air, indoor air pollution and toxic wastes.[23(p1119)]

The following text box lists hazards associated with the urban environment.

Megacities

The term **megacity** denotes an urbanized area that has 10 million or more inhabitants; at the beginning of the 21st century, there were 25 megacities that contained slightly more than 4% of the world's population.[25] Examples of megacities

FIGURE 1-6 Population distribution in urban and rural areas (billions).

and their respective populations in millions are Tokyo (27.9), Mumbai (formerly known as Bombay) (18.1), Sao Paulo (17.8), Shanghai (17.2), and Mexico City (16.4). The two megacities in the United States are New York (16.6) and Los Angeles (13.1). Megacities have major influences upon the environment in a number of ways (e.g., demands for energy, potable water, construction materials, food, sewage processing, and solid waste disposal). Figure 1-7 shows street life in a crowded megacity.

Carrying Capacity

Carrying capacity is "[t]he population that an area will support without undergoing environmental deterioration."[26] Both human and nonhuman populations may be threatened with disastrous consequences when available resources are exhausted. "Like a bacterial colony in a culture medium, we are susceptible to depletion of nutriments and to poisoning by our own waste products."[15(p123)]

Hazards to Health within the Urban Environment

1. Biological pathogens or pollutants within the human environment that impair human health—including pathogenic agents and their vectors (and reservoirs); for instance, the many pathogenic microorganisms in human excreta, airborne pathogens (for instance, those responsible for acute respiratory infections and tuberculosis), and disease vectors such as malaria-carrying (Anopheline) mosquitoes.
2. Chemical pollutants within the human environment including those added to the environment by human activities (e.g., industrial wastes) and chemical agents present in the environment independent of human activities.
3. The availability, cost, and quality of natural resources on which human health depends—for instance, food, water, and fuel.
4. Physical hazards (e.g., high risks of flooding in houses and settlements built on floodplains or of mud slides or landslides for houses on slopes).
5. Aspects of the built environment with negative consequences on physical or psychosocial health (e.g., overcrowding, inadequate protection against noise, inadequate provision of infrastructure, services, and common areas).
6. Natural resource degradation (e.g., of soil and water quality) caused by wastes from city-based producers or consumers that impacts on the health/livelihoods of some urban dwellers.
7. National/global environmental degradation with more indirect but long-term influences on human health.

Source: Adapted and reprinted with permission from D Satterthwaite. The impact on health of urban environments. *Environ Urban.* 1993;5:88.

Animal Populations

In the animal kingdom, the carrying capacity of an environment tends to limit population size. In nature, the factors of food availability, reproductive behavior, and infectious diseases tend to keep animal populations in check. In a given area, the growth of animal populations appears to be sequenced according to the following characteristic patterns:

- "Logistic growth, responding to immediate negative feedback, as carrying capacity is approached
- Domed or capped growth, responding to deferred negative feedback but necessitating a period of excess mortality
- Irruptive growth, with a chaotic post-crash pattern."[18(p978)]

Human Populations

The factors that lead to the crash of animal populations are similar to those that could threaten the survival of the human race. Human life is not possible without adequate food, breathable air, and safe water. Agricultural land must continue to be arable. There needs to be a diversity of plant and animal species. If these components of the human life support system are disrupted by overpopulation of the planet, the species *Homo sapiens* could suffer a population crash. This outcome would be in line with Malthusian predictions.

In 1798, Thomas Malthus authored *First Essay on Population*, which theorized that the human population had the potential to grow exponentially.[16] According to this scenario, the population could outstrip available resources. Malthus suggested that "positive checks" for excessive population growth rates were epidemics of disease, starvation, and population

FIGURE 1-7 Street scene in a crowded megacity (Mexico City).

reduction through warfare. The growth of the population could be constrained also through "preventive checks" such as not allowing people to marry.

Endangerment of the human population through ecological damage is not far-fetched: Previous history has recorded incidents of decimation and collapse of civilizations that were associated with disruption of the environment. It is believed that approximately 5,000 years ago, Mesopotamia, a renowned ancient civilization, declined as a result of agricultural practices that caused soil erosion, buildup of salt in the soil, and the filling of irrigation channels with silt.[27] During medieval times, crowded cities of Europe were devastated by plague and other infectious diseases. In the interval between the 13th and 16th centuries, global temperatures declined by approximately one degree C, contributing to the decimation of societies that were located in the far north (e.g., Viking settlements in Greenland).

Food Insecurity and Famine

The term **food insecurity** refers to a situation in which supplies of wholesome foods are uncertain or may have limited availability. Food insecurity and famine may occur when the carrying capacity in a particular geographic area is exceeded. An illustration of the effect of exceeding the carrying capacity in a local geographic area is the occurrence of a local subsistence crisis, which follows when the ability of land and available water to produce food are overtaxed.[18] In theory, low nutritional levels that accompany local subsistence crises may cause population mortality to increase so that mortality is brought into balance with fertility, stabilizing the population size. Periodically, food insecurity is a reality in some developing regions. For example, food insecurity endangers as much as one-third of Africa, and the prognosis for increasing the food supply in some African countries is poor.[27]

Loss of Biodiversity

The word *biodiversity* is formed from the combination of *biological* and *diversity*. An adequate definition of biodiversity is not readily available. Nevertheless, the term **biodiversity** generally refers to the different types and variability of animal and plant species and ecosystems in which they live.[28] With respect to a particular geographic area, biodiversity involves diversity in the genes of a population of a given species, diversity in the number of species, and diversity in habitats. Biodiversity is considered to be an essential dimension of human health.[29]

The dramatic human population growth during the past few decades and concomitant increases in urbanization and industrialization have caused the physical environment to be degraded substantially; one of the consequences of unchecked population growth is hypothesized to be accelerated loss of biodiversity. Human activities are thought to be related to the spread of harmful insect vectors, extinctions of species, and loss of flora; some of these plants and trees could be the source of new pharmaceuticals. Ultimately, loss of biodiversity may pose a danger to food production as a result of the growth in numbers of invasive species and the eradication of helpful plants and insects. An example of the loss of biodiversity is the destruction of tropical rain forests that has culminated in the extinction of some flowering plants that may have had future medical value.[29]

DEFINITIONS USED IN THE ENVIRONMENTAL HEALTH FIELD

The Environment

The term **environment** refers to "the complex of physical, chemical, and biotic factors (as climate, soil, and living things) that act upon an organism or an ecological community and ultimately determine its form and survival."[30] This definition pertains to the physical environment. Examples of physical environmental factors (as noted previously) that affect human health include toxic chemicals, metallic compounds, ionizing and nonionizing radiation, and physical and mechanical energy. These factors will be discussed in more detail later in the text.

The term *environment* captures the notion of factors that are external to the individual, as opposed to internal factors such as genetic makeup. In contrast to the physical environment, described in the foregoing definition, the **social environment** encompasses influences upon the individual that arise from societal and cultural factors. Among the major determinants of health are the environment (physical and social), personal lifestyle factors, constitutional factors such as heredity and human biology, and healthcare systems dimensions such as access to and quality of medical care and methods for organization of healthcare systems.[31] A model that describes these aspects of health is the **ecological model**, which proposes that the determinants of health (environmental, biological, and behavioral) interact and are interlinked over the life course of individuals. (Refer to Figure 1-8.) From the model it may be inferred that the environment is one component of many interacting dimensions that affect the health of populations.

Ecological System (Ecosystem)

Ecosystems are one of the important dimensions of life in the biosphere. All life on earth survives in the biosphere,

FIGURE 1-8 The ecological model of population health.

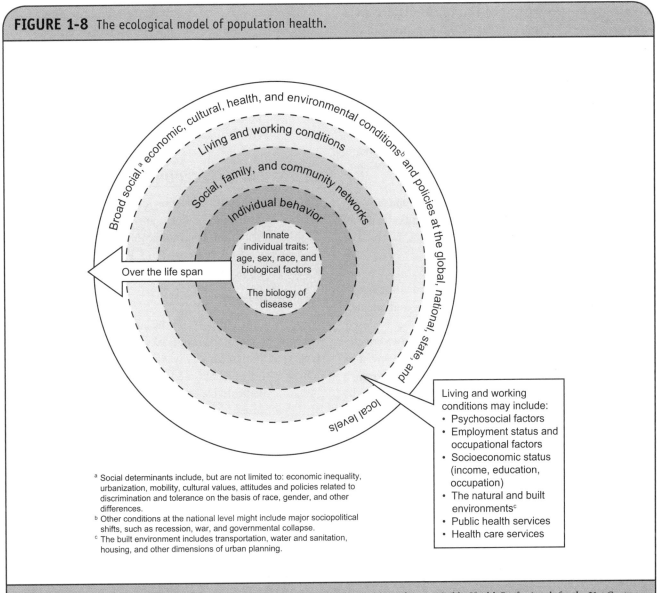

Living and working conditions may include:
- Psychosocial factors
- Employment status and occupational factors
- Socioeconomic status (income, education, occupation)
- The natural and built environments[c]
- Public health services
- Health care services

[a] Social determinants include, but are not limited to: economic inequality, urbanization, mobility, cultural values, attitudes and policies related to discrimination and tolerance on the basis of race, gender, and other differences.
[b] Other conditions at the national level might include major sociopolitical shifts, such as recession, war, and governmental collapse.
[c] The built environment includes transportation, water and sanitation, housing, and other dimensions of urban planning.

Source: Adapted and reprinted with permission from *Who Will Keep the Public Healthy? Educating Public Health Professionals for the 21st Century,* © 2003 by the National Academy of Sciences, courtesy of the National Academies Press, Washington, D.C., p. 33; and from Dahlgren G, Whitehead M. Policies and Strategies to Promote Social Equity in Health. Stockholm, Sweden: Institute for Futures Studies; 1991.

which consists of the atmosphere and the earth's surface and oceans. The biosphere covers a narrow range from about six miles above the earth to the surface of the earth to the deepest ocean trenches, some of which are 36,000 feet deep. One of the crucial aspects of the earth's biosphere is energy flow; the ultimate source of energy for all living beings on earth is the sun. Energy flows from the sun in the form of electromagnetic radiation (e.g., ultraviolet radiation, infrared radiation, and visible light). Only a small percentage of the energy produced by the sun impinges upon the earth. Plants absorb some portions of the sun's electromagnetic radiation and convert them into nutrients and oxygen via the process known as photosynthesis. This energy is then transferred to other life forms through the food chain, for example, via herbivores that eat the plants themselves or carnivores that eat other animals.

"An ecosystem is a dynamic complex of plant, animal, and microorganism communities and the nonliving environment interacting as a functional unit. Humans are an integral part of ecosystems. Ecosystems vary enormously in size: a temporary pond in a tree hollow and an ocean basin can both be ecosystems."[32(p3)] The interconnected components of an **ecosystem** are in a steady state; disrupting one of the components can disrupt the entire ecosystem. Figure 1-9 suggests that the health of the ecosystem is associated with the health of human beings as well as that of domestic animals and wildlife.

Survival of the human population depends upon ecosystems, which aid in supplying clean air and water as part of the earth's life support system.[33] Ecosystems are being degraded with increasing rapidity because of human environmental impacts such as urbanization and deforestation. Degradation of ecosystems poses environmental dangers such as loss of the oxygen-producing capacity of plants and loss of biodiversity.

Environmental Health

The field of **environmental health** has a broad focus and includes a number of subspecializations. For example, occupational health often is regarded as a topic that is closely allied with environmental health and is a subset of broader environmental health concerns. Consequently, in view of its broad reach, the term *environmental health* does not have a single definition, nor is it easy to define. According to the World Health Organization:

Environmental health addresses all the physical, chemical, and biological factors external to a person, and all the related factors impacting behaviours. It encompasses the assessment and control of those environmental factors that can potentially affect health. It is targeted towards preventing disease and creating health-supportive environments.[34]

HISTORICAL BACKGROUND

This section presents a brief review of environmental health history, categorized as follows: ancient history, occupational health (contributions from about 1500 to the mid-1800s), and environmental history post-1800. Figure 1-10 summarizes some of the highlights in environmental health history.

Ancient History

Negative human impacts on the environment are thought to have begun many thousands of years ago. One of the initial targets of human activity was forests, which were cut down for use as timber and burned to clear land for agriculture and human settlements. Deforestation subsequently led to soil erosion that caused rivers and bays to be fouled with silt.

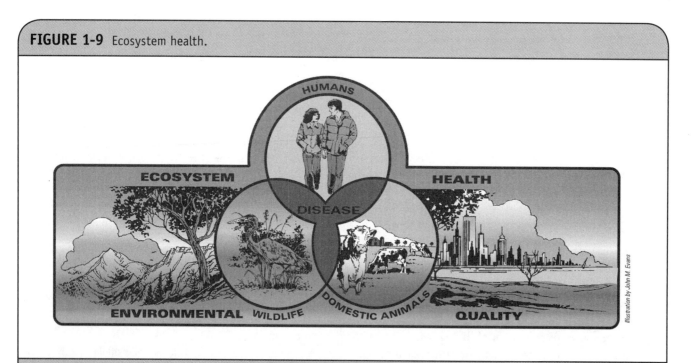

FIGURE 1-9 Ecosystem health.

Source: Reprinted from Friend, Milton. Disease Emergence and Reemergence. The Wildlife-Human Connection. Reston, VA: US Geological Survey, Circular 1285, p. 131. Illustration by John M. Evans.

The observations, insights, and writings of the ancient Greeks are noteworthy for the history of environmental health.[35] Around the fifth century BC, the ancient Greek philosophers had developed the concept of the relationship between environmental factors and human health; instead of advocating for the workings of supernatural factors and the belief that magic potions would have curative powers, their philosophical position linked the influence of environment to disease.

Hippocrates, who lived between 460 and 370 BC, often is referred to as "the father of medicine." (See Figure 1-11.) Hippocrates emphasized the role of the environment as an influence on people's health and health status in his work titled *On Airs, Waters, and Places* (ca. 400 BC). The Greek philosopher proposed that environmental and climatic factors such as the weather, seasons, and prevailing winds; the quality of air, water, and food; and one's geographic location were influential in causing changes in human health. He espoused the doctrine of maintaining equilibrium among the body's four humors, known as yellow bile, black bile, phlegm, and blood; imbalance among the four humors caused by environmental influences led to the onset of infectious diseases.

Many of the principles identified by Hippocrates regarding the impact of the environment on human health and disease remain credible despite the great increases in medical knowledge that have occurred since Hippocrates' time.[35] For example, now it is known that polluted water is associated with many types of waterborne infections (e.g., cholera and cryptosporidiosis [discussed later in this text]). Consistent with the belief that air is a factor in diseases is the origin of the term *malaria* (bad air), a disease that is carried by airborne mosquitoes that dwell in standing pools of water.

The ancient Greeks and Romans both recognized that chemicals used in the production of metals could be poison-

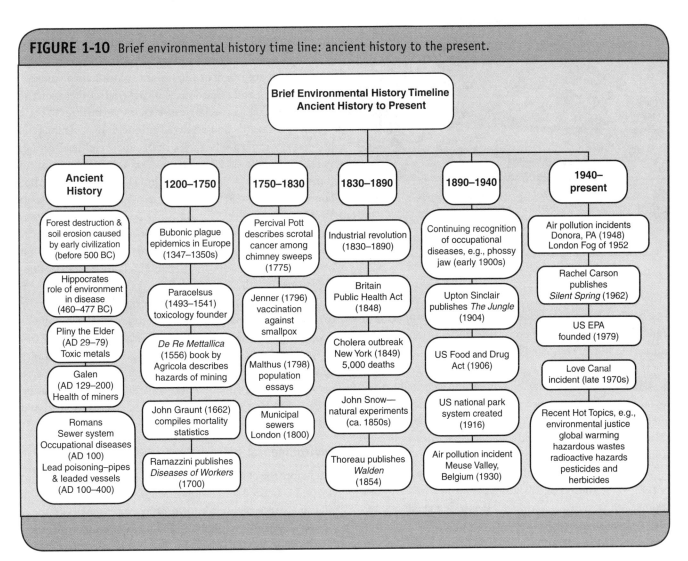

FIGURE 1-10 Brief environmental history time line: ancient history to the present.

FIGURE 1-11 Hippocrates.

Source: Reprinted courtesy of US National Library of Medicine, National Institutes of Health. History of medicine division. Available at: http://ihm.nlm.nih.gov/luna/servlet/view/search?q=B014553. Accessed February 23, 2010.

ous.[36] Also, Hippocrates identified the toxic properties of lead.[37] The toxic properties of sulfur and zinc were pointed out by the Roman scholar Pliny the Elder (AD 29–79) during the first century AD; Pliny invented a mask constructed from the bladder of an animal for protection against dusts and metal fumes. During the second century AD, the renowned Greek physician Galen (AD 129–200) outlined the pathological aspects of lead toxicity and suggested that mists from acids could endanger the health of copper miners.[37]

The ancient Romans designed systems for the transport of water and sewage, heating devices for water and for rooms, and communal baths.[38,39] Beginning about 500 BC, the Etruscans constructed a sewer called the Cloaca Maxima in Rome. As the city grew, a system of aqueducts that sup-plied fresh water and a web of sewers called cloacae were installed.

The Romans brought many of these innovations to their settlements all over Europe. Roman aqueducts and baths can been seen today in many parts of Europe. An example of the Roman baths at Baden-Baden, Germany, is shown in Figure 1-12. The Romans used lead pipes to supply the homes of the affluent, who probably suffered from chronic lead poisoning. After the decline of their empire (possibly due, in part, to chronic lead poisoning), many of the hygiene-related contributions of the Romans were forgotten; for several centuries, the European world endured the abhorrent sanitary conditions of the medieval era, with its periodic outbreaks of epidemics of plague, cholera, and other pestilence.

Occupational Health (Contributions from About 1500 to the Mid-1800s)

The field of occupational health has made numerous contributions to environmental health history. From about 1500 to the mid-1800s, recognition grew regarding the contribution of occupationally related exposures to adverse health conditions. There are many examples of explorations of the impacts of unsafe and hazardous working environments on the health of workers, especially the effects of exposures to toxic metals and hazards that occurred among miners. Among the historically important figures in occupational health were Paracelsus (1493–1541), Agricola (1494–1555), Bernardino Ramazzini (1633–1714), Percival Pott (1714–1788), and Alice Hamilton (1869–1970). See Chapter 3 for information on Paracelsus, Chapter 2 for information about Percival Pott, and Chapter 13 for a discussion of Agricola, Ramazzini, and Hamilton; Chapter 13 also provides information on other historically important individuals in the field of occupational health.

Although his contributions were not limited specifically to occupational health, John Graunt (one of the early compilers of vital statistics data) published *Natural and Political Observations Made upon the Bills of Mortality* in 1662. Sometimes Graunt is referred to as the Columbus of statistics because his book made a fundamental contribution by attempting to demonstrate the quantitative characteristics of birth and death data.

Environmental History Post-1800

Just before the commencement of the 1800s, Jenner (in 1796) devised a method for vaccinating against smallpox; in 1798, Malthus wrote his well-known essays on population, mentioned earlier in this chapter. The history of environmental health since 1800 may be classified into three major eras[40]:

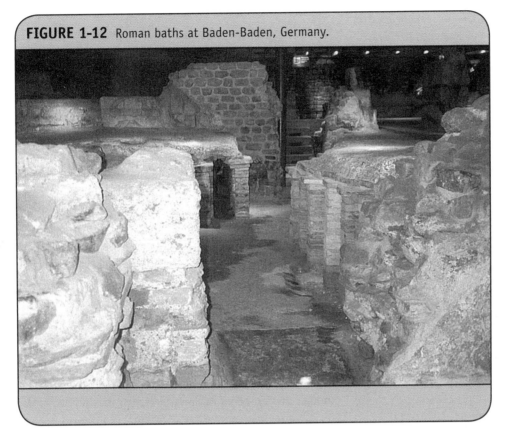

FIGURE 1-12 Roman baths at Baden-Baden, Germany.

The first wave of environmental concern (from the 19th century to mid-20th century), the second wave of environmental awareness (mid-20th century to the 1980s), and the third period of environmental concern (1980s to the present).

The period of approximately 1850 to 1950 was marked by growing awareness of existing threats to public health from unsanitary conditions, detrimental social conditions, and hazardous work environments. For example, a common employment practice in Europe was the use of child labor. This era coincided approximately with the industrial revolution and marked the introduction of public health reforms to improve environmental conditions. In 1800, construction began on sewers that served the city of London. The British Parliament enacted the Public Health Act in 1848 to promote clean water and control infectious diseases. There were major outbreaks of cholera, including an outbreak in New York City in 1849 that killed 5,000 people.

About the same time, John Snow hypothesized that sewage-contaminated water was associated with cholera and conducted a "natural experiment" to demonstrate the cause of an outbreak in the present Soho district of London. John Snow (1813–1858) was an English anesthesiologist who innovated several of the key epidemiologic methods that remain valid

and in use today. In Snow's time, the mechanism for the causation of infectious diseases was largely unknown. The Dutchman Anton van Leeuwenhoek (1632–1723) had used the microscope to observe microorganisms (bacteria and yeast). However, the connection between microorganisms and disease had not yet been ascertained. During Snow's time, one of the explanations for infectious diseases such as cholera was the miasmic theory of disease, which alleged that illnesses were caused by clouds of noxious matter. Snow rejected the miasmatic theory and showed the connection between polluted water and cholera. Because of his pioneering work, Snow is regarded as an icon in the history of public health and continues to be influential during the 21st century. (More information about Snow's work is provided in Chapter 2.)

In the United States, Lemuel Shattuck published the 1850 *Report on the Sanitary Conditions of Massachusetts*. Shattuck argued for the creation of a state health department and local health boards. Among other issues, Shattuck's report dealt in detail with the topic of environmental sanitation and its connection with health. Although not implemented by the state legislature at the time, Shattuck's proposed recommendations were extremely farsighted and innovative and became a major influence in the development of subsequent public health practice. Ultimately, years later, many of Shattuck's proposals were adopted by public health departments and are in use today.

Several additional developments marked the late 19th century and early 20th century. Henry David Thoreau published *Walden* in 1854; this book extolled the virtues of a simple life in a beautiful natural environment. Thoreau suggested that nature enriched the lives of human beings and therefore should be respected.

Beginning in 1900, Walter Reed, who was a US Army medical officer, investigated the causes of yellow fever, which was a scourge of US troops in the Caribbean. He showed that yellow fever was a mosquito-borne affliction. Following this discovery, Major William Gorgas was dispatched to Havana, Cuba, where he implemented a highly successful mosquito eradication program. This action led to a drastic reduction in yellow fever cases in Havana; later Gorgas conducted a mosquito control program in the Panama Canal Zone, making possible the construction of the canal.

In *The Jungle* (1906), Upton Sinclair described the deplorable conditions in the meat processing industry in Chicago. Sinclair's exposé was instrumental in passage of the first Food and Drug Act that was instituted in the United States in 1906. (Some of the US laws regarding food safety are described in Chapter 11.) One other development that reflected the public's concern for the environment was creation of the US National Park System in 1916.

During the second wave of environmental concern, defined approximately from the middle of the 1950s to the 1980s, environmental issues continued to come to the forefront. The period witnessed the occurrence of several noteworthy air pollution incidents, including the fatal 1930 incident in the Meuse Valley, Belgium; an air pollution episode that caused numerous deaths in Donora, Pennsylvania, in 1948; and the deadly London fog of 1952.[41] (More information on these incidents is presented in Chapter 10.)

Awareness increased regarding the potential health hazards of toxic chemicals. In the United States, efforts were made to protect ecologically sensitive areas from toxic hazards and from overdevelopment. Additional legislation in the United States modified food and drug laws designed to regulate toxins and the use of additives in food. Rachel Carson published *Silent Spring*, which highlighted the potential dangers of pesticides. In 1970, the Environmental Protection Agency (EPA) was founded to address environmental concerns at the federal government level (more information on this topic is presented in Chapter 4).

The topic of disposal of toxic wastes also was the focus of much attention during the 1970s. For example, when residents discovered that their homes had been constructed on a former toxic waste site referred to as the Love Canal, they became alarmed about possible adverse health effects that might be linked to the waste site. Love Canal became a cause célèbre for environmental activists. (This topic is covered in more detail in Chapter 12.)

The most recent period in environmental history (the third wave of environmental concern—1980s to the present) has been marked by high population growth rates, industrialization, and urbanization. Specific concerns have continued regarding the effects of toxic chemicals in the environment.

TABLE 1-3 Examples of Hot Topics in Environmental Health

Air quality	Land use
Conservation	Nuclear power
Endangered species/Wildlife impacts	Oceans
	Pesticides and herbicides
Energy resources	Pollution
Environmental justice	Radioactive waste
Environmental protection	Recycling
Forests	Solid waste
Global warming/Global climate change	War and terrorism
	Water resources
Greenhouse gases	Wetlands
Hazardous wastes	

Source: Partial data from LexisNexis, Environment issues. Copyright 2002, LexisNexis, a division of Reed Elsevier Inc. All Rights Reserved.

A new topic has been the emission of greenhouse gases and their possible contribution to global warming.

Table 1-3 presents a compilation of some of the contemporary issues that are relevant to environmental health. Although this list is not exhaustive, it identifies several of the major "hot topics" in the environmental health field.

The topics shown in Table 1-3 will be covered in this textbook. However, let us select four of the issues—global climate change, pesticides and herbicides, air quality, and war and terrorism—and consider them briefly. For example, one issue that commands our attention (and that has generated extensive coverage in the media) is the prospect of global climate change including global warming (and production of greenhouse gases). Among the outcomes believed to be associated with global warming are changes in the distribution of insect vectors that can carry diseases such as malaria and the West Nile virus. Later in this text, in Chapter 10, global warming—its hypothesized causes, extent, and effects—will be considered in more detail.

The impact of toxic pesticides and toxic chemicals is a major issue for environmental health. For example, toxic materials have been introduced into the drinking water supplies of some communities. In mid-November 2005, an explosion at a factory in northeastern China caused about 100 tons of benzene and other hazardous chemicals to be released into the Songhua River. This incident led Chinese officials to shut off the water taps in Harbin because of potential contamination of the water supply in this city. This event in China, as well as many other similar occurrences in which toxic chemicals have intruded into the public water supply, raises the issue of what can be done to prevent and abate such hazards. A related issue concerns the runoff of rainwater that overtaxes sewage processing facilities, resulting in pollution of public beaches and groundwater. Carelessly discarded solvents and other toxic chemicals pose dangers to aquifers; the author will provide more information on toxic pesticides and toxic chemicals in Chapter 7.

Still another issue is the impact of air quality on human health, including the role of air pollution in causing cancer and lung diseases as well as aggravating chronic conditions such as heart disease. Some regions face a continuing and growing threat to the environment from air pollution. Several US cities, such as those located in the Los Angeles basin of Southern California, face occasional episodes of significant air pollution. Fortunately, air quality has shown improvement in Southern California and elsewhere in the United States during the past few decades. In contrast, many cities in the rapidly industrializing nations of the developing world are experiencing declines in air quality due to the increasing use of fossil fuels.

Finally, war and terrorism can have devastating impacts upon the environment. Some of these potential impacts include the destruction of fauna and flora, exposure of the population to hazardous radiation from spent munitions, and water pollution caused by the manufacture of nuclear weapons. (Refer to Chapter 8.) Recently, health officials and the public have been concerned about threats to the environment from the intentional release of infectious biological agents such as the agent that causes anthrax. (Refer to Chapter 5.)

CAREERS IN THE ENVIRONMENTAL HEALTH FIELD

The field of environmental health provides numerous career roles and possible occupations. Private industry, government units, universities, and private research organizations

---

TABLE 1-4 Professions Involved in Environmental Health

Academics, lecturers, teachers, teacher trainers	Hygienists
Agriculturists	Information scientists
Agronomists	Laboratory assistants/technicians
Architects	Marine scientists
Bacteriologists	Materials technologists
Biochemists	Medical specialists (with postgraduate qualifications in the public health area)
Chemical process engineers	
Civil engineers	Meteorologists
Climatologists	Microbiologists
Communications experts	Noise inspectors
Disaster preparedness specialists	Nuclear safety managers
Ecologists	Nutritionists
Economists	Occupational health nurses
Engineering specialists (with postgraduate qualifications)	Occupational health physicians
	Occupational hygienists
Entomologists	Physicists
Environmental biologists	Political scientists
Environmental chemists	Pollution inspectors
Environmental engineers	Psychologists
Environmental health administrators	Public health nurses
Environmental health educators	Public health physicians
Environmental health managers	Public health veterinarians
Environmental health officers	Public relations experts
Environmental health planners	Risk assessors
Environmental health technicians	Rural and urban planners
Environmental lawyers	Safety inspectors
Epidemiologists (with medical degree)	Sanitary engineers
Epidemiologists (without medical degree)	Sanitary officers
Ergonomists	Social scientists
Fire safety officers	Social workers
Food inspectors	Soil scientists
Food safety specialists	Statisticians
Geneticists	Technical assistants
Geographers	Toxicologists
Geologists	Transport planners/managers
Health promotion experts	Water quality inspectors
Hydrogeologists	Zoologists
Hydrologists	

Source: Reprinted with permission from M Fitzpatrick and X Bonnefoy. *Environmental Health Services in Europe 4: Guidance on the Development of Educational and Training Curricula.* Copenhagen, Denmark: World Health Organization Regional Office for Europe; 1999:12. WHO Regional Publications, European Series, No. 84.

employ environmental health workers in diverse functions. Table 1-4 gives an extensive list of occupations that have a connection with environmental health. Although this list is extensive, it is not exhaustive. Following is a description of some of these occupations.

Hygienist

In the work environment, professional industrial hygienists are responsible for control of hazards that may affect the workers as well as hazards that may impact the community. They are involved with the design and installation of control systems for hazards in the occupational and environmental setting. They require training in the epidemiologic and biologic aspects of environmental hazards and also in toxicology. Industrial hygienists work closely with engineers who design and maintain industrial processes.[42]

FIGURE 1-13 Researchers in a toxicology laboratory.

Source: Courtesy of Dr. Arezoo Campbell, Department of Community and Environmental Medicine, University of California, Irvine.

Toxicologist

As a general description of the field, it may be said that toxicology concerns the effects of poisons. Among the many subspecializations in the field of toxicology are medical, veterinary, forensic, and environmental applications. The field of environmental toxicology specializes in the effects of toxic chemicals upon the environment and living creatures such as human beings and wildlife. Occupational and industrial toxicologists investigate the effects of chemicals found in the workplace upon the health of workers. Toxicologists are employed in academia as professors and researchers, by government agencies, by hospitals, and in various private industry settings. (See Figure 1-13).

Environmental Health Inspector

Public health departments provide many job opportunities for environmental health workers. Environmental health inspectors, who work mainly for state and local governments, are responsible for monitoring and enforcing government regulations for environmental quality. This employment category includes pollution inspectors, noise inspectors, and water quality inspectors. Such personnel help to monitor the treatment and disposal of sewage, refuse, and garbage. They also may visit toxic waste dumps, factories, and other sources of pollution in order to collect air, water, and waste samples for testing. They may be sent out to follow up on complaints from the community, attempt to determine the sources and nature of environmental pollution, and provide necessary background data for enforcement actions.

Food Inspector/Food Safety Specialist

Food inspectors and food safety specialists are involved with the cleanliness and safety of foods and beverages consumed by the public. They inspect restaurants, dairies, food processing plants, and other food preparation venues in order to control biological hazards from sources such as *E. coli*, *Salmonella*, and other foodborne agents. Their purview of responsibility also may extend to hospitals and other institutional settings. They may be responsible for examining the methods for handling, processing, and serving of food so that these procedures are in compliance with sanitation rules and regulations.

Vector Control Specialist

Vector control specialists (not listed in Table 1-4) are responsible for the enforcement of various public health laws, sanitary codes, and other regulations related to the spread of disease by vectors. Examples of vectors are insects such as mosquitoes and flies, rodents, and other animals and arthropods that carry disease organisms. Vector control specialists are involved with controlling rabies, mosquito-borne encephalitis, tick-borne diseases, and zoonotic diseases. At the local-government level, vector control specialists may be responsible for conducting community education programs, monitoring animal bites, collecting specimens for testing, and developing other procedures for control of diseases carried by vectors. Figure 1-14 illustrates a vector control specialist at work.

Researcher/Research Analyst

In universities and research units, individuals who have specialized training in environmental health conduct basic research on the risks associated with exposures to certain specific hazards and conduct statistical analyses of the impact of such exposures on human populations. Although this category is not listed in Table 1-4, examples of employment titles found in research settings are laboratory scientist and technician, epidemiologist, and statistician.

Occupational Health Physician/ Occupational Health Nurse

These professionals are involved with the prevention and treatment of occupationally related illnesses and injuries. They investigate hazards in the work environment and develop procedures for their abatement. They also conduct health education programs for the prevention of work-related diseases.

Environmental Lawyer

Beyond the research environment, there is an active field known as environmental health law. Closely linked with environmental health law are environmental policies. Specialists in this field provide input to government agencies, assist in the formulation of environmental policies, and may be involved in litigation concerning environmental health problems.

CONCLUSION AND OVERVIEW OF THE TEXT

The study of environmental health is crucial to one's understanding of the hazards and potential adverse effects posed by environmental agents and the extent to which environ-

FIGURE 1-14 Vector control specialist spraying insecticidal dust for control of plague, 1993.

Source: Reprinted courtesy of the CDC Public Health Image Library, ID#2053. Available at: http://phil.cdc.gov/phil/details.asp. Accessed February 23, 2010.

mental factors play a role in human disease. This foundation is essential for being an effective advocate for preventing environmentally caused diseases and for more advanced study of environmental health issues. Chapter 1 has provided an introduction to the environmental health field: definitions, terminology and concepts, historical background, and career opportunities. The field of environmental health draws heavily upon **epidemiology** and toxicology.[43] As a result, environmental health makes abundant use of terminology from these disciplines. Epidemiologic aspects of environmental health include such well-known methods as case ascertainment, continuous surveillance of hazards, and development of tools for evaluation of intervention programs. Epidemiologic studies have been crucial for delineating the health effects of exposure to pollutants at the population level. Chapter 2 will introduce the topic of environmental epidemiology.

One of the contributions of toxicology to the environmental health field is in assessing **dose–response relationships**, which describe the responses of organisms to exposures to toxic substances. A dose–response relationship can be illustrated by an S-shaped curve known as a dose–response curve.[44] An additional concern of toxicology is exposure assessment, which involves procedures for determining what levels of specific hazards (e.g., a toxic chemical such as DDT) produce symptoms, disease, or other adverse effects. Chapter 3 provides more information on toxicology.

Chapter 4 provides a discussion of environmental policy making and environmental health, including regulatory agencies and specific environmental laws that have been enacted in the United States. Chapters 5 through 9 cover agent factors (e.g., microbes, toxic metals, forms of radiation, and organic chemicals) that are related to risk of disease caused by environmental factors. Chapter 5 focuses on environmental aspects of zoonotic and vector-borne diseases. Chapter 6 describes hazards that arise from toxic metals and elements (e.g., arsenic and chromium). Chapter 7 reveals hazards that arise from toxic chemicals such as pesticides, herbicides, and organophosphates. Chapter 8 focuses on ionizing radiation (for example, radiation emitted during the Chernobyl nuclear power plant accident and from X-ray machines used in body scans) and nonionizing radiation (for example, radio frequency radiation from cell phones and ultraviolet radiation from the sun). Chapter 9 covers water quality and pollution. Chapter 10 focuses on air quality and the impact of climate change. Chapter 11 covers the broad topic of food safety, including foodborne diseases caused by microbial agents and how additives and chemicals affect the food supply. Chapter 12 covers solid waste disposal and sewage processing. Chapter 13 presents information on occupational health. Finally, Chapter 14 demonstrates the role of environmental factors in unintentional injuries, a leading cause of mortality.

Study Questions and Exercises

1. Define the following terms:
   a. Population dynamics
   b. Total fertility rate
   c. Environmental health
   d. Environmental risk transition
   e. Environment, physical and social
   f. Demographic transition
   g. Epidemiologic transition

2. Discuss three of the six major objectives for goal number 8, environmental health, as described in *Healthy People 2010*. What steps can be taken in your community to accomplish the objectives you have selected?

3. Describe the three P's that are principal determinants of health worldwide. Discuss how the three P's could be considered interrelated characteristics. Can you think of other consequences of the three P's that are not discussed in the textbook?

4. Chapter 1 discussed how environmental exposures affect our daily lives.
   a. Discuss the types of environmental health problems that you have in your own community.
   b. Review and summarize at least three articles on environmental health that you have seen in a newspaper during the past week. Are any of these articles relevant to the community where you live?
   c. Why is maintenance of environmental quality important for human health?

5. Discuss the role of population growth in human health. How might recent outbreaks of diseases such as the bird flu or pandemic H1N1 be linked to population growth? In addition to population growth, what other environmental factors could lead to pandemics such as those associated with influenza viruses?

6. Describe the types of environmental health problems that prevail in the developing world. Give at least three examples.

7. Discuss population growth trends over the past two centuries. What is the likelihood that current exponential population growth rates will continue? Take a stand for or against population growth at present high levels.

8. Describe variables that affect the size of a population. What countries or regions of the world are projected to experience stable or declining population sizes? What areas are expected to have the greatest increases in population size?

9. Define and discuss the following terms:
   a. Ecological model of population health
   b. Ecosystem

10. Describe the contributions of the early Greeks to environmental health. How do Hippocrates' explanations of disease etiology compare with current beliefs about the role of the environment in human illness?

11. List and discuss five of today's most pressing environmental health issues ("hot topics"). In addition to the material presented in the text, you also may use your own ideas.

12. Explain why environmental health is an important field of employment. List specific employment roles in environmental health. Consult the World Wide Web for employment listings (e.g., published by state, local, and federal government agencies) and summarize the requirements and functions of three job titles.

REFERENCES

1. US Department of Health and Human Services. *Healthy People 2010: Understanding and Improving Health*. 2nd ed. Washington, DC: U.S. Government Printing Office; November 2000.

2. Winkelstein W Jr. Determinants of worldwide health. *Am J Public Health*. 1992;82:931–932.

3. National Institute of Environmental Health Sciences. Forum: killer environment. *Environ Health Perspect*. 1999;107:A62–A63.

4. Butterfield PG. Upstream reflections on environmental health: an abbreviated history and framework for action. *Adv Nurs Sci*. 2002;25(1):32–49.

5. World Health Organization. HSP glossary. Burden of disease. Available at: http://www.who.int/health-systems-performance/docs/glossary.htm. Accessed February 9, 2010.

6. World Health Organization. WHO to highlight specific health risks to children from environmental dangers. Available at: http://www.who.int/mediacentre/news/notes/note04/en/. Accessed February 9, 2010.

7. Carlson JE. Children's Environmental Health Network, Emeryville, California. *Environ Health Perspect*. 1998;106(Suppl 3):785–786.

8. Goldman LR, Koduru S. Chemicals in the environment and developmental toxicity to children: a public health and policy perspective. *Environ Health Perspect*. 2000;108(Suppl 3):443–448.

9. Chukwuma C Sr. Environmental health concepts and issues—a viewpoint. *Intern J Environ Studies*. 2001;58:631–644.

10. Mellor JW. The intertwining of environmental problems and poverty. *Environ*. 1988;30:8–30.

11. Camp SL. Population pressure, poverty and the environment. *Integration*. June 1992;24–27.

12. Smith KR. Environment and health: issues for the new U.S. administration. *Environ*. 2001;43:34–41.

13. US Census Bureau. *Global Population Profile: 2002*. International Population Reports WP/02. Washington, DC: U.S. Government Printing Office; 2004.

14. Hinrichsen D. The decisive decade: what we can do about population. *Amicus J*. 1990;12(1):30–33.

15. Last JM. *Homo sapiens*—a suicidal species? *World Health Forum*. 1991;12:121–126.

16. Raleigh VS. World population and health in transition. *BMJ*. 1999;319:981–984.

17. Brown LR. Feeding six billion. *World Watch*. September/October 1989;32–40.

18. McMichael AJ, Powles JW. Human numbers, environment, sustainability, and health. *BMJ*. 1999;319:977–980.

19. Downs B. *Fertility of American Women: June 2002*. Current Population Reports, P20-548. Washington, DC: U.S. Census Bureau; 2003.

20. Gelbard A, Haub C. Population "explosion" not over for half the world. *Popul Today*. 1998;26:1–2.

21. PRB staff. World population highlights: Key findings from PRB's 2009 World Population Data Sheet. *Population Bulletin*. 2009;64(3).

22. United Nations Environment Programme. Population and the environment. *Popul Bull UN*. 1987;(21–22):32–44.

23. McMichael AJ. The urban environment and health in a world of increasing globalization: issues for developing countries. *Bull World Health Organ*. 2000;78:1117–1126.

24. Satterthwaite D. The impact on health of urban environments. *Environ Urban*. 1993;5:87–111.

25. Decker EH, Elliott S, Smith FA. Megacities and the environment. *TheScientificWorldJOURNAL*. 2002;2:374–386.

26. The World Bank Group. Youthink. Available at: http://youthink.worldbank.org/glossary.php. Accessed February 9, 2010.

27. McMichael AJ. Ecological disruption and human health: the next great challenge to public health [editorial]. *Aust J Public Health*. 1992;16:3–5.

28. State of California, California Biodiversity Council. Scientific definitions of biodiversity. Available at: http://biodiversity.ca.gov/Biodiversity/biodiv_def2.html. Accessed February 10, 2010.

29. Marwick C. Scientists stress biodiversity-human health links. *JAMA*. 1995;273:1246.

30. Merriam-Webster Online dictionary. Environment. Available at: http://www.merriam-webster.com/dictionary/environment. Accessed February 10, 2010.

31. The National Academies, Institute of Medicine. *Who Will Keep the Public Healthy? Educating Public Health Professionals for the 21st Century*. Washington, DC: The National Academies Press; 2003.

32. Millennium Ecosystem Assessment. *Ecosystems and Human Well-Being: A Framework for Assessment*. Washington, DC: Island Press; 2003.

33. World Health Organization. Damage to ecosystems poses growing threat to human health [press release]. March 29, 2005. Available at: http://www.who.int/globalchange/publications/masynthesis/en/. Accessed February 10, 2010.

34. World Health Organization. Environmental health. Available at: http://www.who.int/topics/environmental_health/en/. Accessed February 22, 2010.

35. Franco DA, Williams CE. "Airs, Waters, Places" and other Hippocratic writings: inferences for control of foodborne and waterborne disease. *J Environ Health*. 2000;62(10):9–14.

36. Lippman M, Cohen BS, Schlesinger RB. *Environmental Health Science: Recognition, Evaluation, and Control of Chemical and Physical Health Hazards*. New York, NY: Oxford University Press; 2003.

37. US Department of Labor, Occupational Safety and Health Administration. Industrial hygiene. Available at: http://actrav.itcilo.org/actrav-english/telearn/osh/hazard/hyg.htm. Accessed February 10, 2010.

38. Environmental history timeline. Ancient civilizations. Available at: http://www.radford.edu/~wkovarik/envhist/1ancient.html. Accessed February 10, 2010.

39. States of Jersey. History of environmental health. Available at: http://www.gov.je/Health/public_health/health_protection/History+of+Environmental+Health.htm. Accessed February 10, 2010.

40. Yassi A, Kjellström T, de Kok T, et al. *Basic Environmental Health*. New York, NY: Oxford University Press; 2001.

41. Bell ML, Davis DL. Reassessment of the lethal London fog of 1952: novel indicators of acute and chronic consequences of acute exposure to air pollution. *Environ Health Perspect*. 2001;109(Suppl 3):389–394.

42. Sherwood RJ. Cause and control: education and training of professional industrial hygienists for 2020. *Am Ind Hyg Assoc J*. 1992;53:398–403.

43. Goldstein BD. Environmental risks and public health. *Ann NY Acad Sci*. 2001;933:112–118.

44. Friis RH, Sellers TA. *Epidemiology for Public Health Practice*. 4th ed. Sudbury, MA: Jones and Bartlett Publishers; 2009.

Environmental Epidemiology

INTRODUCTION

In this chapter you will learn that epidemiology is one of the fundamental disciplines used in the study of environmental health. For example, epidemiology is one of the research tools that seeks answers to the following types of environmental questions, some of which are adapted from a report by the National Institutes of Environmental Health Sciences:[1]

- What is the impact of air pollution on children's lung function?
- Is there a relationship between exposure to agents in the environment and degenerative brain diseases such as Alzheimer's disease?
- What environmental exposures might act in combination with genetic factors to cause breast cancer?
- What are the health effects of consuming seafood contaminated with mercury?
- Is it safe to eat tuna, because it could contain chemical pollutants that were dissolved in the ocean?

- What are the long-term consequences of beach pollution?
- Does secondhand cigarette smoke cause lung cancer in nonsmokers?
- Are death rates higher in geographic regions that have higher air pollution levels in comparison with regions that have lower levels?
- There is considerable concern today about the chronic health hazards of radiation. Would you consider chemicals to be an equal hazard?
- How large an increase in cancer incidence (occurrence) would be necessary before a chemical could be identified as a problem?
- Several years ago, people were concerned that daughters exposed to diethylstilbestrol (DES) would develop cancer. What are the chances that this disease will develop in 10 or 20 years in a DES-exposed daughter who does not have cancer now?

Epidemiology is the method of choice to answer questions such as the foregoing ones. Refer to the following text box for a further discussion of this issue.

Commencing with a definition of the term *environmental epidemiology*, this chapter reviews the scope of this discipline and defines several of the special quantitative measures used to study the occurrence of environmental health problems in populations. Next, the chapter traces the key historical developments in environmental epidemiology. Some of these historical developments include concerns of the ancient Greeks about diseases caused by the environment, the observations of Sir Percival Pott on scrotal cancer among chimney sweeps in

How Do You Study Environmental Health?

How do scientists study the effects of environmental factors—such as man-made and natural substances, and radiation—on human health? Headlines such as, "People in polluted cities have more breathing difficulties" are familiar to most of us. They are likely to be about a study of the occurrence of diseases in people who have been exposed to a natural or man-made factor in the environment. That kind of work is called epidemiology. It is the best known, best understood, and most accepted tool of the environmental health sciences. It is the type of research that most health regulations are based on. The linking of cigarette smoke to lung cancer (and then to many other conditions) was carried out, in large part, by epidemiology. To show that link, which seems so obvious today, researchers not only had to compare smokers with nonsmokers over many years, they had to rule out many other exposures these people might have had.

Source: Modified and reprinted from National Institutes of Health, National Institute of Environmental Health Sciences. How do you study environmental health? NIEHS Fact Sheet #2, 8/96. Available at: http://www.medhelp.cc/NIHlib/GF-298.html. Accessed February 11, 2010.

England, the work of John Snow on cholera, and later work on the role of toxic substances in the etiology of cancer. Closely linked to quantitative measures used by environmental epidemiology are the major study designs: experimental, quasi-experimental, and observational (cross-sectional, ecologic, case-control, and cohort). A special concern of the discipline is causality—whether research findings represent cause-and-effect associations. Environmental epidemiology is a complex field that in some cases provides keen insights into environmentally caused diseases and in others provides unclear results that must be followed up by other types of studies.

DEFINITION OF ENVIRONMENTAL EPIDEMIOLOGY

Epidemiology is concerned with the study of the distribution and determinants of health and diseases, morbidity, injuries, disability, and mortality in populations.[2] Epidemiologic studies are applied to the control of health problems in populations. Epidemiology is one of the core disciplines used to examine the associations between environmental hazards and health outcomes. The term *environmental epidemiology* refers to the study of diseases and health conditions (occurring in the population) that are linked to environmental factors.[3,4] The exposures, which most of the time are outside the control of the individual, usually may be considered involuntary and stem from ambient and occupational environments.[5] According to this conception of environmental epidemiology, standard epidemiologic methods are used to study the association between environmental factors (exposures) and health outcomes. Examples of topics studied include air and water pollution, the occupational environment with its pos-

sible use of physical and chemical agents, and the psychosocial environment.[6]

As noted previously, for an environmentally associated health outcome to be considered a topic of environmental epidemiology, exposure factors must lie outside the individual's immediate control. Hazards associated with smoking can be explored as an exposure dimension that is either under or not under the control of the individual. As an example of the former, studies of the health effects of smoking among individuals who smoke would not be a usual concern of environmental epidemiology. However, exposure of populations to secondhand cigarette smoke would be a concern because nonsmokers and vulnerable groups such as children cannot control whether they are exposed to environmental tobacco smoke.

Thus, traditionally, environmental epidemiology has tended to focus on health effects linked to degradation of the air we breathe, the water we drink, and the food we eat.[7] With the advances achieved during the 20th century in environmental sanitation and control of disease-causing biological organisms, attention to chemical and physical impacts upon the environment has increased. Some of the agents and environmental factors being focused on are lead toxicity, particulates from diesel exhaust, and exposures to pesticides and halogenated compounds. The last category includes **polychlorinated biphenyls (PCBs)**, which through biological processes can become increasingly concentrated in foodstuffs, can pose hazards as potential carcinogens, and can impact the reproductive system. More recent concerns of environmental health include the reemerging infectious diseases (see Chapter 5) and the effects of climate changes due to global warming.

Although the relationship between environmental exposures and their unknown hazards remains a concern of environmental epidemiology, the field has evolved to include a broader approach: identification of previously unrecognized exposures to known hazardous agents and the quantification of such risks; estimation of the amount of exposures that individuals have to environmental hazards; assessment of risks associated with exposures (discussed in Chapter 3); and evaluation of procedures to prevent exposures.[4] Similarly, in the related field of occupational health, the goals of epidemiologic research encompass the description of exposure–response gradients, discovery of how occupational hazards may cause harmful effects, characterization of vulnerable workers, and input into programs for the prevention of occupationally related diseases.[8]

CONTRIBUTIONS OF EPIDEMIOLOGY TO ENVIRONMENTAL HEALTH

Epidemiology aids the environmental health field through:

- Concern with populations
- Use of observational data
- Methodology for study designs
- Descriptive and analytic studies

Epidemiology is important to the study of environmental health problems because (1) many exposures and health effects associated with the environment occur at the population level; (2) the epidemiologic methods of natural experiments and observational techniques are appropriate; (3) the study designs used in epidemiologic research can be applied directly to the study of environmental health issues; and (4) epidemiology aids in the development of hypotheses and the study of causal relationships.

Concern with Populations

In contrast with clinical medicine's traditional focus on the individual, a unique characteristic of epidemiology is that it studies the entire population and hence is sometimes called population medicine. For example, epidemiologic studies of lung disease may examine the occurrence of lung cancer mortality across counties or among regional geographic subdivisions known as census tracts. Investigators may want to determine whether lung cancer mortality is higher in areas with higher concentrations of "smokestack" industries in comparison with areas that have lower levels of air pollution or are relatively free from air pollution. The alternative approach of the clinician would be to concentrate on the diagnosis and treatment of lung cancer among specific individuals.

Use of Observational Data

In examining the occurrence of health and disease in human populations, researchers often are prohibited from using experimental methods because of ethical issues such as potential dangers to subjects. Studies of the population's health present a challenge that is partially met by epidemiology because epidemiology is primarily an observational science that takes advantage of naturally occurring situations in order to study the occurrence of disease.

Methodology for Study Designs

In the realm of environmental health, epidemiologic research generally aims to portray the frequency of disease occurrence in the population or to link disease outcomes to specific exposures.[9] In order to research environmentally caused disease in the population, the field of environmental epidemiology uses characteristic study designs: cross-sectional, ecologic, case-control, and cohort. For example, these methods are useful in and linked closely to the field of risk assessment (discussed in Chapter 3). Smith writes, "The epidemiologic input to environmental risk assessment involves the interpretation of epidemiological studies and their application to estimating the potential health risks to populations from known or estimated environmental exposures."[10(p124)]

Two Classes of Epidemiologic Studies: Descriptive and Analytic

The term **descriptive epidemiology** refers to the depiction of the occurrence of disease in populations according to classification by person, place, and time variables. Examples of person variables are demographic characteristics such as sex, age, and race/ethnicity. Place variables denote geographic locations including a specific country or countries, areas within countries, and places where localized patterns of disease may occur. Some time variables are a decade, a year, a month, a week, or a day. Descriptive studies, regarded as a fundamental approach by epidemiologists, aim to delineate the patterns and manner in which disease occurs in populations.[11]

An example of a pattern derived from descriptive studies is disease clustering, which refers to "A closely grouped series of events or cases of a disease or other health-related phenomena with well-defined distribution patterns in relation to time or place or both. The term is normally used to describe aggregation of relatively uncommon events or diseases, e.g., leukemia, multiple sclerosis."[12]

Clustering may suggest common exposure of the population to an environmental hazard; it also may be purely spuri-

The Texas Sharpshooter Effect

A traveler passing through a small town in Texas noted a remarkable display of sharpshooting. On almost every barn he passed there was a target with a single bullet hole that uncannily passed through the center of the bull's-eye. He was so intrigued by this that he stopped at a nearby gas station to ask about the sharpshooter. With a chuckle, the attendant told him that the shooting was the work of Old Joe. Old Joe would first shoot at the side of a barn and then paint targets centered over his bullet holes so that each shot appeared to pass through the center of the target. . . . In a random distribution of cases of cancer over a geographic area, some cases will appear to occur very close together just on the basis of random variation. The occurrence of a group of cases of a disease close together in time and place at the time of their diagnosis is called a cluster.

Source: Reprinted from S Grufferman. Methodologic approaches to studying environmental factors in childhood cancer. *Environ Health Perspect.* 1998;106(suppl 3):882.

ous—due to the operation of chance. One cause of spurious clustering is called the Texas Sharpshooter Effect, discussed in the text box.

In the field of occupational health—which in many respects is emblematic of the general field of environmental health—"*Descriptive studies* provide information for setting priorities, identifying hazards, and formulating hypotheses for new occupational risk."[13(p944)] A historical example (discussed later in this chapter) is William Farr's work showing that Cornwall metal miners had higher mortality from all causes than the general population.[13]

Analytic epidemiology examines causal (etiologic) hypotheses regarding the association between exposures and health conditions. "Etiologic studies are planned examinations of causality and the natural history of disease. These studies have required increasingly sophisticated analytic methods as the importance of low-level exposures is explored and greater refinement in exposure-effect relationships is sought."[13(p945)] The field of analytic epidemiology proposes and evaluates causal models that employ both outcome variables and exposure variables.

The exposure variables in epidemiologic research include contact with toxic substances, potential carcinogens, or air pollution. In other cases, exposure may be to biological agents or to forms of energy such as ionizing and nonionizing radiation, noise, and extremes of temperature. For an environmental epidemiologic research study to be valid, the level of exposure in a population must be assessed validly.

The outcome variable in epidemiologic studies is usually a specific disease, cause of mortality, or health condition. Accurate clinical assessments of an outcome such as lung cancer are vitally important to the quality of epidemiologic research.

One approach of analytic epidemiology is to take advantage of naturally occurring situations or events in order to test causal hypotheses. These naturally occurring events are referred to as **natural experiments**, defined as "Naturally occurring circumstances in which subsets of the population have different levels of exposure to a supposed causal factor, in a situation resembling an actual experiment where human subjects would be randomly allocated to groups."[12] An example is the work of John Snow, discussed later in this chapter. Many past or ongoing natural experiments are relevant to environmental epidemiology. For example, in some regions of the United States, health legislation prohibits smoking in public areas in order to prevent exposure to secondhand smoke. At the same time, this activity may be considered a natural experiment that impacts human health and that can be studied by environmental epidemiologists.

Measures of Disease Frequency Used in Epidemiology

A number of quantitative terms, useful in environmental epidemiology, have been developed to characterize the occurrence of disease, morbidity, and mortality in populations. Particularly noteworthy are the two terms **prevalence** and **incidence**, which can be stated as frequencies or raw numbers of cases. In order to make comparisons among populations that differ in size, statisticians divide the number of cases by the population size. Several examples follow.

The term *prevalence* refers to the number of existing cases of or deaths from a disease or health condition in a population at some designated time. More specifically, **point prevalence** refers to all cases of or deaths from a disease or health condition that exist at a particular point in time relative to a specific population from which the cases are derived. Prevalence measures are used to describe the scope and distribution of health outcomes in the population. By revealing a snapshot of disease occurrence in the population, prevalence data contribute to the accomplishment of two of the primary functions of descriptive epidemiology: to assess variations in the occurrence of disease in populations and to aid in the development of etiologic hypotheses.

Comparisons among populations that differ in size cannot be accomplished directly by using frequency or prevalence data. In order to make such comparisons, prevalence (usually referring to point prevalence) may be expressed as a proportion formed by dividing the number of cases that occur in a population by the size of the population in which the cases occur.

$$Point\ prevalence = \frac{Number\ of\ persons\ ill}{Total\ number\ in\ the\ group}\ at\ a\ point\ in\ time$$

The term *incidence* refers to the occurrence of new disease or mortality within a defined period of observation (e.g., a week, month, year, or other time period) in a specified population. Those members of the population who are capable of developing the disease or condition being studied are known as the **population at risk**.

The **incidence rate** denotes a rate formed by dividing the number of new cases that occur during a time period by the number of individuals in the population at risk. (Several variations of incidence rates exist, but a discussion of all of them is beyond the scope of this chapter.) Statistically speaking, the incidence rate is a rate because of the specification of a time period during which the new cases occur.

$$Incidence\ rate = \frac{Number\ of\ new\ cases}{Total\ population\ at\ risk}\ over\ a\ time\ period$$
$$\times\ multiplier\ (e.g.,\ 100,000)$$

Incidence measures are central to the study of causal mechanisms with regard to how exposures affect health outcomes. Incidence measures are used to describe the risks associated with certain exposures; they can be used to estimate in a population "the probability of someone in that population developing the disease during a specified period, conditional on not dying first from another disease."[9(p23)]

One additional measure covered in this section is known as the case fatality rate (CFR). (Note that Chapter 5 will refer to the CFR.) The CFR, which provides a measure of the lethality of a disease, is defined as the number of deaths due to a specific disease within a specified time period divided by the number of cases of that disease during the same time period multiplied by 100. The formula is expressed as follows:

$$CFR(\%) = \frac{\begin{array}{c}Number\ of\ deaths\\ due\ to\ disease\ "X"\end{array}}{\begin{array}{c}Number\ of\ cases\\ of\ disease\ "X"\end{array}} \times 100\ during\ a\ time\ period$$

The numerator and denominator refer to the same time period. For example, suppose that 45 cases of hantavirus infection occurred in a western US state during a year of interest. Of these cases, 22 were fatal. The CFR would be:

$$CFR(\%) = \frac{22}{45} \times 100 = 48.9\%$$

BRIEF HISTORY OF ENVIRONMENTAL EPIDEMIOLOGY

Hippocrates

Environmental epidemiology has a long history that dates back 2,000 or more years.[14] For example, in about 400 BC the ancient Greek authority Hippocrates expounded on the role of environmental factors such as water quality and the air in causing diseases.[14] He produced the well-known book *On Airs, Waters, and Places*. Experts in the field posit that these writings form the historical cornerstone of environmental epidemiology. Hippocrates' work and the writings of many of the ancients did not delineate specific known agents involved in the causality of health problems, but referred more generically to air, water, and food. In this respect, early epidemiology shares with contemporary epidemiology the frequent lack of complete knowledge of the specific agents of environmentally associated diseases.

Sir Percival Pott

Sir Percival Pott, a London surgeon, was significant to the history of environmental epidemiology because he is thought to be the first individual to describe an environmental cause of cancer. (See Figure 2-1.)

In 1775, Pott made the astute observation that chimney sweeps had a high incidence of scrotal cancer (in comparison with male workers in other occupations).[1] He argued that chimney sweeps were prone to this malady as a consequence of their contact with soot.[15] (See Figure 2-2.)

In a book entitled *Chirurgical Observations Relative to the Cataract, the Polypus of the Nose, the Cancer of the Scrotum, the Different Kinds of Ruptures, and the Mortification of the Toes and Feet*, published in London in 1775, Pott developed a chapter called "A Short Treatise of the Chimney Sweeper's Cancer." This brief work of only 725 words is noteworthy because

> it provided the first clear description of an environmental cause of cancer, suggested a way to prevent the disease, and led indirectly to the synthesis of the first known pure carcinogen and the isolation of the first carcinogenic chemical to

FIGURE 2-1 Percival Pott, F.R.S., 1714–1788.

PERCIVALL POTT Efq.ʳ

Engraved by Heath, from a Picture
of Sir Joshua Reynolds.

Publish'd March 10ᵗʰ 1790, by J. Johnson, Sᵗ Paul's Church Yard.

Source: © Wellcome Library, London.

singularly hard; in their early infancy, they are most frequently treated with great brutality, and almost starved with cold and hunger; they are thrust up narrow, and sometimes hot chimnies, where they are bruised, burned, and almost suffocated; and when they get to puberty, become peculiary [*sic*] liable to a noisome, painful and fatal disease. Of this last circumstance there is not the least doubt though perhaps it may not have been sufficiently attended to, to make it generally known. Other people have cancers of the same part; and so have others besides lead-workers, the Poictou colic, and the consequent paralysis; but it is nevertheless a disease to which they are particularly liable; and so are chimney-sweepers to the cancer of the scrotum and testicles. The disease, in these people . . . seems to derive its origin from a lodgment of soot in the rugae of the scrotum.[15(pp521–522)]

FIGURE 2-2 A chimney sweep.

Source: © Annamaria Szilagyi/ShutterStock, Inc.

be obtained from a natural product. No wonder therefore that Pott's observation has come to be regarded as the foundation stone on w[h]ich the knowledge of cancer prevention has been built![15(p521)]

In Pott's own words,

[E]very body . . . is acquainted with the disorders to which painters, plummers, glaziers, and the workers in white lead are liable; but there is a disease as peculiar to a certain set of people which has not, at least to my knowledge, been publickly noteced; I mean the chimney-sweepers' cancer. . . . The fate of these people seems

Following his conclusions about the relationship between scrotal cancer and chimney sweeping, Pott established an occupational hygiene control measure—the recommendation that chimney sweeps bathe once a week.

John Snow

During the mid-1800s, English anesthesiologist John Snow (see Figure 2-3) linked a cholera outbreak in London to contaminated water from the Thames River. His methodology for investigating the cholera outbreak of 1849 was known as a "natural experiment," a methodology used currently in the study of environmental health problems. Refer to the text box for more information.

In addition to utilizing the method of natural experiment, John Snow provided expert witness testimony on behalf of industry with respect to environmental exposures to potential disease agents.[17] Snow attempted to extrapolate from the health effects of exposures to high doses of environmental substances what the effects of low doses would be. On January 23, 1855, the Nuisances Removal and Diseases Prevention

The Natural Experiment

The natural experiment: Two water companies, the Lambeth Company and the Southwark and Vauxhall Company, provided water in such a manner that adjacent houses could receive water from two different sources. In 1852, one of the companies, the Lambeth Company, relocated its water sources to a section of the Thames River that was less contaminated. During a later cholera outbreak in 1854, Snow observed that a higher proportion of residents who used the water from the Southwark and Vauxhall Company developed cholera than did residents who used water from the Lambeth Company. The correspondence between changes in the quality of the water supply and changes in the occurrence of cholera became known as a natural experiment. The Lambeth Company provided cleaner water than the Southwark and Vauxhall Company. "The mortality in the houses supplied by the Southwark and Vauxhall Company was therefore between eight and nine times as great as in the houses supplied by the Lambeth Company."[16(p86)]

FIGURE 2-3 John Snow.

Source: © National Library of Medicine.

Amendments bill was introduced in the British Parliament. This bill was a reform of Victorian public health legislation that followed the 1854 cholera outbreak described in the foregoing paragraph.[17] The intent of the bill was to control release into the atmosphere of fumes from operations such as gas works, silk-boiling works, and bone-boiling factories. Snow contended that these odors were not a disease hazard in the community.[18] The thesis of Snow's argument was that deleterious health effects from the low levels of exposure experienced in the community were unlikely, given the knowledge about higher-level exposures among those who worked in the factories. Snow argued that the workers in the factories were not suffering any ill health effects or dying from the exposure. Therefore, it was unlikely that the much lower exposures experienced by the members of the larger community would affect the latter's health.

STRATEGIES OF ENVIRONMENTAL EPIDEMIOLOGY

Study designs used in environmental epidemiology are similar to those developed for general epidemiologic research. Study designs can be arranged on a continuum ranging from hy-

John Snow's Investigation of a Cholera Outbreak in London, Circa 1849

A section of London, designated the Broad Street neighborhood (now part of the Soho district), became the focus of Snow's detective work. Two water companies, the Lambeth Company and the Southwark and Vauxhall Company, provided water in such a manner that adjacent houses could receive water from two different sources. One of the companies, the Lambeth Company, relocated its water sources to a section of the Thames River that was less contaminated. During a later cholera outbreak in 1854, Snow observed that a higher proportion of residents who used the water from the Southwark and Vauxhall Company developed cholera than did residents who used water from the Lambeth Company. Snow's efforts to show a correspondence between changes in the water supply and occurrence of cholera became known as a natural experiment.

Here is Snow's graphic description of the cholera outbreak that occurred in 1849.

The most terrible outbreak of cholera which ever occurred in this kingdom, is probably that which took place in Broad Street, Golden Square, and the adjoining streets, a few weeks ago. . . . The mortality in this limited area probably equals any that was ever caused in this country, even by the plague; and it was much more sudden, as the greater number of cases terminated in a few hours. . . . Many houses were closed altogether, owing to the death of the proprietors; and, in a great number of instances, the tradesmen who remained had sent away their families: so that in less than six days from the commencement of the outbreak, the most afflicted streets were deserted by more than three-quarters of their inhabitants.[16(p38)]

Snow's pioneering approach illustrated the use of both descriptive and analytic epidemiology. One of his first activities was to plot the cholera deaths in relation to a pump that he hypothesized was the cause of the cholera outbreak. Each death was shown on the map (Figure 2-4) as a short line. An arrow in the figure points to the location of the Broad Street pump. "As soon as I became acquainted with the situation and the extent of this irruption of cholera, I suspected some contamination of the water of the much-frequented street-pump in Broad Street, near the end of Cambridge Street; . . . On proceeding to the spot, I found that nearly all the deaths had taken place within a short distance of the pump."[16(pp38–39)] The handle of the pump was later removed—a public health measure to control the outbreak. In Snow's time, many European cities took water for domestic use directly from rivers, which often were contaminated with microorganisms.

Source: Snow J. *Snow on Cholera.* Cambridge, MA: Harvard University Press; 1965.

pothesis-generating designs that provide limited information to complex hypothesis-testing designs.[8] Purely observational study designs include case series, cross-sectional, ecologic, case-control, and cohort studies. Nonobservational and partly observational designs that are used include experimental and quasi-experimental designs.

For the particular problem being investigated, some designs are better than others, depending upon what is to be achieved, the availability of study populations, the disease or health outcome studied, and the need to uncover disease etiology.[8] Examples of the subset of observational designs that are used for hypothesis generation include cross-sectional studies, case series, some types of ecologic correlations, and proportionate mortality comparisons.[8] The subset of observational designs that are used for hypothesis testing includes cohort and case-control studies. One of the distinguishing

characteristics of study designs is whether they involve the individual or group as the unit of analysis. With the exception of ecologic studies, all the designs presented in this chapter use the individual as the unit of analysis.

Experimental Studies

Consider the use of experimental studies in environmental health research; in epidemiology, experimental studies are implemented as intervention studies. An **intervention study** is "[a]n investigation involving intentional change in some aspect of the status of the subjects, e.g., introduction of a preventive or therapeutic regimen, or an intervention designed to test a hypothesized relationship. . . ."[12]

Two experimental methods are randomized controlled trials and quasi-experiments. A simple example of the former is a classic experimental design in which there is manipulation

FIGURE 2-4 Map of cholera cases in the Broad Street area. Each case is indicated by a short line.

Source: Reprinted from Snow J. *Snow on Cholera.* Harvard University Press; © 1965.

of an exposure variable and random assignment of subjects to either a treatment group or a control group. Some uses of randomized controlled trials are to test the efficacy of new medications, medical regimens, and vaccines. A specific application is the use of an experimental trial to test the efficacy of fluoridation of drinking water in preventing tooth decay.[9] In this scenario, communities would be selected at random for the addition of fluoride to the public water supply; those with and those without fluoridated water would be compared with respect to the frequency of dental caries among their residents.

Fluoridation of water also could be conducted as a quasi-experimental study, in which there is manipulation of an exposure variable, but subjects are not randomly allocated to

the study conditions. During the 1940s and 1950s, two comparable New York cities (one having received fluoride for about a decade and the other having received none) were contrasted for the occurrence of tooth decay and related dental problems among children. In the community that added fluoride to the water supply, the frequency of such problems decreased by about one half.[9] This example was a quasi-experiment because the "subjects" (cities) were assigned arbitrarily and not randomly.

For several reasons, the use of experimental methods in environmental epidemiology is difficult to achieve; consequently, observational methods are usually more feasible to implement. Rothman points out:

Randomized assignment of individuals into groups with different environmental exposures generally is impractical, if not unethical; community intervention trials for environmental exposures have been conducted, although seldom (if ever) with random assignment. Furthermore, the benefits of randomization are heavily diluted when the number of randomly assigned units is small, as when communities rather than individuals are randomized. Thus, environmental epidemiology consists nearly exclusively of non-experimental epidemiology. Ideally, such studies use individuals as the unit of measurement; but often environmental data are available only for groups of individuals, and investigators turn to so-called ecologic studies to learn what they can.[6(p20)]

Consequently, in order to study the effects of environmental exposures when dealing with human populations, researchers must use observational methods, and, in fact, the majority of research on health outcomes associated with the environment uses observational methods.[19]

Case Series

A **case series study** is one in which information about patients who share a disease in common is gathered over time. Although this type of study is among the weakest for making causal assertions, a case series can be useful for developing hypotheses for further study. Usually information from a case series study is considered to be preliminary and a starting point for more complex investigations. However, some astute clinicians have used information from series of cases to make important observations. An example comes from the work of Herbst and Scully, who were the first to describe the association between exposure to diethylstilbestrol (DES) during mothers' pregnancies and risk of clear-cell cervicovaginal cancer among six female adolescents and young adults.[20]

Cross-Sectional Studies

A **cross-sectional study** is defined as one

> that examines the relationship between diseases (or other health-related characteristics) and other variables of interest as they exist in a defined population at one particular time. The presence or absence of disease and the presence or absence of the other variables . . . are determined in each member of the study population or in a representative sample at one particular time.[12]

Thus, a cross-sectional study is a type of prevalence study in which the distribution of disease and exposure are determined, although it is not imperative for the study to include both exposure and disease. A cross-sectional study may focus only on the latter.[2] Cross-sectional designs make a one-time assessment of the prevalence of disease in a sample that in most situations has been sampled randomly from the parent population of interest.[9] Cross-sectional studies may be used to formulate hypotheses that can be followed up in analytic studies.

Here is an example of a cross-sectional study: As part of an asthma reduction program conducted in Passaic, New Jersey, during the 1998 through 1999 school year, investigators conducted a survey of a community in which all third graders were targeted.[21] The study children and their parents were given self-report symptom questionnaires. A total of 976 children and 818 parents returned the questionnaire. A respiratory therapist collected spirometry (lung function) readings from 615 children (approximately 58% of the target population). The study demonstrated that about half the children experienced self-reported asthma-related symptoms. However, because self-reports were not associated closely with the results of the spirometry tests, the investigators concluded that the self-reported data from children were not good predictors of asthma risk. From the spirometry results, about 22% of the children had abnormal results, with significant differences occurring by race and ethnicity. More abnormal evaluations were found for blacks and Asians in comparison with other groups. Table 2-1 reports the results of the spirometry evaluation.

Ecologic Studies

Ecologic studies are different from most other types of epidemiologic research in regard to the unit of analysis. An **ecologic study** (also called an ecological study) is "a study in which the units of analysis are populations or groups of people, rather than individuals."[12] For example, the occurrence of an outcome of interest (e.g., a disease, mortality, health effect) might be assessed over different geographic areas—states, census tracts, or counties. To illustrate, one could study the "relationship between the distribution of income and mortality rates in states or counties."[12] The assumption is made that outcome rates would be comparable in exposed and nonexposed groups if the exposure did not take place in the exposed group. In the foregoing example, if the outcome were mortality from

TABLE 2-1 Population Distribution, by Race/Ethnicity, and Percentage of Each Subgroup with Physician-Interpreted Abnormal Spirometry Readings (n = 455)

	Population Distribution >	Abnormal Spirometry, %
Dominican	22.6	28.2
Mexican	19.8	10.0
Puerto Rican	19.3	8.0
Mixed other Hispanic	9.7	4.5
Peruvian	4.0	11.1
Colombian	2.6	8.3
Black	11.2	39.2
White	4.0	27.8
Asian	3.7	47.1
Mixed non-Hispanic	3.1	14.3

Source: Adapted and reprinted with permission from NCG Freeman, D Schneider, and P McGarvey. School-based screening for asthma in third-grade urban children: the Passaic asthma reduction effort survey. *Am J Public Health.* 2002;92:45.

cancer, researchers might hypothesize that persons living in lower-income areas have greater exposure to environmental carcinogens than those who live in higher-income areas, producing differences in cancer mortality.

Ecologic analyses have been used to correlate air pollution with adverse health effects such as mortality. Instead of correlating individual exposure to air pollution with mortality, the researcher measures the association between average exposure to air pollution within a census tract and the average mortality in that census tract. Other types of geographic subdivisions besides census tracts may be used as well. This type of study attempts to demonstrate that mortality is higher in more polluted census tracts than in less polluted census tracts.

A major problem of the ecologic technique for the study of air pollution (and for virtually all ecologic studies) stems from uncontrolled factors. Examples relevant to air pollution include individual levels of smoking and smoking habits, occupational exposure to respiratory hazards and air pollution, differences in social class and other demographic factors, genetic background, and length of residence in the area.[8] Nonetheless, ecologic studies may open the next generation of investigations; the interesting observations gathered in ecologic studies may provide the impetus for more carefully designed studies. The next wave of studies that build on ecologic studies then may attempt to take advantage of more rigorous analytic study designs.

Ecologic studies have examined the association between water quality and both stroke and coronary diseases. A group of studies has demonstrated that hardness of the domestic water supply is associated inversely with risk of cerebrovascular mortality and cardiovascular diseases. However, a Japanese investigation did not support a relationship between water hardness and cerebrovascular diseases. In the latter ecologic study, the unit of analysis was municipalities (population subdivisions in Japan that consisted of from 6,000 to 3 million inhabitants). In analyzing the 1995 death rates from strokes in relationship to the values of water hardness, the researchers did not find statistically significant associations across municipalities.[22]

Other ecologic studies have examined the possible association between use of agricultural pesticides and childhood cancer incidence. For example, a total of 7,143 incident cases of invasive cancer diagnosed among children younger than age 15 were reported to the California Cancer Registry during the years 1988–1994. In this ecologic study, the unit of analysis was census blocks, with average annual pesticide exposure estimated per square mile. The study showed no overall association between pesticide exposure determined by this method and childhood cancer incidence rates. However, a significant increase of childhood leukemia rates was linked to census block groups that had the highest use of one form of pesticide, called propargite.[23]

Case-Control Studies

In a **case-control study**, subjects who participate in the study are defined on the basis of the presence or absence of an outcome of interest. The cases are those who have the outcome or disease of interest, and the controls are those who do not. In a case-control study, cases and controls generally are matched according to criteria such as sex, age, race, or other variables. Exposure to a factor is determined retrospectively, meaning that exposure has already occurred in the past. One method to determine past exposure is for the investigator to interview cases and controls regarding their exposure history. An advantage of case-control studies is that they can examine many potential exposures. For example, subjects may be queried about one or more exposures that they may have had in the past; in some variations of this approach, it may be possible to conduct direct measurements of the environment for various types of exposures. A disadvantage of case-control studies is that, in most circumstances, they can examine only one or a few outcomes.[8]

Researchers have a variety of sources available for the selection of cases and controls. For example, they may use pa-

TABLE 2-2 Table for a Case-Control Study

		Disease Status—Outcome of Interest	
		Yes (Cases)	No (Controls)
Exposure	Yes	A	B
Status	No	C	D
	Total	A + C	B + D

tients from hospitals, specialized clinics, or medical practices. Sometimes, advertisements in media solicit cases. Cases may be selected from disease registries such as cancer registries. Controls can be either healthy persons or those affected by a disease that is etiologically unrelated to the outcome of interest. For example, investigators may identify as controls patients from hospitals or clinics; however, these control patients must not have been affected by the outcome of interest. In other studies, controls may be friends or relatives of the cases or be from the community.

The measure of association between exposure and outcome used in case-control studies is known as the **odds ratio (OR)**. A particular form of OR, the exposure-odds ratio, refers to "the ratio of odds in favor of exposure among the cases [A/C] to the odds in favor of exposure among the non-cases [the controls, B/D]."[12] Table 2-2 illustrates the method for labeling cells in a case-control study. This table is called a 2 × 2 table.

The OR is defined as $\dfrac{\frac{A}{C}}{\frac{B}{D}}$, which can be expressed as $\dfrac{AD}{BC}$.

An odds ratio of more than 1 suggests a positive association between the exposure and disease or other outcome (provided that the results are statistically significant—a concept that will not be discussed here).

Calculation example: Suppose we have the following data from a case-control study: A = 9, B = 4, C = 95, D = 88. The OR is calculated as follows:

$$OR = \frac{AD}{BC} = \frac{(9)(88)}{(4)(95)} = 2.08$$

In this sample calculation, the OR is greater than 1, suggesting that the odds of the disease are higher among the exposed persons than among the nonexposed persons.

Case-control studies are very common in environmental epidemiologic research. For example, environmental health researchers have been concerned about the possible health effects of exposure to electromagnetic fields (EMFs). A case-control study among female residents of Long Island, New York, examined the possible association between exposure to EMFs and breast cancer.[24] Eligible subjects were those who were younger than 75 years of age and who had lived in the study area for 15 years or longer. Cases (n = 576) consisted of women diagnosed with in situ or invasive breast cancer. Controls (n = 585) were selected from the same community by random digit dialing procedures. Several types of measurement of EMFs were taken in the subjects' homes and by mapping overhead power lines. The investigators reported that the odds ratio between EMF exposure and breast cancer was not statistically significantly different from 1; thus, the results suggested that there was no association between breast cancer and residential EMF exposure.

In comparison with cross-sectional study designs, case-control studies may provide more complete exposure data, especially when the exposure information is collected from the friends and relatives of cases who died of a particular cause. Nevertheless, some unmeasured exposure variables as well as methodological biases (a term discussed later in this chapter) may remain in case-control studies. For example, in studies of health and air pollution, exposure levels are difficult to quantify precisely. Also, it may be difficult to measure unknown and unobserved factors, including smoking habits and occupational exposures to air pollution, which affect the lungs.[8]

Cohort Studies

A **cohort study** design classifies subjects according to their exposure to a factor of interest and then observes them over time to document the occurrence of new cases (incidence) of disease or other health events. Cohort studies are a type of longitudinal design, meaning that subjects are followed over an extended period of time. Using cohort studies, epidemiologists are able to evaluate many different outcomes (causes of death) but few exposures.[8]

Cohort studies may be either prospective or retrospective. At the inception of a prospective cohort study, participating individuals must be certified as being free from the outcome of interest. As these individuals are followed into the future, the occurrence of new cases of the disease is noted. A retrospective cohort study (historical cohort study) is "conducted by reconstructing data about persons at a time or times in the past. This method uses existing records about the health or other relevant aspects of a population as it was at some time in the past and determines the current (or subsequent) status of members of this population with respect to the condition of interest."[12] An example of a retrospective cohort study would be one that examined mortality among an occupational cohort such as shipyard workers who were employed at a specific naval yard during a defined time interval (e.g., during World War II).

The measure of association used in cohort studies is called **relative risk (RR)**, the ratio of the incidence rate of a disease or health outcome in an exposed group to the incidence rate of the disease or condition in a nonexposed group. As noted previously, an incidence rate may be interpreted as the risk of occurrence of an outcome that is associated with a particular exposure. The RR provides a ratio of two risks—the risk associated with an exposure in comparison with the risk associated with nonexposure.

Mathematically, the term *relative risk* is defined as A/(A + B) (the rate [incidence] of the disease or condition in the exposed group) divided by C/(C + D) (the rate [incidence] of the disease or condition in the nonexposed group). A 2 × 2 table for the elements used in the calculation of a relative risk is shown in Table 2-3.

$$RR = \frac{\dfrac{A}{A + B}}{\dfrac{C}{C + D}}$$

Calculation example: Suppose that we are researching whether exposure to solvents is associated with risk of liver cancer. From a cohort study of industrial workers, we find that three persons who worked with solvents developed liver cancer (cell A of Table 2-3) and 104 did not (cell B). Two cases of liver cancer occurred among nonexposed workers (cell C) in the same type of industry. The remaining 601 nonexposed workers (cell D) did not develop liver cancer. The RR is:

$$RR = \frac{\dfrac{3}{3 + 104}}{\dfrac{2}{2 + 601}} = 8.45$$

We may interpret relative risk in a manner that is similar to that of the odds ratio. For example, a relative risk greater than 1 (and statistically significant) indicates that the risk of disease is greater in the exposed group than in the nonexposed

group. In other words, there is a positive association between exposure and the outcome under study. In the calculation example, the risk of developing liver cancer is eight times greater among workers who were exposed to solvents than among those who were not exposed to solvents.

Sometimes a relative risk calculation yields a value that is less than 1. If the relative risk is less than 1 (and statistically significant), the risk is lower among the exposed group. This level of risk (i.e., less than 1) sometimes is called a protective effect.

Accurate disease verification is necessary to optimize measures of relative risk; disease misclassification affects estimates of relative risk. The type of disease and method of diagnosis affect accuracy of diagnosis.[8] To illustrate, death certificates are used frequently as a source of information about the diagnosis of a disease. Information from death certificates regarding cancer as the underlying cause of death is believed to be more accurate than the information for other diagnoses such as those for nonmalignant conditions. Nevertheless, the accuracy of diagnoses of cancer as a cause of death varies according to the particular form of cancer.

Cohort studies are applied widely in environmental health. For example, they have been used to examine the effects of environmental and work-related exposures to potentially toxic agents. One concern of cohort studies has been exposure of female workers to occupationally related reproductive hazards and adverse pregnancy outcomes.[25]

A second example is an Australian study that examined the health impacts of occupational exposure to insecticides.[26] The investigators selected a cohort of 1,999 outdoor workers known to be employed as field officers or laboratory staff for the New South Wales Board of Tick Control between 1935 and 1996. Only male subjects were selected for the study. A control cohort consisted of 1,984 men who worked as outdoor field officers at any time since 1935. Occupational monitoring programs demonstrated that members of the exposure cohort had worked with pesticides, including DDT. The investigators carefully evaluated exposure status and health outcomes such as mortality from various chronic diseases and cancer. They reported an association between exposure to pesticides and adverse health effects, particularly for asthma, diabetes, and some forms of cancer including pancreatic cancer.

Study Endpoints Used in Environmental Epidemiologic Research

In evaluating the health effects of occupational exposures to toxic agents, researchers may study various endpoints, including measures derived from self-report questionnaires, results of direct physical examinations, and mortality experience in a

TABLE 2-3 Table for a Cohort Study

		Disease Status		
		Yes	No	Total
Exposure	Yes	A	B	A+B
Status	No	C	D	C+D

population. The endpoints also may be keyed to any of a number of stages in the natural progression of disease (e.g., presymptomatic, symptomatic, or permanent dysfunction).[27]

In some studies, self-reported symptom rates are used as a measure of the effects of low-level chemical exposure. Occupational health investigators can design and administer self-report questionnaires inexpensively. Self-reports to questionnaires, however, may not always be reliable, and although they correlate often with clinical diagnoses they also may differ markedly.[6]

Physiologic or clinical examinations are other means to evaluate adverse health effects. For example, in a study of respiratory diseases, pulmonary function tests, such as forced expiratory volume, may be an appropriate indicator. Although clinical examinations may provide "harder" evidence of health effects than self-reports, such examinations may be expensive or impractical to conduct in the case of workers who have left employment.

In other studies, mortality is the outcome of interest; research on mortality frequently uses a retrospective cohort study design.[7] Mortality experience in an employment cohort can be compared with the expected mortality in the general population (national, regional, state, or county) by using the standardized mortality ratio (SMR), which is defined as "The ratio of the number of deaths observed in the study group or population to the number that would be expected if the study population had the same specific rates as the standard population. Often multiplied by 100."[12] Typically the SMR is denoted by a percentage; when the percentage is greater than 100%, the SMR in the study population is elevated above that found in the comparison population. Conversely, when the SMR is less than 100%, the mortality experience in the study population is lower than that of the comparison population.

One also can contrast the mortality experience of exposed workers with the mortality rate of nonexposed workers in the same industry. For example, production workers might be compared with drivers or office workers. Another option is to identify a second industry or occupation that is comparable in terms of skill level, educational requirements, or geographic location but in which the exposure of interest is not present.

The use of mortality as a study endpoint has several advantages, including the fact that it may be relevant to agents that have a subtle effect over a long time period. Although any fatal chronic disease may be investigated, mortality from cancer often is studied as an outcome variable in occupational exposures. According to Monson, "Cancer specifically tends to be a fatal illness; its presence is usually indicated on the death certificate. Also, cancer is a fairly specific disease and

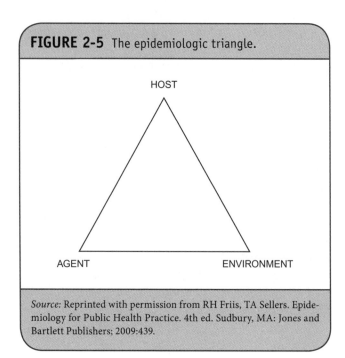

FIGURE 2-5 The epidemiologic triangle.

HOST

AGENT

ENVIRONMENT

Source: Reprinted with permission from RH Friis, TA Sellers. Epidemiology for Public Health Practice. 4th ed. Sudbury, MA: Jones and Bartlett Publishers; 2009:439.

is less subject to random misclassification than, say, one of the cardiovascular diseases."[28(p106)]

CAUSALITY IN EPIDEMIOLOGIC STUDIES

One of the fundamental models of causality used in epidemiologic studies is the **epidemiologic triangle**, which includes three major factors: agent, host, and environment. Although this model has been applied to the field of infectious disease epidemiology, it also provides a framework for organizing the causality of other types of environmental problems. Refer to Figure 2-5 for an illustration.

The term *environment* is defined as the domain in which disease-causing agents may exist, survive, or originate; it consists of "[a]ll that which is external to the individual human host."[12] The **host** is "[a] person or other living animal, including birds and arthropods, that affords subsistence or lodgment to an infectious agent under natural conditions."[12] A human host is a person who is afflicted with a disease; or, from the epidemiologic perspective, the term host denotes an affected group or population. An **agent** (of disease) refers to

> a factor—such as a microorganism, chemical substance, or form of radiation—whose presence, excessive presence, or (in deficiency diseases) relative absence is essential for the occurrence of a disease. A disease may have a single agent, a number of independent alternative agents (at least one of which must be present),

or a complex of two or more factors whose combined presence is essential for the development of the disease.[12]

In environmental health, agent factors can include (but are not limited to) particulate matter from pollution, toxic chemicals and pesticides, and microbes. Examples of agent factors covered in this text are:

- Microbial agents responsible for zoonotic diseases
- Microbial agents linked to foodborne illness
- Toxic chemicals including pesticides
- Toxic metals
- Airborne particulates and gases
- Radiation: ionizing and nonionizing

These agents are relevant to many of the environmental problems discussed in this text, including hazardous waste disposal, zoonotic illnesses, foodborne illnesses, accidents, occupational illnesses, and adverse health outcomes associated with water and air pollution.

Criteria of Causality

The epidemiologic triangle provides a framework for viewing hypothesized relationships among agent, host, and environmental factors in causation of disease. One of the central concerns of environmental health epidemiology is to be able to assert that a causal association exists between an agent factor and a disease in the host. Hill pointed out that in the realm of occupational health, extreme conditions in the physical environment or exposure to known toxic chemicals should be invariably injurious.[29] More commonly the situation occurs in which weaker associations have been observed between certain aspects of the environment and the occurrence of health events. An example would be the development of lung diseases among persons exposed to dusts (e.g., miners who work in dusty, unventilated mines). Hill raised the question of how one moves from such an observed association to the verdict of causation (e.g., exposure to coal dust *causes* coal miner's pneumoconiosis). A second example is the perplexing question of the extent to which studies reveal a causal association between a specific environmental exposure and a particular form of cancer.[20]

Hill proposed a situation in which there is a clear association between two variables and in which statistical tests have suggested that this association is not due to chance. For example, data have revealed that smoking is associated with lung cancer in humans and that chance can be ruled out as being responsible for this observed association. The 1964 US government report *Smoking and Health* stated that

Table 2-4 Hill's Criteria of Causality	
Strength	Biological gradient
Consistency	Plausibility
Specificity	Coherence
Temporality	

the evaluation of a causal association does not depend solely upon evidence from a probabilistic statement derived from statistics, but is a matter of judgment that depends upon several criteria.[30] Similarly, Hill listed nine causal criteria that need to be taken into account in the assessment of a causal association between factor A and disease B. For the purposes of this text, we will consider seven of the criteria, which are included in Table 2-4.

Strength

Strong associations give support to a causal relationship between factor and disease. Hill provided the example of the very large increase in scrotal cancer (by a factor of 200 times) among chimney sweeps in comparison with workers who were not exposed occupationally to tars and mineral oils. Another example arises from the steeply elevated lung cancer mortality rates among heavy cigarette smokers in comparison with nonsmokers (20 to 30 times higher). Hill also cautioned that we should not be too ready to dismiss causal associations when the strength of the association is small, because there are many examples of causal relationships that are characterized by weak associations. One example would be exposure to an infectious agent such as meningococcus that produces relatively few clinical cases of meningococcal meningitis.

Consistency

According to Hill, a consistent association is one that has been observed repeatedly "by different persons, in different places, circumstances and times. . . ."[29(p296)] An example of consistency comes from research on the relationship between smoking and lung cancer, a relationship that was found repeatedly in many retrospective and prospective studies.

Specificity

A specific association is one that is constrained to a particular disease–exposure relationship. In a specific association, a given disease results from a given exposure and not from other types of exposures. Hill gave the example of an association that "is limited to specific workers and to particular sites and types of disease and there is no association between the work and other modes of dying. . . ."[29(p297)] Returning to the smoking–lung cancer example, one may argue that the association is not specific, because "the death rate among smokers is higher than the death rate of non-smokers from many causes of death. . . ."[29(p297)] Nevertheless, Hill argued that one-to-one causation is unusual, because many diseases have more than one causal factor.

Temporality

This criterion specifies that we must observe the cause before the effect; Hill stated that we cannot put the cart before the horse. For example, if we assert that air pollution causes lung cancer, we first must exclude persons who have lung cancer from our study; then we must follow those who are exposed to air pollution to determine whether lung cancer develops.

Biological Gradient

A biological gradient also is known as a dose–response curve (discussed in Chapter 3), which shows a linear trend in the association between exposure and disease. An example arises from the linear association between the number of cigarettes smoked and the lung cancer death rate.

Plausibility

This criterion states that an association must be biologically plausible from the standpoint of contemporary biological knowledge. The association between exposure to tars and oils and the development of scrotal cancer is plausible in view of current knowledge about carcinogenesis. However, this knowledge was not available when Pott made his observations during the 18th century.

Coherence

This criterion suggests that "the cause-and-effect interpretation of our data should not seriously conflict with the generally known facts of the natural history and biology of the disease. . . ."[29(p298)] Examples related to cigarette smoking and lung cancer come from the rise in the number of lung cancer deaths associated with an increase in smoking, as well as lung cancer mortality differences between men (who smoke more and have higher lung cancer mortality rates) and women (who smoke less and have lower rates).

BIAS IN ENVIRONMENTAL EPIDEMIOLOGIC STUDIES

Epidemiologic studies may be impacted by **bias**, which is defined as the "[s]ystematic deviation of results or inferences from the truth. Processes leading to such deviation. An error in the conception and design of a study—or in the collection,

analysis, interpretation, reporting, publication, or review of data—leading to results or conclusions that are systematically (as opposed to randomly) different from the truth."[12] There are many types of bias; particularly important for environmental epidemiology are those that impact study procedures. Examples of such bias are related to how the study was designed, the method of data collection, interpretation and review of findings, and procedures used in data analysis. For example, in measurements of exposures and outcomes, faulty measurement devices may introduce biases into study designs.

A complete discussion of all the kinds of bias is beyond the scope of the text; however, we will consider two types of bias, *recall bias* and *selection bias*. The former is particularly relevant to case-control studies. Recall bias refers to the fact that cases may remember an exposure more clearly than controls.[19] The consequence of recall bias is to reduce the reliability of exposure information gathered from control groups.

Selection bias is defined as "Distortions that result from procedures used to select subjects and from factors that influence participation in the study."[12] The effect of selection bias may be to cause systematic differences in characteristics between participants and nonparticipants in research. An example of selection bias is the **healthy worker effect**, which may reduce the validity of exposure data when employed persons are chosen as research subjects in studies of occupational health. Monson states that the healthy worker effect refers to the "observation that employed populations tend to have a lower mortality experience than the general population."[28(p114)] The healthy worker effect may have an impact on occupational mortality studies in several ways. People whose life expectancy is shortened by disease are less likely to be employed than healthy persons. One consequence of this phenomenon would be a reduced (or attenuated) measure of effect for an exposure that increases morbidity or mortality; that is, because the general population includes both employed and unemployed individuals, the mortality rate of that population may be somewhat elevated in comparison with a population in which everyone is healthy enough to work. As a result, any excess mortality associated with a given occupational exposure is more difficult to detect when the healthy worker effect is operative. The healthy worker effect is likely to be stronger for nonmalignant causes of mortality, which usually produce worker attrition during an earlier career phase, than for malignant causes of mortality, which typically have longer latency periods and occur later in life. In addition, healthier workers may have greater total exposure to occupational hazards than those who leave the workforce at an earlier age because of illness.

Another example of study bias is **confounding**, which denotes "the distortion of a measure of the effect of an exposure on an outcome due to the association of the exposure with other factors that influence the occurrence of the outcome."[12] Confounding factors are associated with disease risk and produce a different distribution of outcomes in the exposure groups than in the comparison groups. The existence of confounding factors that occur in the exposed group may lead to invalid conclusions from a study.

An example of confounding arises from the possible association between exposure of workers to occupational dusts and development of lung cancer. One of the types of dust encountered in the workplace is silica (e.g., from sand used in sandblasting). In a retrospective cohort study, one might compare the workers' mortality rates for lung cancer with those of the general population (by using SMRs). Suppose we find that the SMR for lung cancer of workers exposed to silica is greater than 100% (i.e., exceeds the rate of the nonexposed population). One conclusion is that the workers have a higher risk of lung cancer than the nonexposed population. However, the issue of confounding also should be considered: Employees exposed to silica are usually blue-collar workers who, as a rule, have higher smoking rates than the general population (that might be used as a comparison population). When smoking rates are taken into account, the strength of the association between silica exposure and lung cancer is reduced—suggesting that smoking is a confounder that needs to be considered in the association.[31]

LIMITATIONS AND DEFICIENCIES OF ENVIRONMENTAL EPIDEMIOLOGY

According to Buffler, the three major requirements for the successful epidemiologic investigation of environmental exposures are: "(1) direct and accurate estimates of the exposures experienced by individual members of the study population, (2) direct and accurate determination of the disease status of individual members of the study population, and (3) appropriate statistical summarization and analysis of the individual data pertaining to disease and exposure."[14(p131)] To the extent that these requirements are not met, limitations are introduced into epidemiologic studies. Other limiting factors include the long latency periods and infrequent occurrence that characterize many environmentally associated diseases. (Refer to Table 2-5.)

Long Latency Periods

A consideration that limits one's ability to derive causal inferences from epidemiologic studies is the long **latency** period phenomenon.[9] The term *latency period* refers to the time

TABLE 2-5 Limitations Faced by Epidemiologists in Studying Relationships between Exposure and Disease Outcomes in Relation to Community Environmental Pollution

Limitations in detecting disease
1. Long and variable latency periods between exposure and disease diagnosis
2. Etiologic nonspecificity of disease clinical features
3. Small population size coupled with low disease frequency
4. Observer bias in reporting illness occurrence

Limitations in measuring exposure
1. Dependence on indirect, surrogate estimates of exposure and dose (distance from pollution site, etc.)
2. Uncertainty regarding pathways of exposure
3. Probable low-dose levels in most settings
4. Frequent inability to develop useful dose–response data

Source: Reprinted with permission from CW Heath Jr. Uses of epidemiologic information in pollution episode management. *Arch Environ Health.* 1988;43:76.

interval between initial exposure to a disease-causing agent (e.g., environmental risk factor or exposure) and the appearance of a disease or its manifestations in the host.[12] Note that the occurrence of disease can be conceptualized in a number of different ways depending on the measure used, such as screening tests and observation of clinical signs and symptoms. Environmentally caused diseases, for example, cancer, have latency periods that span many years. These long latency periods reduce the epidemiologist's ability to ascertain definitively the outcomes of exposure.[9] Examples are asbestos-related diseases, which in many cases do not appear until many years after initial exposure.[32]

Low Incidence and Prevalence

Another limiting factor of studies concerns the infrequent occurrence of certain diseases that are the target of environmental epidemiologic studies.[9] An example is the occurrence of childhood cancers, which have been examined in relation to environmental factors such as toxic chemicals.[11] The incidence of cancers among children is only one-twentieth that of adults—143.9 per million and 126.9 per million for white males and females aged 0 to 14 years, respectively, and 330.4 and 277.0 per 100,000 white males and females of all ages, respectively. When diseases are uncommon, one's ability to make precise estimates of exposure–disease associations is reduced. The researcher also may be dependent upon less powerful research designs—descriptive and case-control studies.

Difficulties in Exposure Assessment

Several authorities have stressed the requirement for accurate assessment of exposures in epidemiologic studies of environmental health. Rothman points out that "Atop the list of methodologic problems is the problem of exposure assessment, a problem that extends through all of epidemiologic research but is a towering obstacle in environmental epidemiology."[6(p19)] Gardner points out that "Epidemiological methods of investigation are incomplete without good quality exposure data to parallel information on health. The need for monitoring environmental and biological exposure is paramount to the successful interpretation of results and implementation of any required preventive programs."[33(p108)]

For high levels of exposures to toxic agents that produce clear and immediate effects, causation is clear-cut.[34] Examples are the release of toxic gases in Bhopal, India, in 1984, and the 1986 Chernobyl nuclear reactor disaster in the former Soviet Union. Moreover, although earlier generations of studies led to the control of intense environmental exposures that were strongly correlated with disease outcomes, the focus of contemporary research has shifted. Modern studies examine low levels of exposure that potentially are associated with low levels of risk.[14]

Low-level environmental exposures challenge epidemiologic researchers who when dealing with them have difficulty applying standard laboratory methods used to determine exposure levels. Consequently, researchers are unable to establish definitively whether exposure to a particular agent has occurred. In the ambient environment, not only may several exposures be mixed, but also the levels of exposures may be uncertain.[34]

Examples of exposure measurements used in environmental epidemiology include the following: samples of toxic fumes in a manufacturing plant, ozone readings in the community, and distances of housing tracts from high-tension power lines that emit electromagnetic radiation. All of these measures are prone to error because they are indirect measures of exposure and do not provide direct information on the amount of exposure that an individual may actually receive.[6] As noted, a common method for approximating exposure is the use of proxies (substitutes for direct measures). An example of such a measure is the previously noted distance of a housing tract from the source of an environmental hazard. These proxy or surrogate measures are usually too diffuse to establish exposure definitively.

Nonspecific Effects

A specific health outcome is one that is usually associated with a particular exposure, and only that exposure. When an outcome is nonspecific, it can be associated with several or many different environmental exposures. The majority of diseases and conditions thought to be related to environmental exposures are influenced by many factors.[32] Consequently, any particular environmental exposure probably will not be associated with a specific outcome. Further complicating the picture of exposure determination is the fact that we are exposed to hundreds of chemicals in the environment; these chemicals often are mixed, clouding our knowledge of the level of exposure that took place. Exposures to any of these chemicals could produce outcomes that are similar to one another.

CONCLUSION

Environmental epidemiology is one of the fields that research fundamental questions regarding the role of environmental exposures in human health. The discipline traces its history from the time of Hippocrates and from early studies of occupational cancer during the late 18th century. Also historically significant were Snow's investigations of cholera during the mid-19th century. Epidemiology, with its emphasis on observation as well as focus on populations, contributes important methodological tools—particularly with respect to study design.

Several of the key characteristics, weaknesses, and strengths of environmental epidemiology are shown in Table 2-6. One strength is the ability to deal with "real world"

TABLE 2-6 Characteristics, Weaknesses, and Strengths of Environmental Epidemiology

Characteristics	Weaknesses	Strengths
Deals with nondisease effects	Sample size is insufficient	Engages the real world
Involves numerous variables	Important variables "uncontrolled"	Unique perspective on disease/health
Tends to be community-specific	Exposure estimation invalid	Basis for action despite ignorance of mechanism

Source: Reprinted with permission from JR Goldsmith. Keynote address: improving the prospects for environmental epidemiology. *Arch Environ Health.* 1988;43:71.

problems, for example community exposure to environmental contaminants; a second strength is the possibility of examining complex problems that involve multiple variables (e.g., exposure, demographic, and outcome variables); a third is the capability to impel environmental action, even though the level of exposure and etiologic mechanisms of health effects have not been ascertained definitively. The weaknesses include the fact that exposure levels in environmental epidemiology studies are difficult to measure precisely; also, there may be many uncontrolled variables that can bias the results.[35] In the words of Grandjean, "The quality of environmental epidemiology research can be considered from two perspectives, one representing methodological issues, the other dealing with the usefulness of the work. These two views are connected, because a study of superior quality is likely to be of greater validity and therefore more useful. Still, an imperfect study can be of great relevance, and epidemiologists must therefore tackle the challenging balance between being an advocate for particular policies and being a skeptical ivory-tower scientist."[36(p158)] Nevertheless, these weaknesses do not negate the fact that environmental epidemiology has made, and will continue to make, important contributions to the environmental health field. For more information about epidemiology, consult Friis and Sellers[2] or one of the other introductory texts that is available.

Study Questions and Exercises

1. Define the following terms:
   a. Epidemiology
   b. Environmental epidemiology
   c. Descriptive epidemiology
   d. Natural experiments
   e. Prevalence
   f. Incidence
   g. Case fatality rate
   h. Odds ratio
   i. Relative risk

2. What is meant by a cause in environmental epidemiology? Apply Hill's criteria of causality to an example of an association between a specific environmental exposure and health outcome.

3. Explain the reason why studies of the health effects of smoking among individuals who smoke would not be a concern of environmental epidemiology. Explain the reason why exposure to secondhand cigarette smoke is a concern of this discipline.

4. Define the following terms and discuss how each affects the validity of epidemiologic study designs:
   a. Bias
   b. Confounding
   c. Latency period
   d. Exposure assessment

5. List the reasons why epidemiology is important to research studies of environmental health. What

are some of the important limitations of the epidemiologic approach with respect to the study of environmental health problems?

6. Explain why epidemiology sometimes is called "population medicine." State how epidemiology contrasts with clinical medicine.

7. Explain the difference between descriptive and analytic epidemiology. Give examples of how both types of study design are utilized in the field of environmental health.

8. What does early epidemiology (e.g., Hippocrates) share in common with contemporary epidemiology in terms of examining the causality of health problems?

9. Describe the importance of the contributions of Sir Percival Pott to environmental health, particularly in the area of cancer prevention.

10. Explain the work of John Snow using the methodology of the natural experiment.

11. Name the study designs that are used for hypothesis testing and those that are used for generating hypotheses.

12. Explain why most studies conducted in the field of environmental epidemiology are nonexperimental.

13. Explain how ecologic analysis is used to study the health effects of air pollution. Give examples of uncontrolled factors that may affect ecologic study results.

14. Explain why cross-sectional studies are defined as prevalence studies. Give an example of a cross-sectional study.

15. Explain why cohort studies are an improvement over case-control studies with respect to measurement of exposure data.

REFERENCES

1. National Institutes of Health, National Institute of Environmental Health Sciences. What is environmental health? Available at: http://www.niehs.nih.gov/health/docs/enviro-health-define.pdf. Accessed March 5, 2010.

2. Friis RH, Sellers TA. *Epidemiology for Public Health Practice*. 4th ed. Sudbury, MA: Jones and Bartlett Publishers; 2009.

3. Pekkanen J, Pearce N. Environmental epidemiology: challenges and opportunities. *Environ Health Perspect*. 2001;109:1–5.

4. Terracini B. Environmental epidemiology: a historical perspective. In: Elliott P, Cuzick J, English D, Stern R, eds. *Geographical and Environmental Epidemiology: Methods for Small-Area Studies*. New York, NY: Oxford University Press; 1992.

5. Acquavella JF, Friedlander BR, Ireland BK. Interpretation of low to moderate relative risks in environmental epidemiologic studies. *Ann Rev Public Health*. 1994;15:179–201.

6. Rothman KJ. Methodologic frontiers in environmental epidemiology. *Environ Health Perspect*. 1993;101(suppl 4):19–21.

7. Hertz-Picciotto I, Brunekreef B. Environmental epidemiology: where we've been and where we're going. *Epidemiol*. 2001;12:479–481.

8. Blair A, Hayes RB, Stewart PA, Zahm SH. Occupational epidemiologic study design and application. *Occup Med*. 1996;11:403–419.

9. Morgenstern H, Thomas D. Principles of study design in environmental epidemiology. *Environ Health Perspect*. 1993;101(Suppl 4):23–38.

10. Smith AH. Epidemiologic input to environmental risk assessment. *Arch Environ Health*. 1988;43:124–127.

11. Grufferman S. Methodologic approaches to studying environmental factors in childhood cancer. *Environ Health Perspect*. 1998;106(Suppl 3): 881–886.

12. Porta M. *A Dictionary of Epidemiology*. 5th ed. New York, NY: Oxford University Press; 2008.

13. Wegman DH. The potential impact of epidemiology on the prevention of occupational disease. *Am J Public Health*. 1992;82:944–954.

14. Buffler PA. Epidemiology needs and perspectives in environmental epidemiology. *Arch Environ Health*. 1988;43:130–132.

15. Doll R. Pott and the path to prevention. *Arch Geschwulstforsch*. 1975;45:521–531.

16. Snow J. *Snow on Cholera*. Cambridge, MA: Harvard University Press; 1965.

17. Lilienfeld DE. John Snow: the first hired gun? *Am J Epidemiol*. 2000;152:4–9.

18. Sandler DP. John Snow and modern-day environmental epidemiology. *Am J Epidemiol*. 2000;152:1–3.

19. Prentice RL, Thomas D. Methodologic research needs in environmental epidemiology: data analysis. *Environ Health Perspect*. 1993;101(Suppl 4):39–48.

20. DeBaun MR, Gurney JG. Environmental exposure and cancer in children. A conceptual framework for the pediatrician. *Pediatr Clin North Am*. 2001;48:1215–1221.

21. Freeman NCG, Schneider D, McGarvey P. School-based screening for asthma in third-grade urban children: the Passaic asthma reduction effort survey. *Am J Public Health*. 2002;92:45–46.

22. Miyake Y, Iki M. Ecologic study of water hardness and cerebrovascular mortality in Japan. *Arch Environ Health*. 2003;58:163–166.

23. Reynolds P, Von Behren J, Gunier RB, et al. Childhood cancer and agricultural pesticide use: an ecologic study in California. *Environ Health Perspect*. 2002;110:319–324.

24. Schoenfeld ER, O'Leary ES, Henderson K, et al. Electromagnetic fields and breast cancer on Long Island: a case-control study. *Am J Epidemiol*. 2003;158:47–58.

25. Taskinen HK. Epidemiological studies in monitoring reproductive effects. *Environ Health Perspect*. 1993;101(Suppl 3):279–283.

26. Beard J, Sladden T, Morgan G, et al. Health impacts of pesticide exposure in a cohort of outdoor workers. *Environ Health Perspect*. 2003;111: 724–730.

27. Neutra R, Goldman L, Smith D, et al. Study, endpoints, goals, and prioritization for a program in hazardous chemical epidemiology. *Arch Environ Health*. 1988;43(2):94–99.

28. Monson RR. *Occupational Epidemiology*. Boca Raton, FL: CRC Press; 1990.

29. Hill AB. The environment and disease: association or causation? *Proc R Soc Med*. 1965;58:295–300.

30. US Department of Health, Education, and Welfare, Public Health Service, Centers for Disease Control. *Smoking and Health. Report of the Advisory Committee to the Surgeon General of the Public Health Service*. PHS Publication No. 1103. Washington, DC: US Government Printing Office; 1964.

31. Steenland K, Greenland S. Monte Carlo sensitivity analysis and Bayesian analysis of smoking as an unmeasured confounder in a study of silica and lung cancer. *Am J Epidemiol*. 2004;160:384–392.

32. Grandjean P. Epidemiology of environmental hazards. *Public Health Rev*. 1993–1994;21:255–262.

33. Gardner MJ. Epidemiological studies of environmental exposure and specific diseases. *Arch Environ Health*. 1988;43:102–108.

34. Heath CW, Jr. Uses of epidemiologic information in pollution episode management. *Arch Environ Health*. 1988;43:75–80.

35. Goldsmith JR. Keynote address: improving the prospects for environmental epidemiology. *Arch Environ Health*. 1988;43:69–74.

36. Grandjean P. Seven deadly sins of environmental epidemiology and the virtues of precaution. *Epidemiology*. 2008;19:158–162.

Environmental Toxicology

LEARNING OBJECTIVES

By the end of this chapter the reader will be able to:

- Define the term *toxicology*
- Define three important terms used in the field of toxicology
- State five factors that affect responses to a toxic chemical
- Discuss the steps involved in risk assessment
- Describe methods for human exposure assessment

INTRODUCTION

This chapter will define terms used in environmental toxicology and provide an overview of the discipline in order to establish a foundation for the environmental health applications covered in the remainder of the text. First, let us explore why toxicology is important to the environmental health field and the methods it uses to illuminate environmental health problems. The National Toxicology Program (NTP) emphasizes the central role of toxicology in identifying the potential hazards of the numerous chemicals in use in the United States. The NTP states:

> More than 80,000 chemicals are registered for use in the United States. Each year, an estimated 2,000 new ones are introduced for use in such everyday items as foods, personal care products, prescription drugs, household cleaners, and lawn care products. We do not know the effects of many of these chemicals on our health, yet we may be exposed to them while manufacturing, distributing, using, and disposing of them or

when they become pollutants in our air, water, or soil. Relatively few chemicals are thought to pose a significant risk to human health. However, safeguarding public health depends on identifying both what the effects of these chemicals are and at what levels of exposure they may become hazardous to humans—that is, understanding their toxicology.[1(p4)]

Toxicology, a cornerstone of environmental health, overlaps other disciplines, including physiology, pharmacology, and pathology, and to some extent epidemiology, chemistry, and statistics. A basic assumption in toxicology is that "[a]ll substances are poisons; there is none which is not a poison. The right dose differentiates a poison from a remedy."[2(p4)] We can think of toxicology and epidemiology as working hand in hand, the latter concerned with the occurrence and etiology of disease, and the former studying dose–response relationships and mechanisms of action in order to better understand the adverse health effects linked to chemicals. A recent application is the coupling of toxicology and epidemiology with genomic methods (employed in the study of genes) to perform risk assessment.[3] Toxicology contributes to the armamentarium of tools that are crucial to the description and characterization of environmental chemicals and the responses of living organisms to these chemicals. Related to the functions of toxicology are assessment of exposure, risk, and hazards. **Exposure** is defined as "[p]roximity and/or contact with a source of a disease agent in such a manner that effective transmission of the agent or harmful effects of the agent may occur."[4] The terms **risk** and **hazard** are defined later in the chapter. In the

Epidemiology, Toxicology, and Disease Causation

Toxicologists and epidemiologists often work together to assess the available scientific evidence relating to potential environmental disease-causing hazards. . . . The assessment of available evidence lays the foundation for the problem of complexity: Relevant evidence arises from toxicologic and epidemiological investigations, and reflects the acquisition of knowledge from many levels of scientific understanding: molecular, cellular, tissue, organ systems, complete organisms (man and mouse), relationships between individuals, and on to social and political processes that may impact human health. . . . Consider, as a representative example, the evidence involved in considering whether electrical and magnetic fields are causes of cancer, reproductive and developmental disabilities, and neurobiologic dysfunction (e.g., learning and behavioral disabilities). . . . Studies range along a continuum, starting at the level of atoms, simple molecules, larger molecules such as DNA including adducts and repair mechanisms, proteins and their synthesis, intracellular environments (e.g., calcium levels), cell-signaling pathways and other extracellular phenomena, tissues (cell cultures, bones, nerves, polyps and tumors), and on to the studies in intact individuals (e.g., mice) wherein toxicologists study tumor incidence in rodents and observational studies wherein epidemiologists study the relationship between field exposures and the incidence of diseases and disorders.

Source: Adapted from DL Weed. Environmental epidemiology basics and proof of cause-effect. *Toxicology.* 2002;181–182:399–401.

text box, Weed describes how epidemiology and toxicology are compatible in delving into the complex nature of disease causation.[5]

DESCRIPTION OF TOXICOLOGY

The field of toxicology has been in existence for many centuries, although in its early history the field may have operated under a rubric that is different from its current name. Modern toxicology has evolved a number of subspecializations.

Definition of Toxicology

According to its traditional definition, toxicology is the science of poisons. A more complete definition is "[t]he study of the adverse effects of chemicals on living organisms."[6] The science of toxicology is not confined to the study of humans, but can be applied to other species and organisms as well. Through in vivo (in living organisms) and in vitro (in "glass," e.g., cell culture) studies, toxicologists examine such health effects of chemical exposures as carcinogenesis (production of cancer), and damage to internal organs, to the developing fetus, and to the reproductive system. Several types of cancer have been tied to chemical exposure, including carcinoma of the lung, breast, and prostate gland, and some forms of skin cancer and leukemia.

History of Toxicology

Toxicology may be regarded as a field that, in some respects, has a venerable history, yet it has a short history in the sense that much of the information regarding toxicology has been acquired in the last few decades. Since early history, human beings have been mystified by the nature of chemicals; they also became fascinated with the use of poisons. Ancient civilizations, early cave dwellers, and isolated primitive tribes were aware of the existence of toxic plants and animal venoms. In ancient Greece and Rome, poisons were used for suicides and executions, and to accomplish political aims. Socrates, who lived from 470 to 399 BC, was executed by poison, as was Theophrastus (370–286 BC). Around the fourth century BC, poisonings (especially by use of arsenic) grew more frequent in the Roman Empire; Nero was said to have used arsenic to poison Claudius in order to serve political ambitions.

Poisonings also were employed frequently during the Middle Ages to do away with rivals, including spouses and politicians. Beginning about the 17th century and onward, physicians and others developed a gradually increasing awareness of the toxic effects of exposure to industrial metals and chemicals that were then in common use.

Paracelsus (born Phillippus Theophrastus Aureolus Bombastus von Hohenheim) is considered to be one of the founders of modern toxicology.[7] His image is shown in Figure 3-1. Active during the time of da Vinci and Copernicus, Paracelsus contributed to the discipline during the early 16th century. Among his contributions were several important concepts, including the dose–response relationship, which refers to the observation that the effects of a poison are related to the strength of its dose, and the notion of target organ specificity of chemicals.

FIGURE 3-1 Paracelsus (1493–1541).

1651.
EFFIGIES PARACELSI MEDICI CELEBERRIMI

Source: © National Library of Medicine

Mathieu Orfila was another pioneer in the field of toxicology. In the 1800s, he authored a number of significant works, among them *Trait des poisons* (1813). This work described in great detail various types of poisons and their bodily effects, a development that contributed to the foundations of forensic toxicology.

Fields within Toxicology

What type of work does a toxicologist perform and what are the specializations within toxicology? A **toxicologist** is a scientist who has received extensive training in order to investigate in living organisms "the adverse effects of chemicals . . . (including their cellular, biochemical, and molecular mechanisms of action) and assess the probability of their occurrence."[6(p7)] The field of toxicology comprises approximately nine areas, including regulatory matters (*regulatory toxicology*), medico-legal issues (*forensic toxicology*), and

clinical manifestations of disease related to toxic substances (*clinical toxicology*).[6] In addition, the specializations known as *environmental toxicology*, *reproductive toxicology*, and *developmental toxicology* are particularly relevant to environmental health problems.

The field of **environmental toxicology** is defined as

> the study of how ecological systems—their structure, dynamics, function, etc.—are affected by pollutants. A developing subfield of environmental toxicology is ecotoxicology, in which special concern is placed on the release of toxic pollutants into the environment, especially into aquatic systems, by focusing on how these toxicants may become distributed within food chains and by measuring the toxic responses made within a particular ecosystem to such pollutants.[8]

Environmental toxicology examines how environmental exposures to chemical pollutants may present risks to biological organisms, particularly animals, birds, and fish.

In certain respects, the mission of environmental toxicology overlaps those of reproductive and developmental toxicology. *Reproductive toxicology* examines the association between chemicals and adverse effects upon the reproductive system.[9] Exposure to chemicals may arise from a number of environmental sources including the workplace, the home, and the medications and foods that we consume. On the list of hazardous chemicals and other agents that impact human reproduction negatively are pesticides, drugs, heavy metals, and hormones.[10] *Developmental toxicology* researches the effects of natural and man-made chemicals (some classified as teratogens—substances that cause birth defects) on prenatal development. Other chemicals that can produce developmental toxicity are included in the broad class known as **xenobiotics**, "Chemical substances that are foreign to the biological system. They include naturally occurring compounds, drugs, environmental agents, carcinogens, [and] insecticides. . . . ."[11] Some specific examples of xenobiotics are antibiotics, dioxins, and polychlorinated biphenyls (PCBs).

TERMINOLOGY USED IN THE FIELD OF TOXICOLOGY

One aspect of toxicology is the examination of the mechanisms by which chemicals produce toxic effects on living organisms and their tissues. Virtually all known chemicals (even sodium chloride—common table salt) have the capacity to produce toxic effects, such as injury or death, depending upon their amounts. The **spectrum of toxic dose** describes the toxicity or hazards that are related to exposure to a particular chemical.[6] Measures of lethality (discussed later in this chapter) may not describe fully a chemical's spectrum of toxicity; chemicals that have low acute toxicity may have other effects such as carcinogenicity or teratogenicity. This section introduces a number of terms that are used to describe toxic materials. It should be noted that some of the terms tend to overlap conceptually and are not always differentiated clearly in the literature.

Poison

The term **poison** is "defined as any agent capable of producing a deleterious response in a biological system. Virtually every known chemical has the potential to produce injury or death if it is present in a sufficient amount."[6(p8)] Examples of deleterious responses are death or serious impairment of biological functioning. Some definitions of a poison posit that it is an agent that produces immediate effects such as lethality or sickness even when present in small doses.[12]

Toxic Agent

The term **toxic agent** refers very generally to a material or factor that can be harmful to biological systems.[12] Examples are physical energy (e.g., heat and ionizing and nonionizing radiation), substances derived from biological sources (e.g., black widow spider venom), and almost all chemicals.

Toxicity

Toxicity is defined as "the degree to which something is poisonous."[13] Toxicity is related to a material's physical and chemical properties. Some chemicals have low innate toxicity (e.g., ethyl alcohol, sodium chloride); others have high toxicity (e.g., dioxin and botulinum toxin formed by the bacteria that cause botulism). Substances that have low toxicity must be ingested in large amounts in order for them to have toxic effects; the converse is true of chemicals that have high toxicity. For example, ingestion of large amounts of water (which has low toxicity) is necessary in order to produce water intoxication. In contrast, injection with a small amount of a highly toxic insect venom may be sufficient to cause severe damage to the body or even death.

Toxic Substance

A material that has toxic properties is called a **toxic substance**.[12] This substance can be a single toxic chemical (e.g., arsenic, lead) or a mixture of toxic chemicals (e.g., gasoline). Toxic substances also can be categorized as organic toxins and inorganic toxins. Organic toxins denote substances originally taken from living organisms; such chemicals are carbon-containing, frequently made up of large molecules, and capable of being synthesized. Inorganic toxins refer to specific chemicals, such as minerals, that have not been extracted from living organisms and do not follow the structure of a toxin derived from a living organism; such toxins generally are made up of small molecules.

Toxicant

Toxicants denote toxic substances that are man-made or result from human (anthropogenic) activity.[6] The toxic effect may occur directly or indirectly. The chemical potassium cyanide is directly toxic to the body; in contrast, methanol, a form of alcohol (wood alcohol) that is not poisonous in itself, is indirectly toxic through the action of the liver, which converts it to formaldehyde.[14]

Toxin

A **toxin** usually refers to a toxic substance made by living organisms including reptiles, insects, plants, and microorganisms. To give one illustration, certain bacteria produce toxins that may act directly on the nervous or gastrointestinal system to produce symptoms of toxic effects. Foodborne botulism caused by *Clostridium botulinum* is an environmental hazard associated with improperly canned foods and other unsafe practices in food preparation. Toxin production by microorganisms differs from disease causation by actual invasion and multiplication of microorganisms and consequent organ and cell damage. *Systemic toxins* are those that affect the entire body or multiple organ systems; *target organ toxins* affect specific parts of the body.

Other toxins originate from plants. There are many examples of plants that are toxic:

- Some mushrooms (e.g., *Amanita phalloides*, "death cap")
- Poison hemlock
- Foxglove
- Poison oak/poison ivy
- Rhubarb, especially the leaves, which have high levels of oxalates
- Some houseplants such as dieffenbachia

Refer to the following text box for an example of foodborne disease caused by nicotine, a highly toxic substance derived from the tobacco plant.

THE CONCEPT OF A DOSE AND RELATED TERMS
Dose

The term **dose** refers to "the amount of a substance administered at one time."[15] There are several ways of describing a dose such as exposure dose, absorbed dose, administered

Nicotine Poisoning After Ingestion of Contaminated Ground Beef—Michigan, 2003

On January 3, 2003, the Michigan Department of Agriculture's (MDA) Food and Dairy Division and the US Department of Agriculture (USDA) were notified by a supermarket of a planned recall of approximately 1,700 pounds of ground beef because of customer complaints of illness after eating the product. . . .

The recall was prompted by complaints from four families comprising 18 persons who became ill immediately after eating product sold on December 31 or January 1. Reported symptoms included burning of the mouth, nausea, vomiting, and dizziness. One person reported having been seen in the emergency department (ED) and treated for atrial fibrillation. The recalled product had been ground in the store using ground beef purchased from an out-of-state processor inspected by USDA, Food Safety Inspection Service. . . .

Company officials submitted samples of ground beef provided by the ill families to a private laboratory, where product testing for foodborne pathogens was negative. Additional testing for chemical contamination was conducted at a large regional medical center. On January 10, company officials notified MDA and USDA that nicotine had been presumptively identified in the ground beef samples tested by the second laboratory, which reported an assay result 1 week later of approximately 300 mg/kg nicotine in the submitted samples. The high nicotine concentrations found in the tested meat products prompted concerns of intentional contamination with a pesticide, which sometimes contain nicotine as an additive. . . .

The local health department conducted an epidemiologic investigation, including interviews of persons reporting illness, to assess the consistency of the clinical presentation and to establish a case definition. . . . A total of 148 interviews were conducted with persons who reported they had experienced illness after eating the product and of [sic] family members and friends who also might have eaten the contaminated meat. Of those interviewed, 92 persons had illness consistent with the case definition [of nicotine poisoning]. Patients had a median age of 31 years (range: 1–76 years), and 46 (50%) were female; 65% of the patients lived in the town where the implicated store was located. The majority of illness occurred during the time that the contaminated product was sold. Cases were identified as late as 49 days after the last date of potential sale, indicating that some persons froze and then ate the contaminated product after the first recall was issued. Of the 92 patients, four (3%) sought medical treatment, including two who reported to their personal physicians with complaints of vomiting and stomach pains and two who were evaluated in EDs. The two who were treated in the EDs included a man aged 39 years with atrial fibrillation and a woman aged 31 years who had nausea, vomiting, and complaint of rectal bleeding. Information is being collected on an additional 16 persons to assess whether their illnesses are consistent with the case definition, including a pregnant woman aged 24 years who was hospitalized for 1 day with episodic vomiting.

On February 12, a grand jury returned an indictment for arrest of a person accused of poisoning 200 pounds of meat at the supermarket with an insecticide called Black Leaf 40, which has a main ingredient of nicotine. The person was an employee of the supermarket at the time of the contamination.

Source: Adapted from the Centers for Disease Control and Prevention. Nicotine poisoning after ingestion of contaminated ground beef—Michigan, 2003. *MMWR.* 2003;52:413–415.

dose, total dose, external dose, internal dose, and biologically effective dose. (Refer to Table 3-1.) In practice, dose often is expressed as a concentration of a substance in the body, for example, the concentration per milliliter (ml) of blood.

Toxicologists take into account the total dose, how often each individual dose occurs, and the time period during which the dosing occurs in order to describe the effects of a dose. When a dose is fractionated (broken up over a period of time), the effects may be different from those that transpire when a dose is administered all at one time. For example, poison that is fatal in a single, concentrated dose may no longer be fatal when the same dose is broken down into small units and given over time. Another consideration in the lethality or other effects of a dose relates to the body size of the subject. Young children, who have small body sizes, are more affected by a specific dose than are large adults who are given the same dose. For this reason, environmental exotoxins (those originating from external sources such as lead and mercury) at a given concentration may present a greater hazard to children than to adults.

TABLE 3-1 Ways to Describe a Dose

Term	Definition
Exposure dose	The amount of a substance encountered in the environment
External dose	A dose acquired by contact with contaminated environmental sources
Absorbed dose	The amount of a substance that is available to the internal organs of the body
Internal dose	The portion of a substance that becomes internalized in the body through ingestion, absorption, and other means
Administered dose	The quantity of a substance that is administered
Biologically effective dose	That portion of the internal dose that is required to cause a health outcome
Total dose	The dosage acquired by adding together all of the individual doses

Source: Adapted from RJ Kendall, TA Anderson, RJ Baker, et al. Ecotoxicology. In: CD Klaassen, JB Watkins III, eds. *Casarett & Doull's Essentials of Toxicology.* New York, NY: McGraw-Hill; 2003:422; and National Library of Medicine. *Toxicology Tutor I.* Basic Principles: Dose and Dose Response—Dose. Available at: http://sis.nlm.nih.gov/ToxTutor/Tox1/a21.htm. Accessed February 24, 2010.

Lethal Dose 50 (LD₅₀)

To describe toxic effects, toxicologists use the symbol **LD$_{50}$ (lethal dose 50)**, which is "the dosage (mg/kg body weight) causing death in 50 percent of exposed animals."[6(p8)] One of the applications of LD$_{50}$ is to compare the toxicities of chemicals (i.e., to describe whether one chemical is more or less toxic than another). Other variations of the term *lethal dose* include LD$_{10}$ and LD$_{90}$ (10% and 90% mortality, respectively). Lethality tests are becoming rare in research due to the availability of less destructive methods of study.

Dose–Response Relationships

One of the most basic toxicologic concepts, a dose–response relationship, refers to a type of correlative relationship between "the characteristics of exposure to a chemical and the spectrum of effects caused by the chemical."[16(p61)] The existence of a dose–response relationship may be used to establish the following kinds of information[15]:

- Causal association between a toxin and biological effects
- Minimum dosages needed to produce a biological effect
- Rate of accumulation of harmful effects

Dose–Response Curves

The dose–response curve is a type of graph that is used to describe the effect of exposure to a chemical or toxic substance upon an organism such as an experimental animal. Toxicologists have devised two types of dose–response curves, one for the responses of an individual to a chemical and one for a population. For both types of curves, the dose is indicated along the *x* axis, and the response is shown along the *y* axis.

A typical dose–response curve for an individual exposed to ethyl alcohol is shown in Figure 3-2. The curve, which assumes a one-time exposure, shows a graded and increasing response as the dose of alcohol increases. The spectrum of effects can range from no effect when the dose is zero to death when the dose is increased to a toxic level.

With respect to the population, a dose–response relationship is "[t]he relationship of observed outcomes (responses) in a population to varying levels of a protective or harmful agent such as a form of medication or an environmental contaminant."[4] The response could be measured as the percentage of exposed animals showing a particular effect, or it could reflect the effect in an individual subject.

The population dose–response curve, which has a sigmoid shape (S-shaped), is also a cumulative percentage response curve. (Refer to Figure 3-3.) This type of dose–response curve also is called a quantal curve.[6] At the beginning of the curve, there is a flat portion suggesting that at low levels an increase in dosage produces no effect; this is known as the subthreshold phase. After the threshold is reached, the curve

FIGURE 3-2 Individual dose-response curve.

Source: Reprinted with permission from AE Marczewski, M Kamrin. Toxicology for the Citizen. 2nd ed. East Lansing, Mich: Michigan State University, Center for Integrative Toxicology; 1991:5.

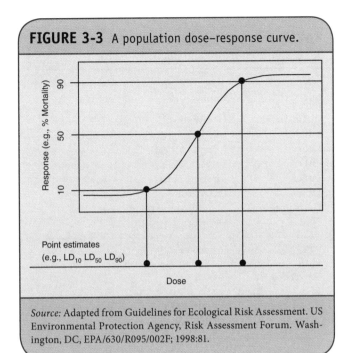

FIGURE 3-3 A population dose–response curve.

Point estimates
(e.g., LD$_{10}$ LD$_{50}$ LD$_{90}$)

Dose

Source: Adapted from Guidelines for Ecological Risk Assessment. US Environmental Protection Agency, Risk Assessment Forum. Washington, DC, EPA/630/R095/002F; 1998:81.

FACTORS THAT AFFECT RESPONSES TO A TOXIC CHEMICAL

Several factors determine whether an individual will respond to exposure to a toxic chemical and the type of response that occurs.[17] The nature of a toxic effect depends on the innate toxicity of the chemical, whether it is in sufficient concentration, and how it impinges upon a somatic location as a consequence of the route and site of exposure. In addition, exposure needs to take place for a sufficient time duration and frequency: The effects of a one-time exposure of short duration are usually different from those of an exposure that happens on several occasions over a long period of time. Other factors are related to a person's sensitivity to a chemical, for example, one's ability to metabolize the chemical (through biological processes that convert the chemical into either less harmful or more harmful substances). The concentration and toxicity of the chemical are affected by the following:

- Route of entry into the body
- Received dose of the chemical
- Duration of exposure
- Interactions that transpire among multiple chemicals
- Individual sensitivity

Route and Site of Entry

The most frequent sites of exposure to environmental (i.e., xenobiotic) chemicals include the gastrointestinal tract, the respiratory system, and the skin. (Refer to Table 3-2.) With respect to route of exposure, chemicals may enter the body in-

rises steeply and then progresses to a linear phase, where an increase in response is proportional to the increase in dose (see Figure 3-4). When the maximal response is reached, the curve flattens out. A dose–response relationship is one of the indicators used to assess a causal effect of a suspected exposure upon a health outcome.

The term **threshold** refers to the lowest dose at which a particular response may occur. It is unclear whether exposure to toxic chemicals at low (sub-threshold) levels may produce any health response. Although society's concern about the health effects of exposure to environmental pollutants has increased, it still remains unclear whether chronic exposures to toxic chemical agents in the environment occur at high enough doses to affect human health. Nevertheless, environmental scientists have had increasing concerns over the long-term effects of low-level exposures to toxic substances, exposures such as those that may take place in the workplace.

FIGURE 3-4 The threshold of a dose–response curve.

Source: Reprinted from National Institutes of Health, National Institute of Environmental Health Sciences. Chemicals, the Environment and You: Explorations in Science and Human Health, p. 63. Available at: http://science.education.nih.gov/supplements/nih2/chemicals/guide/pdfs/lesson3.pdf. Accessed February 25, 2010.

tentionally (as in the example of medical interventions) or unintentionally (through accidents or environmental exposures). Illustrations of the routes of exposure corresponding to the sites of entry are ingestion (e.g., consumption of contaminated food or drink), injections into the bloodstream, contact with the surface of the skin (topical mode), and inhalation. With respect to inhalation, when we breathe contaminated air (for instance, at work), potentially dangerous particles and gases may enter our bodies and be absorbed into the bloodstream by the alveoli of the lungs without producing any warning symptoms. These chemicals later may cause serious lung diseases, including lung cancer. In some cases the absorbed chemicals may affect other organs such as the brain.

As mentioned previously, other routes of exposure include skin contact, eye contact, and ingestion. The skin forms a protective barrier that can be compromised by dehydration, physical damage, caustic chemicals, and organic solvents; the result is that chemicals may bypass the barrier and enter the bloodstream. The eyes are particularly vulnerable to chemical exposure, especially when chemicals splash into the eye during an accident. Finally, employees who work with toxic chemicals may unwittingly ingest such chemicals when they smoke or eat on the job; in addition, workers unintentionally may transport them home on their clothing and skin.

How quickly a chemical produces acute and other effects depends on the site and route of exposure.[6] Among possible sites and routes, contact with the skin generally produces the slowest response, and direct injection into the bloodstream typically yields the fastest and strongest effects. (Refer to Table 3-2.)

List of Terms That Describe Duration of Exposure

- *Acute*—Usually a single exposure for less than 24 hours
- *Subacute*—Exposure for one month or less
- *Subchronic*—Exposure for one to three months
- *Chronic*—Exposure for more than three months

Source: Definitions from DL Eaton, CD Klaassen. Principles of toxicology. In: Klaasen CD, Watkins JB III, eds. *Casarett & Doull's Essentials of Toxicology.* New York, NY: McGraw-Hill, 2003;9.

TABLE 3-2 Ranking of the Relative Speed of Effect According to the Site and Route of Exposure

Site	Route	Relative Speed of Effect[a]
Bloodstream	Intravenous	++++++++
Lungs	Inhalation	+++++++
Other	Intraperitoneal	++++++
Other	Subcutaneous	+++++
Other	Intramuscular	++++
Other	Intradermal	+++
Gastrointestinal	Ingestion (oral route)	++
Skin	Dermal	+

[a] The greater the number of plus signs (+), the faster the effect; e.g., when chemicals enter the bloodstream directly they usually have the fastest effect.

Source: Data from DL Eaton, CD Klaassen. Principles of toxicology. In: CD Klaassen, JB Watkins III, eds. *Casarett & Doull's Essentials of Toxicology.* New York, NY: McGraw-Hill; 2003:9.

Length and Duration of Exposure

Toxicologists describe the duration of exposure in a range from acute to chronic. Relevant terms are defined in the following box.

The duration of exposure is important from the toxicologic point of view because the effects of exposure to many chemicals may vary depending on whether the exposure is minimal and takes place on a single occasion for a short time period or is heavy and long-standing. Some workers (for example, agricultural workers) receive exposures to pesticides in greater concentrations and over much longer time periods than does the general population. Acute exposures may produce acute effects that disappear rapidly, although this outcome is not invariable. In comparison with short-term exposures, chronic exposures may allow for the buildup of effects over time with the resulting accumulation of biological damage. However, such accumulation may not occur if the chemical is excreted before the next exposure happens.

Effects of Chemical Mixtures

In the "real world" of environmental exposures, most exposures are to multiple chemicals rather than to a single chemical. By way of example, the ambient air in a factory may contain a soup of chemicals that impinge upon the production workers. Toxicologists and others have observed that when chemicals mix, they may produce surprising effects—sometimes their combined effects may be greater and sometimes less than expected. When an organism is exposed to two or more chemicals, their combined effects may be additive, synergistic, antagonistic, or coalitive; some chemicals may cause potentiation. **Additive** means that the combination of two chemicals produces an effect that is equal to their individual effects added together. The term **synergism** (from the Greek word *synergos*—working together) indicates that the combined effect of exposures to two or more chemicals is greater than the sum of their individual effects.

There are many examples of synergism in the field of environmental health. One is the interaction between asbestos and smoking in causing lung cancer. Selikoff et al. demonstrated that lung cancer mortality risk among asbestos insulation workers was much higher among those who smoked in comparison with those who did not smoke.[18] A second example pertains to the synergistic effects of solvents (e.g., n-hexane and methyl ethyl ketone [MEK]). These chemicals, when acting simultaneously on the nervous system, produce a much greater combined effect than would be expected from their simple additive individual effects.[19]

Another type of interaction between two chemicals is called **potentiation**, which happens when one chemical that is not toxic causes another chemical to become more toxic.[6] For example, isopropanol by itself is not toxic to the liver but has the capacity to increase the liver toxicity of carbon tetrachloride when exposure of the two chemicals occurs together. In a **coalitive interaction**, several agents that have no known toxic effects interact to produce a toxic effect.[20]

The term **antagonism** means that "two chemicals administered together interfere with each other's actions or one interferes with the action of the other. . . ."[6(p11)] In illustration, supplemental vitamins may reduce the effects of needed prescription medicines such as antibiotics; an example is the antagonistic relationship between calcium and tetracycline.

Individual Responses to Toxic Exposures

The responses of individuals to toxic substances can vary greatly, ranging from no apparent response to severe responses. Responses may vary according to age, sex, race, and health status. Other influences include the person's genetic background, use of medications, consumption of alcohol, and pregnancy status. Some chemicals (e.g., bee venom) produce severe or life-threatening reactions in persons afflicted with allergies.

The term **chemical allergy** refers to "an immunologically mediated adverse reaction to a chemical resulting from previous sensitization to that chemical or to a structurally similar one."[6(p10)] Some of the alternative terms used to describe this response are hypersensitivity, allergic reaction, and sensitization reaction. After initial sensitization, small doses of a chemical may bring about an allergic reaction. Some genetically predisposed persons may be prone to *chemical idiosyncrasy*, meaning that they have either extreme sensitivity to low doses of a chemical or insensitivity to high doses.

Recall that the term *xenobiotics* refers to foreign chemicals that are introduced into the body. Although their effects may be beneficial, they also may produce adverse effects at the same time; these adverse effects may occur either directly or indirectly. A direct effect denotes an immediate impact upon the cells and tissues of the body or upon specific target organs. An indirect effect would be a change in the function of the body's biochemical processes. Examples of direct and indirect adverse effects are shown in Table 3-3.

Direct adverse effects of exposures to chemicals range from local effects to systemic effects to target organ effects. These terms are defined as follows:

- *Local effects*—Damage at the site where a chemical first comes into contact with the body; examples are redness, burning, and irritation of the skin.
- *Systemic effects*—Adverse effects associated with generalized distribution of the chemical throughout the body by the bloodstream to internal organs.
- *Target organ effects*—Some chemicals may confine their effects to specific organs; the most common organs affected by such chemicals are the liver, lungs, heart, kidneys, brain and nervous system, and the reproductive system.

TABLE 3-3 Direct and Indirect Adverse Effects of Xenobiotics

Direct Adverse Effects	Indirect Adverse Effects
Cell replacement, such as fibrosis (buildup of scar tissue)	Modification of an essential biochemical function
Damage to an enzyme system	Interference with nutrition
Disruption of protein synthesis	Alteration of a physiological mechanism
Production of reactive chemicals in cells	
DNA damage	

Source: Adapted from National Library of Medicine, *Toxicology Tutor I. Basic Principles: Toxic Effects.* Available at: http://www.sis.nlm.nih.gov/enviro/toxtutor/Tox1/a31.htm. Accessed March 5, 2010.

Latency and Delayed Responses to Toxic Substances

The term latency refers to the time period between initial exposure and a measurable response. The latency period can range from a few seconds (in the case of acutely toxic agents) to several decades for agents that may be carcinogenic.

One example of a delayed effect of exposure to chemicals is carcinogenesis, the potential to induce cancerous growth of cells. The word **carcinogen** denotes a chemical (or substance) that causes or is suspected of causing cancer, a disease associated with unregulated proliferation of cells in the body. In fact, many forms of cancer are believed to have a latency period of 10 years up to 40 years (counting the time between first exposure to a carcinogen and the subsequent development of cancer). For example, mesothelioma (a rare form of thoracic or abdominal cancer) has a latency period as long as 40 years between first exposure to asbestos and subsequent development of the condition.

The long latency for many of the health events studied in environmental research makes detection of the effects of exposures to toxic substances a methodologically difficult problem. For human exposures, toxicologists may be unable to differentiate among exposures to multiple chemicals and to rule out the impacts of confounding factors (discussed in Chapter 2) that may be implicated in carcinogenesis.

Methods of Testing for Toxicity

The subjects used for testing the toxicity of chemicals include the following[21]:

- Volunteers who have had normal or accidental exposures
- Animals exposed purposively (in vivo experiments)
- Cells derived from human, animal, or plant sources (in vitro experiments)

Toxicity testing that uses these categories of subjects may take the form of epidemiologic investigations (described in Chapter 2), formal clinical trials, or animal studies.

In the United States, randomized controlled clinical trials are regulated by the Food and Drug Administration (FDA). They are used to evaluate the safety of new drugs in humans, following tests in animals. The trials are conducted in three phases, beginning with small groups of patients and gradually expanding to larger patient populations after an earlier phase has demonstrated the safety and efficacy of the drug in question. Before the advent of rigorous clinical trials, new drugs could enter the marketplace without the benefit of evaluation. A notorious example is the drug thalidomide, which, when administered to pregnant women outside the United States (e.g., in Europe, Japan, Australia, and Canada) was found to be a potent teratogen (a drug or other substance that causes birth defects). Not approved for use in the United States, thalidomide was prescribed during the late 1950s to treat morning sickness in pregnant women. As a result, these women gave birth to more than 10,000 children who had severe birth defects, such as missing limbs.[22] Even with the use of clinical trials, new drugs entering the marketplace still may have potential to cause harm. An example that occurred in 2005 involved Vioxx (used to control pain among arthritis patients), which is thought to increase the risk of heart problems.

When highly controlled and standardized conditions are desired, animal models are used in toxicologic testing. Another purpose for the use of animals is in preliminary testing of pharmaceuticals, pesticides, and substances that may present toxic hazards to human subjects. Standard protocols using animals evaluate the acute effects of chemicals, as well as toxicity to specific organs. Another concern of animal assays for toxicity is damage to the reproductive system or offspring. Animal protocols also are applied to measure the carcinogenic potential of chemicals. Research and toxicity testing may require the use of multiple animal species, including rats, mice, rabbits, dogs, and monkeys. Animal studies aid in preventing highly toxic chemicals from being introduced into human populations.

One focus of evaluation is the role of chemicals in causing toxicity to nucleic acids; some results might be mutations, chromosomal abnormalities, and DNA damage. In these studies, tests may be conducted with bacteria, fruit flies, and cell lines from animals or humans.

LINKS BETWEEN TOXICOLOGY AND RISK ASSESSMENT

Once we have obtained toxicologic information regarding the nature and health effects of a chemical, we would like to be able to determine the risks to health that the chemical represents. Let us examine the concept of risk briefly. One can never be free from all risk to health and well-being. Even the most benign activities carry risk: For example, while riding on a busy street, a bicyclist may be struck by a car. Perhaps the person chose to ride a bicycle in order to avoid the financial risk of owning a car. Thus, many aspects of life involve weighing risks (e.g., buying versus renting a house, investing in stocks versus purchasing a certificate of deposit, or choosing a potential life partner) and then making a decision about what action to take.

In simple terms, a risk involves the likelihood of experiencing an adverse effect. The term **risk assessment** refers to "a process for identifying adverse consequences and their associated probability."[23(p611)] Risk assessment is "[t]he process of determining risks to health attributable to environmental or other hazards."[4] "Risk research addresses the identification and management of situations that might result in losses or harm, immediate or delayed, to individuals, groups, or even to whole communities or ecosystems, often as a result of the interaction of human activities with natural processes."[24(px)] Risk assessment provides a qualitative or quantitative estimation of the likelihood of adverse effects that may result from exposure to specified health hazards or from the absence of beneficial influences. "Risk assessment uses clinical, epidemiologic, toxicologic, environmental, and any other pertinent data."[4]

The meaning of the term *risk* varies greatly not only from one person to another, but also between lay persons and professionals; the latter characterize risk mainly in terms of mortality.[25] In a psychometric study, Slovic reported that lay persons classified risk according to two major factors. His methods enabled risks to be portrayed in a two-dimensional space so that their relative positions could be compared. The two factors that Slovic identified were the following:

> Factor 1, labeled "dread risk," is defined at its high (right-hand) end by perceived lack of control, dread, catastrophic potential, fatal consequences, and the inequitable distribution of risks and benefits. . . .
> Factor 2, labeled "unknown risk," is defined at its high end by hazards judged to be unobservable, unknown, new, and delayed in their manifestation of harm.[25(p283)]

Refer to Figure 3-5, which maps the spatial relationships among a large number of risks according to the two major factors shown in the figure. For example, nuclear reactor accidents fall in the space that defines uncontrollable dread factors that are of unknown risk. In other words, nuclear reactor accidents fall in the quadrant defined by both high levels of unknown risk and high levels of dread risk. In contrast, home swimming pools are perceived as falling in the quadrant in which risks are not dread and are known to those exposed.

Risk assessment generally takes place in four steps: (1) hazard identification, (2) dose–response assessment, (3) exposure assessment, and (4) risk characterization.[26,27] Refer to Figure 3-6 for an illustration. The term **risk management** shown in the figure is discussed in Chapter 4.

Hazard Identification

Hazard identification (hazard assessment) "examines the evidence that associates exposure to an agent with its toxicity and produces a qualitative judgment about the strength of that evidence, whether it is derived from human epidemiology or extrapolated from laboratory animal data."[27(p286)] Evidence regarding hazards linked to toxic substances may be derived from the study of health effects among exposed humans and animals. These health effects may range from dramatic outcomes such as mortality or cancer to lower-level conditions such as developmental delays in children and reductions in immune status.[26]

A **hazard** is defined as the "[i]nherent capability of an agent or a situation to have an adverse effect. A factor or exposure that may adversely affect health."[4] Hazards may originate from chemicals, biological agents, physical and mechanical energy and force, and psychosocial influences. We have covered the toxic agents such as organic toxins and chemicals. Examples of other hazards will be covered in more detail later in the book. Some physical hazards arise from ionizing radiation from medical X-rays and naturally occurring background radiation. Other hazards originate from nonionizing radiation—sunlight, infrared and ultraviolet light, and electromagnetic radiation from power lines and radio transmissions. In urban and work environments, mechanical energy is associated with high levels of noise that can be hazardous for hearing and for psychological well-being. Examples of psychosocial hazards are work-related stresses, combat fatigue, and post-traumatic stress disorder (topics not covered in this text).

Dose–Response Assessment

Dose–response assessment is the measurement of "the relationship between the amount of exposure and the occurrence of the unwanted health effects."[26(p38)] According to Russell and Gruber:

> Dose-response assessment examines the quantitative relation between the experimentally administered dose level of a toxicant and the incidence or severity or both of a response in test animals, and draws inferences for humans. The presumed human dosages and incidences in human populations may also be used in cases where epidemiological studies are available.[27(p286)]

Exposure Assessment

Exposure assessment is defined as the procedure that "identifies populations exposed to the toxicant, describes their composition and size, and examines the roots, magnitudes, frequencies, and durations of such exposures."[27(p286)] The

FIGURE 3-5 Location of 81 hazards on factors 1 and 2 derived from the relationships among 15 risk characteristics.

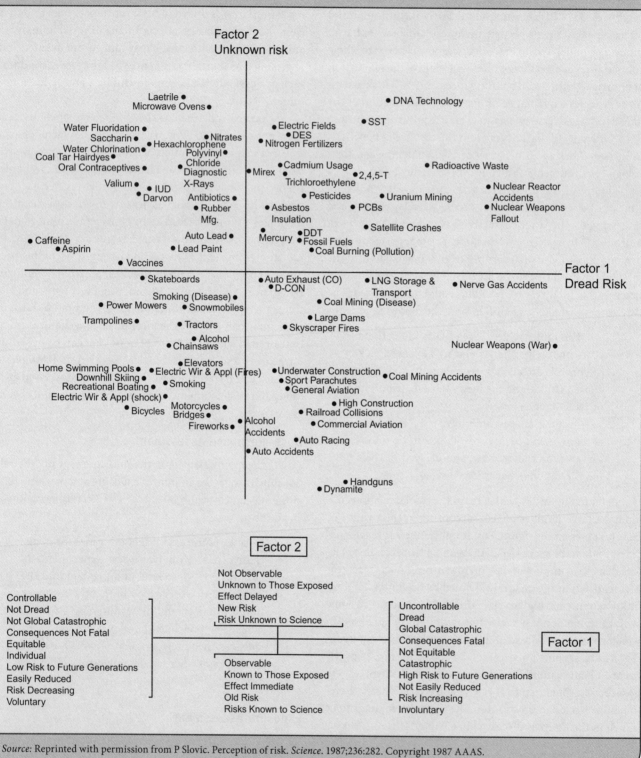

Source: Reprinted with permission from P Slovic. Perception of risk. *Science.* 1987;236:282. Copyright 1987 AAAS.

FIGURE 3-6 Steps in risk assessment.

Research

Laboratory and field observations (including epidemiological studies) of adverse health effects from exposure to particular ages.

Quantitative dose–response studies and extrapolation from high to low dose and from animals to humans.

Field measurements estimating exposures in defined populations.

Risk Assessment

1. Hazard Identification (Which are the health effects that this agent can cause?)

2. Dose–Response Assessment (What is the relationship between dose and occurrence of health effects in humans?)

3. Exposure Assessment (What exposures are currently experienced or anticipated under different conditions?)

4. Risk Characterization (What is estimated occurrence of the adverse effect in a given population?)

5. Risk Management (Development, evaluation, and implementation of regulatory options, aimed at risk reduction and control)

Source: From Basic Environmental Health by Annalee Yassi and Tord Kjellström, Theo de Kok, Tee Guidotti, copyright © 2001 by the World Health Organization. Used by permission of Oxford University Press, Inc.

process of human exposure assessment is believed to be one of the weakest aspects of risk assessment. Available methods are unable to provide adequate quantitative information regarding how much humans are exposed to toxic substances as well as the specific kinds and patterns of exposure.[28] The quality of exposure assessment data determines the accuracy of risk assessments and therefore is a limiting factor in the risk assessment process.[29]

When referring to a toxic substance, exposure assessment must take into account where the exposure occurs, how much exposure occurs, and how the substance is absorbed by the body. The process of human exposure assessment examines "the manner in which pollutants come into actual contact with the human body—the concentration levels at the points of contact and the sources of these pollutants making contact. The key word here is 'contact'—the occurrence of two events at the same location and same time."[30(p449)] The methods by which human beings are exposed to toxic substances include encountering them in water, air, food, soil, and various consumer products and medications.

As noted previously in Chapter 2, high-quality data on exposure are necessary for making valid interpretations of a study's findings.[31] (Refer to the text box for more information on exposure assessment.) Several methods of exposure assessment (e.g., personal exposure monitoring and use of biological

markers) are used in toxicology, environmental epidemiology, and other environmental health disciplines.

During a review of records to assess exposure, the investigator may select a study population from personnel records maintained by a company. If the records of former and retired workers are retained by the company, a complete data set spanning long time periods may be available. Ideally, every previous and current worker exposed to the factor should be included. Selection bias may occur if some workers are excluded because their records have been purged from the company's database.[32] Data collected from employment records may include:

- Personal identifiers to permit record linkage to Social Security Administration files and retrieval of death certificates
- Demographic characteristics, length of employment, and work history with the company
- Information about potential confounding variables, such as the employee's medical history, smoking habits, lifestyle, and family history of disease

Some environmental studies use biomarkers that may be correlated with exposures to potential carcinogens and other chemicals. These biomarkers involve changes in genetic structure that are thought to be the consequence of an exposure.

What Is an Exposure Assessment?

An exposure assessment attempts to answer the following questions for a particular substance or chemical:

- Who or what is exposed (e.g., people, aquatic ecosystems)?
- Does the exposure occur through breathing air, drinking water, skin contact, or any other routes?
- How much exposure occurs?
- How often and for how long does exposure occur, that is, what is its frequency and duration?

Exposure occurs through contact with a chemical. Such contact can occur by inhaling air, drinking water, eating food, or touching a variety of products that contain the chemical. The concentration of the chemical and the extent of the contact are important components of exposure assessment. The results of an exposure assessment are often considered with a hazard assessment of the chemical. A hazard assessment provides an understanding of the potential for the chemical to cause adverse effects to humans and plant and animal life. Together, the exposure assessment and the hazard assessment can be combined into a risk assessment, which reaches conclusions about the likelihood of adverse effects in the exposed population. . . .

Estimating Concentrations in the Environment Using Models: Before environmental concentrations can be predicted, releases to the environment need to be estimated. Chemicals can be released to air, water, or landfill. Release estimates are generated using industrial data, engineering expertise and information on the production process. Manufacturing and processing operations are reviewed to determine potential releases in the work place (e.g., vapors from processing equipment, etc.) that could result in worker exposure and releases to the environment. Releases from consumer products should also be considered.

A number of databases and tools allow the user to gather information about the environment into which the chemical is discharged, and to estimate chemical concentrations in air and water. These tools range from mathematical equations to predict simple dilution in a room to complex computer models which estimate the path of the chemical through the environment over time. Some of these computer models can account for chemical decay in the environment and estimate overlapping concentrations from multiple chemical releases.

Assessing Exposures: The last step in an exposure assessment involves estimating the level of contact of the exposed population with the chemical. For people who live near a discharge location, the level of contact involves two factors: the location of nearby populations and the daily human activities that influence how often people come in contact with the chemical. For consumer product exposures and worker exposures, the frequency of use, duration of exposure and use conditions are important factors.

Assessing Exposures Using Monitoring Data: The most accurate way to obtain environmental concentrations and human exposures is usually to conduct a well-designed exposure monitoring study. Elements of a well-designed exposure monitoring study include: establishing quality assurance objectives that will allow exposure assessors to make estimates of average and high end exposures with a known level of reliability; where possible, using sampling and analytical chemistry methods that have been found acceptable by an independent authoritative body . . . and ensuring that quality control procedures have been employed and documented. [Also, monitors should be placed so that they obtain representative samples that relate to the actual exposure of the population under study.]

Assessing Exposures Using Models: The screening level tools often make simplifying assumptions which are protective by design (for example, assuming that people live near chemical discharge locations). Higher tier tools are more complex and allow for more realistic exposure assessments, such as using census data and a measure of the distance between the location of the chemical release and the populations living nearby. Daily activities include the amount of time people spend at home as well as the amount of air they breathe and the amount of water they drink. For workers, daily activities include the amount of time they spend handling the chemical during the day. The amount of chemical that an individual breathes, comes into contact [with] via the skin, or drinks via water is the final product of an exposure assessment.

Source: Adapted and reprinted from US Environmental Protection Agency. Exposure assessment tools and models: What is an exposure assessment? Available at: http://www.epa.gov/oppt/exposure/pubs/exposurep.htm. Accessed February 25, 2010.

One marker is called a **sister chromatid exchange (SCE)**. SCEs refer to reciprocal exchanges of DNA between pairs of DNA molecules.[33] In a study of exposure to styrene gas (involved in boat-building and plastics manufacture), researchers examined the utility of SCEs in comparison with environmental monitoring, and exhaled styrene levels as alternative measures of styrene exposure.[34] The use of biomarkers such as SCEs is growing in the environmental health field.

Risk Characterization

Risk characterization develops "estimates of the number of excess unwarranted health events expected at different time intervals at each level of exposure."[26(p38)] Risk characterization follows the three foregoing steps by integrating the information from hazard identification, dose–response assessment, and exposure assessment.[35] The process of risk characterization yields "[a] synthesis and summary of information about a hazard that addresses the needs and interests of decision makers and of interested and affected parties. Risk characterization is a prelude to decision making and depends on an iterative, analytic-deliberative process."[36(p216)] "Risk characterization presents the policy maker with a synopsis of all the information that contributes to a conclusion about the nature of the risk and evaluates the magnitudes of the uncertainties involved and the major assumptions that were used."[27(p286)]

Risk Management

Oriented toward specific actions, risk management "consists of actions taken to control exposures to toxic chemicals in the environment. Exposure standards, requirements for premarket testing, recalls of toxic products, and outright banning of very hazardous materials are among the actions that are used by governmental agencies to manage risk."[26(p37)] This topic is covered more fully in Chapter 4 (Environmental Policy and Regulation).

CONCLUSION

Toxicology, the science of poisons, is a powerful and important discipline for protecting human health and the environment. Often, toxicologists work collaboratively with specialists in other overlapping fields, such as epidemiology. Toxicology has a lengthy and distinguished history, beginning with ancient civilizations. This chapter has covered some of the important terminology used to characterize the effects of xenobiotics on biological systems. Two of these concepts are the lethal dose and dose–response curves. Environmental chemicals have differing effects upon humans, depending upon a number of factors that include route of entry into the body, received dose, duration of exposure, interactions among chemicals, and individual sensitivity. Toxicology is an important component of risk assessment.

Despite the many helpful applications of toxicology, the field has some limitations as well. First, the laboratory models used (in vivo and in vitro) may not completely represent environmental conditions, which often are more complex than those conditions found in controlled settings. Also, toxicology, by looking only at adverse effects, ignores benefits important to human health and welfare that may also be present.

Study Questions and Exercises

1. Define environmental toxicology. Give an example of a study that would be relevant to this field.

2. What were the contributions of Paracelsus to toxicology?

3. Define the terms *teratogen*, *xenobiotic*, and *carcinogen*.

4. Explain the difference between toxins and toxicants. Give an example of each. How does a toxin differ from a poison?

5. State what is meant by the term LD_{50}.

6. What determines the toxicity of a chemical? To what extent do you agree with the assumption that "all substances are poisons"?

7. Describe methods for testing the toxicity of chemicals.

8. Explain the significance of duration of exposure from a toxicity point of view. What are the terms used to describe the different ranges of exposure?

9. What is latency? How does the issue of latency challenge environmental researchers who are trying to detect hazards associated with specific exposures?

10. Describe the typical shape of the population dose–response curve and explain why it is shaped this way.

11. Define the terms *dose* and *threshold*. Draw a figure to illustrate a threshold.

12. Explain the differences among synergism, antagonism, and potentiation. Give specific examples of each.

13. What is meant by the term *risk assessment*? Describe the steps that constitute risk assessment. Give an example of each step.

14. What is human exposure assessment? Describe some of the methods of exposure assessment.

REFERENCES

1. US Department of Health and Human Services, Public Health Service, National Toxicology Program. Current directions and evolving strategies: good science for good decisions; 2004. Available at: http://ntp.niehs.nih.gov/ntp/Main_Pages/PUBS/2004CurrentDirections_Press.pdf. Accessed February 24, 2010.

2. Gallo MA. History and scope of toxicology. In: Klaassen CD, Watkins JB III, eds. *Casarett & Doull's Essentials of Toxicology*. New York, NY: McGraw-Hill; 2003.

3. Henry CJ, Phillips R, Carpanini F, et al. Use of genomics in toxicology and epidemiology: findings and recommendations of a workshop. *Environ Health Perspect*. 2002;110:1047–1050.

4. Porta M, ed. *A Dictionary of Epidemiology*. 5th ed. New York, NY: Oxford University Press; 2008.

5. Weed DL. Environmental epidemiology basics and proof of cause-effect. *Toxicol*. 2002;181–182:399–403.

6. Eaton DL, Klaassen CD. Principles of toxicology. In: Klaassen CD, Watkins JB III, eds. *Casarett & Doull's Essentials of Toxicology*. New York, NY: McGraw-Hill; 2003.

7. Borzelleca JF. Profiles in toxicology. Paracelsus: herald of modern toxicology. *Toxicol Sci*. 2000;53:2–4.

8. Environmental Studies Virtual Library, University of Illinois at Urbana-Champaign. Ecotoxicology. Available at: http://www.library.uiuc.edu/envi/toxigateway.htm. Accessed February 14, 2010.

9. Briggs GB. Risk assessment policy for evaluating reproductive system toxicants and the impact of responses on sensitive populations. *Toxicol*. 1996;111:305–313.

10. Schwetz BA. Noncancer risk assessment: reproductive toxicology. *Drug Metab Rev*. 1996;28(1–2):77–84.

11. Webster's Online Dictionary. Xenobiotics. Available at: http://www.websters-online-dictionary.org/definition/english/Xe/Xenobiotics.html. Accessed February 14, 2010.

12. National Library of Medicine. *Toxicology Tutor I*. Basic principles: introduction—basic toxicology terminology. Available at: http://sis.nlm.nih.gov/enviro/toxtutor/Tox1/a12.htm. Accessed February 14, 2010.

13. Hyperdictionary. Meaning of toxicity. Available at: http://www.hyperdictionary.com/dictionary/toxicity. Accessed February 24, 2010.

14. WordiQ.com. Definition of toxicology. Available at: http://www.wordiq.com/definition/Toxicology. Accessed February 24, 2010.

15. National Library of Medicine. *Toxicology Tutor I*. Basic principles: dose and dose response—dose. Available at: http://sis.nlm.nih.gov/enviro/toxtutor/Tox1/a21.htm. Accessed March 5, 2010.

16. National Institutes of Health, National Institute of Environmental Health Sciences. *Chemicals, the Environment, and You: Explorations in Science and Human Health*. Dose-response relationships. Available at: http://science.education.nih.gov/supplements/nih2/chemicals/guide/pdfs/lesson3.pdf. Accessed February 15, 2010.

17. Health Evaluation System and Information Service (HESIS), Occupational Health Branch, California Department of Public Health. Understanding toxic substances: an introduction to chemical hazards in the workplace. 2008 edition. Richmond, CA: HESIS; 2008.

18. Selikoff IJ, Cuyler HE, Chung J. Asbestos exposure, smoking, and neoplasia. *JAMA*. 1968;204:106–112.

19. Australian Government, National Occupational Health and Safety Commission. Synergism and potentiation. Available at: www.safeworkaustralia.gov.au/swa/AboutUs/Publications/NationalStandards/. Accessed March 5, 2010.

20. Suk WA, Olden K. Multidisciplinary research: strategies for assessing chemical mixtures to reduce risk of exposure and disease. *Int J Occup Med Environ Health*. 2004;17:103–110.

21. National Library of Medicine. *Toxicology Tutor I*. Basic principles: toxicity testing methods. Available at: http://sis.nlm.nih.gov/enviro/toxtutor/Tox1/a51.htm. Accessed February 15, 2010.

22. March of Dimes. Professionals & researchers quick reference: fact sheets. Thalidomide. Available at: http://www.marchofdimes.com/professionals/14332_1172.asp. Accessed March 5, 2010.

23. McKone TE. The rise of exposure assessment among the risk sciences: an evaluation through case studies. *Inhal Toxicol*. 1999;11:611–622.

24. Amendola A, Wilkinson DR. Risk assessment and environmental policy making. *J Hazard Mater*. 2000;78:ix–xiv.

25. Slovic P. Perception of risk. *Science*. 1987;236:280–285.

26. Landrigan PJ, Carlson JE. Environmental policy and children's health. *The Future of Children*. 1995;5(2):34–52.

27. Russell M, Gruber M. Risk assessment in environmental policy-making. *Science*. 1987;236:286–290.

28. Department of Health and Human Services, National Toxicology Program. Human exposure assessment. Available at: http://webharvest.gov/peth04/20041020135705/ntp.niehs.nih.gov/index.cfm?objectid=06F6F41D-9B12-8FD0-63E4048B173CC36A. Accessed February 15, 2010.

29. Lippmann M, Thurston GD. Exposure assessment: input into risk assessment. *Arch Environ Health*. 1988;43:113–123.

30. Ott WR. Human exposure assessment: the birth of a new science. *J Expos Anal Environ Epidem*. 1995;5:449–472.

31. Gardner MJ. Epidemiological studies of environmental exposure and specific diseases. *Arch Environ Health*. 1988;43:102–108.

32. Monson RR. *Occupational Epidemiology*. Boca Raton, FL: CRC Press; 1990.

33. Hyperdictionary. Meaning of sister chromatid exchange. Available at: http://www.hyperdictionary.com/dictionary/sister+chromatid+exchange. Accessed February 15, 2010.

34. Rappaport SM, Symanski E, Yager JW, et al. The relationship between environmental monitoring and biological markers in exposure assessment. *Environ Health Perspect*. 1995;103(Suppl 3):49–54.

35. Duffus JH. Risk assessment terminology. *Chemistry International*. 2001;23(2):34–39.

36. Stern PC, Fineberg HV, eds. National Academy of Sciences' National Research Council, Committee on Risk Characterization. *Understanding Risk: Informing Decisions in a Democratic Society*. Washington, DC: National Academy Press; 1996.

CHAPTER 4

Environmental Policy and Regulation

LEARNING OBJECTIVES

By the end of this chapter the reader will be able to:

- Describe key environmental health regulatory agencies at the international, national, state/provincial, and local levels
- State four principles that guide environmental policy development
- Discuss five major environmental laws that have been introduced within the past 10 years
- Describe environmental policies designed to protect vulnerable groups
- List the steps in the policy-making process

INTRODUCTION

During the current century, human illness and death linked to environmental exposures represent one of the most significant challenges to the world's inhabitants. To date, extensive resources have been expended in the implementation of public policies, regulations, and laws that are designed to protect the health of the public from environmentally caused diseases. Nevertheless, much more work needs to be completed. Referring specifically to the United States, Bailus Walker, the past president of the American Public Health Association, noted:

> Despite these investments—which amount to billions of dollars—we have not at all completed the task of preventing environmentally provoked disease and of providing more protection for the ecological system. Even an abbreviated list will show how many problems remain to be solved:

an epidemic of childhood lead poisoning, the increasing incidence of genetic diseases exacerbated by environmental stressors, pesticides in food and water, too much ozone at ground level and too little in the stratosphere, global temperature warming, slow implementation of national toxic waste policies, and flaws in the institutions and processes the nation relies on to reduce environmental risks. Obviously, environmental health activities cannot be narrowly focused but must recognize the critical interrelationships between environmental media and between policies and programs.[1(p1395)]

Increasingly, protection from environmentally associated health hazards is regarded as a fundamental human right; policy making will need to take into account the reduction of disparities in health status that result from environmental sources. Momentum is gathering for the development of policies that protect the health of vulnerable population groups such as children, who may be even more susceptible to the actions of environmental toxins than adults. For example, data have shown an increasing occurrence of childhood asthma, which may be linked to air pollution.

This chapter presents terminology and concepts related to the **environmental policy** process. Also described are some of the major US governmental and international agencies charged with the development, adoption, and enforcement of environmental policies and regulations. The chapter also will cite some of the US laws and regulations that have been developed to protect air and water quality and natural resources and to guard the public from hazards that originate from toxic substances and wastes.

OVERVIEW OF THE ENVIRONMENTAL POLICY PROCESS

This overview will define and explain the following terms and concepts related to the policy process:

- Environmental policy
- Principles of environmental policy development
- The policy cycle
- The interplay between the evaluation process and policy development

Some argue that a systems approach—holistic thinking—is essential for policy development in the arena of the environment, which may be thought of as a set of interconnected elements or subsystems.[2] These include scientific, economic, cultural, and political dimensions that are relevant to the formulation and implementation of particular environmental policies. An example relates to the problem of agricultural pollution, which poses health hazards from animal wastes, fertilizers, and pesticides. Farming practices are designed to maximize output, using economic, climatic, and land use criteria. In addition to taking into account the health consequences of agricultural pollution, environmental policies also need to consider economic factors such as market costs that influence agricultural practices.[3] Another economic factor concerns stakeholders' willingness to pay for the costs necessitated by policy programs. Good policy decisions can be made if data on the economic costs and benefits of the policy package and its components are available.[4]

The environmental policy process takes place within the political context and reflects tension between political considerations and scientific knowledge. In some instances, the public may reject environmental policies that are justified scientifically. In illustration, research has suggested that logging of the nation's forests contributes to increases in greenhouse gases; as a result, some municipalities may decide to prohibit logging in order to protect the natural environment. However, in communities supported by lumber production, residents may oppose restrictions on logging because such prohibitions cause widespread unemployment. In other instances, politics may be instrumental in the adoption of environmental policies that might not be scientifically justified. For example, scientific findings may demonstrate that the low levels of some pollutants in the water supply are unlikely to have adverse human health impacts. Nevertheless, consumers may demand that such pollutants be removed completely from the water supply even if their removal is very costly.

Definition of Environmental Policy

An **environmental policy** is "[a] statement by an organization [either public, such as a government, or private] of its intentions and principles in relation to its overall environmental performance. Environmental policy provides a framework for action and for the setting of its environmental objectives and target."[5] The goal of environmental policy is "to reduce human risks or environmental damages resulting from pollution. Policy analysis facilitates social valuation of these risks and damages, by clarifying the costs of reducing environmental damages in terms of foregone economic returns."[3(pp244–245)] An example of an environmental policy in the United States is the National Environmental Policy Act of 1969, which sought to benefit the human population by preventing damage to the environment. The act is written, in part, as follows:

> **Congressional Declaration of National Environmental Policy**
>
> **Sec. 101 [42 USC § 4331].**
>
> (a) The Congress, recognizing the profound impact of man's activity on the interrelations of all components of the natural environment, particularly the profound influences of population growth, high-density urbanization, industrial expansion, resource exploitation, and new and expanding technological advances and recognizing further the critical importance of restoring and maintaining environmental quality to the overall welfare and development of man, declares that it is the continuing policy of the Federal Government, in cooperation with State and local governments, and other concerned public and private organizations, to use all practicable means and measures, including financial and technical assistance, in a manner calculated to foster and promote the general welfare, to create and maintain conditions under which man and nature can exist in productive harmony, and fulfill the social, economic, and other requirements of present and future generations of Americans.[6]

Principles of Environmental Policy Development

In the environmental health arena, a number of environmental principles or philosophies may guide the work of those who are charged with creation of policy (formal and informal policy actors, policy researchers, and policy analysts):

- The precautionary principle
- Environmental justice
- Environmental sustainability
- The polluter-pays principle

A significant ethical issue for policy developers involves setting an acceptable level of risk associated with a potential environmental hazard. There needs to be a "moral consensus regarding the level of risk that is sufficient to regard a substance in the environment as a potential threat to human and ecologic health."[7(p1786)]

The **precautionary principle** states that "preventive, anticipatory measures . . . [should] be taken when an activity raises threats of harm to the environment, wildlife, or human health, even if some cause-and-effect relationships are not fully established."[8(p263)] The practice of risk assessment is a science of uncertainty, so environmental toxins often present risks that have not been ascertained completely. The precautionary principle suggests that policy makers should err on the side of "an ounce of prevention" and take protective measures even when full scientific certainty is lacking.

A specific case that could merit the application of the precautionary principle relates to endocrine disruptors. The term *endocrine disruptor* refers to "exogenous substances that alter function(s) of the endocrine system and consequently cause adverse health effects in an intact organism, or its progeny, or (sub)populations."[9] For example, some chemicals are believed to have an estrogenic effect (acting as female hormones); two of the many varieties of these chemicals are DDT and the family of pesticides known as organochlorines. Scientists have speculated that endocrine-disrupting chemicals may be related to human sexual abnormalities such as low sperm counts in boys and animal abnormalities such as changes in the sexual functioning of aquatic animals.

The precautionary principle would advocate for the control of potential endocrine-disrupting chemicals, even though the focus of most research has been on whether or not they cause cancer (carcinogenesis). The absence of demonstrated carcinogenic effects does not rule out the possibility of other health hazards (e.g., endocrine disruption). Environmental research that focuses on risks of carcinogenic effects should not exclude from consideration other effects such as damage to the endocrine and immune systems; these health effects are overlooked frequently in environmental research. Further, exposures to such chemicals that occur early in life may pose greater health risks than exposures that occur later in life. Policies developed by the European Union adhere to the precautionary principle and advocate that preventive action be taken to reduce risks from potential environmental hazards.[10]

The principle is applied when the weight of scientific evidence suggests that a chemical is suspected of having adverse health consequences, even though such health effects have not been established definitively.

The concept of **environmental justice** denotes the equal treatment of all people in society irrespective of their racial background, country of origin, and socioeconomic status. The presence of an environmental hazard may be the end product of disparities of power and privilege within a community. Consequently, unequal toxic exposures of adults and children from different racial, ethnic, or socioeconomic groups may occur. Children of color may receive especially high exposures to environmental toxins.

Here is a statement on environmental justice by the US Environmental Protection Agency (EPA):

> Environmental Justice is the fair treatment and meaningful involvement of all people regardless of race, color, national origin, or income with respect to the development, implementation, and enforcement of environmental laws, regulations, and policies. Fair treatment means that no group of people should bear a disproportionate share of the negative environmental consequences resulting from industrial, governmental and commercial operations or policies. Meaningful involvement means that: (1) people have an opportunity to participate in decisions about activities that may affect their environment and/or health; (2) the public's contribution can influence the regulatory agency's decision; (3) their concerns will be considered in the decision-making process; and (4) the decision makers seek out and facilitate the involvement of those potentially affected. EPA has this goal for all communities and persons across this Nation. It will be achieved when everyone enjoys the same degree of protection from environmental and health hazards and equal access to the decision-making process to have a healthy environment in which to live, learn, and work.[11]

As a goal of environmental policy, **environmental sustainability** adheres to the philosophical viewpoint "that a strong, just, and wealthy society can be consistent with a clean environment, healthy ecosystems, and a beautiful planet."[12(p5383)] The three components of sustainable development are materials and energy use, land use, and human development. Environmental sustainability means that resources should not be depleted faster than they can be regenerated;

the concept also specifies that there should be no permanent change to the natural environment. Critics of sustainable development argue that the definition of the term is not entirely clear and is open to interpretation.[13]

A crucial aspect of any environmental policy concerns who should bear the costs of eliminating environmental hazards. As defined by the Organisation for Economic Co-operation and Development (OECD), the **polluter-pays principle** "means that the polluter should bear the expenses of carrying out the pollution prevention and control measures introduced by public authorities in Member countries, to ensure that the environment is in an acceptable state."[14] The principle, implemented by the OECD in November 1974, applies to pollution that originates from a variety of sources including accidental releases during manufacturing processes and from installations that handle hazardous materials. The costs of controlling pollution generated during manufacturing and consumption are to be incorporated into the prices of associated goods and services.

The Policy Cycle

The **policy cycle** refers to the distinct phases involved in the policy-making process.[15] (Refer to Figure 4-1.) The policy cycle comprises several stages: (1) problem definition, formulation, and reformulation; (2) agenda setting; (3) policy establishment (i.e., adoption and legislation); (4) policy implementation; and (5) policy assessment.

The terms subsumed under the policy cycle are illustrated in Table 4-1.

Problem definition, *formulation*, and *reformulation* are terms that denote the processes of defining the problem for which the policy actors believe that policies are necessary. This early stage—problem definition and development of alternative solutions—often is regarded as the most crucial phase of the policy development process. The problems chosen should be significant for the health of the environment and have realistic and practical solutions. Poorly defined problems are unlikely to lead to successful policy implementation. Note that Figure 4-1 (the policy cycle) shows that following a process of assessment, problem definitions may need to be reformulated and the steps in the policy cycle repeated.

Agenda setting refers to setting priorities, deciding at what time to deal with the environmental problem, and determining who will deal with the problem. Policy makers need to establish priorities in order to reconcile budgetary constraints, resource restrictions, and the complexity of environmental problems against the need to develop those policies that are most feasible, realistic, and workable. Public support for protecting the environment is strong; opinion polls suggest that environmental policies are likely to gain acceptance in many sectors of society.

Barriers and difficulties in establishing priorities stem from the lack of information on risks[16] and lack of coordination among government agencies.[17] When the nature of the risks associated with an environmental hazard or toxin is uncertain, planners are left in a quandary about what aspects of the exposure require policy interventions. In addition, a criticism levied against the US Congress, which is a crucial policy-formulating body for the government of the United States, is its inability to set priorities due to fragmentation of authority among numerous committees and subcommittees that are involved with environmental policy.

A successful approach in developing priorities (and environmental policies in general) is to involve the community and stakeholders. This statement is especially true for the development of policies that impact arctic native territories and tribal lands. For such policies to be successful, planners should respect the cultural traditions of potentially affected indigenous peoples.[18]

Policy establishment involves the formal adoption of policies, programs, and procedures that are designed to protect the public from environmental hazards. A factor that impedes policy establishment is the unavailability of empirical information on the scope of risks associated with environmental

FIGURE 4-1   The policy cycle.

Start
Policy definition/
Formulation/
Reformulation

Agenda
Setting

The Policy Cycle

Assessment Policy

Policy
Establishment

Policy
Implementation

Source: Adapted from data presented in D@dalos, Policy Cycle: Teaching Politics. Available at: http://www.dadalos.org/politik_int/ politik/policy-zyklus.htm. Accessed March 9, 2010.

TABLE 4-1 Components of the Environmental Policy Cycle

	Problem Definition, Formulation, and Reformulation	Agenda Setting	Policy Establishment	Policy Implementation	Assessment/ Evaluation
What happens?	Define problems and alternatives	Set priorities; Involve stakeholders	Formally adopt public policy; Legitimization	Putting the policy into practice	Assess or evaluate effectiveness
Who performs the function?	Formal and informal policy actors	Formal and informal policy actors	Formal decision makers	Government agencies	Arm of government responsible for assessment
What factors influence policy?	Research and science; Interest groups; Public opinion; Social and economic factors	Research and science; Interest groups; Public opinion; Social and economic factors	Research and science; Interest groups; Public opinion; Social and economic factors	Research and science; Interest groups; Public opinion; Social and economic factors	Research and science; Interest groups; Public opinion; Social and economic factors
What problems are encountered?	Poorly defined problems	Lack of information on risk; Lack of coordination	Inability to coordinate and assess research information	Lack of government support	Lack of sound scientific data

hazards. According to Walker, "Limitations on our ability to coordinate, assess, and disseminate research information hampers efforts to translate policy into programs and services designed to reduce environmental risk."[16(p190)]

Policy implementation is the phase of the policy cycle that "focuses on achieving the objectives set forth in the policy decision."[16(p186)] Often this phase of the policy cycle is neglected in favor of the earlier phases of policy development. Barriers to policy implementation can arise from the government administration in power. In the case of the United States, whatever administration is in power may choose to weaken policy prescriptions due to political considerations. Organizations such as environmental groups, trade associations, and professional associations may be able to stimulate public opinion and influence elected government officials with respect to environmental health policy.[19] In order for a policy to be implemented successfully, policy developers may include economic incentives. For example, some policies for control of environmental pollutants use a market-based trading scheme.[20] This method assigns limits for pollution. Companies that fall below their assigned limits can accumulate credits for pollution control. These credits can be "banked" or resold to other companies that exceed their pollution limits.[21]

The political and social contexts may stimulate or impede the creation and implementation of environmental policy.[22] In many situations, public concern over a perceived hazard may provide the impetus to new environmental policies, regardless of whether scientific evidence supports their adoption. Research conducted in China has demonstrated the linkage among the social, environmental, and political elements as they affect policy goals and the implementation mechanisms for policy. (Refer to Figure 4-2.)

Assessment/evaluation, the final stage in the policy cycle, refers to assessment of the effectiveness of the policy. In order to facilitate assessment, environmental policies may incorporate **environmental objectives**, which "are statements of policy . . . intended to be assessed using information from a monitoring program. An environmental monitoring program has to be adequate in its quality and quantity of data so that the environmental objectives can be assessed."[23(p144)] An example of an environmental objective is the statement that the amount of particulate matter in an urban area (e.g., Mexico City) will be reduced by 10% during the next 5 years.

Interplay between the Evaluation Process and Policy Development

Underlying the policy development cycle is environmental health research, which includes the identification of toxic substances and other hazards, assessment of mechanisms of environmental toxicity, and establishment of evaluations

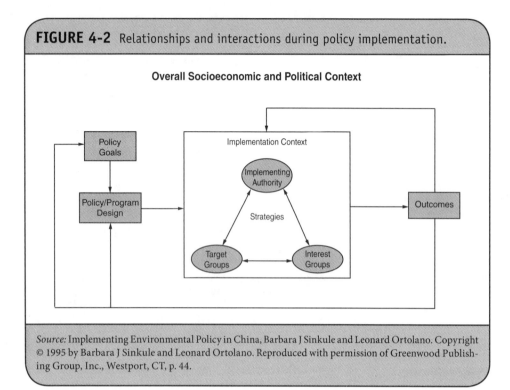

FIGURE 4-2 Relationships and interactions during policy implementation.

Overall Socioeconomic and Political Context

Policy Goals

Policy/Program Design

Implementation Context

Implementing Authority

Strategies

Target Groups

Interest Groups

Outcomes

Source: Implementing Environmental Policy in China, Barbara J Sinkule and Leonard Ortolano. Copyright © 1995 by Barbara J Sinkule and Leonard Ortolano. Reproduced with permission of Greenwood Publishing Group, Inc., Westport, CT, p. 44.

of interventions to mitigate hazards.[7] Some recent US governmental initiatives have emphasized the importance of research on pollutants as a specific component of environmental policies.[20]

Scientific data are linked closely to the policy cycle. "The creation of sound policy requires a foundation of sound data. It is through fundamental, mechanistically based research that environmental and public health officials can improve their understanding of risk and translate this knowledge into prevention strategies."[18(p118)] Epidemiologic studies provide the source of much valuable data for construction of environmental health policies. Figure 4-3 demonstrates the interface between science and policy development. The linkage begins with creation of hypotheses, moves to review of scientific evidence, and proceeds to development of models of exposures and health effects, and assessments of risks associated with exposures. The linkage concludes with the decision-making process in setting priorities and, ultimately, with formulation of specific policies.

RISK ASSESSMENT AND POLICY DEVELOPMENT

In Chapter 3, risk assessment was defined as a process for determining health risks associated with environmental and other hazards. Risk assessment is closely aligned with the policy process through the balancing of economic and other costs with health and societal benefits that may ac-

crue through specific policy alternatives. It should be obvious that the adoption of new environmental policies may involve the expenditure of considerable public and private funds, with potentially adverse economic consequences. For example, imagine the expense incurred when the United States and other countries implemented the policy decision to switch from leaded to unleaded gasoline. However, removal of lead from gasoline carried numerous health benefits that justified the high economic cost of this policy decision.

In some instances, the risks associated with exposure to hazardous substances may be so minimal as to obviate the need for policies to control exposure to them, although this issue is controversial. At some point the net economic and social costs of a policy may exceed the social benefits of pollution controls. An example is the presence of trace levels of pollutants in drinking water that has already undergone purification.

Policy adoption is difficult when an environmental issue is complex. An example comes from policies to control the potential environmental impacts of agricultural pesticide use.[24] Policy developers are confronted with several complex and often interrelated issues:

1. Pesticide use involves multiple contaminants that have differing characteristics.
2. Exposure of the population (both the general public and agricultural workers) to contaminants can arise from unspecified sources as well as clearly delineated sources; sometimes it is difficult to identify the sources of pesticide emissions.
3. The costs incurred to measure pesticide emissions are high.
4. There may be interactions among different types of pesticides.

The complicated nature of measuring pesticide exposures muddies the development of policies to limit the population's exposure to pesticides and to promote the appropriate uses of pesticides.

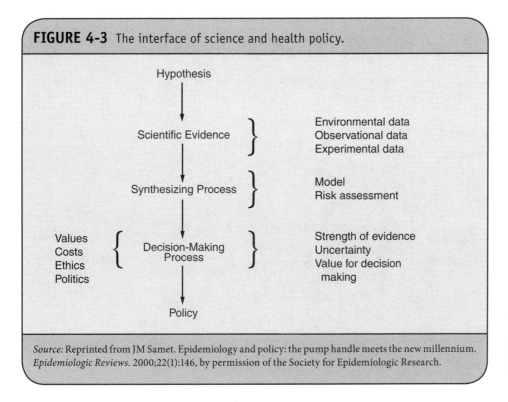

FIGURE 4-3 The interface of science and health policy.

Source: Reprinted from JM Samet. Epidemiology and policy: the pump handle meets the new millennium. *Epidemiologic Reviews.* 2000;22(1):146, by permission of the Society for Epidemiologic Research.

markers of contaminant exposures in children and adults. A biomarker is "[a] specific biochemical in the body which has a particular molecular feature that makes it useful for measuring the progress of disease or the effects of treatment."[26] The participatory process aims "at eliciting the 'values' and the perspectives of the community involved so that the multiple dimensions of risk can be taken into account early on in the assessment."[10(pxi)]

Risk Management

The process of risk management involves the adoption of steps to eliminate identified risks or lower them to acceptable levels (often as determined by a government agency that has taken into account input from the public).[25] After a risk assessment has been completed, public policy mandates may be adopted for the management of the identifiable risk. Suppose, for example, that a risk assessment shows that exposure to lead is harmful to children. A government agency has adopted a policy that states that children shall be protected from environmental exposures to lead. The risk management plan involves the adoption and implementation of procedures that are designed to protect children from lead exposure. Refer to Figure 4-5 for more information.

Falconer has presented a model for the development of policies regarding the use of pesticides; this model consists of four components: hazard, risk, impacts, and social costs.[24] The term *hazard* relates to chemical and physical properties (e.g., color, boiling point, volatility) of pesticides; *risk* refers to the probability of exposure; the term *impacts* pertains to the actual effects (e.g., harm) of pesticide usage; *social cost* refers to society's perception of the importance of harm to the environment. The interrelationships among these terms are shown in Figure 4-4. Planners need to take into account the entire panel of variables when developing appropriate environmental policies.

Risk assessment should occur at the inception of the environmental policy-making process.[25] Risk assessment should be "a participatory procedure, in which the different stake-holders are involved early in the risk analysis process to 'characterize' risks, even before they are given a formal assessment."[10(px)] An example would be incorporating community-based participatory methods designed to assess bio-

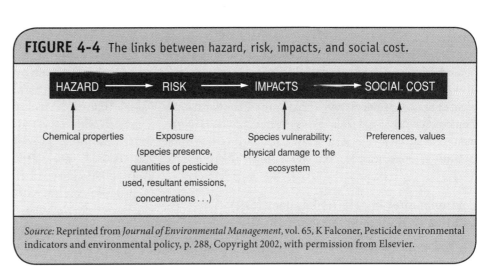

FIGURE 4-4 The links between hazard, risk, impacts, and social cost.

HAZARD → RISK → IMPACTS → SOCIAL COST

Chemical properties

Exposure (species presence, quantities of pesticide used, resultant emissions, concentrations . . .)

Species vulnerability; physical damage to the ecosystem

Preferences, values

Source: Reprinted from *Journal of Environmental Management*, vol. 65, K Falconer, Pesticide environmental indicators and environmental policy, p. 288, Copyright 2002, with permission from Elsevier.

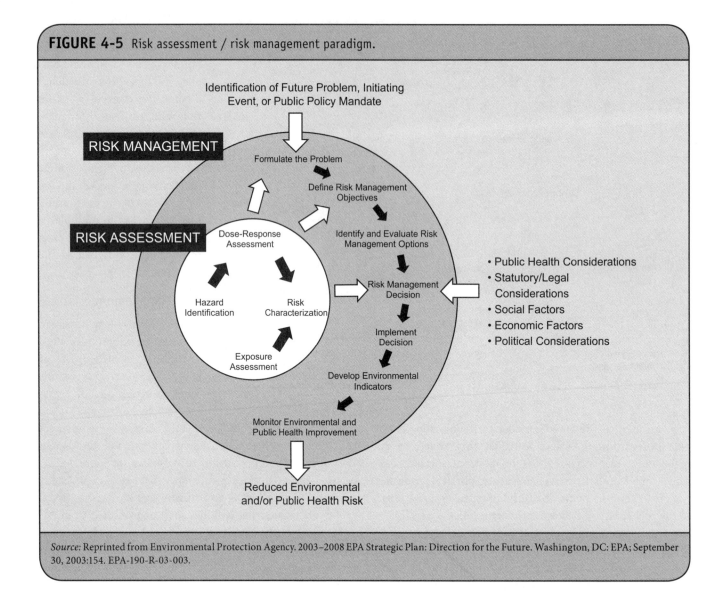

FIGURE 4-5 Risk assessment / risk management paradigm.

Source: Reprinted from Environmental Protection Agency. 2003–2008 EPA Strategic Plan: Direction for the Future. Washington, DC: EPA; September 30, 2003:154. EPA-190-R-03-003.

Other examples of risk management include the development of regulations that control the production, use, and disposal of toxic chemicals. In the United States, risk management of toxic substances is governed by the Toxic Substances Control Act (discussed later in this chapter). Methods of risk management include licensing laws, standard-setting laws, control-oriented measures, and monitoring.[25] (Refer to Table 4-2.)

Environmental Impact Assessment (EIA) and Health Impact Assessment (HIA)

An *environmental impact* is defined as "[a]ny change to the environment, whether adverse or beneficial, wholly or partially resulting from an organization's activities, products or services."[5] An **environmental impact assessment (EIA)** is a process that reviews the potential impact of anthropogenic (human-related) activities (e.g., a proposed construction project) with respect to their general environmental consequences. To give an example, an EIA might consider whether a proposed residential development would increase water and air pollution beyond acceptable limits or endanger threatened species of animals and plants. An EIA seeks abatement measures for pollution before it is produced; procedures for control of pollution should be feasible and cost-effective.[22] An example of an abatement procedure is the construction of catch basins for containment of water runoff from new

TABLE 4-2 Examples of Risk Management

Risk Management Procedure	Description
Licensing laws	Require licensing and registration for new and existing chemicals; include requirements for toxicity testing, including the Federal Insecticide, Fungicide, and Rodenticide Act (FIFRA).
Standard-setting laws	Establish standards of exposure for chemicals used in specific situations; an example is the Clean Air Act.
Control-oriented measures	Deal with explicitly identified chemicals, groups of chemicals, or chemical processes; an example is the design of packages so that they are childproof and prevent young children's access to harmful substances
Monitoring	Measures of the level of an environmental toxin so that regulations can be enforced. Monitoring programs are in place for ozone and smog and for pesticide levels in foods, to name several examples.

Source: Data from PJ Landrigan, JE Carlson. Environmental policy and children's health. *The Future of Children.* 1995;5(2):41–43.

TABLE 4-3 Applications of Health Impact Assessment

Activity	Examples
"Traditional" project EIA	Large dams, mines, power plants, airports
Regional or local project EIA	Development corridors, urban redevelopment
"Cumulative" environmental assessment	Air/watershed management
"Sectoral" environmental assessment	Energy/water sector planning
"Policy" environmental assessment	Infrastructure planning
Economic policy/structural adjustment	Country level impacts/ mitigation
International treaties	Climate/biodiversity
Special cases	Private sector/budget planning

Source: Reprinted from LB Lerer, How to do (or not to do) . . . health impact assessment. *Health Policy and Planning.* 1999;14(2):199, by permission of Oxford University Press.

housing developments in order to prevent polluted water from reaching the ocean.

Although it is similar to an environmental impact assessment, a **health impact assessment (HIA)** refers to "a method for describing and estimating the effects that a proposed project or policy may have on the health of a population."[27(p198)] Refer to Table 4-3 for a list of the types of projects that may require an HIA. Major construction projects can have a damaging effect upon the health of human populations and, accordingly, should require an HIA. An example would be the construction of a giant water reservoir in a densely populated, tropical country that has high levels of tropical diseases. The large body of standing water created by the reservoir could encourage the multiplication of disease-causing vectors such as mosquitoes.

Six stages have been identified for the completion of an HIA.[28] Although not all of the stages are presented here, among them are the following: An HIA makes an in-depth appraisal of data relevant to a project. The appraisal should consider how a project affects health-related and sociodemographic variables (e.g., population displacement). The HIA incorporates a plan for the meticulous evaluation and continuous monitoring of possible adverse outcomes such as increases in poverty, undue damage to the environment, detriments to the social fabric, and increases in morbidity from infectious and other diseases.[27]

CASE STUDIES: ENVIRONMENTAL POLICIES TO PROTECT HUMAN HEALTH

The 2009–2014 EPA Strategic Plan

The US EPA has developed a strategic plan that, according to the requirements of the Government Performance and Results Act of 1993, must be updated every three years.

> As in prior EPA *Strategic Plans*, the 2009–2014 update provides a framework for Agency annual planning, budgeting, and accountability by identifying the measureable environmental and human health outcomes the public can expect over the next five years and describing how we intend to achieve those results. . . . The Agency is focusing on a limited number of target areas . . . [that] are most critical in helping the Agency

to better achieve and measure environmental and human health outcomes. These targeted areas include:

- Reduction of Greenhouse Gas (GHG) Emissions
- Sustainable Agriculture
- Impacts of Global Climate Change
- Contaminants
- Import Safety
- Improving Program Implementation in Indian Country
- Enforcement/Compliance Measurement Approach
- Research Strategic Directions and Targets
- Environmental Indicators, Monitoring, and Related Information[29(pp3–4)]

Protection of the Arctic and Antarctic Environments

Significant contamination of the arctic environment with organic materials, toxic metals, and radioactivity has occurred as a result of pollution that originates in the industrialized areas of the world. The list of contaminants found in the traditional foods used by indigenous arctic peoples (and in their tissue samples) is extensive. (See Table 4-4; refer to Chapters 6 through 8 for definitions of the terms used in the table.)

In view of the future potential health impacts of toxic substances in the arctic environment, policies will need to be developed to protect this region. The use of a community advisory board working in conjunction with environmental scientists to protect the arctic environment has been recommended. The Arctic Monitoring and Assessment Program, with the input of community advisory boards, will aid in

---

TABLE 4-4 Environmental Contaminants Detected in Traditional Food Items and Human Tissue Samples

Industrial chemicals and by-products (e.g., dioxins, polychlorinated biphenyls, flame retardants)
Pesticides (e.g., DDT)
Polycyclic aromatic hydrocarbons (e.g., benzo(a)pyrene)
Heavy metals (e.g., mercury, lead)
Products of nuclear radiation

Source: Adapted and reproduced with permission from WA Suk, MD Avakian, D Carpenter, et al. Human exposure monitoring and evaluation in the Arctic: the importance of understanding exposures to the development of public health policy. *Environmental Health Perspectives.* 2004;112:115.

---

the development of appropriate policies. The Antarctic environment is also at risk and requires protection from pollution generated by military activities, tourism, and scientific exploration.[30]

Water Policy Reform in South Africa

South Africa has developed new policies—the National Water Act (1998) and the Water Services Act (1997)—to increase the equitability of water distribution and to protect aquatic ecosystems in the country.[31] Historically, before the introduction of these acts, water rights were held almost exclusively by large landowners. The purposes of the acts are to bring water rights under the control of the South African central government; to ensure that all citizens have sufficient water supplies to meet their basic needs; to make water affordable; to introduce controls over pollution; and to make sufficient water available for the maintenance of the aquatic environment.

Environmental Policies in Economies in Transition

In the Baltic and nearby regions of Central and Eastern Europe, former Soviet economies have changed to market economies as a result of the collapse of the Soviet Union. (Estonia, Poland, Hungary, and the Czech Republic are examples.) Previously, emphasis in these economies was placed on heavy industries that contributed greatly to the burden of pollution. Environmental protections were not enforced vigorously, resulting in heavy pollution of some regions. These economies inherited barriers to implementation of environmental policies that included economic and governmental inefficiencies and absence of environmental policy principles. New and effective environmental policies have been implemented that gradually have brought pollution under control. These policies include adoption of the polluter-pays principle and reduction in subsidies to inefficient heavy industries that cause pollution. Consequently, many of these countries have had substantial remediation of stationary sources of pollution such as those related to the coal mining industry.[32]

Control of Pollution across International Boundaries

Environmental impacts caused by the release of greenhouse gases such as carbon dioxide are global in scope. Control of such problems may not necessarily be confined to a single country but may involve actions at the international level. The New York Convention (1992) and Kyoto Protocol (1997) are two multilateral agreements that set forth international policies to reduce the emission of so-called greenhouse gases into the atmosphere. Other examples of environmental problems that have an international scope are climate change, ozone layer depletion, loss of **biodiversity**, and radioactive emergencies. Thus, international cooperation should be a feature of a single country's environmental policy. For example, three Baltic countries—Estonia, Latvia, and Lithuania—have designed multinational environmental agreements to control pollution in this region.[33]

Industrialization of Rural China

The shift from an agricultural economy to rapid industrialization, with consequential environmental quality degradation, is an increasingly common feature of rural China. Some of the causes of pollution are use of low-quality coal, energy inefficiencies, and lack of wastewater treatment facilities. Although strong environmental policies exist in China, numerous social, political, and economic barriers (e.g., insufficient funding) restrict their implementation or prevent their enforcement. Awareness is increasing among the general public regarding the adverse consequences of pollution. Nevertheless, environmental degradation remains a compelling issue in China.[22]

Protecting the Rights of Children and Special and Vulnerable Populations

Those who may be especially sensitive to environmental hazards include children, persons with genetic vulnerability, and minority groups such as African Americans and American Indians. Although efforts are under way to intervene in childhood asthma, birth defects, and lead poisoning, increased attention needs to be given to other environmental issues such as exposure to carcinogens, neurotoxins, and endocrine disruptors.[34] Despite this need, according to some experts, the United States lacks a coherent policy to assure that the environment is free from children's exposure to environmental toxicants. African Americans in many cases reside in urban centers where they are exposed to high levels of air pollution and toxic metals such as lead. Many American Indians live on sovereign lands that have serious environmental problems. American Indian groups sometimes face difficulty in reaching consensus about the appropriate action steps needed to reduce environmental hazards on their lands.

Landrigan and Carlson state that "[u]nderstanding the differences in the effects of environmental contamination on children and adults is an important part of environmental policymaking; however, unless environmental health policies reflect the differences between adults and children, this knowledge will have little practical effect."[25(p34)] Children's vulnerability to environmental toxins is related to their reduced ability to metabolize and excrete toxicants, rapid growth and development that increase vulnerability to toxicants, and the fact that children have more time to develop chronic diseases than do adults.[35]

Nowadays children are exposed to thousands of new chemicals. As a result of medical advances, infectious diseases are taking a reduced toll in the developed world. Consequently, chronic diseases of noninfectious origin are replacing infectious diseases as major causes of death among children in the developed world. (This shift is known as the epidemiologic transition.) Long-term exposure to environmental toxicants may play a role in causing some of these chronic conditions. Note that asthma and lead poisoning are increasingly important examples of the new morbidity among children. Some researchers believe that asthma may be associated with factors such as outdoor and indoor air pollution and insect contamination; lead poisoning is associated with exposure to environmental lead from painted surfaces in older buildings and from leaded fuels (which presently are banned from use in the United States and most developed countries).

One method for controlling and intervening in children's exposures to environmental hazards is known as the lifecycle approach to identifying exposure pathways.[34] (See Figure 4-6.) Environmental policies can be directed toward the various lifestyle exposure pathways shown in the figure (e.g., prevention of children's oral, dermal, and inhalations exposures to toxicants in the home and outdoor environments).

Turning from the developed world, consider the less developed regions such as parts of Southeast Asia and the Pacific, where numerous environmental threats confront children. These regions comprise the most rapidly industrializing areas of the world and contain half the world's children.[35] The quantity and severity of threats are increasing due to rapid industrialization and the epidemiologic transition. Examples of environmental hazards are smoke from wood used in home cooking and heating, arsenic in ground water, pesticides, lead emissions, and methyl isocyanate.[35] (Methyl isocyanate is a highly poisonous chemical used in the manufacture of pesticides. On December 3, 1984, 40 tons of the gas were released in Bhopal, India, causing many fatalities.)

The Built Environment

The term **built environment** refers to urban areas and structures (e.g., roads, parks, and buildings) constructed by human beings, as opposed to undeveloped, rural areas. From the world perspective, the built environment is increasing dramatically as formerly rural and agricultural economies transition to industrialized economies. In many sections of the United States, cities have taken over farmland and forests as metropolitan areas have expanded.

FIGURE 4-6 Pathways of children's exposure to environmental pollutants and hazards vary according to stage of development.

Prenatal

A stage when the developing fetus is very susceptible to the effects of pollutants; exposures can be transplacental and external.

Neonatal (birth to < 3 months)

Oral and dermal exposures: breast and bottle feeding; hand-to-mouth activity.
Inhalation exposures: time spent sleeping; time spent in sedentary activities.

Infant/Crawler (3 to 12 months)

Oral and dermal exposures: consumption of solid food, increased floor mobility, hand-to-mouth activity.
Inhalation exposures: breathing close to floor; development of personal dust clouds.

Toddler (1 to < 2 years)

Oral and dermal exposures: consumption of range of solid foods; increased play activity and curiosity.
Inhalation exposure: time spent sleeping; time spent in sedentary activities.

Preschool (2 to < 6 years)

Oral and dermal exposures: wearing adult-style clothing; decreased hand-to-mouth activities.
Inhalation exposures: increased time spent outdoors.

School-Age (6 to < 11 years)

Oral and dermal exposures: decreased oral contact with hands and objects; decreased contact with surfaces.
Inhalation exposures: time spent in school environments; participation in sports.

| Exposure Pathways During Stages of Childhood |

Source: Photographs and data from United States Environmental Protection Agency. A Decade of Children's Environmental Health Research: Highlights from EPA's Science to Achieve Results Program. EPA/600/S-07/038. December 2007.

Policies for design of the built environment have great potential for influencing public health.[36] Examples of design features with implications for health consequences are land development, community design, and transportation patterns. Some land development methods inadvertently cause people to drive cars by increasing the distances that people must travel. Encouraging the use of cars by making them affordable and installing free parking lots may have the indirect consequences of increasing air pollution and a sedentary lifestyle. Adoption of innovative public policies may stimulate people to walk more and use public transportation. An example is the colocating of business facilities, shopping centers, and residences so that city inhabitants are able to walk to work, ride bicycles, or take public transportation. Finally, development policies should foster the protection of open space and the creation of public parks.

AGENCIES INVOLVED IN THE ADOPTION, IMPLEMENTATION, AND ENFORCEMENT OF ENVIRONMENTAL POLICIES

A constellation of international, national, state/territorial, and local agencies maintain responsibility for development and enforcement of environmental health regulations, and for investigation of incidents that affect environmental health.

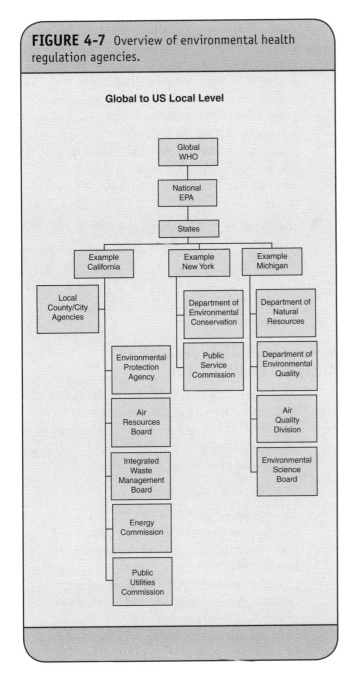

FIGURE 4-7 Overview of environmental health regulation agencies.

Global to US Local Level

prevention. More information about WHO is presented later in this chapter.

At the national level, many countries have a federalist system of government. The concept of federalism implies a type of government "that is structured around a strong central (i.e., federal) government, with specified authorities retained by lower levels of government, such as states and local governments."[19(p34)] This situation characterizes the United States, where the legislative and judicial branches of government perform important functions in environmental policy formulation. The Congress of the US government (Senate and House of Representatives) retains significant responsibility for creation of environmental laws. Judicial bodies in the United States (i.e., the court system) support interpretation, strengthening, and enforcement of environmental laws; an example is the interpretation of relevant environmental policies that are the focus of lawsuits.

At the national level, many government agencies regulate environmental health hazards in their respective countries. For example, in the United States, the EPA is responsible for protecting human health and safeguarding the natural environment, including air, land, and water. The EPA develops and enforces environmental regulations, which bring about cleaner air and purer water as well as protect the land. In addition, other national agencies (discussed later in this chapter) are charged with the responsibility of protecting the environment.

Within the United States, individual states and local governments also maintain responsibility for control of environmental health issues. Figure 4-7 shows some examples of agencies involved in environmental health regulation in three representative states—California, New York, and Michigan. As an example of one state agency's function, California's Air Resources Board (ARB) states as its mission: "To promote and protect public health, welfare and ecological resources through the effective and efficient reduction of air pollutants while recognizing and considering the effects on the economy of the state."[37] In large urban areas such as California's major cities, air pollution has continued to be a significant health and aesthetic issue. The ARB has had a significant role in reducing air pollution in California.

Local government agencies such as health departments also are closely connected with enforcement of environmental laws. For example, the City of Long Beach Department of Health and Human Services (DHHS), one of the city health departments in California, operates an environmental health division. This division is responsible for water quality, hazardous materials management, community sanitation, vector control, lead poisoning, food inspection, and housing quality

Figure 4-7 shows a flow chart of some of the agencies involved with environmental health regulations.

Referring to Figure 4-7, you can see that the World Health Organization (WHO) is a major international agency that is responsible for environmental health at the global level. WHO provides leadership in minimizing adverse environmental health outcomes associated with pollution, industrial development, and related issues. Although WHO's primary mission is to control and prevent disease, its reach extends to environmental health, which is closely related to disease

TABLE 4-5 Some Major Environmental Regulatory Agencies: US and Other

United States	Other
US Environmental Protection Agency (EPA)	European Environment Agency (EEA)
National Institute for Occupational Safety and Health (NIOSH)	World Health Organization (WHO)/Regional Office for Europe
Agency for Toxic Substances and Disease Registry (ATSDR)	
National Institute of Environmental Health Sciences (NIEHS)	

(e.g., through lead abatement). County and local government agencies in other states perform similar functions, although their exact organizational configurations may differ from one another. The remainder of this section identifies some of the agencies in the US that are responsible for environmental regulation. (Refer to Table 4-5.)

US Environmental Protection Agency (EPA)

EPA leads the nation's environmental science, research, education and assessment efforts. The mission of the Environmental Protection Agency is to protect human health and the environment. Since 1970, EPA has been working for a cleaner, healthier environment for the American people. . . .

In July of 1970, the White House and Congress worked together to establish the EPA in response to the growing public demand for cleaner water, air and land. Prior to the establishment of the EPA, the federal government was not structured to make a coordinated attack on the pollutants that harm human health and degrade the environment. . . .

EPA employs 17,000 people across the country, including our headquarters offices in Washington, DC, 10 regional offices, and more than a dozen labs. Our staff are highly educated and technically trained; more than half are engineers, scientists, and policy analysts. In addition, a large number of employees are legal, public affairs, financial, information manage-

ment and computer specialists. [Note that EPA is led by an administrator, who is appointed by the president of the United States]. . . .

When Congress writes an environmental law, we implement it by writing regulations. Often, we set national standards that states and tribes enforce through their own regulations. If they fail to meet the national standards, we can help them. We also enforce our regulations, and help companies understand the requirements. . . .

[Other functions of the EPA are to:]

- Give Grants . . .
- Study Environmental Issues . . .
- Sponsor Partnerships . . .
- Teach People About the Environment . . .
- Publish Information . . .[38]

National Institute for Occupational Safety and Health (NIOSH)

The National Institute for Occupational Safety and Health (NIOSH) is the federal agency responsible for conducting research and making recommendations for the prevention of work-related injury and illness.

Mission

The mission of the NIOSH is to generate new knowledge in the field of occupational safety and health and to transfer that knowledge into practice for the betterment of workers. To accomplish this mission, NIOSH conducts scientific research, develops guidance and authoritative recommendations, disseminates information, and responds to requests for workplace health hazard evaluations.

NIOSH provides national and world leadership to prevent work-related illness, injury, disability, and death by gathering information, conducting scientific research, and translating the knowledge gained into products and services, including scientific information products, training videos, and recommendations for improving safety and health in the workplace.

Origin

The Occupational Safety and Health Act of 1970 . . . created both NIOSH and the Occupational

Safety and Health Administration (OSHA). OSHA is in the US Department of Labor and is responsible for developing and enforcing workplace safety and health regulations. NIOSH is part of the Centers for Disease Control and Prevention (CDC) . . . in the Department of Health and Human Services. . . . NIOSH is an agency established to help assure safe and healthful working conditions for working men and women by providing research, information, education, and training in the field of occupational safety and health. . . .

Locations

NIOSH headquarters are in Washington, D.C. and Atlanta, GA with staff in Anchorage, AK; Cincinnati, OH; Denver, CO; Morgantown, WV; Pittsburgh, PA; and Spokane, WA. NIOSH has a professionally diverse staff of 1,200 scientists from the fields of epidemiology, medicine, industrial hygiene, safety, psychology, engineering, chemistry, statistics, economics and administration.[39]

Agency for Toxic Substances and Disease Registry (ATSDR)

The Agency for Toxic Substances and Disease Registry (ATSDR) is the nation's public health agency for chemical safety. The agency's mission is to use the best science, take responsive action, and provide trustworthy health information to prevent and mitigate harmful exposures [to] toxic substances and related disease.

The discovery of contamination in New York State's Love Canal during the 1970s first brought the problem of hazardous wastes to national attention. Similarly, the health threat from sudden chemical releases came into focus in December 1984, when a cloud of Methyl isocyanate gas released from a Union Carbide facility in Bhopal, India, seriously injured or killed thousands of people.

Both events represent the kinds of issues at the core of ATSDR's congressional mandate. First organized in 1985, ATSDR was created by the Comprehensive Environmental Response, Compensation, and Liability Act (CERCLA) of 1980, more commonly known as the Superfund law. In 1986, Congress passed the Superfund

Amendments and Reauthorization Act (SARA). Through these and other pieces of legislation, Congress responded to the public's demand for a more complete accounting of toxic chemicals and releases. In addition, Congress was—and remains—concerned by other pathways of potential exposure, including food, water, air, and consumer goods.

Since the creation of ATSDR, thousands of hazardous sites have been identified around the country. The Superfund program remains responsible for finding and cleaning up the most dangerous hazardous waste sites in the country. ATSDR has also been at the forefront in protecting people from acute toxic exposures that occur from hazardous leaks and spills, environment-related poisonings, and natural and terrorism-related disasters.

Under its CERCLA mandate, ATSDR's work falls into four functional areas:

- Protecting the public from toxic exposures;
- Increasing knowledge about toxic substances;
- Delivering health education about toxic chemicals; and
- Maintaining health registries.

Through our work in these areas, ATSDR continues to prevent and mitigate exposures and related health effects at hazardous waste sites across the nation.[40(p9)]

National Institute of Environmental Health Sciences (NIEHS)

The National Institute of Environmental Health Sciences (NIEHS) is one of 27 Institutes and Centers of the National Institutes of Health (NIH), which is a component of the US Department of Health and Human Services (HHS).

Unlike the other NIH institutes, the NIEHS is located in Research Triangle Park (RTP), North Carolina. RTP is a science and technology hub located between Raleigh, Durham, and Chapel Hill.

The NIEHS is home to the National Toxicology Program (NTP), the nation's premier program for the testing and evaluation of agents in our environment. . . . The NTP is a federal, interagency program, headquartered at the NIEHS, whose goal is to safeguard the public by identifying substances in the environment that may affect human health. Current NTP initiatives are examining the effects of cell phone radiation, endocrine disruptors, and nanomaterials, as well as developing new approaches to advance high throughput (high speed and high quantity) screening of chemicals, and to reduce the number of animals used in research. The NTP also works to understand individual susceptibility—why some people get sick when exposed to an environmental agent and others don't. . . .

The mission of the NIEHS is to reduce the burden of human illness and disability, by understanding how the environment influences the development and progression of human disease.

NIEHS's broad focus on the environmental causes of disease makes the institute a unique part of the NIH. . . .

Since 1966, the NIEHS has made many health research advances, and has been an important source of meaningful information for the public and decision makers.

The pioneering work of NIEHS researchers and grantees has shown the deadly effects of asbestos exposure, the developmental impairment of children exposed to lead, and the health effects of air pollution.

Federal and state regulatory, environmental, and public health agencies use NIEHS research to calculate new standards to protect health of people throughout the world. Thousands of lives are saved and diseases prevented in the US every year as a result of standards created under the Clean Air Act and the Safe Drinking Water Act. Actions taken by other agencies, such as the Centers for Disease Control and Prevention's recognition that even lower levels of lead in the blood are cause for concern and intervention, and the US Food and Drug Administration's 2010 update on the chemical bisphenol A (BPA) expressing some concern for its effects on human health, help protect the health of the public and are based on NIEHS/NTP research results.[41]

European Union (EU) and European Environment Agency (EEA)

The European Environment Agency (EEA), which is located in Copenhagen, Denmark, is an arm of the European Union. The EEA is tasked with the mission of supplying information to 32 member countries regarding the environment. This information is used for environmental policy development, adoption, implementation, and evaluation.

"The EU plays an important role in environmental policymaking. Environmental problems, such as air and water pollution, climate change and the decline in biodiversity, do not respect borders, so cooperation at EU level is necessary and well developed."—Stavros Dimas, EU Environment Commissioner

The EU's environmental laws help protect against water, air and noise pollution and control risks related to chemicals, biotechnology and nuclear energy within the Union.

The overall direction of EU environment policy is laid out in the latest action program—"Environment 2010: Our Future, Our Choice." It concentrates on 4 priority areas: climate change; nature and biodiversity; environment and health; and natural resources and waste. Also, an Environment and Health Action Plan for 2004–2010 promotes a close relationship between health, environment and research policy.

How the EU protects the environment

The EU is a leader in global efforts to protect the environment. The EU, for instance, is one of the initiators of the United Nations Environment Program (UNEP) creating a strategic approach to the international management of chemicals. The EU is a signatory and active participant in the Kyoto Protocol on Climate Change, which entered into force in February 2005. Moreover, the EU is party to a number of international agreements and partnerships, including the UN Framework Convention on Climate Change and the UN Montreal Protocol on Ozone Depletion.

Internally, the EU has established a comprehensive system of environmental protection covering emissions into the air and water, noise, waste disposal, conservation of natural habitats, chemicals and industrial accidents. An example of such domestic actions is the EU Emission Trading Scheme (EU ETS) on CO_2 emissions from industrial installations. In general, the EU's environmental policy is underpinned by the "precautionary principle." It is based on the "polluter pays" concept and the management and control of pollution at source.

The EU's treaty-based notion of "sustainable development" adheres to this practice by integrating environmental requirements into the definition and implementation of other EU policies and activities. The ultimate goal of sustainable development is to achieve a form of development that meets the needs of the present without compromising the ability of future generations to meet their own needs.[42]

World Health Organization (WHO)/ Regional Office for Europe

Environment is responsible for as much as 24% of the total burden of disease, which could be prevented through well-targeted interventions. . . .

In 1989, concerned about the growing evidence of the impact of hazardous environments on human health, WHO/Europe initiated the environment and health process to raise awareness and start collaboration between sectors, particularly the health and environment sectors. Sectors are brought together through ministerial conferences, to work on common issues and to shape the European agenda on health and environment. . . .

The European Environment and Health Committee (EEHC) . . . , which brings together representatives from health ministries, environment ministries, intergovernmental and civil-society organizations, monitors and reports on countries' work to implement their commitments. Its second key role is promotion and advocacy, by sharing experience and best practice and building partnerships with a range of stakeholders.[43]

Beyond the Regional Office for Europe, WHO's global environmental health activities cover a broad range of issues in many countries. These public health and environmental topics include:

- Air pollution, including indoor air pollution
- Children's environmental health
- Environmental health impact assessment
- Climate change and human health
- Environmental health in emergencies
- Quantifying environmental health impacts
- Water, sanitation, and health

For more information, refer to the WHO website: http://www.who.int.

Environmental Advocacy Organizations

Although they are not components of government, environmental advocacy organizations constitute an important part of the fabric of environmental policy formulation and are a significant force in influencing public policy. Environmental advocacy organizations help to educate people and seek to mold public opinion regarding the organizations' positions on specific topics, including global warming; reduction of air pollution; and protection of consumers from potential carcinogens in food, water, and cosmetics. One of the recent concerns of environmental advocacy groups is the development of alternative and green energy sources. Refer to Figure to 4-8, which shows the use of wind turbines for generation of electric power.

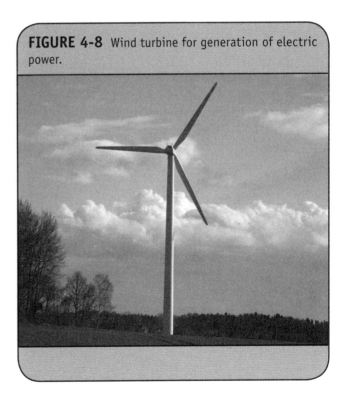

FIGURE 4-8 Wind turbine for generation of electric power.

Many organizations lobby local, state, and federal governmental bodies in support of particular environmental causes such as protection of endangered species and purchase of wilderness areas for public access. Numerous organizations in the United States and worldwide function at various levels, from grassroots to national and international. Some examples of the multitude of environmental advocacy groups are the following:

- Greenpeace
- National Resources Defense Council
- National Wildlife Federation
- The Nature Conservancy
- Sierra Club
- Union of Concerned Scientists

MAJOR US ENVIRONMENTAL HEALTH LAWS

Several of the major environmental health laws adopted by the United States are presented in Table 4-6.

Clean Air Act (42 U.S.C. § 7401 et seq. [1970])

The Clean Air Act (CAA) is the comprehensive federal law that regulates air emissions from stationary and mobile sources. Among other things, this law authorizes EPA to establish National Ambient Air Quality Standards (NAAQS) to protect public health and public welfare and to regulate emissions of hazardous air pollutants.

TABLE 4-6 Major US Environmental Health Laws

Name of Law	Date Enacted
Clean Air Act	1970
Clean Water Act	1977, and later amendments
Safe Drinking Water Act	1974
National Environmental Policy Act (NEPA)	1969
Federal Insecticide, Fungicide, and Rodenticide Act (FIFRA)	1996
Toxic Substances Control Act (TSCA)	1976
Comprehensive Environmental Response, Compensation, and Liability Act (CERCLA-Superfund)	1980
Resource Conservation and Recovery Act (RCRA)	1976
Occupational Safety and Health Act	1970
Endangered Species Act	1973

One of the goals of the Act was to set and achieve NAAQS in every state by 1975 in order to address the public health and welfare risks posed by certain widespread air pollutants. The setting of these pollutant standards was coupled with directing the states to develop state implementation plans (SIPs), applicable to appropriate industrial sources in the state, in order to achieve these standards. The Act was amended in 1977 and 1990 primarily to set new goals (dates) for achieving attainment of NAAQS since many areas of the country had failed to meet the deadlines. [See Figure 4–9.]

Section 112 of the Clean Air Act addresses emissions of hazardous air pollutants. Prior to 1990, CAA established a risk-based program under which only a few standards were developed. The 1990 Clean Air Act Amendments revised Section 112 to first require issuance of technology-based standards for major sources and certain area sources. "Major sources" are defined as a stationary source or group of stationary sources that emit or have the potential to emit 10 tons per year or more of a hazardous air pollutant or 25 tons per year or more of a combination of hazardous air pollutants. An "area source" is any stationary source that is not a major source.

For major sources, Section 112 requires that EPA establish emission standards that require the maximum degree of reduction in emissions of hazardous air pollutants. These emission standards are commonly referred to as "maximum achievable control technology" or "MACT" standards. Eight years after the technology-based MACT standards are issued for a source category, EPA is required to review those standards to determine whether any residual risk exists for that source category and, if necessary, revise the standards to address such risk.[44]

Clean Water Act (33 U.S.C. § 1251 et seq. [1972]) (Comprises Several Related Acts)

The Federal Water Pollution Control Act of 1948 was the first major US law to address water pollution. Growing public awareness and concern for controlling water pollution led to sweeping amendments in 1972. As amended in 1977,

FIGURE 4-9 The 1990 Clean Air Act.

Source: Reprinted from United States Environmental Protection Agency. The Plain English Guide to the Clean Air Act. EPA 400-K-93-001. 1993. Cover page.

Funded the construction of sewage treatment plants under the construction grants program.

Recognized the need for planning to address the critical problems posed by nonpoint source pollution.

Subsequent amendments modified some of the earlier CWA provisions. Revisions in 1981 streamlined the municipal construction grants process, improving the capabilities of treatment plants built under the program. Changes in 1987 phased out the construction grants program, replacing it with the State Water Pollution Control Revolving Fund, more commonly known as the Clean Water State Revolving Fund. This new funding strategy addressed water quality needs by building on EPA-state partnerships.

Over the years, many other laws have changed parts of the Clean Water Act. Title I of the Great Lakes Critical Programs Act of 1990, for example, put into place parts of the Great Lakes Water Quality Agreement of 1978, signed by the US and Canada, where the two nations agreed to reduce certain toxic pollutants in the Great Lakes. That law required EPA to establish water quality criteria for the Great Lakes addressing 29 toxic pollutants with maximum levels that are safe for humans, wildlife, and aquatic life. It also required EPA to help the States implement the criteria on a specific schedule.[45]

the law became commonly known as the Clean Water Act (CWA). The 1977 amendments:

Established the basic structure for regulating pollutants discharges into the waters of the United States.

Gave EPA the authority to implement pollution control programs such as setting wastewater standards for industry.

Maintained existing requirements to set water quality standards for all contaminants in surface waters.

Made it unlawful for any person to discharge any pollutant from a point source into navigable waters, unless a permit was obtained under its provisions.

Safe Drinking Water Act (42 U.S.C. § 300f et seq. [1974])

The Safe Drinking Water Act (SDWA) was established to protect the quality of drinking water in the US This law focuses on all waters actually or potentially designed for drinking use, whether from above ground or underground sources.

The Act authorizes EPA to establish minimum standards to protect tap water and requires all owners or operators of public water systems to comply with these primary (health-related) standards. The 1996 amendments to SDWA require that EPA consider a detailed risk and cost assessment, and best available peer-reviewed science, when developing these standards. State governments, which can be approved to implement these rules for EPA, also encourage attainment of secondary standards (nuisance-related). Under the Act, EPA also establishes minimum standards for state programs to protect underground sources of drinking water from endangerment by underground injection of fluids.[46]

Refer to the text box for provisions of the Safe Drinking Water Act as amended in 1996.

National Environmental Policy Act (42 U.S.C. § 4321 et seq. [1969])

The National Environmental Policy Act (NEPA) was one of the first laws ever written that establishes the broad national framework for protecting our environment. NEPA's basic policy is to assure that all branches of government give proper consideration to the environment prior to undertaking any major federal action that significantly affects the environment.

NEPA requirements are invoked when airports, buildings, military complexes, highways, parkland purchases, and other federal activities are proposed. Environmental Assessments (EAs) and Environmental Impact Statements (EISs), which are assessments of the likelihood of impacts from alternative courses of action, are required from all Federal agencies and are the most visible NEPA requirements.[47]

Federal Insecticide, Fungicide, and Rodenticide Act (7 U.S.C. § 136 et seq. [1996])

The Federal Insecticide, Fungicide, and Rodenticide Act (FIFRA) provides for federal regulation of pesticide distribution, sale, and use. All pesticides distributed or sold in the United States must be registered (licensed) by EPA. Before EPA may register a pesticide under FIFRA, the applicant must show, among other things, that using the pesticide according to specifications "will not generally cause unreasonable adverse effects on the environment."

FIFRA defines the term "unreasonable adverse effects on the environment" to mean: "(1) any unreasonable risk to man or the environment, taking into account the economic, social, and environmental costs and benefits of the use

1996 SDWA Amendment Highlights

Consumer Confidence Reports All community water systems must prepare and distribute annual reports about the water they provide, including information on detected contaminants, possible health effects, and the water's source.

Cost-Benefit Analysis US EPA must conduct a thorough cost-benefit analysis for every new standard to determine whether the benefits of a drinking water standard justify the costs. . . .

Microbial Contaminants and Disinfection Byproducts US EPA is required to strengthen protection for microbial contaminants, including Cryptosporidium, while strengthening control over the byproducts of chemical disinfection. . . .

Operator Certification Water system operators must be certified to ensure that systems are operated safely. . . .

Public Information and Consultation SDWA emphasizes that consumers have a right to know what is in their drinking water, where it comes from, how it is treated, and how to help protect it. . . .

Small Water Systems Small water systems are given special consideration and resources under SDWA, to make sure they have the managerial, financial, and technical ability to comply with drinking water standards.

Source Water Assessment Programs Every state must conduct an assessment of its sources of drinking water (rivers, lakes, reservoirs, springs, and ground water wells) to identify significant potential sources of contamination and to determine how susceptible the sources are to these threats.

Source: Reprinted from US Environmental Protection Agency, Office of Water (4606). Understanding the Safe Drinking Water Act. EPA 816-F-04-030. Washington, DC: US EPA; June 2004, p. 2.

of any pesticide, or (2) a human dietary risk from residues that result from a use of a pesticide in or on any food inconsistent with the standard under section 408 of the Federal Food, Drug, and Cosmetic Act."[48]

Toxic Substances Control Act (15 U.S.C. § 2601 et seq. [1976])

The Toxic Substances Control Act of 1976 provides EPA with authority to require reporting, record-keeping and testing requirements, and restrictions relating to chemical substances and/or mixtures. Certain substances are generally excluded from TSCA, including, among others, food, drugs, cosmetics and pesticides.

TSCA addresses the production, importation, use, and disposal of specific chemicals including polychlorinated biphenyls (PCBs), asbestos, radon and lead-based paint.

Various sections of TSCA provide authority to:

- Require, under Section 5, pre-manufacture notification for "new chemical substances" before manufacture.
- Require, under Section 4, testing of chemicals by manufacturers, importers, and processors where risks or exposures of concern are found.
- Issue Significant New Use Rules (SNURs), under Section 5, when it identifies a "significant new use" that could result in exposures to, or releases of, a substance of concern.
- Maintain the TSCA Inventory, under Section 8, which contains more than 83,000 chemicals. As new chemicals are commercially manufactured or imported, they are placed on the list.[49]

[Note: The foregoing list is abstracted from a list of nine items.]

Comprehensive Environmental Response, Compensation, and Liability Act (Superfund) (42 U.S.C. § 9601 et seq. [1980])

The Comprehensive Environmental Response, Compensation, and Liability Act—otherwise known as CERCLA [pronounced "SIR-cla"] or Superfund—provides a Federal "Superfund" to clean up uncontrolled or abandoned hazardous-waste sites as well as accidents, spills, and other emergency releases of pollutants and contaminants into the environment. Through CERCLA, EPA was given power to seek out those parties responsible for any release and assure their cooperation in the cleanup.

EPA cleans up orphan sites when potentially responsible parties cannot be identified or located, or when they fail to act. Through various enforcement tools, EPA obtains private party cleanup through orders, consent decrees, and other small party settlements. EPA also recovers costs from financially viable individuals and companies once a response action has been completed.

EPA is authorized to implement the Act in all 50 states and US territories. Superfund site identification, monitoring, and response activities in states are coordinated through the state environmental protection or waste management agencies.[50]

Resource Conservation and Recovery Act (42 U.S.C. § 6901 et seq. [1976])

The Resource Conservation and Recovery Act (RCRA) [pronounced "rick-rah"] gives EPA the authority to control hazardous waste from the "cradle-to-grave." This includes the generation, transportation, treatment, storage, and disposal of hazardous waste. RCRA also set forth a framework for the management of non-hazardous solid wastes. The 1986 amendments to RCRA enabled EPA to address environmental problems that could result from underground tanks storing petroleum and other hazardous substances.

HSWA—the Federal Hazardous and Solid Waste Amendments—are the 1984 amendments to RCRA that focused on waste minimization and phasing out land disposal of hazardous waste as well as corrective action for releases. Some of the other mandates of this law include increased enforcement authority for EPA, more stringent hazardous waste management standards, and a comprehensive underground storage tank program.[51]

Occupational Safety and Health Act (29 U.S.C. §651 et seq. [1970])

Congress passed the Occupational Safety and Health Act to ensure worker and workplace safety. Their goal was to make sure employers provide their workers a place of employment free from recognized hazards to safety and health, such as exposure to toxic chemicals, excessive noise levels, mechanical dangers, heat or cold stress, or unsanitary conditions.

In order to establish standards for workplace health and safety, the Act also created the National Institute for Occupational Safety and Health (NIOSH) as the research institution for the Occupational Safety and Health Administration (OSHA). OSHA is a division of the US Department of Labor that oversees the administration of the Act and enforces standards in all 50 states.[52]

Endangered Species Act (16 U.S.C. §1531 et seq. [1973])

The Endangered Species Act (ESA) provides a program for the conservation of threatened and endangered plants and animals and the habitats in which they are found. [Endangered species are those at risk of extinction; threatened species are those at risk of becoming endangered in the future.] The lead federal agencies for implementing ESA are the US Fish and Wildlife Service (FWS) and the US National Oceanic and Atmospheric Administration (NOAA) Fisheries Service. The FWS maintains a worldwide list of endangered species. Species include birds, insects, fish, reptiles, mammals, crustaceans, flowers, grasses, and trees.

The law requires federal agencies, in consultation with the US Fish and Wildlife Service and/or the NOAA Fisheries Service, to ensure that actions they authorize, fund, or carry out are not likely to jeopardize the continued existence of any listed species or result in the destruction or adverse modification of designated critical habitat of such species. The law also prohibits any action that causes a "taking" of any listed species of endangered fish or wildlife. Likewise, import, export, interstate, and for-

eign commerce of listed species are all generally prohibited.[53]

CONCLUSION

This chapter defined issues and principles that pertain to the development and implementation of public policies, regulations, and laws designed to protect the health of the public from environmentally caused diseases. The chapter presented terminology and concepts such as the policy cycle and risk assessment that are related to the environmental policy process. Also described were some of the major US and international agencies charged with the development, adoption, and enforcement of environmental policies and regulations. Some of the specific US laws and regulations designed to reduce air pollution, maintain water quality, and protect natural resources also were reviewed. It was noted that a significant ethical issue for policy developers involves setting acceptable levels of risk associated with potential environmental hazards and balancing these risks against societal benefits that may accrue through specific policy alternatives. Despite the efforts made to develop and implement appropriate environmental policies, much more work is required in order to protect the population from environmental hazards. Particularly in need of greater protection from environmental hazards are vulnerable groups such as children, as well as residents of less developed countries that do not have adequate environmental protections in place.

Although such efforts will be essential, promotion of human health in some cases may run counter to safeguarding the environment. Bioethicist David Resnik wrote that "Policies that protect the environment, such as pollution control and pesticide regulation, also benefit human health. In recent years, however, it has become apparent that promoting human health sometimes undermines environmental protection. Some actions, policies, or technologies that reduce human morbidity, mortality and disease [e.g., increasing food production and draining swamps] can have detrimental effects on the environment. Since human health and environmental protection are sometimes at odds, political leaders, citizens, and government officials need a way to mediate and resolve conflicts between these values."[54(p261)]

Study Questions and Exercises

1. Define and give examples of the following terms:
   a. Risk assessment
   b. Risk management
   c. Environmental impact assessment
   d. Health impact assessment
   e. The built environment

2. What is meant by the term *environmental policy*? Give two examples of environmental policies that have been developed in the United States.

3. Discuss the precautionary principle. Describe the types of environmental situations to which this principle might apply.

4. Cite the EPA's statement on environmental justice. What does the term *fair treatment* mean?

5. List the components of meaningful involvement; indicate how they are correlated with equal access of communities to the decision-making process that leads to a healthful environment.

6. Define the term *environmental sustainability*. List the three components of sustainable development.

7. Describe the rationale for the polluter-pays principle.

8. List and define the stages of the policy cycle. Explain how environmental health research is a component of the policy cycle. How does environmental health research contribute to the implementation of sound environmental policies?

9. Explain how risk assessment aligns with policy development. Give an example.

10. Why is it important to incorporate community-based participatory methods into the process of environmental policy development?

11. Name some environmental problems that have an international scope. What policy initiatives have been developed to bring them under control?

12. Explain why children are more vulnerable to environmental toxins than adults. What types of policies are needed to protect vulnerable populations from environmental hazards?

13. Describe the role of each of the following agencies in policy formation and in protecting the environment:
    a. US Environmental Protection Agency (EPA)
    b. National Institute for Occupational Safety and Health (NIOSH)
    c. National Institute of Environmental Health Sciences (NIEHS)
    d. European Environment Agency (EEA)
    e. World Health Organization (WHO)

14. Define the following environmental acts and explain how they have helped to ensure a safe environment in the United States:
    a. Clean Water Act
    b. Safe Drinking Water Act
    c. National Environmental Policy Act
    d. Federal Insecticide, Fungicide, and Rodenticide Act
    e. Toxic Substances Control Act
    f. Comprehensive Environmental Response, Compensation, and Liability Act
    g. Resource Conservation and Recovery Act
    h. Occupational Safety and Health Act
    i. Endangered Species Act

REFERENCES

1. Walker B Jr. Environmental health and African Americans. *Am J Public Health.* 1991;81:1395–1398.

2. Edgens JG. Environmental policy through a systems approach. *J Med Assoc Georgia.* 1995;84:225–227.

3. House R, McDowell H, Peters M, et al. Agriculture sector resource and environmental policy analysis: an economic and biophysical approach. *Novartis Found Symp.* 1999;220:243–261.

4. Christie M. A comparison of alternative contingent valuation elicitation treatments for the evaluation of complex environmental policy. *J Environ Manage.* 2001;62:255–269.

5. Sturm A. The Global Development Research Center. Glossary of environmental terms. Available at: http://www.gdrc.org/uem/ait-terms.html. Accessed March 17, 2010.

6. Executive Office of the President of the United States. Council on Environmental Quality. A Citizen's Guide to the NEPA: Having Your Voice Heard. National Environmental Policy Act Sec. 101. Available at: http://www.gc.energy.gov/NEPA/documents/Citizens_Guide_Dec07.pdf. Accessed March 17, 2010.

7. Sharp RR. Ethical issues in environmental health research. *Environ Health Perspect.* 2003;111:1786–1788.

8. Smith C. The precautionary principle and environmental policy: science, uncertainty, and sustainability. *Int J Occup Environ Health.* 2000;6:263–265.

9. EUROPA—European Commission. Endocrine disrupter research. What is endocrine disruption? What are endocrine disrupters? Available at: http://ec.europa.eu/research/endocrine/background_disruption_en.html. Accessed March 6, 2010.

10. Amendola A, Wilkinson DR. Risk assessment and environmental policy making. *J Hazard Mater.* 2000;78:ix–xiv.

11. US Environmental Protection Agency. Environmental justice: basic information. Available at: http://www.epa.gov/compliance/basics/ej.html. Accessed February 15, 2010.

12. Thomas VM, Graedel TE. Research issues in sustainable consumption: toward an analytical framework for materials and the environment. *Environ Sci Technol.* 2003;37:5383–5388.

13. Maddox J. Positioning the goalposts: the best environmental policy depends on how you frame the question. *Nature.* 2000;403:139.

14. Organization for Economic Cooperation and Development. Recommendation of the council concerning the application of the polluter-pays principle to accidental pollution. 7 July 1989–C(89)88/Final. Available at: http://webdomino1.oecd.org/horizontal/oecdacts.nsf/Display/AC74CADF13 B9FE74C12570880057D85E?OpenDocument. Accessed February 15, 2010.

15. D@dalos. Policy cycle: teaching politics. Available at: http://www.dadalos.org/politik_int/politik/policy-zyklus.htm. Accessed March 9, 2010.

16. Walker B Jr. Impediments to the implementation of environmental policy. *J Public Health Policy.* 1994;15:186–202.

17. Rabe BG. Legislative incapacity: the congressional role in environmental policy-making and the case of Superfund. *J Health Polit Policy Law.* 1990;15:571–589.

18. Suk WA, Avakian MD, Carpenter D, et al. Human exposure monitoring and evaluation in the Arctic: the importance of understanding exposures to the development of public health policy. *Environ Health Perspect.* 2004;112:113–120.

19. Johnson BJ. *Environmental Policy and Public Health.* Boca Raton, FL: Taylor & Francis Group, CRC Press; 2007.

20. Kaiser J. EPA gives science a bigger voice. *Science.* 2002;296:1005.

21. Schmidt CW. The market for pollution. *Environ Health Perspect.* 2001;109:A378–A381.

22. Swanson KE, Kuhn RG, Xu W. Environmental policy implementation in rural China: a case study of Yuhang, Zhejiang. *Environ Manage.* 2001;27:481–491.

23. Goudey R, Laslett G. Statistics and environmental policy: case studies from long-term environmental monitoring data. *Novartis Found Symp.* 1999;220:144–157.

24. Falconer K. Pesticide environmental indicators and environmental policy. *J Environ Manage.* 2002;65:285–300.

25. Landrigan PJ, Carlson JE. Environmental policy and children's health. Future Child. 1995;5(2):34–52.

26. Hyperdictionary. Meaning of biomarker. Available at: http://www.hyperdictionary.com/dictionary/biomarker. Accessed February 15, 2010.

27. Lerer LB. How to do (or not to do) . . . health impact assessment. *Health Policy Plan.* 1999;14(2):198–203.

28. Lock K, Gabrijelcic-Blenkus M, Martuzzi M, et al. Health impact assessment of agriculture and food policies: lessons learnt from the Republic of Slovenia. *Bull World Health Organ.* 2003;81:391–398.

29. US Environmental Protection Agency. *2009–2014 EPA Strategic Plan Change Document for Public Review.* Washington, DC: U.S. Environmental Protection Agency, Office of the Chief Financial Officer; September 30, 2008.

30. Ensminger JT, McCold LN, Webb JW. Environmental impact assessment under the National Environmental Policy Act and the Protocol on Environmental Protection to the Antarctic Treaty. *Environ Manage.* 1999;24:13–23.

31. Tarmann A. South Africa's water policy champions rights of people and ecosystem. *Popul Today.* 2000;28(5):1–2.

32. Zylicz T. Environmental policy in economies in transition. *Scand J Work Environ Health.* 1999;25(suppl 3):72–80.

33. Kratovits A, Punning J-M. Driving forces for the formation of environmental policy in the Baltic countries. *Ambio.* 2001;30:443–449.

34. Goldman L, Falk H, Landrigan PJ, et al. Environmental pediatrics and its impact on government health policy. *Pediatrics.* 2004;113: 1146–1157.

35. Suk WA, Ruchirawat KM, Balakrishnan K, et al. Environmental threats to children's health in Southeast Asia and the Western Pacific. *Environ Health Perspect.* 2003;111:1340–1347.

36. Pollard T. Policy prescriptions for healthier communities. *Am J Health Promot.* 2003;18(1):109–113.

37. California Air Resources Board. ARB mission and goals. Available at: http://www.arb.ca.gov/html/mission.htm. Accessed February 15, 2010.

38. US Environmental Protection Agency. About EPA. Available at: http://www.epa.gov/epahome/aboutepa.htm. Accessed February 27, 2010.

39. Centers for Disease Control and Prevention. About NIOSH. Available at: http://www.cdc.gov/niosh/about.html. Accessed February 15, 2010.

40. Department of Health and Human Services, Agency for Toxic Substances and Disease Registry. *FY 2008 ATSDR Annual Performance Report: Safer Healthier People.* Atlanta, GA: Agency for Toxic Substances and Disease Registry; 2008.

41. National Institutes of Health. National Institute of Environmental Health Sciences. NIEHS Overview. Available at: http://www.niehs.nih.gov/health/docs/niehs-overview.pdf. Accessed March 7, 2010.

42. European Union. Environment. Available at: http://www.eurunion.org/policyareas/environment.htm. Accessed March 12, 2010.

43. World Health Organization, Regional Office for Europe. Environment and health. What is environmental health? Available at: http://www.euro.who.int/envhealth/20060609_1. Accessed March 8, 2010.

44. US Environmental Protection Agency. Summary of the Clean Air Act. Available at: http://www.epa.gov/lawsregs/laws/caa.html. Accessed March 8, 2010.

45. US Environmental Protection Agency. History of the Clean Water Act. Available at: http://www.epa.gov/lawsregs/laws/cwahistory.html. Accessed March 8, 2010.

46. US Environmental Protection Agency. Summary of the Safe Drinking Water Act. Available at: http://www.epa.gov/lawsregs/laws/sdwa.html. Accessed February 26, 2010.

47. US Environmental Protection Agency. Summary of the National Environmental Policy Act. Available at: http://www.epa.gov/lawsregs/laws/nepa.html. Accessed February 26, 2010.

48. US Environmental Protection Agency. Summary of the Federal Insecticide, Fungicide, and Rodenticide Act. Available at: http://www.epa.gov/lawsregs/laws/fifra.html. Accessed February 26, 2010.

49. US Environmental Protection Agency. Summary of the Toxic Substances Control Act. Available at: http://www.epa.gov/lawsregs/laws/tsca.html. Accessed February 26, 2010.

50. US Environmental Protection Agency. Summary of the Comprehensive Environmental Response, Compensation, and Liability Act (Superfund). Available at: http://www.epa.gov/lawsregs/laws/cercla.html. Accessed February 26, 2010.

51. US Environmental Protection Agency. Summary of the Resource Conservation and Recovery Act. Available at: http://www.epa.gov/lawsregs/laws/rcra.html. Accessed February 26, 2010.

52. US Environmental Protection Agency. Summary of the Occupational Safety and Health Act. Available at: http://www.epa.gov/lawsregs/laws/osha.html. Accessed February 26, 2010.

53. US Environmental Protection Agency. Summary of the Endangered Species Act. Available at: http://www.epa.gov/lawsregs/laws/esa.html. Accessed February 26, 2010.

54. Resnik DB. Human health and the environment: In harmony or in conflict? *Health Care Anal.* 2009;17:261–276.

PART II

Agents of Environmental Disease

CHAPTER 5

Zoonotic and Vector-Borne Diseases

LEARNING OBJECTIVES

By the end of this chapter the reader will be able to:

- Discuss the impact of human environmental change on emerging infectious diseases in animals and man
- Indicate how a disease may be transmitted from an animal reservoir to humans
- Define what is meant by a vector-borne disease and a zoonotic disease
- List three human diseases transmitted by arthropod vectors and three caused by zoonoses
- Discuss methods used to control vector-borne and zoonotic diseases

INTRODUCTION

This chapter covers zoonotic and vector-borne diseases, both of which have substantial environmental components and contribute greatly to society's burdens of morbidity and mortality. Medicine and public health made great strides toward the control of infectious diseases during the late 19th century and the 20th century. In fact, by the mid-1960s, some health authorities proclaimed that society was moving toward the virtual elimination of infectious diseases as significant causes of morbidity and mortality.[1] Medical advances included immunizations, the use of antibiotics for the treatment of infectious diseases, declines in mortality from infectious and parasitic diseases, and the eradication of smallpox during the late 1970s. Public health advances included improved environmental sanitation, disinfection of drinking water, and advances in methods of food storage. Despite these notable achievements, infectious diseases once again have come to the forefront, with the increasing incidence of these conditions leading to the popularization of the phrase "emerging and re-emerging infections."

Emerging and re-emerging infectious diseases include conditions that may have been unrecognized as well as those reappearing after a decline in incidence. Several factors may have contributed to the resurgence of these conditions: migration of human populations within tropical and semitropical areas, increases in international travel, population growth with attendant crowding and urbanization, overuse of antibiotics and pesticides, lack of clean drinking water, and climate changes attributed to human activity.[1] In the northern hemisphere, rising temperatures and increasing rainfall promote the growth and northward migration of mosquito populations, with corresponding increases in diseases transmitted by mosquitoes. Notable examples are malaria, dengue fever, and viral hemorrhagic fevers—conditions that are discussed in this chapter.

TERMINOLOGY USED IN THE CONTEXT OF ZOONOTIC AND VECTOR-BORNE DISEASES

The pathogenic agents for diseases in this category may involve prions, viruses, bacteria, protozoa, and helminths. For example, a total of more than 200 zoonotic pathogens may cause disease in human beings. Refer to Table 5-1 for a list of some of the diseases in this category.

Zoonosis

The term **zoonosis** refers to "An infection or infectious disease transmissible under natural conditions from vertebrate animals to humans."[2] The definition of *zoonosis* varies to

TABLE 5-1 Examples of Zoonoses and Vector-Borne Diseases

Bacterial
  Anthrax
  Cat scratch disease
  E. coli O157:H7 infection (discussed in Chapter 11)
  Lyme disease
  Plague
  Psittacosis
  Salmonellosis (discussed in Chapter 11)
  Tularemia

Viral
  Dengue fever
  Encephalitis
      Eastern equine encephalitis (EEE)
      Japanese encephalitis (JE)
      St. Louis encephalitis (SLE)
      Tick-borne viral encephalitis
      Venezuelan equine encephalitis (VEE)
      Western equine encephalitis (WEE)
  Foot and mouth disease
  Hantavirus
  Human monkeypox
  Influenza
  Avian influenza (discussed in Chapter 1)
  Swine flu
  Rabies
  Rift Valley fever
  West Nile virus
  Yellow fever

Parasitic
  Cryptosporidiosis (discussed in Chapter 9)
  Cysticercosis and taeniasis (discussed in Chapter 11)
  Giardia (discussed in Chapter 9)
  Leishmaniasis
  Malaria (vector-borne, but not a zoonosis)
  Trichinellosis (discussed in Chapter 11)

Rickettsial
  Q fever
  Rocky Mountain spotted fever (RMSF)

Nonconventional (e.g., Prions)
  Variant Creutzfeldt-Jakob disease (v-CJD); mad cow disease (discussed in Chapter 11)

include several different situations.[3] In some cases a zoonosis may be a disease-causing pathogen that maintains an infection cycle in a host that is independent from humans, who can become inadvertent hosts. Other definitions refer to organisms that can infect both humans and animals during their life cycles. Conceptions of zoonotic agents may also include pathogens that cause disease in a nonhuman host or situations in which an infected animal remains free from symptoms of the disease. Contact with the skin, the bite or scratch of an animal, direct inhalation or ingestion (e.g., eating contaminated foods such as infected meat), or the bite of an arthropod vector are some of the methods for transmission of zoonotic pathogens. Note that immunocompromised persons, infants, and children younger than five years old may be at increased risk of morbidity from zoonotic diseases (e.g., toxoplasmosis) transmitted by cats and dogs. Table 5-2 provides examples of zoonotic diseases and animals that are associated with those diseases.

Vector

In the context of infectious diseases, a **vector** is defined as "an insect or any living carrier that transports an infectious agent from an infected individual or its wastes to a susceptible individual or its food or immediate surroundings."[2] Part of the chain in transmission of infectious disease agents, vectors include various species of rodents (rats and mice) and arthropods (mosquitoes, ticks, sand flies, biting midges).

Vector-Borne Infection

The term **vector-borne infection** refers to "[s]everal classes of vector-borne infections . . . each with epidemiological features determined by the interaction between the infectious agent and the human host on the one hand and the vector on the other. Therefore, environmental factors, such as climatic and seasonal variations, influence the epidemiologic pattern by virtue of their effects on the vector and its habits."[2] Vector-borne infections spread by biological transmission, which refers to "[t]ransmission of the infectious agent to [a] susceptible host by bite of blood-feeding (arthropod) vector, as in malaria, or by other inoculation, as in *Schistosoma* infection."[2]

EXAMPLES OF VECTOR-BORNE DISEASES

Names of diseases in this group are malaria, leishmaniasis, plague, Lyme disease, and Rocky Mountain spotted fever. Malaria is a disease of great significance for environmental health, even though it does not usually occur in developed regions such as North America, Europe, and Australia. Leishmaniasis affects residents of Middle Eastern countries, where it is endemic, and has been a particular concern of US military personnel stationed in endemic areas. The plague remains a serious threat to the world's population; during the Middle Ages, the "black death" (caused by plague) wiped out millions of people in Europe. Lyme disease, with an epidemic focus in the eastern and upper Midwest United States and an expanding focus in the western United States, also occurs in other parts of the world.

TABLE 5-2 Examples of Zoonotic Diseases (and Associated Animals)

Name/Type of Animal	Zoonotic Disease
Domestic Animals	
Cats	Rabies, parasites such as tapeworm, cat scratch fever, toxoplasmosis
Cattle	Anthrax, *Escherichia coli* O157:H7, Q fever, cryptosporidiosis, mad cow disease (BSE)
Dogs	Rabies, parasites such as tapeworm, leptospirosis, campylobacteriosis
Horses	Anthrax, salmonellosis, cryptosporidiosis, rabies (unusual)
Poultry, e.g., chickens and ducks	Influenza, salmonellosis
Reptiles, e.g., pet turtles and snakes	Salmonellosis
Sheep and goats	Anthrax, Q fever
Swine	Trichinosis, tapeworm, influenza, yersiniosis
Wild Animals	
Bats	Rabies (Bats are the major source of human rabies cases in the United States)
Birds	Psittacosis, cryptococcosis
Mammals, e.g., raccoons, skunks, foxes, deer	Rabies, giardiasis, brucellosis
Rodents	Hantavirus, plague, tularemia

Source: Data from the Centers for Disease Control and Prevention, National Center for Infectious Diseases. Healthy Pets Healthy People. Available at: http://www.cdc.gov/healthypets/browse_by_animal.htm. Accessed March 1, 2010.

Malaria

According to the Centers for Disease Control and Prevention (CDC), malaria is a disease that is found in more than 100 countries, with more than 40% of the world's population at risk.[4] Typically, malaria is endemic to the warmer geographic areas of the globe. Endemic regions include Central and South America, Africa, India, Southeast Asia, the Middle East, and Oceania. The worldwide annual death toll for malaria is more than 1 million persons, with an estimated 300–500 million cases occurring each year.[4]

The health impacts of malaria can be severe, as demonstrated by Figure 5-1, which shows a child who has developed edema (swelling) brought on by nephrosis associated with malaria. Nephrosis is a disease that impairs kidney function, resulting in a syndrome that produces edema, protein in the urine, and elevated levels of cholesterol in the blood.[5]

Developing countries located in economically disadvantaged tropical and subtropical regions are especially affected by malaria. At greatest risk of dying are young children.[4] In addition to its human toll, malaria also exacts devastating economic impacts.[6] Highly affected developing countries may experience up to a 1.3% annual reduction in their economic growth rates.[7]

The average global, direct economic costs incurred by malaria are estimated to be $12 billion US annually. The direct costs include those for treatment and prevention of the disease (e.g., medicine, hospitalization, and pesticide use). Other economic costs include lost productivity and earnings as well as negative impacts upon travel and tourism and agricultural labor.

The name *malaria* originates from the Italian *mala aria*, which referred to "bad air."[8] Originally, it was believed that malaria originated from the dank atmosphere around swamps. Now it is known that malaria is transmitted by mosquitoes that carry a unicellular parasite known as a plasmodium. Ronald Ross, an Indian Medical Service Officer (portrait shown in Figure 5-2), is credited with discovering the malaria parasite in 1897 when he dissected mosquitoes and found the organism in their stomachs. He reported that he "saw a clear and almost perfectly circular outline before me of about 12 microns in diameter. The outline was much too sharp, the cell too small to be an ordinary stomach-cell of a mosquito. I looked a little further. Here was another, and another exactly similar cell."[9]

The four human forms of malaria are: *Plasmodium falciparum* (*P. falciparum*), *P. vivax*, *P. ovale*, and *P. malariae*. Infection with plasmodia, the causative agent, can be life-threatening; malaria symptoms include the occurrence of fever and flu-like symptoms such as headache, muscle aches, fatigue, and shaking chills. In some instances vomiting and diarrhea may accompany the disease. Other symptoms of malaria are jaundice due to anemia, which is caused by the loss

FIGURE 5-1 The edema exhibited by this African child was brought on by nephrosis associated with malaria (1975).

Source: Reprinted courtesy of the CDC Public Health Image Library. ID# 3894. Dr. Myron Schultz Content Provider. Available at: http://phil.cdc.gov/phil/details.asp. Accessed March 1, 2010.

FIGURE 5-2 Ronald Ross, one of the discoverers of the malaria parasite.

Source: Reprinted courtesy of the CDC Public Health Image Library. ID# 1441. Available at: http://phil.cdc.gov/phil/details.asp. Accessed March 1, 2010.

of red blood cells. *P. falciparum*, the most deadly type, may produce kidney failure, seizures, mental confusion, coma, and ultimately death.[4] *P. falciparum* is the most common variety in Africa south of the Sahara desert.

The *Anopheles* mosquito is the principal vector for malaria. The transmission of malaria involves the complex life cycle of mosquitoes (the vector) and human hosts (with human liver and human blood stages). The first stage in transmission involves the bite of an infected mosquito of the anopheles type. (Refer to Figure 5-3.)

During the transmission cycle the malaria parasite (called the sporozoite form) is transferred to the human host when the mosquito takes a blood meal. In the human host the organism multiplies in the liver (exo-erythrocytic cycle) and red blood cells (erythrocytic cycle) and later develops into a form (game-

tocytic) that can be transmitted from the infected person to another host after a mosquito feeds on the infected host. In the sporogenic cycle in the mosquito, oocysts are produced that can be transmitted to a human host, continuing the life cycle of malaria. Symptoms of malaria occur approximately 9 to 14 days after the bite of an infected mosquito. Figure 5-4 illustrates the cycle of transmission. (Malaria also may be transmitted by contaminated syringes or through blood transfusions.)

In the United States, malaria was endemic until the end of the 1940s. An antimalaria campaign was launched on July 1, 1947; one of the major activities consisted of spraying homes with DDT. By 1949, malaria was declared as having been brought under control as a major public health challenge in the United States.[10]

FIGURE 5-3 Female *Anopheles gambiae* mosquito feeding.

Source: Reprinted courtesy of the CDC Public Health Image Library. ID# 1662. Jim Gathany Content Provider. Available at: http://phil.cdc. gov/ phil/details.asp. Accessed March 1, 2010.

During the mid-20th century, efforts to control malaria by spraying with DDT and administering synthetic antimalaria drugs were found to be efficacious. Consequently, the World Health Organization (WHO) submitted a plan to the World Health Assembly in 1955 for the global eradication of malaria.[11] The plan involved spraying, drug treatment, and surveillance. These efforts at eradication were successful in countries that had temperate climates and seasonal transmission of malaria but had limited success in other countries such as Indonesia, Afghanistan, Haiti, and Nicaragua.

DDT was highly effective in controlling the mosquito that can transmit malaria. For example, Figure 5-5 and Figure 5-6, respectively, illustrate the use of bi-planes to spray for mosquitoes over wide areas and hand spraying methods to apply insecticide. At one time insecticides such as DDT were applied directly to military personnel (Figure 5-7). Over a period of several decades, environmental observers began to gather suggestive evidence that DDT was harmful to bird

FIGURE 5-4 The life cycle of the parasites of the genus *Plasmodium*, causal agents of malaria.

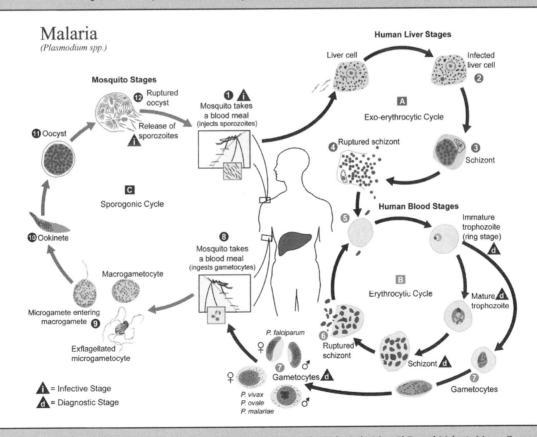

Source: Reprinted courtesy of the CDC Public Health Image Library. ID# 3405. Alexander J. da Silva, PhD, and Melanie Moser Content Providers. Available at: http://phil.cdc.gov/phil/details.asp. Accessed March 1, 2010.

FIGURE 5-5 A Stearman bi-plane spraying an insecticide during malaria control operations in Savannah, GA.

Source: Reprinted courtesy of the CDC Public Health Image Library. ID# 2622. Available at: http://phil.cdc.gov/phil/details.asp. Accessed March 1, 2010.

FIGURE 5-6 In 1958, the National Malaria Eradication Program used an entirely new approach, implementing DDT for spraying of mosquitoes.

Source: Reprinted courtesy of the CDC Public Health Image Library. ID# 4684. Available at: http://phil.cdc.gov/phil/details.asp. Accessed March 14, 2010.

FIGURE 5-7 A US soldier is demonstrating DDT hand spraying equipment while applying the insecticide.

Source: Reprinted courtesy of the CDC Public Health Image Library. ID# 2620. Available at: http://phil.cdc.gov/phil/details.asp. Accessed March 14, 2010.

species and other species of wildlife; the use of DDT was eventually opposed by many developed nations, especially the United States. This opposition led to withdrawal of funding for malaria spraying programs.

Discontinuance of outdoor DDT spraying and mosquitoes' development of insecticide resistance are among the factors that are believed to have contributed to the resurgence of malaria-bearing mosquitoes. As an alternative to outdoor spraying, South Africa has used annual spraying of DDT inside of homes, a procedure that appears to reduce the number of malaria cases.[12] Another means to control malaria is the use of bed nets that are impregnated with insecticides.

In addition to the use of insecticides, other methods of malaria control include the regular use of suppressive drugs in endemic areas and the avoidance of blood from donors who reside in endemic areas. Sanitary improvements such as the filling and draining of swamps and removal of standing water help to reduce the breeding areas for malaria-carrying mosquitoes. More information on the topic of mosquito control is provided later in the chapter.

The equatorial and southern areas of the continent of Africa form one of the endemic regions for malaria, as shown in Figure 5-8. In Africa, which accounts for a total of 89% of the world's malaria deaths,[6] evidence points to the movement of malaria from the low-lying areas where it is usually found to higher elevations where it is uncommon. In the late 1980s and early 1990s, Kenya experienced an upward movement of malaria cases, possibly due to small changes in climate that provided suitable conditions for malaria to survive.[13]

Malaria cases are not confined to endemic areas, because they may be imported into nonendemic areas by refugees and immigrants.[14] For example, the US state of Minnesota saw an increase in the number of reported cases of malaria from 5 in 1988 to 76 in 1998. The sources of these cases were persons native to Minnesota who had traveled to foreign areas and returned home as well as immigrants whose travel originated in a foreign country. Importation of cases of malaria presents a significant challenge to healthcare providers in nonendemic areas, who may not be familiar with the symptoms of diseases that they may not ordinarily see in clinical practice or during their training.

Leishmaniasis

Three forms of leishmaniasis are the visceral, muco-cutaneous, and cutaneous varieties; the latter is the focus of this section. Cutaneous leishmaniasis is transmitted by the bite of an infected sand fly.[15,16] After being bitten by the fly, the human host develops a characteristic sore on the skin that forms after an incubation period of several weeks or months. Figure 5-9 illustrates a lesion due to leishmaniasis. Near the site of the bite, a localized reaction occurs that forms a papule, which is "a small, raised, solid pimple or swelling, often forming part of a rash on the skin and typically inflamed."[17] Subsequently, ulceration, healing, and a scar form at the site.

The reservoir for the cutaneous form of leishmaniasis includes wild rodents, human beings, and carnivores (e.g., domestic dogs). The disease is transmitted from the reservoir to the human host by a sand fly known as the phlebotomus fly. (See Figure 5-10.)

Figure 5-11 shows the cycle of transmission from the sand fly to the human host and vice versa, during the sand fly and human stages. The causative agent for leishmaniasis is a protozoal organism, which exists in two forms—promastigotes and amastigotes. These two organisms are shown in Figure 5-11. Promastigotes are an extracellular form of the organism that has flagella (whip-like appendages that enable the organism

FIGURE 5-8 Malaria mortality rates per 100,000 in Africa, 2006.

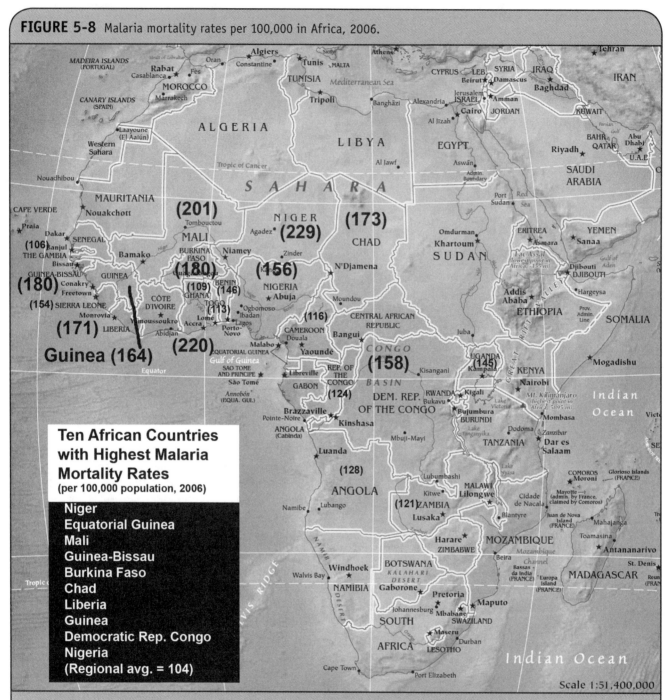

Ten African Countries with Highest Malaria Mortality Rates
(per 100,000 population, 2006)

Niger
Equatorial Guinea
Mali
Guinea-Bissau
Burkina Faso
Chad
Liberia
Guinea
Democratic Rep. Congo
Nigeria
(Regional avg. = 104)

Mortality rates for countries above the regional average are shown in parentheses; large type denotes the countries with the ten highest rates.

Source: Data from the World Health Organization, *World Health Statistics 2010*, Geneva, Switzerland: World Health Organization, 2010, p. 36. Map from the Central Intelligence Agency, The World Factbook. Available at: https://www.cia.gov/library/publications/the-world-factbook/index.html. Accessed August 1, 2010.

to move), whereas amastigotes are nonflagellated intracellular forms. Following the bite of an infected sand fly, promastigotes are injected into the host. The promastigotes are phagocytized by macrophages; phagocytization refers to the process whereby the macrophages in bodily fluids scavenge for foreign materials and, in this case, capture the promastigotes. The promastigotes transform into amastigotes within the macrophages, multiply and later explode out of the macrophages, and then may be ingested by sand flies through a blood meal that contains infected macrophages. Subsequently, amastigotes are transformed in the gut of the sand fly into promastigotes, continuing the cycle of transmission.

The various forms of leishmaniasis, present in the countries surrounding the Mediterranean and also endemic in a total of 82 countries, are showing an increasing incidence. For example, Syria, Tunisia, and Israel have reported increasing numbers of cases. Among 350 million persons at risk for leishmaniasis, the annual incidence is approximately 600,000 cases. The environmental factors hypothesized to be responsible for increases in leishmaniasis include movement of the human population into endemic areas, increasing urbanization, extension of agricultural projects into endemic areas, and climate change due to global warming.

Cutaneous leishmaniasis is a concern of US military personnel stationed in endemic areas (e.g., Afghanistan, Iraq, and Kuwait). Of a total of 22 cases reported in these three countries during 2002 and 2003, 19 occurred in Iraq. (Refer to Figure 5-12.) The condition has been subjected to extensive epidemiologic investigations in Israel, where leishmaniasis affects both military personnel and the general population.

Methods of control of leishmaniasis include the following:

- Periodic application of long-acting insecticides to dwelling units
- Use of screens to prevent sand flies from entering housing
- Elimination of breeding areas (e.g., rubbish heaps) for the phlebotomus fly
- Destruction of rodent burrows and control of domestic dogs

Plague

The bacterium *Yersinia pestis* is the infectious agent for plague, a condition that infects both animals and humans. Plague may be transmitted by the bite of a flea harbored by rodents

FIGURE 5-9 Skin ulcer due to leishmaniasis; hand of Central American adult.

Source: Reprinted courtesy of the CDC Public Health Image Library. ID# 352. Dr. D.S. Martin Content Provider. Available at: http://phil.cdc.gov/ phil/details.asp. Accessed March 14, 2010.

FIGURE 5-10 This is a female *Phlebotomus sp.* sand fly, a vector of the parasite responsible for leishmaniasis.

Source: Reprinted courtesy of the CDC Public Health Image Library. ID# 3811. W.H.O. Content Provider. Available at: http://phil.cdc.gov/ phil/ details.asp. Accessed March 14, 2010.

FIGURE 5-11 This is an illustration of the life cycle of *Leishmania spp.*, the causal agents of leishmaniasis.

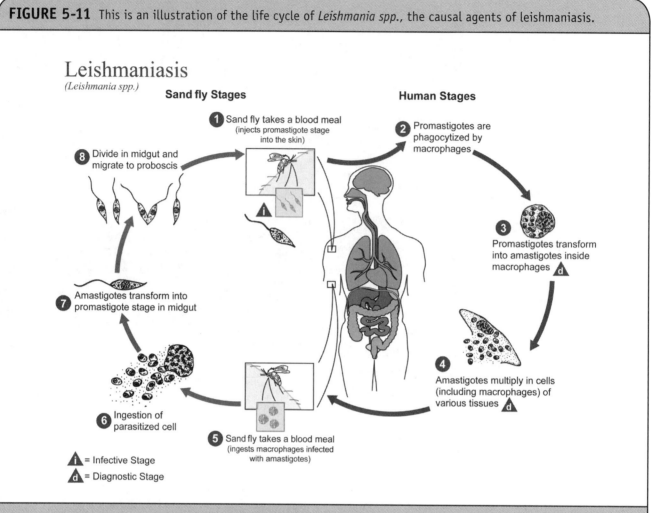

Leishmaniasis
(Leishmania spp.)

Sand fly Stages   **Human Stages**

1. Sand fly takes a blood meal (injects promastigote stage into the skin)
2. Promastigotes are phagocytized by macrophages
3. Promastigotes transform into amastigotes inside macrophages [d]
4. Amastigotes multiply in cells (including macrophages) of various tissues [d]
5. Sand fly takes a blood meal (ingests macrophages infected with amastigotes)
6. Ingestion of parasitized cell
7. Amastigotes transform into promastigote stage in midgut
8. Divide in midgut and migrate to proboscis

[i] = Infective Stage
[d] = Diagnostic Stage

Source: Reprinted courtesy of the CDC Public Health Image Library. ID# 3400. Alexander J. da Silva, PhD, and Blaine Mathison Content Providers. Available at: http://phil.cdc.gov/phil/details.asp. Accessed March 14, 2010.

(see Figure 5-13). Historians believe that the plague epidemic during the Middle Ages (the "black death") was caused by fleas from infested rats. Although morbidity and case fatality rates among persons infected with the disease remain high, prompt treatment with antibiotics is efficacious.[18] Nevertheless, human infections with *Y. pestis* remain a matter of great concern for authorities. Plague is distributed widely across the world, including the United States, South America, Asia, and parts of Africa (see Figure 5-14). In some regions, plague is a zoonotic disease.

One of the natural reservoirs for plague is wild rodents, such as the ground squirrels that are at home in the western United States. Pets, such as house cats and dogs, may bring the wild rodents' fleas into homes or may even transmit plague

on rare occasions from their bites or scratches. The condition known as bubonic plague begins with nonspecific symptoms such as fever, chills, and headache and then progresses into lymphadenitis (infected lymph nodes) at the site of the initial flea bite. There may be secondary involvement of the lungs known as pneumonic plague. The epidemiologic significance of this form of plague is that respiratory droplets from an infected person can transfer *Y. pestis* to other individuals. The case fatality rate for untreated bubonic plague is high, ranging from about 50%–60%. Patients who are infected with the disease need to be placed in strict isolation and their clothing and other personal articles disinfected. Persons who have had contact with the patient should be placed under quarantine.

FIGURE 5-12 Number* of cases of cutaneous leishmaniasis in US military personnel, by self-reported onset of skin lesions—Afghanistan, Iraq, and Kuwait, May 2002–August 2003.

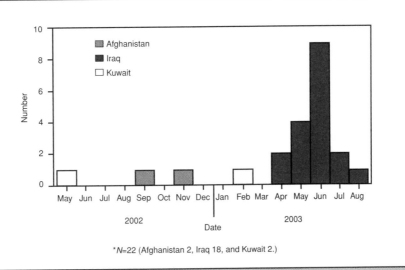

*N=22 (Afghanistan 2, Iraq 18, and Kuwait 2.)

Source: Reprinted from the Centers for Disease Control and Prevention. Cutaneous leishmaniasis in US military personnel—Southwest/Central Asia, 2002-2003. *MMWR.* 2003;52:1009.

FIGURE 5-13 Male *Xenopsylla cheopis* (oriental rat flea) engorged with blood. This flea is the primary vector of plague in most large plague epidemics in Asia, Africa, and South America. Both male and female fleas can transmit the infection.

Actual size→

Source: Reprinted from the Centers for Disease Control and Prevention. Plague: CDC Plague Home Page. Available at: http://www.cdc.gov/ncidod/dvbid/plague/index.htm. Accessed February 28, 2010.

FIGURE 5-14 World distribution of plague, 1998.

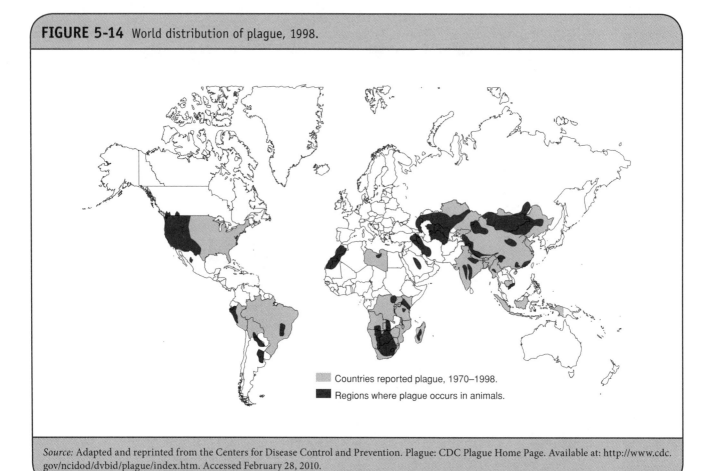

Countries reported plague, 1970–1998.

Regions where plague occurs in animals.

Source: Adapted and reprinted from the Centers for Disease Control and Prevention. Plague: CDC Plague Home Page. Available at: http://www.cdc.gov/ncidod/dvbid/plague/index.htm. Accessed February 28, 2010.

Environmental control of the disease may be accomplished by encouraging the public to avoid enzootic areas, especially rodent burrows, and direct contact with rodents. Unfortunately, some people ignore posted warning signs in nature parks and risk contracting plague when they feed squirrels and chipmunks. Also, the number of rodents needs to be kept in check. Public health officials should inform the public of the importance of preventing rats from entering buildings and should encourage the removal of food sources that could enable rats to multiply. Shipping areas and docks need to be patrolled because rats can be transferred to and from cargo containers and ships. Hunters and persons who handle wildlife should take care to wear gloves.[19]

Lyme Disease

Lyme disease is a condition that was identified in 1977 when a cluster of arthritis cases occurred among children around the area of Lyme, Connecticut. The causative agent for the disease is a bacterium (bacterial spirochete) known as *Borrelia burgdorferi*,[20] shown in Figure 5-15.

FIGURE 5-15 *Borrelia burgdorferi*, the spirochetal bacteria that cause Lyme disease.

Source: Reprinted from the Centers for Disease Control and Prevention, Division of Vector-Borne Infectious Diseases. Lyme Disease. Available at: http://www.cdc.gov/ncidod/dvbid/lyme/bburgdorferi_sm.htm. Accessed March 14, 2010.

FIGURE 5-16 (Top) From left to right: The black-legged tick (*Ixodes scapularis*) adult female, adult male, nymph, and larva.

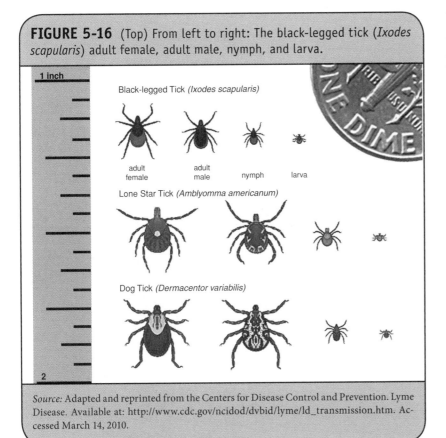

Black-legged Tick (*Ixodes scapularis*)

adult female   adult male   nymph   larva

Lone Star Tick (*Amblyomma americanum*)

Dog Tick (*Dermacentor variabilis*)

Source: Adapted and reprinted from the Centers for Disease Control and Prevention. Lyme Disease. Available at: http://www.cdc.gov/ncidod/dvbid/lyme/ld_transmission.htm. Accessed March 14, 2010.

be at risk of infection with Lyme disease. Antibiotic therapy exists for successful treatment of most patients who are diagnosed in the early stages of the disease. Preventive measures are directed at reducing exposure to the ticks that carry the bacterium. For example, people who venture into endemic areas should be inspected for the presence of ticks. Wearing light-colored clothing helps to disclose the presence of ticks.

Rocky Mountain Spotted Fever (RMSF)

RMSF, among the most acute infectious diseases, is caused by *Rickettsia rickettsii*, a rickettsial agent. (Rickettsia are agents that are similar to viruses in that they reproduce within living cells and are similar to some bacteria in that they require oxygen and are susceptible to antibiotics.) It is a febrile disease with sudden onset of moderate to high fevers that may last up to three weeks when untreated. Other symptoms include rash, headache, and chills. The case-fatality rate can range up to 25% among untreated patients, but drops dramatically when patients are treated with antibiotics early in the course of the disease. The bite of an infected tick (e.g., the American dog tick or the Rocky Mountain wood tick) is associated with transmission of RMSF. These species of ticks form the reservoir for *R. rickettsii*. Ticks also can transmit RMSF to wild animals and domestic animals such as dogs.

VIRAL HEMORRHAGIC FEVERS (VHFS)

According to the Centers for Disease Control and Prevention, viral hemorrhagic fevers (VHFs) denote

> a group of illnesses that are caused by several distinct families of viruses. In general, the term "viral hemorrhagic fever [VHF]" is used to describe a severe multisystem syndrome.... Characteristically, the overall vascular system is damaged, and the body's ability to regulate itself is impaired. These symptoms are often accompanied by hemorrhage (bleeding); however, the bleeding is itself rarely life-threatening. While some types of hemorrhagic fever viruses can cause relatively mild illnesses, many of these viruses cause severe, life-threatening disease.[21]

Transmission of Lyme disease to humans is associated with infected black-legged ticks (*Ixodes scapularis*) that ingest blood by puncturing the skin of the host. (Refer to Figure 5-16.) In the Pacific coastal region of the United States, the western black-legged tick (*Ixodes pacificus*) has been identified as the vector. Also shown in the figure are the Lone Star tick and the dog tick, which are not known to be transmitters of the Lyme disease bacterium to human beings.

The geographic distribution for Lyme disease covers northeastern, mid-Atlantic, and upper central regions of the United States as well as several counties in northwestern California. (Refer to Figure 5-17.)

A total of 28,921 confirmed cases were reported to the CDC in 2008. From 1992 to 2006, the CDC received reports of 248,074 cases of Lyme disease. The vast majority (93%) were from 10 states (Connecticut, Delaware, Rhode Island, Maryland, Massachusetts, Minnesota, New Jersey, New York, Pennsylvania, and Wisconsin).[20] Those at risk of developing Lyme disease include people who work in or come into contact with tick-infested areas. For example, persons who engage in recreational activities that take them outdoors into infested areas or who clear brush or landscape their own backyards may

FIGURE 5-17 Number of reported cases of Lyme disease by county—United States, 2007.

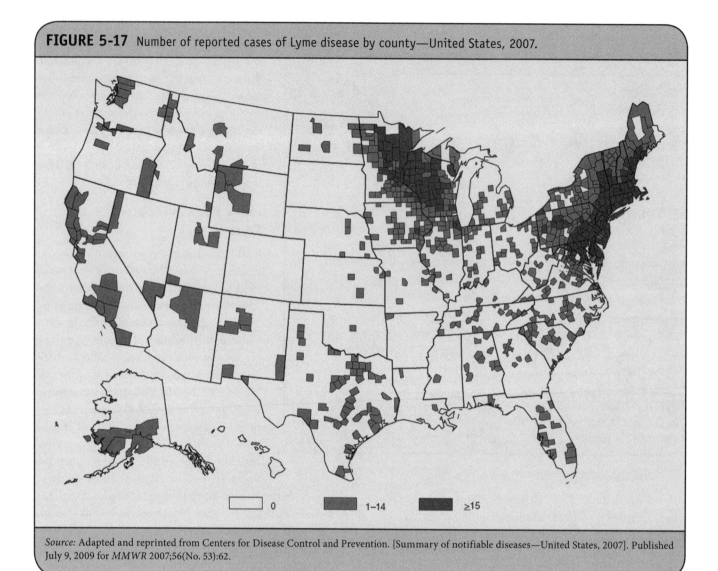

Source: Adapted and reprinted from Centers for Disease Control and Prevention. [Summary of notifiable diseases—United States, 2007]. Published July 9, 2009 for *MMWR* 2007;56(No. 53):62.

Of particular interest to the field of environmental health are the characteristics that VHFs share. The viruses that cause most VHFs are zoonoses, referring to the fact that they require an animal or insect host as a natural reservoir; the viruses reside and multiply in their hosts and are dependent upon their hosts for survival. The principal reservoirs for VHFs are rodents and arthropods. Examples of rodents that form the animal host reservoir for VHFs include certain species of rats such as the cotton rat, mice including the deer mouse and house mouse, and field rodents. Mosquitoes and ticks serve as the main arthropod vectors, whereas other forms of VHFs have unknown hosts.

The causative viruses for VHFs can be found throughout much of the world. Nevertheless, many of the viruses responsible for VHFs tend to be localized to those geographic areas in which the host species reside. Humans may become infected when they encounter an infected host (e.g., through contact with excreta from rodents) or are bitten by an arthropod. Sometimes, person to person transmission of the viruses can occur; examples of viruses in this category are Ebola and Marburg viruses. In most instances, there are no known cures for viral hemorrhagic fevers with the exception of supportive therapy. Viruses that cause VHFs and are spread by arthropods are also classified as arboviruses (discussed in the next section).

Examples of VHFs discussed in this chapter are:

- Hantavirus pulmonary syndrome (see emerging zoonoses)
- Dengue hemorrhagic fever (covered in the section on emerging and re-emerging infections)

ARTHROPOD-BORNE VIRAL DISEASES (ARBOVIRAL DISEASES)

The term **arboviral disease** (abbreviated from arthropod-borne viral disease) denotes viral diseases that can be acquired when blood-feeding arthropod vectors infect a human host. Typically, the complex cycle of transmission involves a non-human vertebrate (reservoir host) and an arthropod vector. The arthropod vectors that transmit arboviruses include ticks, sand flies, biting midges, and mosquitoes; however, most arboviruses are spread by mosquitoes. A total of more than 100 viruses are known at present as arboviruses that produce disease in humans. For some arboviral diseases (e.g., West Nile virus and Japanese encephalitis virus), humans are not usually an important component of the cycle of infection; other arboviruses (e.g., dengue fever virus and yellow fever virus) involve humans in virus amplification and infection of vectors.[19] The four main clinical symptoms or illnesses caused by arboviruses are:

1. Acute central nervous system (CNS) illness ranging in severity from mild aseptic meningitis to encephalitis or flaccid paralysis
2. Acute self-limited fevers, with and without exanthum [rash], and often accompanied by headache; some may give rise to more serious illness with CNS involvement or hemorrhages
3. Hemorrhagic fevers, often associated with capillary leakage, shock and high case-fatality rates (these may be accompanied by liver damage with jaundice, particularly in cases of yellow fever)
4. Polyarthritis and rash, with or without fever and of variable duration, self-limited or with arthralgic sequelae lasting several weeks to years.[19(p34)]

Examples of diseases caused by arboviruses are arboviral encephalitides (e.g., mosquito-borne and tick-borne viral encephalitis) and West Nile virus.

Arboviral Encephalitides

This group of viral illnesses (encephalitis) is associated with acute inflammation of sections of the brain, spinal cord, and meninges. Generally of short duration, the majority of infections are asymptomatic. Other cases present as a mild illness with fever, headache, or aseptic meningitis. Severe illness also can occur, with headache, high fever, disorientation, coma, and, occasionally, convulsions and paralysis, and death.[19]

Among the etiologic agents (four main viruses in the United States) are the viruses associated with St. Louis encephalitis (SLE), western equine encephalitis (WEE), Venezuelan equine encephalitis (VEE), eastern equine encephalitis (EEE), Lacrosse virus, and other California serogroup viruses.[22] EEE is found in the eastern and north-central United States, nearby Canada, parts of Central and South America, and the Caribbean islands. WEE occurs primarily in the western and central United States. The condition also occurs in Canada and parts of South America. An additional form known as Japanese encephalitis (JE) affects the western Pacific islands ranging from the Philippines to Japan, parts of eastern Asia including Korea and China, as well as India.[19]

Most arboviral encephalitides are transmitted by the bite of an arthropod vector (primarily mosquitoes), but other vectors include midges or sandflies.[19] The reservoir hosts for some forms of encephalitis viruses consist of nonhuman vertebrate hosts (e.g., wild birds and small animals). According to the Centers for Disease Control and Prevention, the cost of arboviral encephalitides is approximately $150 million per year, including vector control and surveillance activities. In the United States, the incidence of these forms of encephalitis varies from 150 to 3,000 cases per year.[22] Figure 5-18 shows the components in the transmission and maintenance of arboviral encephalitis.

Tick-borne viral encephalitides refer to a group of viral encephalitides transmitted by ticks.[19] These forms of encephalitides, also caused by arboviruses, produce diseases that bear a similarity to mosquito-borne encephalitides; the geographic range for tick-borne encephalitides includes parts of the former Soviet Union, Eastern and Central Europe, Scandinavia, and the United Kingdom. They are found also in eastern Canada and the United States. The reservoir for this group of encephalitides consists of ticks, or ticks in combination with some mammalian species, rodents, and birds.

Other Mosquito-Borne Viral Fevers—West Nile Virus (WNV)

The West Nile virus (WNV), an example of an arboviral disease, is classified as a type of mosquito-borne viral fever; the etiologic agent is a *Flavivirus*.[19] WNV has gained much notoriety in the United States because of its ability to spread rapidly across wide geographic regions. In addition, WNV caused the deaths of many wild birds and some humans. During summer 2004, WNV spread to the US state of California, having been associated previously with outbreaks in New York and other areas of the eastern United States. People most at risk of contracting WNV are those who spend a great deal of time outdoors, where they could be bitten by infected mosquitoes.

FIGURE 5-18 Arbovirus transmission cycle.

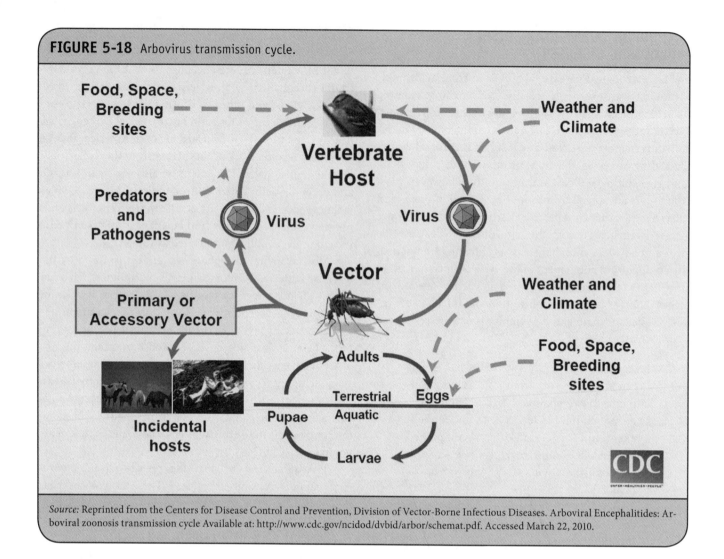

Source: Reprinted from the Centers for Disease Control and Prevention, Division of Vector-Borne Infectious Diseases. Arboviral Encephalitides: Arboviral zoonosis transmission cycle Available at: http://www.cdc.gov/ncidod/dvbid/arbor/schemat.pdf. Accessed March 22, 2010.

Older people (age 50+) are more likely than younger people to develop serious symptoms from WNV infection. Refer to the text box for more information.

Figure 5-19 shows the distribution of West Nile virus infection in the United States during 2009. The three states with the greatest number of human cases were Texas, California, and Colorado.

EMERGING ZOONOSES

The term **emerging zoonoses** refers to zoonotic diseases that are caused by either apparently new agents or by known agents that occur in locales or species that previously did not appear to be affected by these known agents.[23] (See Figure 5-20 for the geographic locations where emerging and reemerging infections have been identified; note that the figure shows both zoonotic and nonzoonotic conditions.) Among the most com-

monly identified factors associated with the rise of emerging zoonoses are ecological changes that result from agricultural practices (e.g., deforestation, conversion of grasslands, and irrigation).[23] Other factors include changes in the human population and human behavior (e.g., wars, migration, and urbanization). Table 5-3 presents examples of emerging zoonoses and lists conditions that may be linked to their occurrence. In the following sections, some of these emerging zoonoses will be covered in more detail.

Hantaviruses and Hantavirus Pulmonary Syndrome (HPS)

The hantavirus pulmonary syndrome (HPS) represents a highly fatal condition that is transmitted by rodent vectors.[24] The causative agent is the hantavirus, part of the viral family known as Bunyaviridae.[25] HPS may be transmitted when

West Nile Virus: What You Need to Know

What Is West Nile Virus?

West Nile virus (WNV) is a potentially serious illness. Experts believe WNV is established as a seasonal epidemic in North America that flares up in the summer and continues into the fall. . . .

What Can I Do to Prevent WNV?

The easiest and best way to avoid WNV is to prevent mosquito bites.

- When you are outdoors, use insect repellent containing an EPA-registered active ingredient. Follow the directions on the package.
- Many mosquitoes are most active at dusk and dawn. Be sure to use insect repellent and wear long sleeves and pants at these times or consider staying indoors during these hours.
- Make sure you have good screens on your windows and doors to keep mosquitoes out.
- Get rid of mosquito breeding sites by emptying standing water from flower pots, buckets and barrels. Change the water in pet dishes and replace the water in bird baths weekly. Drill holes in tire swings so water drains out. Keep children's wading pools empty and on their sides when they aren't being used.

What Are the Symptoms of WNV?

- **Serious Symptoms in a Few People.** About one in 150 people infected with WNV will develop severe illness. The severe symptoms can include high fever, headache, neck stiffness, stupor, disorientation, coma, tremors, convulsions, muscle weakness, vision loss, numbness and paralysis. These symptoms may last several weeks, and neurological effects may be permanent.
- **Milder Symptoms in Some People.** Up to 20 percent of the people who become infected have symptoms such as fever, headache, and body aches, nausea, vomiting, and sometimes swollen lymph glands or a skin rash on the chest, stomach and back. Symptoms can last for as short as a few days, though even healthy people have become sick for several weeks.
- **No Symptoms in Most People.** Approximately 80 percent of people (about 4 out of 5) who are infected with WNV will not show any symptoms at all.

How Does West Nile Virus Spread?

- **Infected Mosquitoes.** Most often, WNV is spread by the bite of an infected mosquito. Mosquitoes become infected when they feed on infected birds. Infected mosquitoes can then spread WNV to humans and other animals when they bite.
- **Transfusions, Transplants, and Mother-to-Child.** In a very small number of cases, WNV also has been spread through blood transfusions, organ transplants, breastfeeding and even during pregnancy from mother to baby.
- **Not through touching.** WNV is not spread through casual contact such as touching or kissing a person with the virus.

How Soon Do Infected People Get Sick?

People typically develop symptoms between 3 and 14 days after they are bitten by the infected mosquito.

How Is WNV Infection Treated?

There is no specific treatment for WNV infection. In cases with milder symptoms, people experience symptoms such as fever and aches that pass on their own, although even healthy people have become sick for several weeks. In more severe cases, people usually need to go to the hospital where they can receive supportive treatment including intravenous fluids, help with breathing and nursing care.

Source: Reprinted from the Centers for Disease Control and Prevention. West Nile Virus: What You Need to Know. CDC Fact Sheet. Available at: http://www.cdc.gov/ncidod/dvbid/westnile/wnv_factsheet.htm. Accessed March 3, 2010.

FIGURE 5-19 2009 West Nile virus activity in the United States (Reported to the CDC as of December 8, 2009). Map shows the distribution of avian, animal, or mosquito infection occurring during 2009 with number of human cases, if any, by state.

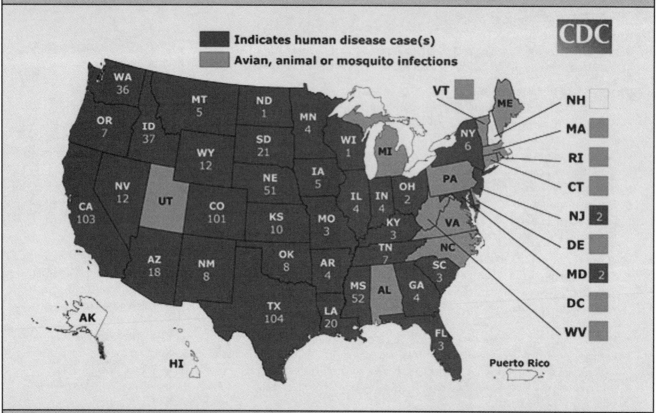

Source: Adapted and reprinted from the Centers for Disease Control and Prevention, Division of Vector-Borne Infectious Diseases. West Nile Virus: Statistics, Surveillance, and Control. Available at: http://www.cdc.gov/ncidod/dvbid/westnile/mapsactivity/surv&control09Maps.htm. Accessed March 22, 2010.

aerosolized (airborne) urine and droppings from infected rodents are inhaled. For example, vacationers who return to a mountain cabin after an extended absence may cause rodent droppings to be aerosolized when they sweep up in order to make the cabin habitable. Or they may stir up virus particles when they walk across a floor contaminated with urine from rodents. The primary known vectors for transmission of the hantavirus are four species of rodents: the cotton rat, the rice rat, the white-footed mouse, and the deer mouse (shown in Figure 5-21). One of the most widely distributed vectors and the main host for the hantavirus is the deceptively cute deer mouse—*Peromyscus maniculatus*—which is found throughout North America. (Refer to Figure 5-22.)

Hantaviruses have existed for many years, yet they gained public attention in 1993 when a mysterious case (a so-called

first outbreak) occurred. The CDC reports that "[i]n May 1993, an outbreak of an unexplained pulmonary illness occurred in the southwestern United States, in an area shared by Arizona, New Mexico, Colorado and Utah known as 'The Four Corners.' A young, physically fit Navajo man suffering from shortness of breath was rushed to a hospital in New Mexico and died very rapidly."[26] This case created an environmental health mystery in which an unknown causative agent also was believed to have caused the death of the man's fiancée and an additional five people. Epidemiologic investigations ruled out a new type of influenza or pesticide exposure. Eventually the deaths were linked to a heretofore unknown form of hantavirus, which was traced to the deer mouse via extensive rodent-trapping programs. To avoid a panic situation, the trappers did not wear protective devices. However, in the laboratory,

FIGURE 5-20 Range and recognized site(s) of origin of a variety of emerging and re-emerging infections. v-CJD = variant Creutzfeldt-Jakob disease; E. coli = *Escherichia coli*.

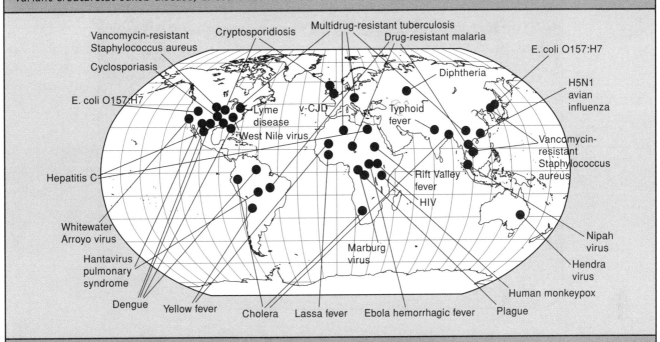

Source: Adapted and reprinted from AS Fauci. Infectious diseases: considerations for the 21st century. *Clinical Infectious Diseases.* 2001;32:677, with permission from the University of Chicago Press, © 2001 by the Infectious Diseases Society of America.

TABLE 5-3 Examples of Emerging Zoonoses and Factors Contributing to Emergence

Infection or Agent	Factor(s) Contributing to Emergence
Non-conventional agent	
Bovine spongiform encephalopathy [BSE—mad cow disease][a]	Changes in rendering process
Viral	
Argentinian, Bolivian hemorrhagic fever	Changes in agriculture favoring rodent host
Dengue, dengue hemorrhagic fever	Transportation, travel and migration; urbanization
Ebola	Unknown, nosocomial
Hantaviruses	Ecological/environmental changes, increasing rodent contacts
Lassa fever	Urbanization favoring rodent host, increasing exposure
Rift Valley fever	Dam building, agriculture, irrigation; possible change in virulence or pathogenicity
Bacterial	
Heliobacter pylori (gastric ulcers)	Probably has been long widespread, now recognized
Escherichia coli O157:H7 (hemolytic-uremic syndrome)	Mass food processing technology allowing contamination of meat
Borrelia burgdorferi (Lyme disease)	Reforestation around homes, suburbanization, and other conditions favoring tick vector and deer population
Parasitic	
Cryptosporidium and other pathogens	Contaminated surface water, faulty water purification

[a] Discussed in Chapter 11.

Source: Adapted and reprinted from BB Chomel. New emerging zoonoses: a challenge and an opportunity for the veterinary profession. *Comparative Immunology, Microbiology & Infectious Diseases.* 1998;21:4. Copyright 1998; used with permission from Elsevier.

FIGURE 5-21 This is a deer mouse, *Peromyscus maniculatus,* a hantavirus carrier that becomes a threat when it enters human habitation in rural and suburban areas.

Source: Reprinted from the CDC Public Health Image Library, ID# 1183. Photo credit: James Gathany. Available at: http://phil.cdc.gov/Phil/details.asp. Accessed March 18, 2010.

FIGURE 5-22 Distribution of the *Peromyscus maniculatus* and location of hantavirus pulmonary syndrome cases, January 27, 1997 (map).

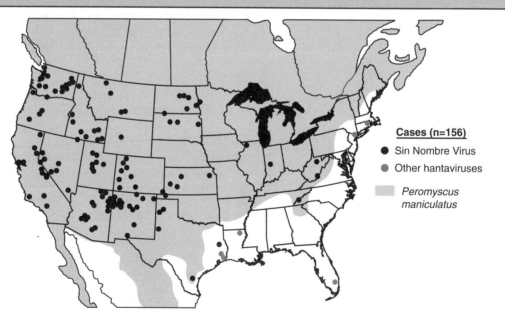

Cases (n=156)
● Sin Nombre Virus
● Other hantaviruses
Peromyscus maniculatus

(Rodent distributions from: Burt WH, Grossenheider RP. *A Field Guide to the Mammals.* 3rd ed. New York, NY: Houghton Mifflin Company; 1980.)

Source: Adapted and reprinted from the CDC Public Health Image Library, ID# 90. NCID Content Provider. Available at: http://phil.cdc.gov/phil/details.asp. Accessed March 18, 2010.

FIGURE 5-23 Three CDC health officials inspecting specimens suspected of being connected with a hantavirus outbreak.

Source: Reprinted courtesy of the CDC Public Health Image Library, ID# 7271. Available at: http://phil.cdc.gov/phil/details.asp. Accessed March 18, 2010.

researchers who dissected the trapped rodents wore special clothing, masks, and goggles as protection against biohazards (see Figure 5-23).

Further study suggested that rodents may have entered the households where the victims lived. During 1993, the deer mouse population increased to higher levels than normal. This population increase was attributed to heavy snows and rainfall in early 1993 that followed a lengthy drought in the Four Corners area. Because of the increased availability of food following the heavy precipitation, the mouse population increased by a factor of 10 between May 1992 and May 1993. Thus it was more likely that humans could contract hantavirus carried by the mice.

Although HPS is known to cause potentially deadly infections, fortunately the syndrome is rare. According to the CDC, "Through December 1, 2009, a total of 534 cases of hantavirus pulmonary syndrome have been reported in the United States. Of these, 503 cases occurred from 1993, onward, following identification of hantavirus pulmonary syndrome, whereas 31 cases were retrospectively identified."[27] The epidemiologic features of these 534 cases in 31 states were as follows: 63% male, 78% white, 18% American Indian, and mean age 37 years; the case fatality rate for the disease was 36%.[27] As of January 26, 2010, a total of 538 cases had been reported. (See Figure 5-24.) Among the states with the largest number of cases—more than 30 cases in each state—were New Mexico

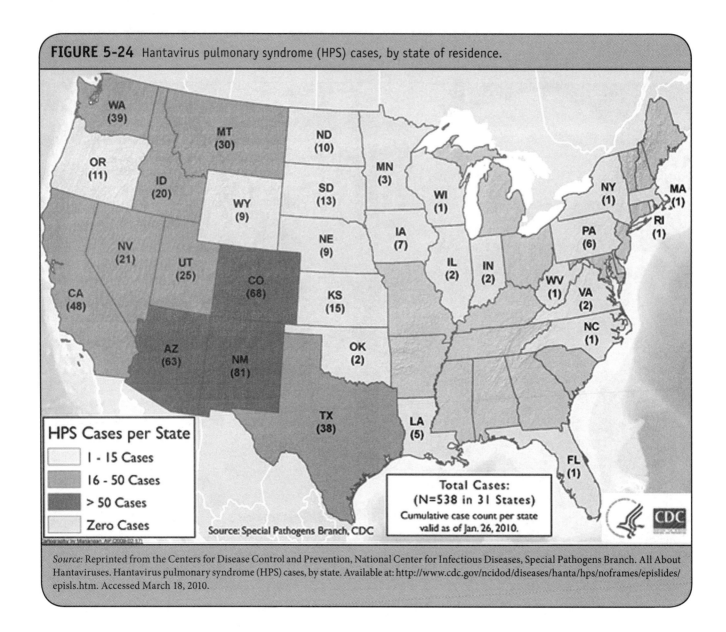

FIGURE 5-24 Hantavirus pulmonary syndrome (HPS) cases, by state of residence.

Source: Reprinted from the Centers for Disease Control and Prevention, National Center for Infectious Diseases, Special Pathogens Branch. All About Hantaviruses. Hantavirus pulmonary syndrome (HPS) cases, by state. Available at: http://www.cdc.gov/ncidod/diseases/hanta/hps/noframes/epislides/episls.htm. Accessed March 18, 2010.

(81), Colorado (68), Arizona (63), California (48), Washington (39), and Texas (38).

Dengue Fever (DF), Dengue Hemorrhagic Fever (DHF), and Dengue Shock Syndrome (DSS)

Four dengue viruses (flavivirus serotypes) cause dengue infection, which produces a spectrum of illness that ranges from mild to severe. The mildest form of dengue causes a low-level illness with a nonspecific fever. Classic dengue fever (DF) is also a rather benign, self-limited disease; symptoms may include high fever, severe headache, eye pain, muscle pain, joint pain, rash, and mild bleeding. Dengue hemorrhagic fever (DHF) results in a life-threatening illness with fever (that lasts 2–7 days), abdominal pain, and bleeding phenomena. Dengue shock syndrome (DSS) includes the symptoms of DHF and is associated with shock (e.g., hypotension and rapid, weak pulse). When shock is not treated promptly, the proportion of deaths among victims of DSS can be as high as 40% to 50%.[28,19]

As shown in Figure 5-25, the primary locations for dengue fever are the tropical and subtropical areas of the world, for example, Southeast Asia, tropical Africa, and South America. The virus is thought to have existed among monkeys, and

FIGURE 5-25 World distribution of dengue—2008.

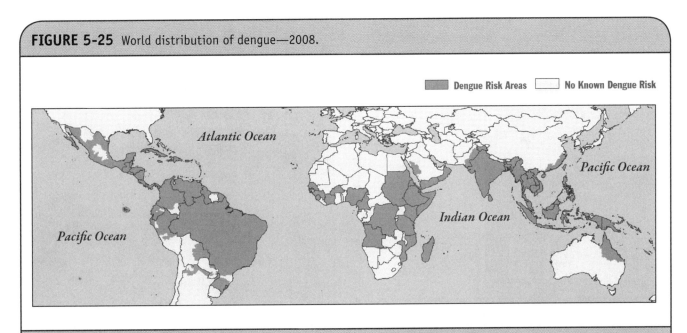

Dengue Risk Areas   No Known Dengue Risk

Source: Reprinted from the Centers for Disease Control and Prevention. Dengue and dengue hemorrhagic fever, p. 4. Available at: http://www.cdc.gov/dengue/resources/Dengue&DHF%20Information%20for%20Health%20Care%20Practitioners_2009.pdf. Accessed March 21, 2010.

several centuries ago moved to humans in Africa and Asia. Dengue was uncommon until after the mid-20th century, with outbreaks occurring in the Philippines and Thailand in the 1950s and later in the Caribbean and Latin America.

The vector for transmission of the disease is a type of domestic day-biting mosquito known as the *Aedes aegypti*, a mosquito that prefers to feed on human hosts. (Refer to Figure 5-26.) The spread of the vector was linked to transport ships during World War II. At present, dengue is among the most significant mosquito-borne viral diseases that afflict humans. Each year, an estimated 50–100 million cases of dengue fever occur.[28]

In the United States, most reported cases of dengue usually are imported by travelers who are returning from endemic areas or by immigrants. Although very uncommon, cases of dengue fever that originated in the continental United States have been documented. Southern Texas and the southeastern United States are at theoretical risk for transmission of dengue and for sporadic outbreaks.

Public health authorities have attributed the dramatic global emergence of dengue fever to lack of effective mosquito control in endemic areas, rapid population growth and urbanization, and poor or nonexistent systems for the treatment of water and human wastes. International travel is also thought to have contributed to increases in dengue fever by transmit-

FIGURE 5-26 A female *Aedes aegypti* mosquito, which is the primary vector for the spread of dengue fever.

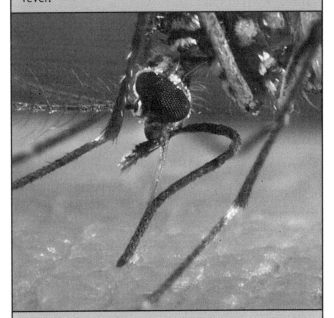

Source: Reprinted courtesy of the CDC Public Health Image Library. ID# 7633. James Gathany Content Provider. Available at: http://phil.cdc.gov/phil/details.asp. Accessed March 21, 2010.

FIGURE 5-27 Transmission Electron Micrograph of the Ebola Virus.

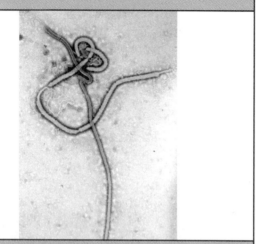

Source: Reprinted courtesy of the CDC Public Health Image Library. ID# 1833. Dr. Frederick A. Murphy Content Provider. Available at: http://phil.cdc.gov/phil/details.asp. Accessed March 21, 2010.

FIGURE 5-28 Electron micrograph of the Rift Valley Fever virus.

Source: Reprinted courtesy of the CDC Public Health Image Library. ID# 1870. Dr. Fred Murphy Content Provider. Available at: http://phil.cdc.gov/phil/details.asp. Accessed March 15, 2010.

ting the viruses from endemic to nonendemic areas. Mosquito eradication programs that involved the use of DDT have been discontinued, causing the resurgence of *Aedes aegypti*. For example, between 1930 and 1970, the range of *Aedes aegypti* declined greatly in much of Central and South America; then, by 1998, the mosquito had reinvaded previous habitats.

Ebola Virus Hemorrhagic Fever (HF)

This condition refers to a dramatic, highly fatal, and acute disease associated with infection with Ebola virus (shown in Figure 5-27). Ebola HF is one of a group of viral diseases known as Ebola-Marburg viral diseases.[19] Symptoms of infection with the virus can include sudden onset of fever, headache, diarrhea, and vomiting and may also involve external and internal bleeding. Ebola disease was first recognized in 1976 in the Sudan and in Zaire (now called the Democratic Republic of Congo—DRC). In 1995, Kikwit, DRC, experienced an outbreak of 315 cases that caused 244 deaths. Outbreaks associated with a subtype of Ebola virus have occurred among monkeys housed in quarantine facilities in the United States.

Rift Valley Fever (RVF)

The causative agent for Rift Valley fever (RVF) is a virus from the genus *Phlebovirus* in the family of Bunyaviridae.[29] Figure 5-28 presents an electron micrograph of the virus.

RVF can produce epizootic or widespread disease among domestic animals including cattle, buffalo, sheep, goats, and camels. Mosquitoes transmit the disease to domestic animals that can then spread the disease to one another. The disease is transmissible to humans and can produce epidemics among human populations. Infected mosquitoes are able to transmit RVF to humans, who also may contract the disease if they encounter the blood or body fluids of infected animals through slaughtering or handling infected meat. In humans, infection with RVF most typically produces either no obvious symptoms or mild illness characterized by fever and liver abnormality. Some patients may develop a more severe form in which they experience a hemorrhagic fever, encephalitis, or ocular diseases. An outbreak of Rift Valley fever in Kenya in 1950 through 1951 caused the death of approximately 100,000 sheep.

FIGURE 5-29 Rift Valley fever distribution map.

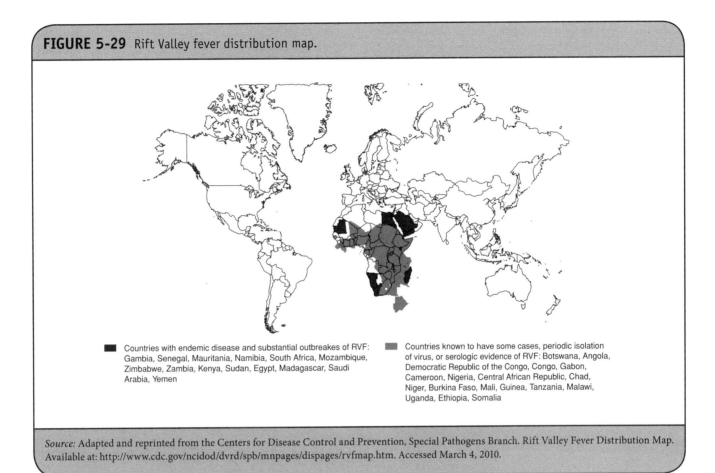

Countries with endemic disease and substantial outbreakes of RVF: Gambia, Senegal, Mauritania, Namibia, South Africa, Mozambique, Zimbabwe, Zambia, Kenya, Sudan, Egypt, Madagascar, Saudi Arabia, Yemen

Countries known to have some cases, periodic isolation of virus, or serologic evidence of RVF: Botswana, Angola, Democratic Republic of the Congo, Congo, Gabon, Cameroon, Nigeria, Central African Republic, Chad, Niger, Burkina Faso, Mali, Guinea, Tanzania, Malawi, Uganda, Ethiopia, Somalia

Source: Adapted and reprinted from the Centers for Disease Control and Prevention, Special Pathogens Branch. Rift Valley Fever Distribution Map. Available at: http://www.cdc.gov/ncidod/dvrd/spb/mnpages/dispages/rvfmap.htm. Accessed March 4, 2010.

The endemic areas for RVF include southern Africa, most countries of sub-Saharan Africa, and Madagascar. (Refer to Figure 5-29.)

Increases in Rift Valley fever follow periods of heavy rainfall when large numbers of mosquitoes develop. In West Africa in 1987, an outbreak of Rift Valley fever was linked to construction of the Senegal River project. This project modified the usual interactions between animals and humans when flooding occurred in the lower Senegal River area.

OTHER ZOONOTIC DISEASES

Monkeypox

According to the CDC, "Monkeypox is a rare viral disease that occurs mostly in central and western Africa. It is called 'monkeypox' because it was first found in 1958 in laboratory monkeys. . . . The disease is caused by *Monkeypox virus*. It belongs to a group of viruses that includes the smallpox virus (variola), the virus used in the smallpox vaccine (vaccinia), and the cowpox virus. . . . In humans, the signs and symptoms

of monkeypox are like those of smallpox, but usually they are milder. Another difference is that monkeypox causes the lymph nodes to swell."[30] Refer to the text box for a description of an outbreak that occurred in the midwestern United States during 2003.

Tularemia

Also known as rabbit fever, tularemia is a bacterial disease associated with *Francisella tularensis*. The disease is broadly distributed in the United States, and occurs in all states except Hawaii. It is a disease found in rural areas and is linked with wild animals such as rodents, rabbits, and hares. The bacterium may be transmitted in several ways, including the bite of an arthropod (e.g., tick or deer fly), coming into contact with infected animal carcasses, consuming food or water that has been contaminated with the bacterium, or even breathing in the bacterium.[31] The condition presents with a range of possible symptoms that are related to how the organism enters the body. Often, symptoms include skin ulcers, swollen lymph glands, painful eyes, and sore throat. Inhalation of the bacterium may cause sudden fever, chills, headaches, muscle aches, joint pain, dry cough, and progressive weakness; in some cases, pneumonia may occur.[19] Tularemia, which is treatable with antibiotics, may be a severe or fatal condition when untreated.

Rabies (Hydrophobia)

Rabies is an acute and highly fatal disease of the central nervous system caused by a virus transmitted most often through saliva from the bites of infected animals; globally, dog bites are the principal source of transmission of rabies to humans.[19] A disease that affects mammals, it causes encephalopathy and paralysis of the respiratory system. In the early stages of the disease, symptoms of rabies are nonspecific, consisting of apprehension, fever, headache, and malaise. The disease then progresses to paralysis, hallucinations, swallowing difficulties, and fear of water (called hydrophobia). After a period of days, death ensues. Only a few cases of survival from rabies have been documented worldwide.

In the United States, human cases of rabies are rare. A case of abortive human rabies occurred in Texas beginning in early 2009. The case was termed "abortive" because that patient recovered without ever having received intensive care. The patient was a 17-year-old female who was seen in a hospital emergency room for symptoms that included severe headache, photophobia (sensitivity to light), neck pain, and fever. The patient was discharged after three days, when the symptoms resolved. Subsequently, after the headaches returned, she was rehospitalized and treated for suspected infectious encephalitis. During subsequent examinations, the patient revealed that while on a camping trip she had been bitten by flying bats. After serological tests were found to be positive for rabies, the patient was administered rabies immune globulin and rabies vaccine. Following these steps, the young woman was given supportive care until the symptoms resolved and she was discharged. Refer to Figure 5-30 for a time line of the patient's illness.

The hosts for rabies are wild animals—carnivores and bats. The CDC estimates that more than 90% of rabies cases occur in wild animals (e.g., skunks, raccoons, foxes, and coyotes) and the remainder in domestic animals. The locations of wild animal rabies reservoirs in the United States

---

FIGURE 5-30 Timeline of course for a patient with presumptive abortive human rabies—Texas, 2009.

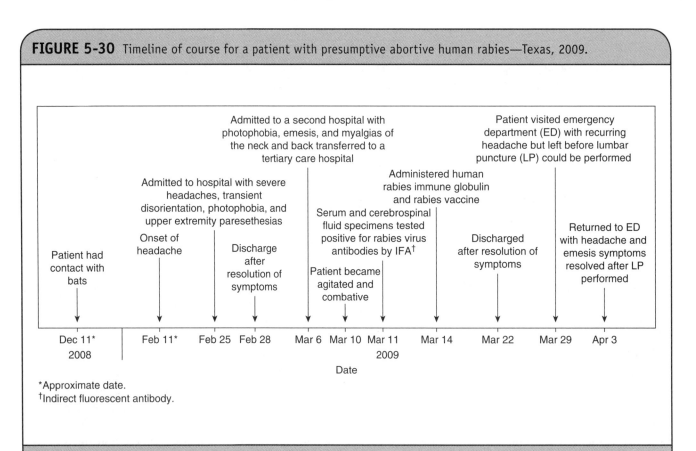

Source: Reprinted from the Centers for Disease Control and Prevention. Presumptive abortive human rabies—Texas, 2009. *MMWR* 2010;59:187.

Multistate Outbreak of Monkeypox—Illinois, Indiana, and Wisconsin, 2003

The CDC has received reports of patients with a febrile rash illness who had close contact with pet prairie dogs and other animals. . . . A total of 51 patients reported direct or close contact with prairie dogs (*Cynomys* sp.), and one patient reported contact with a Gambian giant rat (*Cricetomys* sp.). One patient had contact with a rabbit (Family *Leporidae*) that became ill after exposure to an ill prairie dog at a veterinary clinic. Traceback investigations have been initiated to identify the source of monkeypox virus introduced into the United States and have identified a common distributor where prairie dogs and Gambian giant rats were housed together in Illinois. A search of imported animal records revealed that Gambian giant rats were shipped from Ghana in April to a wildlife importer in Texas and subsequently were sold to the Illinois distributor. The shipment contained approximately 800 small mammals of nine different species that might have been the actual source of introduction of monkeypox.[pp537–538]

BIOHAZARD

Source: Centers for Disease Control and Prevention. Multistate outbreak of monkeypox—Illinois, Indiana, and Wisconsin, 2003. *MMWR.* 2003;52:537–540.

FIGURE 5-31 Map of terrestrial rabies in the United States during 2008.

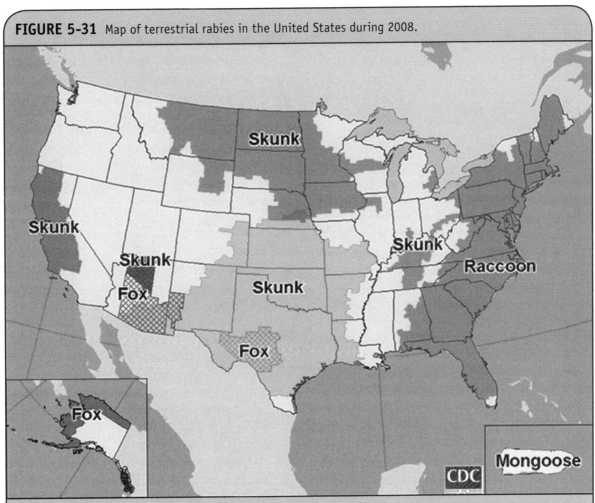

Source: Reprinted from the Centers for Disease Control and Prevention. Rabies: Epidemiology. Available at: http://www.cdc.gov/rabies/images/2008_surveillance_maps/2008_geographic_boundaries_reservoirs-lg.gif. Accessed March 21 2010.

are shown in Figure 5-31. Figure 5-32 presents the number of reported cases of rabies that occurred among wild and domestic animals during 1997 to 2007 (in the United States and Puerto Rico). The two most commonly affected species were raccoons and bats. Before 1960, the majority of US rabies cases occurred among domestic animals—dogs, cats, and cattle—although now most cases occur in the wild. In the United States, vaccination programs for domestic animals, measures to control animals, and public health laboratories for conducting rabies tests have changed the prevalence of rabies.

Environmental health programs have prevented human cases of rabies very successfully through postexposure prophylaxis (PEP). In the United States, one reason that fatal human rabies cases have declined from about 100 annually in the early 1900s to about 1 to 2 cases annually at the end of the 20th century has been the introduction of PEP, which is nearly 100% successful; the remaining fatal cases usually can be attributed to failure to seek medical attention. PEP consists of a series of vaccinations that should be given as soon as possible after the occurrence of an animal bite from a suspected rabid animal. Outside the United States, rabid dogs—which

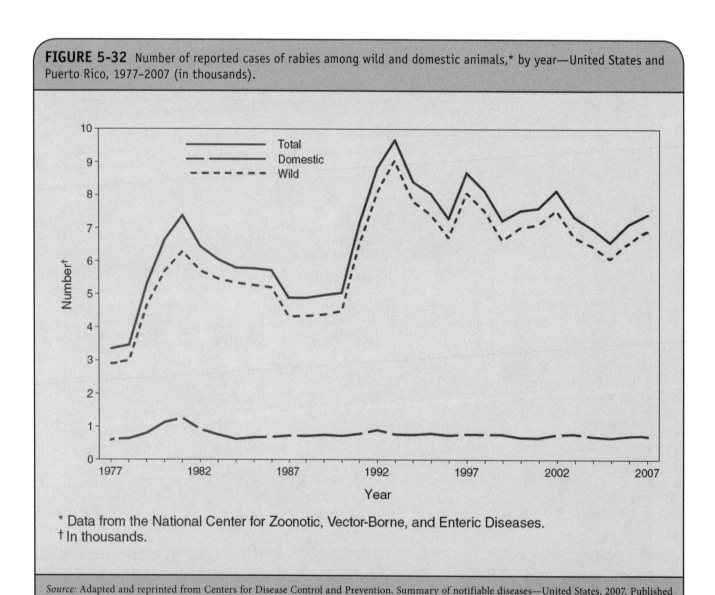

FIGURE 5-32 Number of reported cases of rabies among wild and domestic animals,* by year—United States and Puerto Rico, 1977–2007 (in thousands).

* Data from the National Center for Zoonotic, Vector-Borne, and Enteric Diseases.
† In thousands.

Source: Adapted and reprinted from Centers for Disease Control and Prevention. Summary of notifiable diseases—United States, 2007. Published July 9, 2009 for *MMWR* 2007;56(No. 53):66.

FIGURE 5-33 Spores from the Sterne strain of Bacillus anthracis bacteria.

Acc.V Spot Magn   Det WD   Exp |———————————| 5 µm
20.0 kV 3.0 12483x   SE   25.2 0

Source: Reprinted courtesy of the CDC Public Health Image Library. ID# 10122. Laura Rose Content Provider. Available at: http://phil.cdc.gov/phil/details.asp. Accessed March 20, 2010

The causative agent for anthrax, an acute infectious disease, is *Bacillus anthracis*, a spore-forming bacterium. (Refer to Figure 5-33.) Anthrax is a disease that most commonly occurs among cattle, sheep, goats, and other herbivores.[35] Those normally at risk of anthrax are veterinarians, agricultural workers who come into contact with cattle, and those who are involved with the processing of animal products: hides, wool, and hair.[19] The general population is unlikely to become infected (with the exception of those who work on ranches or farms where livestock are present).

The three forms of anthrax are cutaneous, inhalational, and gastrointestinal. In humans, the cutaneous form is characterized by itching, skin lesions, development of a black eschar, and possible spread to lymph nodes. Although the case fatality rate for untreated cutaneous anthrax ranges from 5% to 20%, the disease can be treated effectively with antibiotics.[19]

The inhalational form of anthrax begins with nonspecific symptoms that mimic upper respiratory infections and then deepen into respiratory distress, fever, and shock. This form of anthrax is very severe and has a high case fatality rate.

The gastrointestinal form may be acquired from infected animals by eating contaminated meat that is undercooked. Gastrointestinal anthrax is the least common form of anthrax in the United States. Symptoms of gastrointestinal anthrax include nausea, anorexia, and abdominal pain; from 25% to 60% of cases are fatal. All three forms of anthrax are treatable with antibiotics that should be administered as soon as possible after suspected exposure. Anthrax infections can develop largely undetected until the patient becomes very ill and nearly dies. When the case is very advanced, treatment with antibiotics is not likely to be effective.

Before the use of anthrax as a terrorist weapon, environmental health experts were concerned mainly about

cause 99% of human rabies deaths—constitute the most common source of rabies exposure. For this reason, an important component of rabies prevention is the control and vaccination of stray dogs. Within the United States, people are most likely to be exposed to rabies from bats.[19]

Anthrax

Anthrax gained notoriety in 2001 when it was distributed intentionally via the US mail system. Approximately one week after the September 11 terrorist attacks on the World Trade Center in New York City and the Pentagon in Washington, DC, letters containing anthrax spores were mailed to NBC news anchor Tom Brokaw and to the editor of the *New York Post* in New York City, exposing employees to the spores. These exposures resulted in five confirmed cases of anthrax among media company employees or visitors. An isolated case was a 61-year-old hospital worker who subsequently died. Additional exposures also were reported in Washington, DC; Virginia; New Jersey; and Florida. Ultimately, there were a total of 22 confirmed cases of anthrax and 5 resulting deaths.[32–34] outbreaks of the disease among cattle and other herbivores and among people who have contact with these animals and their products. Subsequently, public health departments were spurred to action by the potential threat from a terrorist-incited anthrax epidemic. The anthrax bacterium has the capacity to spread across a wide area and cause many cases of illness and numerous deaths. A challenge to environmental health professionals will be the development of effective methods to recognize a terrorist attack, respond to it in an appropriate and timely manner, and bring the threat under control.

Psittacosis

Psittacosis, a disease associated with the bacterial agent *Chlamydia psittaci*, is conveyed by dried bird droppings (refer to the text box for a description).

Influenza: Animal to Human Transmission of Influenza A Viruses

Influenza A viruses associated with human influenza epidemics and pandemics are linked to animal reservoirs (especially birds and swine). An example of an influenza A pandemic was the "Spanish flu" pandemic of 1918 to 1920 (responsible for the deaths of more than 20 million people). Other influenza A pandemics were the outbreaks of the Asian flu in 1957 and the Hong Kong flu in 1968. Lesser outbreaks were the swine flu of 1976 and the chicken flu of 1997.

The three types of influenza viruses are A, B, and C, which have the following characteristics:

- Influenza A viruses—wild and aquatic birds are considered to be the main natural reservoir. In addition to humans, influenza A viruses can infect a variety of

Psittacosis

Clinical Features	In humans, fever, chills, headache, muscle aches, and a dry cough. Pneumonia is often evident on chest X-ray.
Etiologic Agent	*Chlamydia psittaci*, a bacterium
Incidence	Since 1996, fewer than 50 confirmed cases were reported in the United States each year. Many more cases may occur that are not correctly diagnosed or reported.
Sequelae	Endocarditis, hepatitis, and neurologic complications may occasionally occur. Severe pneumonia requiring intensive-care support may also occur. Fatal cases have been reported.
Transmission	Infection is acquired by inhaling dried secretions from infected birds. The incubation period is 5 to 19 days. Although all birds are susceptible, pet birds (parrots, parakeets, macaws, and cockatiels) and poultry (turkeys and ducks) are most frequently involved in transmission to humans.
Risk Groups	Bird owners, pet shop employees, and veterinarians. Outbreaks of psittacosis in poultry processing plants have been reported.
Surveillance	Psittacosis is a reportable condition in most states.
Trends	Annual incidence varies considerably because of periodic outbreaks. A decline in reported cases since 1988 may be the result of improved diagnostic tests that distinguish *C. psittaci* from more common *C. pneumoniae* infections.
Challenges	Diagnosis of psittacosis can be difficult. Antibiotic treatment may prevent an antibody response, thus limiting diagnosis by serologic methods. Infected birds are often asymptomatic. Tracebacks of infected birds to distributors and breeders often is not possible because of limited regulation of the pet bird industry.

Source: Reprinted from the Centers for Disease Control and Prevention. Psittacosis. Content source: National Center for Immunization and Respiratory Diseases: Division of Bacterial Diseases. Available at: http://www.cdc.gov/ncidod/dbmd/diseaseinfo/psittacosis_t.htm. Accessed March 18, 2010 animals such as ducks, chickens, pigs, whales, horses, and seals. "However, certain subtypes of influenza A virus are specific to certain species, except for birds, which are hosts to all known subtypes of influenza A. . . . Influenza A viruses normally seen in one species sometimes can cross over and cause illness in another species."[36] Examples are the transfer of influenza viruses from humans to pigs or from horses to dogs. Influenza A viruses can be transmitted indirectly from pigs (intermediate hosts) to humans or directly from birds to humans.

Direct infection of humans with avian influenza A is unusual. Human infections with avian influenza A viruses have been linked to direct contact with infected poultry. The spread of these influenza viruses may be promoted by the close proximity of live animals such as poultry and swine to residents of densely populated areas. In order to prevent epidemics, environmental health authorities need to maintain surveillance programs and conduct routine investigations of influenza outbreaks in animals and humans.

Influenza A viruses are categorized into subtypes according to the arrangement of two proteins on the surface of the virus. An example of a subtype is the 2009 H1N1 influenza virus (discussed in Chapter 1); another example is the H5N1 avian influenza A virus that occurred as early as 1997 in Hong Kong (Special Administrative Region).

- Influenza B viruses—confined to humans, who form the primary reservoir for these viruses.
- Influenza C viruses—a cause of mild illnesses and sporadic outbreaks among humans; they are not considered to be responsible for widespread epidemics.

CONTROL AND PREVENTION OF MOSQUITO-BORNE DISEASES

One method to control mosquito-borne diseases is to monitor for the presence of viruses in sentinel chickens and birds. Some health departments position small flocks of chickens and other birds in strategic locations where mosquitoes may be active. These birds are tested periodically for the presence of viral antibodies. Examples of sentinel birds are shown in Figure 5-34.

Mosquitoes are dependent upon water to lead and complete their life cycle. Accordingly, one method for mosquito control consists of removing standing sources of water in which mosquitoes can multiply. Vector control experts advise homeowners to remove standing water from around their households, for example, water standing in buckets,

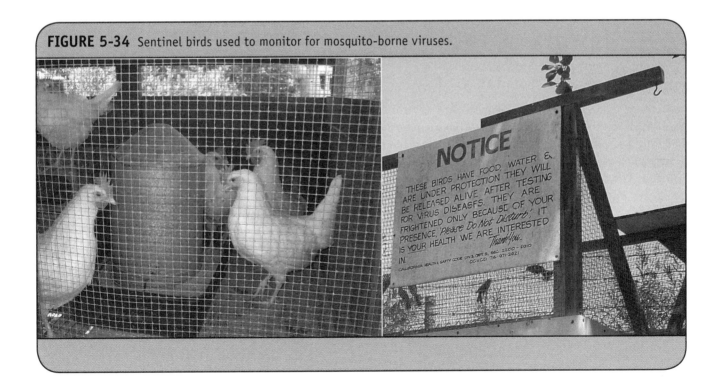

FIGURE 5-34 Sentinel birds used to monitor for mosquito-borne viruses.

FIGURE 5-35 Check for *Aedes* mosquito breeding in your home.

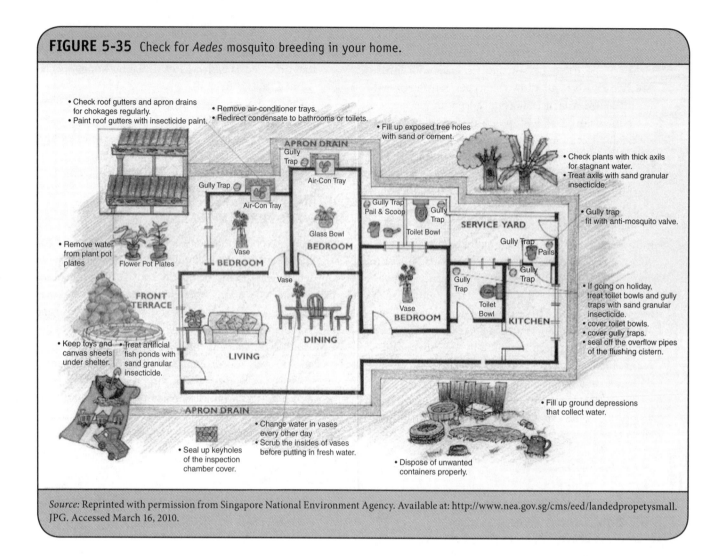

- Check roof gutters and apron drains for chokages regularly.
- Paint roof gutters with insecticide paint.
- Remove air-conditioner trays.
- Redirect condensate to bathrooms or toilets.
- Fill up exposed tree holes with sand or cement.
- Check plants with thick axils for stagnant water.
- Treat axils with sand granular insecticide.

APRON DRAIN
Gully Trap
Gully Trap
Air-Con Tray
Air-Con Tray

Gully Trap
Pail & Scoop
Gully Trap
Toilet Bowl

SERVICE YARD

- Gully trap fit with anti-mosquito valve.

Gully Trap   Pails

Glass Bowl
BEDROOM

Vase
BEDROOM

Gully Trap
Gully Trap

- Remove water from plant pot plates   Flower Pot Plates

Vase

Vase
BEDROOM

Toilet Bowl   KITCHEN

- If going on holiday, treat toilet bowls and gully traps with sand granular insecticide.
- cover toilet bowls.
- cover gully traps.
- seal off the overflow pipes of the flushing cistern.

FRONT TERRACE

DINING

LIVING

- Keep toys and canvas sheets under shelter.
- Treat artificial fish ponds with sand granular insecticide.

APRON DRAIN

- Fill up ground depressions that collect water.

- Change water in vases every other day
- Scrub the insides of vases before putting in fresh water.

- Seal up keyholes of the inspection chamber cover.

- Dispose of unwanted containers properly.

Source: Reprinted with permission from Singapore National Environment Agency. Available at: http://www.nea.gov.sg/cms/eed/landedpropetysmall. JPG. Accessed March 16, 2010.

old tires, or flowerpots. (Refer to Figure 5-35.) They also introduce mosquito-eating fish into small ponds and other bodies of standing water. Other preventive efforts include wearing long clothing to prevent being bitten by mosquitoes, using insect repellent, closing open windows, and repairing broken screens.

CONCLUSION

Zoonotic and vector-borne diseases represent a continuing and growing challenge. Among the recent conditions that have gained the attention of environmental health experts are the emerging and reemerging infections (e.g., dengue fever and hantavirus). In addition, scourges first observed and notorious during early historical times, such as plague, present hazards to modern society. Diseases brought under control during the mid-20th century (e.g., malaria) are showing resurgence. Several factors are responsible for the emergence of new diseases and the reemergence of formerly uncommon ones. Some of these factors are reduction in funding for environmental control programs, movement of human populations, increasing urbanization, and possible climatic changes. It is likely that zoonotic and vector-borne diseases will continue to challenge experts in the field of environmental health.

Study Questions and Exercises

1. Define the following terms:
   a. Emerging infectious disease
   b. Reemerging infectious disease
   c. Emerging zoonosis
   d. Zoonotic disease
   e. Vector
   f. Vector-borne infection

2. State three factors that have contributed to the development of emerging infectious diseases. Give one example of an emerging disease and another example of a reemerging disease.

3. Give an example of some major zoonotic diseases. Explain how zoonotic diseases can be transmitted.

4. Describe how vectors play a role in the transmission of disease.

5. List three characteristics of viral hemorrhagic fevers.

6. Discuss the impact of malaria on environmental health. Give an example of the economic impact this disease has on the developing world.

7. Summarize briefly the life cycle of malaria, describing the human and insect phases of the disease.

8. In what respects is leishmaniasis a vector-borne disease? Name some of the countries in the world where leishmaniasis is endemic and state why the disease is of particular concern to US military personnel.

9. Discuss the vector and agent factors involved in the transmission and causation of plague. Distinguish between bubonic and pneumonic plague. Describe procedures for control and prevention of plague.

10. What factors are involved in the chain of causation of Lyme disease? From the environmental health perspective, describe how the condition can be controlled and prevented.

11. What are arboviral encephalitides? Describe the reservoirs and modes of transmission of this group of diseases to humans.

12. What are the primary symptoms of West Nile virus (WNV)? List some of the ways that individuals can avoid being infected with WNV. Describe methods that environmental health officials might use to control the condition.

13. For the conditions listed below, provide the following information: (a) causative agent; (b) symptoms; (c) geographic distribution; (d) host factors; (e) responsible vectors, if any; (f) potential hazards to the human population; and (g) methods of control.
    - Dengue fever and dengue hemorrhagic fever
    - Rift Valley fever
    - Rabies
    - Anthrax

REFERENCES

1. Nicastri E, Girardi E, Ippolito G. Determinants of emerging and re-emerging infectious diseases. *J Biol Regul Homeost Agents.* 2001;15:212–217.

2. Porta M, ed. *A Dictionary of Epidemiology.* 5th ed. New York: Oxford University Press; 2008.

3. Sellman J, Bender J. Zoonotic infections in travelers to the tropics. *Prim Care Clin Office Pract.* 2002;29:907–929.

4. Centers for Disease Control and Prevention. Malaria: frequently asked questions about malaria. Available at: http://www.cdc.gov/malaria/faq.htm. Accessed February 28, 2010.

5. Hyperdictionary. Meaning of nephrosis. Available at: http://www.hyperdictionary.com/search.aspx?define=nephrosis. Accessed February 28, 2010.

6. Centers for Disease Control and Prevention. Impact of malaria. Available at: http://www.cdc.gov/malaria/malaria_worldwide/impact.html. Accessed February 28, 2010.

7. World Health Organization. Fact Sheet: Malaria. Available at: http://www.who.int/mediacentre/factsheets/fs094/en/index.html. Accessed February 28, 2010.

8. *The American Heritage Dictionary of the English Language.* 4th ed. Boston, MA: Houghton Mifflin Company; 2000.

9. The Wellcome Trust. The mosquito: Ronald Ross and the transmission of malaria. Available at: http://malaria.wellcome.ac.uk/print/WTD023869_print.html. Accessed February 28, 2010.

10. Centers for Disease Control and Prevention. Malaria: History. Eradication of malaria in the United States (1947–1951). Available at: http://www.cdc.gov/malaria/history/eradication_us.htm. Accessed February 28, 2010.

11. Centers for Disease Control and Prevention. Malaria: History. Eradication efforts worldwide: Success and failure (1955–1978) Available at: http://www.cdc.gov/malaria/history/index.htm. Accessed February 28, 2010.

12. Rosenberg T. What the world needs now is DDT. *New York Times*; April 11, 2004;sec.6:38.

13. Hay SI, Noor AM, Simba M, et al. Clinical epidemiology of malaria in the highlands of western Kenya. *Emerg Infect Dis.* 2002;8:543–548.

14. Seys SA, Bender JB. The changing epidemiology of malaria in Minnesota. *Emerg Infect Dis.* 2001;7:993–995.

15. Anis E, Leventhal A, Elkana Y, et al. Cutaneous leishmaniasis in Israel in the era of changing environment. *Public Health Rev.* 2001;29:37–47.

16. Wasserberg G, Abramsky Z, Anders G, et al. The ecology of cutaneous leishmaniasis in Nizzana, Israel: infection patterns in the reservoir host, and epidemiological implications. *Int J Parasitol.* 2002;32:133–143.

17. *The Oxford College Dictionary.* 2nd ed. New York: Spark Publishing, by arrangement with Oxford University Press, Inc.; 2007.

18. Centers for Disease Control and Prevention. Plague: CDC plague home page. Available at: http://www.cdc.gov/ncidod/dvbid/plague/index.htm. Accessed February 28, 2010.

19. Heymann DL ed. *Control of Communicable Diseases Manual.* 19th ed. Washington, DC: American Public Health Association; 2008.

20. Bacon RM, Kugeler KJ, Mead PS. Surveillance for Lyme disease—United States, 1992–2006. Centers for Disease Control and Prevention. *MMWR Surveillance Summaries.* 2008;57(SS10):1–9.

21. Centers for Disease Control and Prevention. Special Pathogens Branch. Viral hemorrhagic fevers. Available at: http://www.cdc.gov/ncidod/dvrd/spb/mnpages/dispages/vhf.htm. Accessed March 16, 2010.

22. Centers for Disease Control and Prevention, Division of Vector-Borne Infectious Diseases. Arboviral encephalitides. Fact sheet: arboviral encephalitis. Available at: http://www.cdc.gov/ncidod/dvbid/arbor/. Accessed March 16, 2010.

23. Chomel BB. Control and prevention of emerging zoonoses. *J Vet Med Educ.* 2003;30(2):145–147.

24. Centers for Disease Control and Prevention, National Center for Infectious Diseases, Special Pathogens Branch. All about hantaviruses: hantavirus pulmonary syndrome (HPS). Available at: http://www.cdc.gov/ncidod/diseases/hanta/hps/index.htm. Accessed March 1, 2010.

25. Centers for Disease Control and Prevention, National Center for Infectious Diseases, Special Pathogens Branch. All about hantaviruses: hantaviruses. Available at: http://www.cdc.gov/ncidod/diseases/hanta/hps/noframes/hanta.htm. Accessed March 1, 2010.

26. Centers for Disease Control and Prevention, National Center for Infectious Diseases, Special Pathogens Branch. All about hantaviruses. Tracking a mystery disease: the detailed story of hantavirus pulmonary syndrome. Available at: http://www.cdc.gov/ncidod/diseases/hanta/hps/noframes/printgenlsection.htm. Accessed March 16, 2010.

27. Centers for Disease Control and Prevention, National Center for Infectious Diseases, Special Pathogens Branch. All about hantaviruses. Case information: Hantavirus pulmonary syndrome case count and descriptive statistics. Available at: http://www.cdc.gov/ncidod/diseases/hanta/hps/noframes/caseinfo.htm. Accessed March 19, 2010.

28. Centers for Disease Control and Prevention. Dengue. Available at: http://www.cdc.gov/dengue/. Accessed March 1, 2010.

29. Centers for Disease Control and Prevention, Special Pathogens Branch. Rift Valley fever. Available at: http://www.cdc.gov/ncidod/dvrd/spb/mnpages/dispages/rvf.htm. Accessed March 1, 2010.

30. Centers for Disease Control and Prevention. Monkeypox. Fact sheet: What you should know about monkeypox. Available at: http://www.cdc.gov/ncidod/monkeypox/factsheet2.htm. Accessed March 1, 2010.

31. Centers for Disease Control and Prevention, Emergency Preparedness & Response. Frequently asked questions (FAQ) about tularemia. Available at: http://www.bt.cdc.gov/agent/tularemia/faq.asp. Accessed March 1, 2010.

32. Centers for Disease Control and Prevention. Update: investigation of bioterrorism-related anthrax, 2001. *MMWR.* 2001;50:1008–1010.

33. Jernigan DB, Raghunathan PL, Bell BP, et al. Investigation of bioterrorism-related anthrax, United States, 2001: epidemiologic findings. *Emerg Infect Dis.* 2002;8:1019–1028.

34. Hughes JM, Gerberding JL. Anthrax bioterrorism: lessons learned and future directions. *Emerg Infect Dis.* 2002;8:1013–1014.

35. Centers for Disease Control and Prevention, Division of Foodborne, Bacterial and Mycotic Diseases (DFBMD). Disease listing: anthrax. Available at: http://www.cdc.gov/nczved/dfbmd/disease_listing/anthrax_gi.html. Accessed March 1, 2010.

36. Centers for Disease Control and Prevention. Avian influenza (bird flu). Transmission of influenza A viruses between animals and people. Available at: http://www.cdc.gov/flu/avian/gen-info/pdf/transmission.pdf. Accessed March 16, 2010.

Toxic Metals and Elements

INTRODUCTION

Heavy metals (e.g., lead, mercury, and nickel) and other metallic compounds (e.g., aluminum, iron, and tin) are widely dispersed in the environment and arise from both natural and man-made sources. The entire human population is exposed to low levels of heavy metals from naturally occurring deposits of these elements in the earth's crust. Other sources of human exposure to metals are emissions from smelters and coal-fired power plants, contact with contaminants that are leaching from hazardous waste sites, ingestion of contaminated food and water, and contact with metals in occupations related to metal working.

Two examples of metals that pose hazards for human health are lead and mercury. The latter has elicited much public controversy as a cause of fish contamination that may be of special concern to women who are pregnant, nursing, or may become pregnant. Such women, according to guidelines from the EPA and reports in the media, should avoid certain types of fish that contain high levels of mercury (examples are shark and swordfish) and limit intake of tuna, especially white tuna. It was also recommended that children should have a restricted intake of fish. These guidelines generated heated controversy: Fish is a low-fat source of protein; tuna fish is the popular staple of many people's lunches.

Lead is a cause for alarm because of its potential to harm children's development. Not only do lead-based paints continue to pose a hazard to inner-city children, but lead also can present dangers to creatures in the rural environment. A newspaper article reported that lead bullets used by hunters remain in the game animals that they shoot and abandon. Scavengers such as endangered California condors may develop paralyzed digestive systems when they feed on the remains.

This chapter is a companion to Chapter 7, which covers pesticides, herbicides, and organophosphates. The current chapter will begin by presenting a list of hazardous substances of metallic and chemical origin. The chapter will provide an overview of the major categories of metallic compounds and their possible sources and effects; then it will cover pathways of metallic compounds into the human body. A detailed review of some of the most important compounds will follow, in addition to an explanation of their potential health effects. Chapter 7 will continue with a discussion of chemical hazards.

THE CERCLA PRIORITY LIST OF HAZARDOUS SUBSTANCES

The Agency for Toxic Substances and Disease Registry (ATSDR) has developed a rank-ordered list of hazardous substances, known as the CERCLA Priority List of Hazardous Substances. The acronym CERCLA refers to the Comprehensive Environmental Response, Compensation, and

Liability Act. A provision of the Superfund Amendments and Reauthorization Act (SARA) mandates that ATSDR and the EPA prioritize a list of hazardous substances. These are substances that "are most commonly found at facilities on the National Priorities List (NPL) and which are determined to pose the most significant potential threat to human health due to their known or suspected toxicity and potential for human exposure at these NPL sites."[1] The NPL, or Superfund List, is defined as "EPA's list of the most serious uncontrolled or abandoned hazardous waste sites [in the United States] identi-

fied for possible long-term remedial action under Superfund. The list is based primarily on the score a site receives from the Hazard Ranking System. EPA is required to update the NPL at least once a year. A site must be on the NPL to receive money from the Trust Fund for remedial action."[2] Refer to the following text box for the 2007 list, which presents the top 20 hazardous substances. Note that list numbers 1, 2, 3, 7, 18, and 19 are heavy metals or metallic compounds discussed in the present chapter. Many of the remaining compounds are covered in Chapter 7.

CERCLA Priority List of Hazardous Substances

The Comprehensive Environmental Response, Compensation, and Liability Act (CERCLA) section 104(i), as amended by the Superfund Amendments and Reauthorization Act (SARA), requires ATSDR and the EPA to prepare a list, in order of priority, of substances that are most commonly found at facilities on the National Priorities List (NPL) and which are determined to pose the most significant potential threat to human health due to their known or suspected toxicity and potential for human exposure at these NPL sites. CERCLA also requires this list to be revised periodically to reflect additional information on hazardous substances.

This CERCLA priority list is revised and published on a 2-year basis, with a yearly informal review and revision. Each substance on the CERCLA Priority List of Hazardous Substances is a candidate to become the subject of a toxicological profile prepared by ATSDR and subsequently a candidate for the identification of priority data needs. This priority list is based on an algorithm that utilizes the following three components: frequency of occurrence at NPL sites, toxicity, and potential for human exposure to the substances found at NPL sites.

It should be noted that this priority list is not a list of "most toxic" substances, but rather a prioritization of substances based on a combination of their frequency, toxicity, and potential for human exposure at NPL sites.

Thus, it is possible for substances with low toxicity but high NPL frequency of occurrence and exposure to be on this priority list. The objective of this priority list is to rank substances across all NPL hazardous waste sites to provide guidance in selecting which substances will be the subject of toxicological profiles prepared by ATSDR.

The list below contains the top 20 hazardous substances from the CERCLA Priority List of Hazardous Substances for 2007. The complete list contains 275 substances.

Top 20 Hazardous Substances from the 2007 CERCLA Priority List of Hazardous Substances

1. Arsenic
2. Lead
3. Mercury
4. Vinyl chloride
5. Polychlorinated biphenyls
6. Benzene
7. Cadmium
8. Polycyclic aromatic hydrocarbons
9. Benzo(a)pyrene
10. Benzo(b)fluoranthene
11. Chloroform
12. DDT, p, p'-
13. Aroclor 1254
14. Aroclor 1260
15. Dibenzo(a,h)anthracene
16. Trichloroethylene
17. Dieldrin
18. Chromium, hexavalent
19. Phosphorus, white
20. Chlordane

Source: Adapted and reprinted from ATSDR. CERCLA Priority List of Hazardous Substances: What is the CERCLA list? Available at: http://www.atsdr.cdc.gov/cercla/index.html. Accessed March 24, 2010; and ATSDR. 2007 CERCLA Priority List of Hazardous Substances. Available at: http://www.atsdr.cdc.gov/cercla/07list.html. Accessed March 24, 2010.

OVERVIEW OF SOURCES AND EFFECTS OF EXPOSURE TO METALS

This chapter will use a common four-category method for classifying metals.[3] This scheme is shown in Table 6-1, which classifies metals according to whether they are (1) major toxic metals with multiple effects; (2) **essential metals** with potential for toxicity; (3) metals related to medical therapy; or (4) minor toxic metals.

The first group shown in Table 6-1, "Major Toxic Metals with Multiple Effects," comprises the toxic heavy metals, which are toxic to life-forms and are not necessary to sustain life. Examples of metals in this category are arsenic, lead, and mercury. A heavy metal is one that has a high atomic weight with a specific gravity that exceeds the specific gravity of water by five or more times. (Specific gravity is defined as "The ratio of the mass of a solid or liquid to the mass of an equal volume of distilled water at 4°C (39°F) or of a gas to an equal volume of air or hydrogen under prescribed conditions of temperature and pressure.")[4] The second group consists of metals that are considered to be essential for life when present in trace amounts; examples are iron, copper, manganese, and zinc. However, concentrations greater than trace amounts have the potential for toxicity. The third group includes metals used in medical therapy such as aluminum and lithium (e.g., used in lithium therapy for depression). The fourth group is known as minor toxic metals and includes silver and uranium. This chapter will focus primarily on groups one through three.

Let's examine the first group of metals shown in Table 6-1—major toxic metals with multiple effects—in more detail. They not only are toxic at low concentrations (beyond trace amounts), but they also have the capacity to bioaccumulate (sometimes called **biomagnification**), which means that they become more concentrated and potentially more harmful as they move up the food chain. For example, lower organisms may ingest mercury-containing compounds in the water. These lower organisms are consumed by snails and then by small fish. Finally, the smaller fish provide a food source for larger fish that are harvested for human consumption.

Another example is the **bioaccumulation** of toxic substances such as heavy metals by zebra mussels. This species of mussels, which was introduced accidentally into the Great Lakes system of the United States, reproduces in great numbers. Concern has been raised about the ability of the mussels to filter out and concentrate pollutants in the water; some areas of the Great Lakes are known to be polluted with toxic contaminants. In the Great Lakes, biomagnification of toxic substances by zebra mussels could affect other life-forms such as freshwater fish and wildlife.

Sources of Exposure to Metals

There are several possible modes of exposure to metals, corresponding to the human portals and sites of entry that come into contact with the metals. These portals and sites include the lungs (through inhalation of dusts, metal fumes, and vapors), skin (through contact with dusts), and the mouth (by ingestion). Contact with high concentrations of toxic metals is most likely to occur in an occupational setting (e.g., among persons who work with metals). Lower-level exposures may result from contact with the ambient environment. For example, children may ingest toxic metals that are present in paints in

---

TABLE 6-1 Classification of the Toxic Effects of Metals

Major Toxic Metals with Multiple Effects	Essential Metals with Potential for Toxicity	Metals Related to Medical Therapy	Minor Toxic Metals
Arsenic (As)	Cobalt (Co)	Aluminum (Al)	Antimony (Sb)
Beryllium (Be)	Trivalent chromium, Cr(III)	Bismuth (Bi)	Barium (Ba)
Cadmium (CD)	Copper (Cu)	Gallium (Ga)	Germanium (Ge)
Chromium (Cr)	Iron (Fe)	Gold (Au)	Indium (In)
Lead (Pb)	Magnesium (Mg)	Lithium (Li)	Silver (Ag)
Mercury (Hg)	Manganese (Mn)	Platinum (Pt) and related metals	Tellurium (Te)
Nickel (Ni)	Molybdenum (Mo)		Thallium (Tl)
	Selenium (Se)		Tin (Sn)
	Zinc (Zn)		Titanium (Ti)
			Uranium (U)
			Vanadium (V)

Source: Data from RA Goyer and TW Clarkson. Toxic effects of metals. In: Klaassen CD, ed. *Casarett and Doull's Toxicology: The Basic Science of Poisons.* 6th ed. New York, NY: McGraw Hill; 2001:811–812.

homes and playgrounds. Also, people may be exposed to levels of toxic metals in the foods that they eat.

Four major types of media have potential for exposure of the population to heavy metals. As shown in Table 6-2, these media are air, soil/dust, water, and biota (animal and plant life)/food. Some media are more relevant to the transport of a given type of heavy metal than are other media. For example, water is a medium for exposure of the population to arsenic and lead. Food is a medium for exposure of the population to mercury.

Industrial facilities, metal smelters, and power plants that burn coal have the potential to release heavy metals into the environment. Examples of heavy metals emitted from these sources include cadmium and arsenic. In some communities, incinerators constructed to dispose of waste may disperse toxic heavy metals such as mercury and cadmium. Mines are another source of toxic heavy metal wastes, examples being arsenic leaching from gold mines and mercury from cinnabar mines. **Preservatives** used in wood may contain arsenic, which is an occupational hazard to carpenters. Residues that persist from some pesticides that contain chromium and mer-

cury and from fertilizers that are contaminated with cadmium present toxic threats to the environment. Finally, residents of older houses may be exposed to lead in paint and in plumbing systems. Many heavy metals are natural constituents of the earth's crust. One such heavy metal is arsenic, which is present in the groundwater in many areas of the world and poses a hazard to the residents who drink the groundwater. Other sources of exposure to heavy metals include air pollution, water that has been contaminated with wastes, contact with industrial wastes in the soil, and ingestion of contaminated food. Previously, the author noted that toxic metals can bioaccumulate in shellfish and pose a hazard when these mollusks are consumed.

Another example of a source of exposure of a population to toxic heavy metals comes from the disposal of used automobile tires. Worldwide, millions of used automobile tires are discarded every year. These tires are known to contain a number of toxic metals, including zinc, cadmium, and lead. When the tires are deposited in landfills, they degrade and may release toxic metals into the soil; in turn, the toxic metals may find their way into groundwater and also poison the

---

TABLE 6-2 Relevance of Different Media to Metal Exposures[a]

	Air	Soil/dust	Water	Biota/food
Arsenic	+ Occupational Smelters	+ + Mining Smelting	+ + + + Natural	+ +
Mercury	+ Occupational Cultural	+ + + +	+ + + + Methylation in sediments	+ + + + Biomagnification MeHg in fish[b]
Iron	+ + Occupational Mining	+ + Mine tailings	+ + Rust in pipes	+
Tin	+ Occupational smelters	0	+	+ Organotin pesticides[c], TBT in fish[d]
Lead	+ + Occupational Smelters Leaded gasoline	+ + + Toddlers ingestion	+ + Lead pipes and solder	+ + + Leaded glaze and glass Paprika Wheat (Cairo)
Chromium	+ Occupational	+ +	+	+

[a] + + + + Highly relevant; + + + medium relevant; + + relevant; + less or infrequently relevant; 0 not relevant.

[b] MeHg, methylmercury; [c] Organotin, a compound that contains both tin and carbon; [d] TBT, tributyltin.

Source: Adapted and reprinted from D Caussy, M Gochfeld, E Gurzau, et al. Lessons from case studies of metals: investigating exposure, bioavailability, and risk. *Ecotoxicology and Environmental Safety.* 2003;56:46. Copyright 2003; used with permission from Elsevier.

air. Sometimes tires may catch on fire and cause a serious air pollution hazard. The toxic materials released from degrading automobile tires may persist for many years.

Common industrial processes may release toxic metals into the air, which impinges upon nearby residents and passersby who are unaware that they are breathing fumes that contain toxic metals. The jewelry districts found in many large US cities can produce toxic fumes during the smelting of metals and soldering operations that are connected with the manufacture of jewelry. These processes can release significant amounts of pollution into the surrounding areas.

Unsafe disposal of electronic equipment also has raised concerns about the release of toxic metals into the environment. Increasingly, electronic wastes are being tossed into the garbage without further thought about what happens to them when they are deposited in landfills. Examples of items that are being discarded with increasing frequency are fluorescent light bulbs, lithium ion batteries, cell phones, outmoded computers, computer monitors, and nonworking television sets. The toxic metals contained in these devices are lead, mercury, cadmium, chromium, lithium, arsenic, copper, and zinc. In addition, these devices contain toxic organic chemicals that may persist in the environment. (The topic of toxic organic chemicals will be discussed in Chapter 7.) Two important reasons could explain why used electronic equipment is disposed of in an unsafe manner: There are few recycling programs for reuse or remanufacture of the equipment and little information is available to the consumer regarding the proper disposal of these devices. Unfortunately, Third World countries increasingly are being selected as the dumping grounds for electronic waste, which is scavenged by unwitting individuals who are not aware of the hazardous nature of this waste.

Effects of Exposure to Metals

The effects of acute poisoning from high levels of exposure to toxic metals can be differentiated from the effects of chronic low-level exposure. The symptoms of acute poisoning from exposure to metals generally have rapid onset—from a few minutes to approximately one hour. Depending upon the portal of entry, these symptoms may consist of gastrointestinal effects (vomiting and stomach pain) and neurological effects (headaches, suppression of normal breathing, and convulsions). In most cases, the symptoms are likely to be dramatic and severe when the person has had high levels of exposure.

Instances of acute poisoning from toxic metals have occurred when contaminated foodstuffs were consumed. For example, copper from copper cooking vessels may leach into foods that are left standing during meal preparation. Some-

times, errors in food manufacturing may accidentally introduce toxic metals into foods and beverages. An instance of such accidental poisoning occurred when Iraqi residents consumed homemade bread contaminated with mercury.[5] The source of the poisoning was methylmercury (one of the forms of mercury) used as a fungicide to treat grain intended for planting. In this incident more than 6,000 persons had to be hospitalized, and at least 500 died.

The effects of long-term exposure to lower levels of toxic metals typically are more subtle than those of acute exposure. Often, the effects of exposure over extended time periods are difficult to differentiate from those of chronic medical conditions. In addition, it may be impossible to determine the specific source of exposure. Symptoms of chronic exposure can include reduced cognitive functioning, such as learning impairment, as well as lethargy. Sometimes the symptoms show a pattern of symptom remission that causes the victim not to seek medical care.

Heavy Metal Exposure among Women and Children

The health effects of exposure to heavy metals (e.g., nickel, cadmium, lead, and mercury) are different for women than they are for men. These differences in effects have been attributed to hormonal and metabolic processes related to menstruation, pregnancy, and menopause. Women usually have smaller body sizes than men, causing women to be more affected by a given amount of a metal than are men. As an example of different responses to toxic metals, women are known to develop allergies to nickel and rashes from skin contact with nickel more frequently than men. In comparison to men, women are known to accumulate higher internal concentrations of cadmium and lead than men. During pregnancy, exposure to mercury is a particular hazard for the neurodevelopment of the fetus.[6]

The health effects of women's general environmental and occupational exposures to smelters have been studied.[7] In an investigation conducted in the north of Sweden, researchers examined the impact of emissions from the Rönnskär smelter, which is known to release heavy metals such as lead, mercury, and arsenic. Female smelter employees and a sample of female residents in the neighborhood surrounding the smelter were studied with respect to the occurrence of spontaneous abortions. No association between spontaneous abortions and employment in the smelter or residence near the smelter was reported.

For fetuses, infants, and children (especially young children), heavy metals are known to present serious hazards, which can include impairment of physical and mental development, damage to internal organs and the nervous system, some forms of cancer, and even mortality. For example, lead and mercury have the capacity to cross the placental barrier, with the potential to cause fetal brain damage. According to researchers, during growth of various body systems, children have increased sensitivity to heavy metals; this increased sensitivity may result in an increased frequency of adverse health effects.

Symptoms of exposure to heavy metals among children include nervous system damage as reflected in memory impairment and difficulty in learning, and a range of behavioral problems such as hyperactivity syndrome and overt aggressiveness. When children are exposed to high levels of toxic heavy metals, the effects may be irreversible. Because their body weight is smaller than that of adults, children consume more food in proportion to their body weight and consequently receive higher doses of heavy metals that may be present in their food.

One of the outcomes associated with exposure to toxic chemicals, including heavy metals, is the occurrence of de-velopmental disabilities, which have trended upward in frequency during recent years.[8] "Such exposures are of particular concern for genetically susceptible individuals exposed during periods of developmental vulnerability."[8(pS14)] As an example of a particular disability associated with exposure to heavy metals, consider the effect that elevated blood lead levels have on intelligence. For example, doubling the blood lead level from 10 to 20 micrograms per deciliter would increase the demand for special programs for persons who have impaired cognitive ability by almost 60%. Due to recognition of the adverse health effects of lead, especially on children, authorities in the United States have lowered the standard for blood lead levels periodically since the 1960s. In 1990, the toxic threshold for lead was set at 10 micrograms per deciliter of blood for children age six years and younger (this level remains the current standard, although even levels below 10 micrograms are considered unsafe). Thus, reduction of blood lead levels to the lowest level possible is important for the population, especially children. (See the section titled *Lead* for more information.)

TABLE 6-3 Potential Sources of Arsenic Exposure[a]

Source	Examples
Natural environmental sources	Ground water, mineral ore, geothermal processes
Industrial sources	Smelting processes for cobalt, gold, lead, nickel, zinc
Arsenic-containing products	Insecticides such as ant killers and animal dips, algaecides[b]; wood preservatives used to pressure treat lumber for outdoor installations and playground equipment[c]
Arsenic in drugs	Some drugs used for cancer chemotherapy; some traditional medicines; Salvarsan (an arsenic compound) to treat syphilis before antibiotics became available
Component uses of arsenicals	Some microwave devices, lasers, light-emitting diodes, photoelectric chemical cells, semiconductor devices
Other industrial processes that use arsenic	Generating electricity in coal-fired power plants, hardening metal alloys, purifying industrial gases
Foods that may contain arsenic	Seafood (e.g., clams, oysters, scallops, mussels, crabs, lobsters, certain bottom-feeding finfish, seaweed[d])
Drinking water in some regions	Artesian and tube wells supplied by geologically contaminated aquifers; contamination from mineral ores; contamination from mine and mill tailings

Notes:

[a]There has been no domestic production of arsenic since 1985, although the US was the world's largest consumer of arsenic in 2003.

[b]Regulatory restrictions for arsenic, especially for home products, have reduced its use.

[c]In 2003, production of wood preservatives accounted for more than 90% of domestic consumption of arsenic trioxide, one of the forms of arsenic. Since December 2003, residential lumber may no longer be treated with arsenic.

[d]The forms of arsenic found in seafood are generally considered to be nontoxic and are excreted in urine with 48 hours of ingestion.

Source: Data from Agency for Toxic Substances and Disease Registry. Case Studies in Environmental Medicine: Arsenic Toxicity. Available at: http://www.atsdr.cdc.gov/csem/arsenic/docs/arsenic.pdf. Accessed July 2, 2010.

TOXIC HEAVY METALS

The metals in the group known as "major toxic metals with multiple effects" include arsenic, beryllium, cadmium, chromium, lead, mercury, and nickel. (Refer to Table 6-1.)

Arsenic

Arsenic in its pure form is a crystalline metalloid, an element with properties that are intermediate between those of a metal and a nonmetal. It is able to combine with other substances, metallic and nonmetallic, and also to form stable organic compounds.[9] An acutely poisonous material that is ubiquitous in nature—in soils and water—arsenic varies in toxicity depending upon its chemical form; it is also the by-product of refining gold and other metals. Although at one time arsenic was used for medicinal purposes, at present it is no longer widely used for that application. Presently, arsenic has commercial applications as a pesticide and wood preservative, and in manufacturing processes.[10]

As shown in Table 6-3, arsenic exposure can come from many environmental sources, including industrial processes that release arsenic, products that contain arsenic, certain foods, and drinking water in some geographic areas. Ingestion of 100 mg of arsenic produces acute poisoning; however, many people are exposed to lower levels of arsenic in sources such as drinking water and food. Some areas of the world (e.g., Taiwan, Mexico, western South America [Chile and Argentina], Bangladesh, and Inner Mongolia) have high levels of naturally occurring arsenic in the drinking water. In some of these areas, the arsenic levels are as high as 1,000 μg per liter of water. Arsenic levels that range from 50 to 100 μg per liter are found in the drinking water in sections of the United States, for example, New Mexico, Arizona, Nevada, Utah, Southern California, Idaho, and Nebraska.[11] Figure 6-1 shows the distribution of arsenic in groundwater samples in the United States.

The federal government has established standards for the amounts of arsenic that are permitted in the public drink-

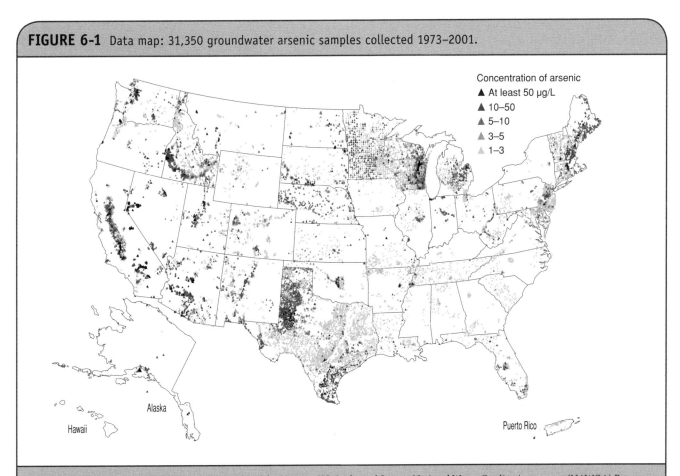

FIGURE 6-1 Data map: 31,350 groundwater arsenic samples collected 1973–2001.

Concentration of arsenic
▲ At least 50 μg/L
▲ 10–50
▲ 5–10
▲ 3–5
▲ 1–3

Alaska

Hawaii

Puerto Rico

Source: Adapted and reprinted from US Department of the Interior, US Geological Survey, National Water-Quality Assessment (NAWQA) Program. Available at: http://water.usgs.gov/nawqa/trace/pubs/geo_v46n11/fig1.html. Accessed March 16, 2010.

ing water supply. In 2001, the EPA announced the standard of 10 μg of arsenic per liter of drinking water, with the year 2006 set as the compliance date for this standard. Previously, a higher standard of 50 μg of arsenic per liter of water was permitted, but this standard was made more stringent when officials realized that arsenic at this level of concentration was a risk factor for cancer. Table 6-4 provides a chronology of US standards for arsenic in drinking water.

Several massive arsenic poisoning incidents, due to the contamination of foodstuffs with arsenic, have been documented.[9] Arsenic-contaminated beer killed 6,000 people in England in 1900; several thousand people were poisoned in Japan in the mid-20th century due to arsenic-contaminated dry milk and soy sauce. Particularly at risk of arsenic exposure are some groups of mining and smelter workers as well as agricultural workers who come into contact with pesticides that contain arsenic.

Low-level chronic exposure to arsenic is associated with **melanosis**, a dermatologic condition that can cause the darkening of the skin of the entire body (diffuse melanosis). Other forms of melanosis are spotted melanosis, which causes spotted pigmentation of the skin, and buccal membrane melanosis, which appears on the tissues of the inside of the mouth, including the tongue. Figure 6-2 shows a case of melanosis of the hand. Melanosis is a problem in some areas of Bangladesh and West Bengal, India, where the levels of arsenic in the groundwater exceed the World Health Organization standard of a maximum permissible limit of 50 μg per liter.[12]

Accumulated evidence suggests that arsenic is a **carcinogen**. It is a cause of skin cancer when ingested and lung cancer when inhaled. Ingestion of arsenic has been linked with internal cancers such as bladder, kidney, and liver cancers.[13] Geographic regions that have high levels of naturally occurring arsenic in the drinking water (e.g., Taiwan and Argentina) also have elevated levels of bladder cancer mortality.[14] Some data suggest that there is a dose–response relationship between exposure to inorganic arsenic in drinking water and bladder cancer. Because many of the findings of an association between arsenic in drinking water and bladder cancer have used ecologic study designs, there is a need for additional analytical research on this topic. A factor that has impeded research on the carcinogenic aspects of arsenic is the absence of a clearly defined animal model of the effects of arsenic exposure; the use of laboratory animals would make possible studies that cannot be carried out with humans.[15]

In addition to the foregoing health outcomes, arsenic exposure has been connected with peripheral vascular disease, cerebrovascular disease, and cardiovascular disease (e.g., hypertensive heart disease). There also may be an association

TABLE 6-4 History of US Standards for Arsenic in Drinking Water

1942	US Public Health Service (USPHS) sets an interim drinking water standard of 50 μg As/liter.[a]
1962	USPHS identifies 10 μg As/liter as the goal.[b]
1975	EPA adopts the interim standard of 50 μg As/liter set by the USPHS in 1942.[a]
1986	Congress directs EPA to revise the standard by 1989.[c]
1988	EPA estimates that the ingestion of 50 μg As/liter results in a skin cancer risk of 1 in 400.[d]
1992	Internal cancer risk estimated to be 1.3 per 100 persons at 50 μg As/liter.[e]
1993	World Health Organization recommends lowering arsenic in drinking water to 10 μg As/liter.[f]
1996	Congress directs the EPA to propose a new drinking water standard by January 2000.[c]
1999	National Research Center (NRC) estimates cancer mortality risks to be about 1 in 100 at 50 μg As/liter.[g]
2000	EPA proposes a standard of 5 μg As/liter and requests comment on 3, 10, and 20 μg As/liter.[c]
2001	(January) Clinton EPA lowers the standard to 10 μg As/liter.[c]
2001	(March) Bush EPA delays lowering the standard.[c]
2001	(September) New NRC report concludes that EPA underestimated cancer risks.[h]
2001	(October) EPA announces it will adopt the standard of 10 μg As/liter.[c]
2002	(February) The effective date for new standard of 10 μg As/liter.[c]
2006	Compliance date for the new arsenic standard.[c]

[a]See www.epa.gov/safewater/ars/ars1.html.

[b]USPHS. *Federal Regist.* 1962;42:2152.

[c]See www.house.gov/science/ets/oct04/ets_charter_100401.htm.

[d]EPA. *Special Report on Ingested Inorganic Arsenic: Skin Cancer; Nutritional Essentiality.* Washington, DC: EPA Risk Assessment Forum; 1988.

[e]AH Smith et al. *Environ Health Perspect.* 1992;97:259.

[f]World Health Organization. *Guidelines for Drinking-Water Quality, Vol. 1, Recommendations.* Geneva: World Health Organization; 1993.

[g]NRC. *Arsenic in Drinking Water.* Washington, DC: National Academy Press; 1999.

[h]NRC. *Arsenic in Drinking Water 2001 Update.* Washington, DC: National Academy Press; 2001.

Source: Adapted and reprinted with permission from AH Smith, PA Lopipero, MN Bates, et al. Arsenic epidemiology and drinking water standards. *Science.* 2002;296:2145. Copyright 2002 AAAS.

FIGURE 6-2 Melanosis of the hand from arsenic poisoning.

Source: Reprinted with permission from R Wilson, Harvard University. Chronic arsenic poisoning: history, study and remediation. Available at: http://phys4.harvard.edu/~wilson/arsenic/pictures/5.%20Melanosis%20hand.jpg. Accessed March 24, 2010.

is inhalation. Exposure to beryllium can result in the disease berylliosis, also known as chronic beryllium disease (CBD). This condition can be extremely debilitating and in some cases fatal. Two factors that affect the development of CBD are beryllium exposure itself and genetic susceptibility, which has been shown to be associated with a specific gene.[17] Beryllium is classified as a class A carcinogen, the most hazardous level for a cancer-causing substance. Exposure of the human population to beryllium may result from the burning of coal, which contains beryllium compounds. Beryllium residues from emissions from coal-burning power plants may contaminate agricultural products.

Cadmium

Cadmium is found in all soils and rocks as well as coal and fertilizers derived from minerals. Typically cadmium occurs as a mineral in combination with other elements, such as oxygen (as in cadmium oxide). As a result of absorption from environmental sources, fish, plants, and animals contain cadmium.[18] It is released as a by-product of the mining industry, electroplating, iron and steel production, combustion of coal, and manufacture of fertilizers and pesticides.[19] Among the general population the primary sources of cadmium exposure are cigarette smoke and dietary cadmium. Other sources include smelting operations, as in the smelting of cadmium-containing zinc ores, and production of batteries. Cadmium also is known to bioaccumulate in shellfish and is found in some species of mushrooms.[20] Cadmium may be ingested from vegetables that are grown in cadmium-containing soil. For example, gardens near installations such as battery factories may contain soil that is contaminated with cadmium.

Occupational exposure to cadmium comes from the production of nickel cadmium batteries, zinc smelting, manufacture of paint pigments, soldering, and employment in metal factories. In occupational settings, the modes for entry of cadmium into the body are primarily through inhalation and, secondarily, through the gastrointestinal tract.[21]

Cadmium is not regarded as essential for life processes. Moreover, various adverse health effects have been attributed to cadmium. Some of these are shown in Table 6-5.

The OSCAR study (Osteoporosis with Cadmium as a Risk Factor) involved the investigation of 1,000 persons who were exposed to cadmium from the environment or from an occupation. This study demonstrated that there was a relationship between environmental and occupational exposure to cadmium and kidney damage (renal tubular damage). Two other adverse health effects that have been attributed to cadmium exposure are osteoporosis in women and loss of height in men.[20]

between long-term arsenic exposure and diabetes mellitus. Women exposed to arsenic in drinking water have demonstrated adverse pregnancy outcomes including spontaneous abortions, stillbirths, and preterm births.[16]

Beryllium

Beryllium is used widely in industry because of its special properties. It is not only lighter than aluminum, but also much stronger than steel. Beryllium also can be alloyed with other metals such as copper. Among those likely to be exposed to beryllium are employees in the metal processing industry. One of the most frequent methods of exposure to beryllium

TABLE 6-5 Health Effects Potentially Associated with Cadmium Exposure

- Renal damage and renal dysfunction
- Bone disease
- Some forms of cancer
- Hypertension
- Cardiovascular diseases
- Genotoxicity
- Circulatory diseases
- Prostate and lung cancers
- Reproductive toxicity
- Reduced life expectancy
- Osteoporosis

Cadmium has been studied in relation to elevated blood pressure and the occurrence of cardiovascular diseases. "The cadmium hypothesis postulates that long-term environmental exposure to cadmium may lead to hypertension . . . and that cadmium via blood pressure elevation, or possibly via other mechanisms, may contribute to the pathogenesis of cardiovascular diseases in industrialized countries. . . ."[22(p257)] However, not all studies have been able to corroborate this hypothesis.

One of the conditions attributed to cadmium is known as **itai-itai disease**. Cases of this disease began occurring in the Jinzu River basin in Japan as early as 1912 and gradually increased until the number of cases peaked in the period of 1955 through 1959. A description of the disease is as follows: "The strange disease that appeared in the downstream basin of the Jinzu River around 1912 was called by locals 'itai-itai byo' ('itai' being what Japanese people say when inflicted with pain and 'byo' literally meaning disease). It came by this name because of the way victims cried out 'itai-itai' under the excruciating pain they endured. Women were mostly afflicted with pain across their entire body and more severe cases suffered broken bones when trying to move on their own."[23]

Various causes of the disease were studied, including malnutrition, infectious disease agents, and the effects of aging. Subsequent investigations revealed that the disease was caused by chronic cadmium poisoning due to the presence of the metal in the water of the Jinzu River. The cadmium contamination of the river was related to discharges from the Kamioka Mining Company, located upstream.[23,24]

Chromium

Found as a naturally occurring element in the earth's crust (e.g., in rocks, soils, and materials of volcanic origin), chro-mium occurs in various forms.[25] The most common forms are chromium(0), chromium(III), and chromium(VI). Found naturally in the environment, chromium(III) is regarded as an essential nutrient. The other two forms result from human activities such as industry. In view of its numerous industrial applications, chromium, particularly chromium(VI) and chromium(0), is a widespread environmental pollutant.

Human exposure to chromium in its various forms can occur as a result of occupational exposure (e.g., breathing chromium-contaminated air) and ingestion of food and drinking water. Early in the 20th century, occupational health specialists observed that employees in the chromium ore industry in Germany had higher rates of lung cancer than the general population. This finding has been replicated in numerous studies, which have suggested that chromium(VI) is a human carcinogen. Because of its potential to cause lung cancer, chromium(VI) has been classified by the World Health Organization and the EPA as a human carcinogen.

Regarding the environment, hexavalent chromium—chromium(VI)—seems to cause the greatest concern. Much attention has been given to chromium(VI), which can leach into drinking water. Consequences of ingestion of chromium(VI) are digestive problems and damage to organs such as the kidneys and liver. Chromium(VI) also may produce skin ulcers when it is applied to the skin. The consequences of breathing chromium(VI) in high concentrations include respiratory problems, for example, nose bleeds, perforation of the nasal septum, and runny nose.

The film *Erin Brockovich* called attention to the potential hazards associated with groundwater pollution from chromium. The text box discusses the successful advocacy efforts of Erin Brockovich, an employee of a California law firm, to win claims against a power company for groundwater pollution by chromium(VI)—shown in the text box as Cr(VI). The film is noteworthy because it brought the issue of environmental contamination with heavy metals such as chromium before the general public.

Mercury

Mercury is a naturally occurring metal that is highly toxic and exists in three major forms: metallic mercury (elemental mercury), inorganic mercury, and organic mercury. At room temperature metallic mercury is a silvery liquid metal. Inorganic mercury refers to compounds of mercury such as mercury oxide or mercury sulfide. The combination of carbon and mercury produces the so-called organic mercury compounds, the most common of which is methyl mercury.[26]

Mercury has been used medically to treat syphilis, as an agricultural fungicide, and in dental amalgams for filling

Hexavalent Chromium: One Town's Story

On 7 December 1987, officials from Pacific Gas and Electric Company (PG&E), the world's largest utility, advised California regulatory authorities that they'd detected hexavalent chromium (Cr[VI]) at levels of 580 micrograms per liter (μg/L)—over 10 times the state's 50-μg/L limit for total chromium—in a groundwater monitoring well. Cr(VI) was being used as an anticorrosive in the cooling towers of a PG&E gas compressor station in the Mojave Desert town of Hinkley.

People who lived in Hinkley had experienced a disturbing array of health problems: liver, heart, respiratory, and reproductive failure, cancer of the brain, kidney, breast, uterus, and gastrointestinal system, Hodgkin disease, frequent miscarriages, and more. Were these problems related to the compressor station's wastewater ponds? PG&E officials said no. But until 1972, PG&E had knowingly released 370 million gallons of Cr(VI)-contaminated wastewater into the unlined ponds, and the toxic compound had made its way into Hinkley's groundwater.

In 1993, 77 Hinkley plaintiffs filed a lawsuit against PG&E. The suit was a direct result of a massive communications effort mounted by Erin Brockovich (Figure 6-3), an employee in a local law firm. She had uncovered the utility's environmental misconduct and launched a personal investigation that ended in the largest settlement on record for a civil class-action lawsuit. PG&E filed a motion to strike all claims for preconception injuries (fear of cancer) as speculative. But the plaintiffs—648 by the end—ended up recovering for injury claims and settling with PG&E for $333 million. In addition, PG&E agreed to stop using Cr(VI) and clean up the contamination.

The case remains controversial among chromium experts because most of the Hinkley exposures involved drinking Cr(VI)-laced water. This route of exposure is widely believed to cause much less toxicity than inhalational exposures because ingested Cr(VI) is converted to inactive trivalent chromium in the stomach. Many experts also claim that the exposures were too low to cause health effects, and that there are few data linking Cr(VI) exposures to the Hinkley residents' symptoms. But others counter that there are too many gaps in the data on chromium to dismiss the Hinkley residents' case. They believe the fact that this toxic form of chromium can enter all types of cells means that scientists may yet discover that it can damage many organ systems. Until more is known about how different doses and routes of exposure of Cr(VI) affect different populations, it is too soon to rule out high drinking water exposures as a health risk.

FIGURE 6-3 The advocacy efforts of Erin Brockovich, an employee of a California law firm (Masry & Vititoe), culminated in a successful lawsuit against a power company for groundwater pollution by chromium(VI). The plaintiffs were residents of Hinkley, California.

Source: © Larry Downing/Reuters

Source: Adapted and reprinted from C Pellerin and SM Booker. Reflections on hexavalent chromium: health hazards of an industrial heavyweight. *Environ Health Perspect.* 2000;108:A407.

cavities. It is released into the environment as a by-product of industrial processes. Even at low levels, when it becomes deposited in the beds of lakes, rivers, and other bodies of water, mercury represents a potential hazard to human health. Low levels of mercury can be magnified to higher levels as a result of methylation and bioaccumulation.

Through the process of methylation, microorganisms (bacteria and fungi) that ingest small amounts of mercury from sediments convert elemental mercury into methyl mercury; the process of bioaccumulation causes mercury levels to increase as the metal moves up the food chain and becomes more concentrated in aquatic invertebrates. Fish used for food may develop high levels of mercury in their tissues when they feed on these lower organisms. Bioaccumulation of mercury may result in mercury levels in fish that are unacceptably high for human consumption. For example, government agencies have warned that certain types of fish, such as shark, swordfish, tilefish, and king mackerel, may contain dangerously high levels of mercury. Canned albacore is suspected to contain unhealthful levels of mercury. As noted, mercury contamination is a particular hazard to the unborn children of pregnant women.

Mercury is extracted from cinnabar, a reddish ore composed of mercuric sulfide. (Refer to Figure 6-4.) Conversion of cinnabar into elemental mercury, a silvery liquid metal called quicksilver, involves crushing the ore and heating it at high temperatures in retorts in which the metal is distilled by condensation. During cinnabar processing, mercury fumes may be disseminated into the ambient environment and also may affect workers who breathe the fumes. Sediments from the mining operation can be transported into nearby bodies of water and persist as an environmental hazard. For more information, refer to the text box titled "The New Almaden Mine, California."

High levels of mercury contamination from the effluents of factories have produced environmental disasters. In 1956, an environmental catastrophe occurred in Minamata Bay, Japan, where approximately 3,000 cases of neurologic disease resulted among people who ate fish contaminated with methyl mercury.[27] The neurologic condition, which became known as **Minamata disease**, was characterized by numbness of the extremities, deafness, poor vision, and drowsiness; the condition was unresponsive to medical intervention and frequently culminated in death. (Refer to Figure 6-6.) The cause was attributed to discharges of mercury compounds into the bay by a plastics factory.

Lead

Sources of environmental lead include leaded gasoline, tap water from soldered pipes, and painted surfaces in older buildings. Figure 6-7 illustrates these common sources of environmental lead. In the past, lead was added to gasoline in order to improve the performance of internal combustion engines and to paint in order to increase the coatings' durability and adhesive properties. Some of the paints used before the 1950s contained as much as 50% or more lead. Since 1978, the use of lead as an additive to paints has been outlawed in the United States. Also, lead has been banned as an additive in gasoline in the United States and other developed countries. The reason for this policy decision was the widespread environmental dissemination of lead by the combustion products of automobile engines. As a result of these measures, the number of children who have elevated blood lead levels has declined gradually.

Figure 6-8A illustrates how lead may peel from walls endangering the health of infants and children living in the house. Another common source of household lead exposure is imported pottery that is used in food service. Some countries still permit the use of lead as a component of paints and glazes for decorating pottery. Over time, this lead may leach into foods and be consumed; Figure 6-8B presents examples of pottery that may contain lead.

Figure 6-9 demonstrates the transfer of lead particles from the environment of workers to the home, where children and other family members may be exposed. Careful hand

FIGURE 6-4 Cinnabar ore.

Source: Courtesy of the Almaden Quicksilver Mining Museum, Almaden, California.

The New Almaden Mine, California

Named after the famous Almaden mines of Spain, the New Almaden Quicksilver Mine is located in the San Francisco Bay area of Northern California. From the late 18th century until 1976 when mining operations terminated, large quantities of mercury were extracted from the mine. However, the legacy of the mining operation lives on: Mercury contamination from this former mining operation poses a continuing hazard to fish and aquatic life in the affected geographic area; signs have been posted to warn persons not to consume fish caught in nearby streams and lakes due to potentially toxic levels of mercury. Figure 6-5 shows different aspects of the mercury mining operations at the New Almaden mine.

FIGURE 6-5 The New Almaden Mine area. A: Sign advising against consumption of mercury-contaminated fish. B: Defunct equipment used for mercury mining and extraction. C: Cinnabar ware crafted by Chinese artisans.

Source: Courtesy of the Almaden Quicksilver Mining Museum, Almaden, California.

washing, personal hygiene, and laundering of clothing will prevent heavy metal–bearing dusts from leaving the workplace and endangering the health of family members.

Lead exposure is associated with serious central nervous system effects and other adverse health consequences, even when ingested at low levels. Lead poisoning is one of the most common environmental pediatric health problems in the United States. Especially damaging to the growing neurologic systems of young children, lead is a neurotoxin.[28] Acutely elevated blood lead levels (BLLs)—defined as 70 μg/dL of blood or higher—are associated with severe neurologic effects, including coma and death. The US DHEW has promulgated the goal of eliminating by 2010 BLLs that exceed 10 μg/dL among children younger than six years of age. Since the period 1976 to 1980, the percentage of children who had BLLs that exceeded 10 μg/dL has declined markedly. The National Health and

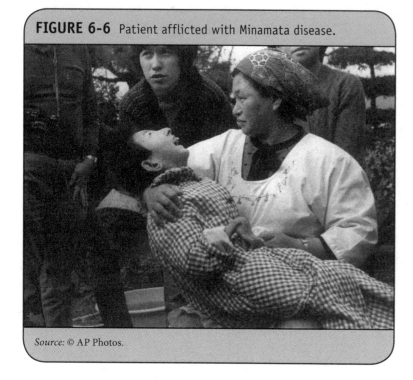

FIGURE 6-6 Patient afflicted with Minamata disease.

Source: © AP Photos.

tion. Cadmium pollution is often the byproduct of smelting of lead-containing ores. A gigantic lead refinery located along the Ribeira River valley in the far south of the state of Sao Paulo, Brazil, produced lead for a period of 50 years until it was closed in 1995. The refinery disseminated large amounts of lead and cadmium into the environment nearby as well as more distant areas. Children who lived close to the refinery were shown to have elevated BLLs.[32]

A German study demonstrated that cadmium and lead may be transported into people's houses through airborne dust.[33] Lead and cadmium concentrations in dust were followed in the German city of Hettstedt, a region in which mining and smelting activities were conducted. Normal household activities were associated with the movements of heavy metals into the home environment in the city, which had been contaminated with lead and cadmium.

Nutrition Examination Survey (NHANES) estimated that during 1976 to 1980, the prevalence was more than 80%. By 1999–2000, the prevalence had dropped to 2.2% or 434,000 children in all. In 1997, a President's Task Force reported that approximately 775,000 children under age six were estimated to have blood lead levels above 10 μg/dL; the corresponding prevalence for blood lead levels above 15 μg/dL was about 190,000.[29] Among children who have blood lead levels above 15 μg/dL, lead toxicity is associated with maladaptive behavior.[30] A study of inner-city pregnant women, nonpregnant women of childbearing age, and their children found a high prevalence of elevated blood lead levels compared with the general US population of whites and African Americans.[31] Evidence suggests that adverse effects of lead exposure occur at BLLs below 10 μg/dL; the threshold for harmful effects of lead exposure has not been determined.[28] The text box on page 144 presents a personal story of how elevated blood lead levels affected one family's child.

Cadmium and Lead

Because cadmium is a common contaminant in lead ores, environmental health researchers often study lead pollution paired with cadmium pollu-

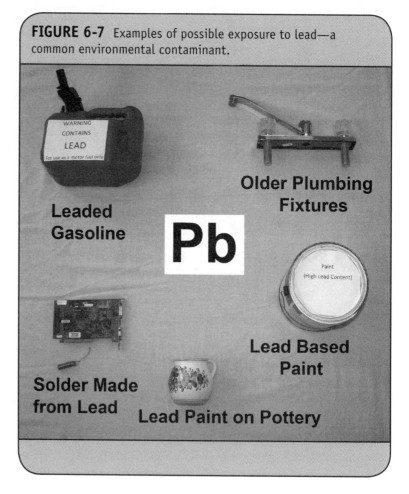

FIGURE 6-7 Examples of possible exposure to lead—a common environmental contaminant.

WARNING
CONTAINS
LEAD
For use as a motor fuel only

Leaded Gasoline

Older Plumbing Fixtures

Pb

Paint
(High Lead Content)

Lead Based Paint

Solder Made from Lead

Lead Paint on Pottery

FIGURE 6-8 A: Lead from peeling paint may compromise the health of infants and children. B: Lead-containing glazes pose a danger if used on dishes or containers intended for food use as lead may leach into the food itself.

A.
Source: © Lowe Chris/Index Stock Imagery, Inc./Alamy Images.

B.
Source: © Photos.com.

Other research has examined the association between lead and cadmium exposure and human reproduction.[34,35] Some studies have reported the occurrence of increased rates of spontaneous abortions and preterm labor among women who live in areas contaminated with lead and cadmium. In sections of eastern Poland known as the Suwalki area, the soil contains high concentrations of lead and cadmium.[34] In addition, residents may be exposed to these heavy metals from air pollution. Nevertheless, the findings regarding the relationship between exposure to lead and cadmium and the

FIGURE 6-9 Transfer of lead from the workplace to the home.

Source: Reprinted from California Department of Health Services, Occupational Lead Poisoning Prevention Program, Childhood Lead Poisoning Branch. Don't Carry Lead into Your House. June 2004.

One Family's Story

In April of 1996, my family and I managed to save enough to buy our own home. Within four months of moving in, our pride and joy evaporated when Samuel, then 10 months old, was diagnosed with a blood lead level of 32 micrograms per deciliter (μg/dL). I soon learned that my son's blood lead level was three times above the limit thought to cause future learning problems. A greater shock was that the lead paint, dust, and soil in and around our treasured home was the culprit.

Worse yet, a month later, Samuel's lead level had risen to 50 μg/dL. He was hospitalized that same afternoon and for three long, agonizing days he stayed in the hospital and began treatment. During Samuel's hospitalization, my husband and I spent many hours attempting to make our home lead safe, all the while keeping vigil over Sam. For nearly 4 years, Sam had his blood tested every two months. We continued to improve our home through repair loans to make it safe. Today, our house has new windows, and lead abatement has been completed on the interior and exterior of our home. Samuel's blood lead level has dropped below 10 μg/dL. To see Samuel, now 4 years old, you would never know what this happy, beautiful little boy has had to endure.

Source: Reprinted from President's Task Force on Environmental Health Risks and Safety Risks to Children. *Eliminating Childhood Lead Poisoning: A Federal Strategy Targeting Lead Paint Hazards.* Washington, DC: US Department of Housing and Urban Development; 2000:3.

frequency of spontaneous abortions have not been established definitively.

Another area where high levels of pollution from lead and cadmium have occurred is in the Asua Valley, which is on the outskirts of Bilbao, Spain.[36] This territory is in the Basque country located in northern Spain. There, during the 1960s through the 1980s, many industries such as foundries and metal-working plants produced air pollution laden with heavy metals. These heavy metals contaminated soil in the food-growing areas. Consequently, residents, both children and adults, ingested very high levels of cadmium and lead,

ranging from almost 200% to almost 700% of the tolerable daily intake of lead for children.

Children who live in areas heavily contaminated with lead and cadmium show concentrations of these metals in their hair and blood.[37] Children from a region known as Upper Silesia in southern Poland were studied for their blood and hair concentrations of lead and cadmium. This region, one of the most highly polluted in the country, contained Poland's largest zinc plant, which was responsible for heavy contamination of the locality with heavy metals. Very high concentrations of heavy metals were found in the bodily tissues of local children, especially among boys. Thought to spend more time outdoors than girls, boys were more likely to have high exposures to heavy metals. Because of high levels of lead and cadmium contamination of the soil in Poland, authorities have recommended that the consumption of foods produced locally, for example, vegetables and potatoes, be reduced.[38]

A Spanish epidemiologic study investigated whether job-related exposure to lead or cadmium was associated with elevated blood pressure levels among two groups of workers in Barcelona.[39] One group was employees who were exposed to lead (e.g., welders); the second group consisted of workers who were exposed to cadmium in pigment and resin factories. Researchers found that workers exposed to lead showed a significant increase in blood pressure, whereas those exposed to high levels of cadmium did not show such an increase. Apparently, in this research, high levels of exposure to these two heavy metals had differential effects upon blood pressure.

Nickel

Classified as a heavy metal, nickel is one of the constituents of the earth's crust. Because of its omnipresence, human exposure to low levels of nickel is probably universal and unavoidable. Nickel has a number of important qualities that make it a valuable metal for use in industry. One of nickel's useful qualities is that it can be machined and polished readily and resists corrosion from nonoxidizing acids and alkalis. It is employed in the production of many of the appliances and tools that are common in everyday life, such as nickel cadmium batteries. Environmental exposures to nickel wastes may occur when nickel cadmium batteries and other nickel-containing metals are discarded.

The occupational environment is a source for significant exposure to nickel. For example, some metal workers risk exposure to nickel and nickel compounds through inhalation or skin contact. One of the common reactions to skin contact with nickel is nickel allergy, manifested as contact dermatitis. Other effects of nickel exposure include cardiovascular-related and renal diseases as well as fibrosis of the lungs. One of the concerns about nickel is its potential carcinogenic action. For example, epidemiologic studies have suggested that nickel miners have a higher incidence of nasal cancer as well as lung cancer than the nonexposed population. Other occupational exposures to nickel occur in the production of nickel through refining, as well as processing the metal via electroplating and welding.

Nickel is present in many different chemical forms, some of which are compounds of nickel and other elements. These compounds are classified as either water-soluble or water-insoluble. The role of nickel compounds as a causal factor in carcinogenesis or as having a role in enhancing the exposure to other carcinogens has not been clearly established.[40] Overall, researchers believe that exposure to low doses of nickel is probably not harmful to human beings.[41]

ESSENTIAL METALS WITH POTENTIAL FOR TOXICITY

Copper, zinc, and iron, examples of metals that are essential for human nutrition, can be toxic if ingested in excessive amounts. An optimal range of these essential metals is necessary to maintain health. When insufficient amounts of these **trace metals** are consumed, dietary deficiencies can result. In fact, if these trace metals are absent from the diet, human beings and other organisms can fail to thrive. The middle range of consumption of essential nutrients is associated with normal health. At the other end of the continuum, when these levels are exceeded, toxic effects and lethality can occur.

Copper

A red-colored metal, copper is present naturally in the earth's rocks and soil. In trace amounts, copper is an essential nutrient. Sometimes copper combines with other elements to form compounds such as copper sulfate, which is characterized by a blue-green color. Elemental copper does not decompose readily in the environment.[42]

Because of its many applications, copper and its various forms have been distributed widely in the environment. Copper appears in electrical wires, pipes, in combination with other metals to form alloys, as a mildew inhibitor, and as a wood and leather preservative. The ATSDR estimates that in the year 2000 alone, approximately 1.4 billion pounds of copper were released into the environment during industrial processing. In addition to the foregoing sources of environmental contamination by copper, others are metal smelting, mining, and waste disposal sites.

Avenues for human exposure to copper include inhalation, ingestion of copper-containing foods and water, and direct contact with the skin. Copper (along with lead) is a potential contaminant of tap water. When tap water stands in copper pipes overnight, small amounts of copper dissolve, causing copper levels to become more concentrated than when the water flows freely. By running the water for approximately half a minute in the morning before use, one can reduce the concentration of copper in the tap water. Workplace exposures to copper arise from breathing dust stirred up by mining and processing copper-rich ore. Other exposures result from inhalation of fumes and dust generated during the welding and grinding of copper metal.

Although copper is an essential nutritional element, at higher levels it is known to produce toxic effects. Exposure to concentrated amounts of copper (far above trace levels) can produce respiratory and gastrointestinal disturbances. The respiratory effects from copper dust include irritation of the respiratory tract (e.g., nose and mouth). The gastrointestinal effects associated with ingestion of copper include vomiting, diarrhea, nausea, and stomach cramping. Very high levels of copper are known to cause liver damage, renal damage, and death. Although it is associated with toxic effects, copper has not been classified as a human carcinogen.

Zinc

A frequently occurring element found in the earth's crust, zinc permeates air, soil, water, and, to some degree, all foods.[43] Zinc is used commercially as a coating for rust inhibition, as a component of batteries, and in combination with other metals to make brass, bronze, and other alloys. Refer to the following text box, which presents possible means of human exposure to zinc. In addition to its commercial uses, zinc is a nutritional element that is important for maintaining health. Among children, inadequate dietary intake of zinc is correlated with low socioeconomic status.[44] In comparison with children from well-to-do families, some poor children have a higher incidence of infectious diseases and other forms of morbidity, which may be related to inadequate intake of zinc.

The metal is believed to play a role in reducing the occurrence of common infections; it is theorized to be necessary for children's growth and for maintaining the health of pregnant women. Also, zinc is thought to influence fetal neurobehavioral development.[44] Inadequate zinc intake during pregnancy may affect the health of the developing fetus adversely, for example, by causing growth retardation. Among adults, insufficient intake of zinc is associated with anorexia, loss of the senses of taste and smell, dermatologic problems, and damage to the immune system.

Excessive levels of zinc exposure, which can have toxic effects, result from the ingestion of contaminated food and

How Might I Be Exposed to Zinc?

- Ingesting small amounts present in your food and water.
- Drinking contaminated water or a beverage that has been stored in metal containers or flows through pipes that have been coated with zinc to resist rust.
- Eating too many dietary supplements that contain zinc.
- Working in any of the following jobs: construction, painting, automobile mechanics, mining, smelting, and welding; manufacture of brass, bronze, or other zinc-containing alloys; manufacture of galvanized metals; and manufacture of machine parts, rubber, paint, linoleum, oilcloths, batteries, some kind[s] of glass, ceramics, and dyes.

Source: Reprinted from Agency for Toxic Substances and Disease Registry (ATSDR). ToxFAQs for Zinc. August 2005 (updated on 02/18/2010). Available at: http://www.atsdr.cdc.gov/tfacts60.html. Accessed March 16, 2010.

water and from inhalation of zinc dusts in occupational environments. Excessive amounts of zinc, defined as beginning at 10 to 15 times the levels required to maintain health, are thought to affect the normal functioning of blood-forming organs, biochemical processes, and the endocrine system. The consumption of large quantities of zinc is associated with gastrointestinal problems such as stomach cramps, nausea, and vomiting. Zinc also can cause anemia and damage to the pancreas. Children and pregnant women are at special risk for the toxic effects of zinc. These groups should use care in taking zinc as a nutritional supplement or for self-medication.[45] Breathing high concentrations of zinc in the workplace causes a disease known as metal fume fever. This condition appears to be an immune-mediated response that originates in the lungs.

Iron

Iron is one of the most ubiquitous metals in the earth's crust. Vital to human health, iron is important to the growth of cells and the transport of oxygen within the circulatory system. About 66% of the iron in the body is used in hemoglobin, the red blood cell protein responsible for transporting oxygen. Well-known symptoms of anemia (deficiency of hemoglobin) include fatigue and lowered immunity. Figure 6-10 demonstrates the lower eyelid (conjunctiva) of a child suspected of having anemia, a condition that causes the conjunctiva to appear white.

Iron has the capacity to accumulate in the body, because little is excreted during metabolic processes. The disease known as hemachromatosis is associated with iron toxicity from excessive buildup of iron. Excessive amounts of iron can have toxic effects, such as vomiting, diarrhea, and damage to the intestines. Iron toxicity also may produce low blood pressure, lethargy, neurologic effects including seizures, and liver injury. Among those at greatest risk of iron toxicity are children. Acute iron intoxication (accidental iron poisoning) is among the most common childhood poisonings. Poisoning incidents sometimes occur when children accidentally swallow mineral supplements that contain concentrated amounts of iron. Other groups at risk from iron overload (iron toxicity) include adult men and postmenopausal women.

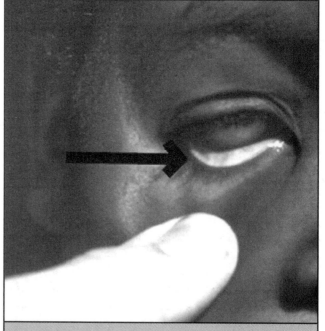

FIGURE 6-10 An EIS officer examining the palpebral conjunctiva of a Nigerian child suspected of having anemia.

Source: Adapted and reprinted courtesy of the CDC Public Health Image Library. ID#6900. CDC/Dr. Lyle Conrad content provider. Available at: http://phil.cdc.gov/Phil/detail.asp. Accessed August 28, 2010.

METALS FOR USE IN MEDICAL THERAPY

Metals in this group, which include aluminum, bismuth, gold, and lithium, are used for medical and other purposes. Aluminum is contained in medicines, for example, certain antacids. Because of its numerous useful properties and possible association with Alzheimer's disease, aluminum is discussed more fully in the following section.

Aluminum

The silver-white metal aluminum is used widely in food and beverage containers, in pots and pans, and in construction sites. Aluminum is an ingredient in various medicines and cosmetics, for example, to buffer aspirin and in antiperspirants. As a result of its widespread use, human exposure to aluminum is almost universal. One of the direct effects of exposure to aluminum dust is respiratory problems such as coughing or exacerbation of asthma. Low levels of aluminum exposure are not thought to be harmful.[46] The following text box provides information on sources of exposure to aluminum.

Aluminum has been studied as a factor that may be linked to Alzheimer's disease. Aluminum is known to be a powerful neurotoxicant.[47] The role of aluminum as a factor in the pathogenesis of Alzheimer's disease remains unconfirmed. One study reported an association between aluminum concentration in drinking water and Alzheimer's disease. The authors of this report suggested that the amount of residual aluminum in public drinking water supplies should be limited.[48] Another study reported an association between exposure to aluminum contained in intravenous feeding solutions and impaired neurologic development among preterm infants.[49] The ATSDR states, "Some people with kidney disease store a lot of aluminum in their bodies and sometimes develop bone or brain diseases which may be caused by the excess aluminum. Some studies show that people exposed to high levels of aluminum may develop Alzheimer's disease, but other studies have not found this to be true. We do not know for certain whether aluminum causes Alzheimer's disease."[46] There also have been some associations of large doses of aluminum with skeletal problems and the development of rashes among people who use deodorants containing aluminum compounds.

CONCLUSION

Many heavy metals and other metallic compounds occur almost universally in the environment, either in the earth's crust or as a result of human activities. Consequently, the entire

How Might I Be Exposed to Aluminum?

- Virtually all food, water, air, and soil contain some aluminum.
- The average adult in the US eats about 7–9 mg aluminum per day in his or her food.
- Breathing higher levels of aluminum dust in workplace air.
- Living in areas where the air is dusty, where aluminum is mined or processed into aluminum metal, near certain hazardous waste sites, or where aluminum is naturally high.
- Eating substances containing high levels of aluminum (such as antacids) especially when eating or drinking citrus products at the same time.
- Children and adults may be exposed to small amounts of aluminum from vaccinations.
- Very little enters your body from aluminum cooking utensils.

Source: Adapted and reprinted from Agency for Toxic Substances and Disease Registry (ATSDR). ToxFAQs for Aluminum. September 2008 (updated 02/18/2010). Available at: http://www.atsdr.cdc.gov/tfacts22.html. Accessed March 16, 2010.

human population is exposed at one time or another to these metals. Although some metals in trace levels are essential for human nutrition, the same metals are toxic at higher levels. Other metals are toxic even at low levels of exposure. For example, arsenic, lead, and mercury are among the top three hazardous substances identified in ATSDR's CERCLA Priority List of Hazardous Substances. Arsenic, a potential carcinogen, is found in high concentrations in the drinking water of some areas of the world. Lead is of concern because of its adverse impact upon the health of children. Mercury, which is associated with neurologic disease, has been identified increasingly as a contaminant of fish and other foodstuffs. An important role for environmental policy makers is to reduce the level of toxic metals in the environment (e.g., air, water, and soil) and in foods, which may constitute an important avenue of exposure of the human population to these metals.

Study Questions and Exercises

1. Define and give examples of the following terms:
   a. Heavy metal
   b. "Itai-itai byo"
   c. Minamata disease
   d. Trace metals

2. Name the four categories of metals. Give an example of a metal from each category.

3. Why is lead contamination a concern for environmental health experts?

4. Name some of the portals of entry into the human body for toxic metals. Describe the methods by which these toxic metals may access specific portals of entry.

5. Give some examples of environmental sources of exposure of populations to toxic heavy metals.

6. Exposure to heavy metals presents a serious hazard to children.
   a. Give an example of a heavy metal that children commonly are exposed to in our environment.
   b. List the symptoms of exposure to this heavy metal among children.
   c. List the long-term effects of this heavy metal on children.

7. State two incidents of mass poisonings of humans that involved arsenic.

8. Provide the following information regarding cadmium:
   a. Possible sources of exposure
   b. Modes of entry into the body
   c. Two major health effects
   d. Name of an associated disease

9. Provide the following information regarding chromium:
   a. Where it occurs in the environment
   b. Its effects on human health
   c. Who is Erin Brockovich?

10. What are some of the medical uses of mercury?

11. Provide the following information regarding lead:
   a. Sources of exposure in the environment
   b. Adverse health effects of exposure to lead

12. Provide the following information regarding nickel:
   a. Two uses of nickel
   b. Two adverse effects of exposure to nickel

13. Name the metals that are essential for human nutrition.

14. How can you reduce your exposure to copper in tap water?

15. Describe the importance of iron to human health. Describe the side effects of ingesting excessive amounts of iron.

16. List at least three sources of exposure to aluminum. Describe the hypothesized association of aluminum and Alzheimer's disease.

REFERENCES

1. Agency for Toxic Substances and Disease Registry (ATSDR). CERCLA priority list of hazardous substances. Available at: http://www.atsdr.cdc.gov/cercla/index.html. Accessed March 24, 2010.

2. US Environmental Protection Agency. Terms of Environment: Glossary: N. Available at: http://www.epa.gov/OCEPAterms/nterms.html. Accessed March 5, 2010.

3. Goyer RA, Clarkson TW. Toxic effects of metals. In: Klaassen CD, ed. *Casarett and Doull's Toxicology: The Basic Science of Poisons.* 6th ed. New York, NY: McGraw-Hill; 2001:811–867.

4. Answers.com. Dictionary: specific gravity. Available at: http://www.answers.com/topic/specific-gravity. Accessed February 16, 2010.

5. Mercury Safety Products Ltd. Mercury toxicity and how it affects our health. Available at: http://www.mercurysafety.co.uk/hlthinfo.htm. Accessed February 16, 2010.

6. Vahter M, Berglund M, Akesson A, et al. Metals and women's health. *Environ Res.* 2002;88(3):145–155.

7. Wulff M, Högberg U, Stenlund H. Occupational and environmental risks of spontaneous abortions around a smelter. *Am J Ind Med.* 2002;41:131–138.

8. Stein J, Schettler T, Wallinga D, et al. In harm's way: toxic threats to child development. *J Dev Behav Pediatr.* 2002;23:S13–S22.

9. Peters GR, McCurdy RF, Hindmarsh JT. Environmental aspects of arsenic toxicity. *Crit Rev Clin Lab Sci.* 1996;33:457–493.

10. Jager JW, Ostrosky-Wegman P. Arsenic: a paradoxical human carcinogen. *Mutat Res.* 1997;386:181–184.

11. Brown KG, Ross GL. Arsenic, drinking water, and health: a position paper of the American Council on Science and Health. *Regul Toxicol Pharmacol.* 2002;36:162–174.

12. Rahman MM, Chowdhury UK, Mukherjee SC, et al. Chronic arsenic toxicity in Bangladesh and West Bengal, India—a review and commentary. *J Toxicol Clin Toxicol.* 2001;39:683–700.

13. Cantor KP. Arsenic in drinking water: how much is too much? [Editorial] *Epidemiol.* 1996;7:113–115.

14. Hopenhayn-Rich C, Biggs ML, Fuchs A, et al. Bladder cancer mortality associated with arsenic in drinking water in Argentina. *Epidemiol.* 1996;7:117–124.

15. Abernathy CO, Liu Y-P, Longfellow D, et al. Arsenic: health effects, mechanisms of actions, and research issues. *Environ Health Perspect.* 1999;107:593–597.

16. Ahmad SA, Sayed SU, Barua S, et al. Arsenic in drinking water and pregnancy outcomes. *Environ Health Perspect.* 2001;109:629–631.

17. Taylor TP, Ding M, Ehler DS, et al. Beryllium in the environment: a review. *J Environ Sci Health.* 2003;A38:439–469.

18. Agency for Toxic Substances and Disease Registry (ATSDR). ToxFAQs for cadmium. September 2008. Available at: http://www.atsdr.cdc.gov/tfacts5.html. Accessed February 16, 2010.

19. Great Lakes Environmental Center. 2000 update of ambient water quality criteria for cadmium (draft). Prepared for US Environmental Protection Agency. EPA Contract No. 68-C-98-134; 2000.

20. Järup L. Cadmium overload and toxicity. *Nephrol Dial Transplant.* 2002;17(suppl 2):35–39.

21. Staessen JA, Lauweyrs RR, Ide G, et al. Renal function and historical environmental cadmium pollution from zinc smelters. *Lancet.* 1994;343:1523–1527.

22. Staessen J, Amery A, Bernard A, et al. Blood pressure, the prevalence of cardiovascular diseases, and exposure to cadmium: a population study. *Am J Epidemiol.* 1991;134:257–267.

23. ICETT. Preventative measures against water pollution: 2. Itai-itai disease. Available at: http://www.icett.or.jp/lpca_jp.nsf/0/b30e2e489f4b4ff1492567ca0011ff90?OpenDocument. Accessed February 16, 2010.

24. Morikawa Y, Nakagawa H, Tabata M, et al. Study of an outbreak of itai-itai disease. [In Japanese] *Nippon Eiseigaku Zasshi.* 1992;46:1057–1062.

25. Agency for Toxic Substances and Disease Registry (ATSDR). ToxFAQs for chromium. September 2008. Available at: http://www.atsdr.cdc.gov/tfacts7.html. Accessed February 16, 2010.

26. Agency for Toxic Substances and Disease Registry (ATSDR). Public health statement for mercury. March 1999. Available at: http://www.atsdr.cdc.gov/toxprofiles/phs46.html. Accessed February 16, 2010.

27. Powell PP. Minamata disease: a story of mercury's malevolence. *South Med J.* 1991;84:1352–1358.

28. Meyer PA, Pivetz T, Dignam TA, et al. Surveillance for elevated blood lead levels among children—United States, 1997–2001. In: *Surveillance Summaries,* September 12, 2003. *MMWR.* 2003;52(No. SS-10):1–9.

29. President's Task Force on Environmental Health Risks and Safety Risks to Children. *Eliminating Childhood Lead Poisoning: A Federal Strategy Targeting Lead Paint Hazards.* Washington, DC: US Department of Housing and Urban Development; 2000.

30. Sciarillo WG, Alexander G, Farrell KP. Lead exposure and child behavior. *Am J Public Health.* 1992;82:1356–1360.

31. Flanigan GD Jr, Mayfield R, Blumenthal HT. Studies on lead exposure in patients of a neighborhood health center: Part II. A comparison of women of childbearing age and children. *J Natl Med Assoc.* 1992;84:23–27.

32. Paoliello MM, De Capitani EM, da Cunha FG, et al. Exposure of children to lead and cadmium from a mining area of Brazil. *Environ Res.* 2002;88(2):120–128.

33. Meyer I, Heinrich J, Lippold U. Factors affecting lead and cadmium levels in house dust in industrial areas of eastern Germany. *Sci Total Environ.* 1999;234:25–36.

34. Laudanski T, Sipowicz M, Modzelewski P, et al. Influence of high lead and cadmium soil content on human reproductive outcome. *Int J Gynecol Obstet.* 1991;36:309–315.

35. Fagher U, Laudanski T, Schütz A, et al. The relationship between cadmium and lead burdens and preterm labor. *Int J Gynecol Obstet.* 1993;40:109–114.

36. Alonso E, Cambra K, Martinez T. Lead and cadmium exposure from contaminated soil among residents of a farm area near an industrial site. *Arch Environ Health.* 2001;56:278–282.

37. Chlopicka J, Zachwieja Z, Zagrodzki P, et al. Lead and cadmium in the hair and blood of children from a highly industrial area in Poland. *Biol Trace Elem Res.* 1998;62:229–234.

38. Gzyl J. Assessment of Polish population exposure to lead and cadmium with special emphasis to the Katowice province on the basis of metal concentrations in environmental compartments. *Cent Eur J Public Health.* 1997;5(2):93–96.

39. Schuhmacher M, Bosque MA, Domingo JL, et al. Effects of chronic lead and cadmium exposure on blood pressure in occupationally exposed workers. *Biol Trace Elem Res.* 1994;41:269–278.

40. Oller AR. Respiratory carcinogenicity assessment of soluble nickel compounds. *Environ Health Perspect.* 2002;110(suppl 5):841–844.

41. Denkhaus E, Salnikow K. Nickel essentiality, toxicity, and carcinogenicity. *Crit Rev Oncol Hematol.* 2002;42:35–56.

42. Agency for Toxic Substances and Disease Registry (ATSDR). Public health statement for copper. September 2004. Available at: http://www.atsdr.cdc.gov/toxprofiles/phs132.html. Accessed February 16, 2010.

43. Agency for Toxic Substances and Disease Registry (ATSDR). ToxFAQs for zinc. August 2005. Available at: http://www.atsdr.cdc.gov/tfacts60.html. Accessed February 16, 2010.

44. Hotz C, Lowe NM, Araya M, et al. Assessment of the trace element status of individuals and populations: the example of zinc and copper. *J Nutr.* 2003;133(5 suppl 1):1563S–1568S.

45. Piao F, Yokoyama K, Ma N, et al. Subacute toxic effects of zinc on various tissues and organs of rats. *Toxicol Lett.* 2003;145(1):28–35.

46. Agency for Toxic Substances and Disease Registry (ATSDR). Tox-FAQs for aluminum. September 2008 (updated 02/18/2010). Available at: http://www.atsdr.cdc.gov/tfacts22.html. Accessed March 5, 2010.

47. Flaten TP. Aluminum as a risk factor in Alzheimer's disease, with emphasis on drinking water. *Brain Res Bull*. 2001;55:187–196.

48. McLachlan DRC, Bergeron C, Smith JE, et al. Risk for neuropathologically confirmed Alzheimer's disease and residual aluminum in municipal drinking water employing weighted residential histories. *Neurology*. 1996;46:401–405.

49. Bishop NJ, Morley R, Day JP, et al. Aluminum neurotoxicity in preterm infants receiving intravenous-feeding solutions. *New Engl J Med*. 1997;336:1557–1561.

CHAPTER 7

Pesticides and Other Organic Chemicals

LEARNING OBJECTIVES

By the end of this chapter the reader will be able to:

- List common substances that are included in the organophosphate group
- Name three commonly used insecticides and one commonly used herbicide
- Discuss the health effects of exposure to pesticides
- Name one chemical used in the manufacture of plastics
- Describe the potential health effects of exposure to household cleaning products

---

INTRODUCTION

This chapter covers **pesticides** and other **organic chemicals**, which include many types of solvents, substances used in the manufacture of plastics, and home cleaning products. The category of solvents alone encompasses a great number of chemicals[1] as does the category of pesticides. Throughout this chapter you will learn about some of these chemicals and examine their impact on the environment. We will review situations in which first responders to chemical accidents are confronted with the practical issue of how to protect the environment, the public, and themselves from potentially toxic substances.

Hazardous chemicals, omnipresent in the environment, are vital to society yet simultaneously raise the specter of potential harm to all living organisms on earth. One expert has stated, "The ubiquity of toxic substances in the environment continues to be a significant public health concern. Body burdens of chemicals such as dioxins, methyl mercury, PCBs, and

a range of the 'usual suspects' are the increasingly represented norm rather than the exception in the US population."[2(pA374)] The National Center for Environmental Health, a branch of the Centers for Disease Control and Prevention (CDC), developed an inventory of biomonitoring exposure data for 212 environmental chemicals to which the noninstitutionalized, civilian US population was exposed over a six-year period ranging from 1999 through 2004.[3] Although it would seem that the population has had declining levels of exposure to environmental chemicals, "serious concerns remain regarding the exposure of the population to a wide spectrum of chemicals in the environment."[2(pA374)] The Fourth National Report on Human Exposure to Environmental Chemicals reported widespread exposure to chemicals found in fire retardants, bisphenol A (BPA), plastics, and nonstick coatings used in cookware.[3]

Advantages and Disadvantages of Hazardous Chemicals

One should take a balanced view of the advantages and disadvantages of hazardous chemicals. First consider the advantages: Although chemicals have the potential to cause harm, they are essential to the functioning of modern society. In fact, humanity could not live without them. According to the National Institute of Environmental Health Sciences (NIEHS):

> Chemicals are the basis of our way of life—and health—today. There are about 15,000 chemicals made and used in high volume in the United States. (. . . when we roast coffee for our morning jump-start, we end up with more than 1,000

Surveillance for Emergency Events Involving Hazardous Substances—United States, 1990–1992

State health departments in selected states collect and each quarter transmit information about the events, substances released, and the public health consequences of hazardous substance releases (i.e., morbidity, mortality, and evacuations) to the Agency for Toxic Substances and Disease Registry (ATSDR). Five state health departments (Colorado, Iowa, Michigan, New Hampshire, and Wisconsin) began data collection on January 1, 1990. On January 1, 1992, the reporting state health departments included those from Colorado, Iowa, New Hampshire, New York, North Carolina, Oregon, Rhode Island, Washington, and Wisconsin. . . .

During 1990–1992, 3,125 events were reported from participating states to ATSDR's Hazardous Substances Emergency Events Surveillance (HSEES) system. Of these events, 2,391 (77%) were fixed-facility events (i.e., occurred at stationary facilities), and 723 (23%) were transportation-related. In 88% of events, a single chemical was released. The most frequently released hazardous substances were **volatile organic compounds** (18% of the total 4,034 substances released), herbicides (15%), acids (14%), and ammonias (11%). In 467 events (15% of all events), 1,446 persons were injured; 11 persons died as a result of these injuries. Respiratory irritation (37%) and eye irritation (23%) were the most frequently reported health effects. A total of 457 (15%) events resulted in evacuations; of these, 400 (88%) were ordered by an official (e.g., a police officer or firefighter). The median number of persons evacuated was 25 (range: from 12 to greater than 9,999 persons). Evacuations lasted an average of 9.4 hours (median: 3 hours; range: 1–240 hours). [Refer to Table 7-1 for a list of substances released during emergency events that involved hazardous substances.]

TABLE 7-1 Substances Released during All Hazardous Substances Emergency Events and during All Such Events Resulting in Personal Injury,[a] by Chemical Category—Selected States,[b] Hazardous Substances Emergency Events Surveillance, 1990–1992

| | Substances released | | | | |
| | During all events | | During events resulting in personal injury | | |
Substance category	No.	(%)[c]	No.	(%)[d]	(%)[e]
Volatile organic compounds	727	(18)	93	(12)	(13)
Herbicides	588	(15)	126	(16)	(21)
Acids	553	(14)	148	(19)	(27)
Ammonias	448	(11)	103	(13)	(23)
Metals	261	(7)	21	(3)	(8)
Insecticides	217	(5)	80	(10)	(37)
Polychlorinated biphenyls	212	(5)	6	(1)	(3)
Bases	152	(4)	40	(5)	(26)
Chlorine	157	(4)	43	(6)	(27)
Cyanides	21	(1)	9	(1)	(43)
Unclassified	698	(17)	108	(14)	(15)
Total	4,034	(100)	777	(100)	

[a]Refers to injuries and all other adverse health effects.

[b]During 1990–1991, participating states included Colorado, Iowa, Michigan, New Hampshire, and Wisconsin. During 1992, participating states included Colorado, Iowa, New Hampshire, New York, North Carolina, Oregon, Rhode Island, Washington, and Wisconsin.

[c]Percentage of all substances released.

[d]Percentage of all substances released during events that resulted in personal injury.

[e]Within the substance category, the percentage of substances released during events that resulted in personal injury.

Source: Adapted and reprinted from Centers for Disease Control and Prevention. *CDC Surveillance Summaries*, Surveillance for emergency events involving hazardous substances—United States, 1990–1992. *MMWR.* 1994;43(SS-2):1,4.

chemicals right there in our cup!) And there are many natural products—herbal products, for example—that have become widely marketed and used without testing.

Synthetic chemicals, used on our farms, not only help feed us cheaply and well, they help feed much of the rest of the world as well. Chemical fibers clothe us. Chemicals cure us. They form key parts of our cars and our phones and computers, many building materials, rugs and other furnishings—you name it. Little wonder that US production of these synthetic chemicals has climbed, almost without pause, from 10 million pounds in 1918 to well over 300 billion pounds in recent years.[4]

Regarding the disadvantages of hazardous chemicals, some (e.g., those called PCBs and dioxins) have been implicated as human health hazards, for example, in the etiology of cancer and adverse birth outcomes. As another, more extreme, example, consider the public's anxiety surrounding the alleged use of chemical weapons during the 1991 Persian Gulf War. Some of the returning soldiers developed symptoms of what came to be known as the "Gulf War Syndrome." Were the symptoms (e.g., multiple chemical sensitivity, chronic fatigue syndrome, and fibromyalgia) reported by afflicted veterans attributable to exposure to chemical weapons, or could other explanations account for those symptoms?

Silent Spring, the classic work by Rachel Carson, is credited with sensitizing the public to the potential hazards of chemicals that were being disseminated into the environment.[5] This issue continues to be a cause for alarm. On a typical day, people encounter numerous chemicals, many of which are known to be injurious to human health and the environment. A large percentage of these chemicals have not been tested at all. Possible adverse health consequences that have been linked to those chemicals that have been tested include impairment of fertility and reproductive outcomes, psychological and behavioral deficits such as autism, and carcinogenesis. The Environmental Protection Agency (EPA) expanded its effort to measure the blood and urine concentrations of chemicals by increasing the number from 116 to 148 chemicals; these include several of the major pesticides and organic chemicals. According to a 2005 report from EPA, the levels of three organochlorine pesticides (aldrin, endrin, and dieldrin) are low or undetectable in the United States population.[6] The fact that the levels of these three pesticides are low (due to their discontinued use) reflects progress in the control of toxic chemicals. Another

concern relates to the impact of accidental spills and releases of toxic chemicals (for example, by illegal methamphetamine labs) and how first responders must be prepared to cope with these events (refer to the text box "Illicit Methamphetamine Laboratories").

Terms Used to Describe Organic Chemicals

Table 7-2 lists some definitions that will be helpful in reading the chapter.

CHEMICALS AMONG THE TOP 20 IN THE ATSDR LIST OF 275 HAZARDOUS SUBSTANCES

Referring back to the list of hazardous substances presented in Chapter 6, among the most important chemical hazards identified by the ATSDR are:

- Polychlorinated biphenyls (PCBs)—Used in electrical cable insulation and transformers.
- Benzene—Used as a solvent in the manufacture of plastics and other materials and as a constituent of fuels.
- Polycyclic aromatic hydrocarbons (PAHs)—Individual members of the ATSDR list; they include benzo(a)pyrene (BaP), benzo(b)fluoranthene, and dibenzo(a,h)anthracene. PAHs are not used commercially. As noted previously, they result from incomplete combustion of petroleum-based chemicals and other organic substances.
- Chloroform—Formerly used as an anesthetic; now used to manufacture other chemicals.
- DDT; DDT, p, p' (DDT, p, p' is one of the synonyms for DDT)—Used as an insecticide. (DDT no longer is used as an insecticide in the United States.)
- Aroclor 1254 and Aroclor 1260—Both are a type of polychlorinated biphenyl (PCB); used in electrical transformers and other applications such as hydraulic fluids, plastics manufacture, and pesticide extenders.
- Trichloroethylene (TCE)—A solvent used by industries and the military.
- Dieldrin—Used as a pesticide.
- Chlordane—Used as a pesticide.

PESTICIDES

Until the middle of the 18th century, control of insects was accomplished by manually removing them or by using inorganic poisons that frequently were not very effective. Inorganic chemicals used in the past included compounds of sulfur, zinc, copper, mercury, lead, and arsenic (i.e., arsenicals) in addition to boric acid. These substances formed the arsenal of **pest** control weapons.

TABLE 7-2 30-Second Organic Chemistry Lesson

Term	Definition
Aromatic compound	An organic molecule that contains a benzene ring, for example, benzene and toluene.[a]
Hydrocarbon	An organic compound (as acetylene, benzene, or butane) containing only carbon and hydrogen and often occurring in petroleum, natural gas, coal, and bitumens.[b]
Organic chemicals/compounds	Naturally occurring (animal or plant-produced or synthetic) substances containing carbon, hydrogen, nitrogen, and oxygen.[c] Example: table sugar
Persistent organic pollutants (POPs)	Toxic chemicals that adversely affect human health and the environment around the world. Because they can be transported by wind and water, most POPs generated in one country can and do affect people and wildlife far from where they are used and released. They persist for long periods of time in the environment and can accumulate and pass from one species to the next through the food chain.[d] Example: the pesticide DDT
Polycyclic aromatic hydrocarbons (PAHs)	A group of over 100 different chemicals that are formed during the incomplete burning of coal, oil and gas, garbage, or other organic substances like tobacco or charbroiled meat.[e]
Volatile organic compounds (VOCs)	Organic compounds that evaporate readily into the air. VOCs include substances such as benzene, toluene, methylene chloride, and methyl chloroform.[f]

Source: [a]About.com. Chemistry. Aromatic compound definition. Available at: http://chemistry.about.com/od/chemistry/glossary/a/aromaticcmpndef.htm. Accessed March 30, 2010.

[b]Medline Plus */Merriam-Webster. Medical Dictionary. Available at: http://www.merriam-webster.com/medlineplus/hydrocarbon. Accessed March 30, 2010.

[c]US Environmental Protection Agency. Terms of environment: Glossary. Available at: http://www.epa.gov/OCEPAterms/oterms.html. Accessed March 30, 2010.

[d]US Environmental Protection Agency. Persistent organic pollutants: A global issue, a global response. Available at: http://www.epa.gov/international/toxics/pop.htm. Accessed March 30, 2010.

[e]Agency for Toxic Substances and Disease Registry (ATSDR). ToxFAQs: Polycyclic Aromatic Hydrocarbons (PAHs). Available at http://www.atsdr.cdc.gov/toxfaq.html. Accessed March 30, 2010.

[f]Agency for Toxic Substances and Disease Registry (ATSDR). Glossary of terms. Available at: http://atsdr.cdc.gov/glossary.html. Accessed March 30, 2010.

Chapter 7 will cover pesticides that are derived from organic chemicals; an example is organophosphate pesticides. The "Golden Age of Discovery" of insecticides occurred in the mid-1900s, with the invention of neuroactive chemicals, such as chlorinated hydrocarbons, organophosphates, methylcarbamates, and pyrethroids.[7] (These terms are defined later in the chapter.) About the middle of the 20th century, use of the pesticide DDT was purported to have led to a complete victory over harmful insects. However, by the 1970s, use of DDT was restricted in the United States because of concerns about this chemical's effects on health and the environment. A significant question for environmental policy is "How should society regulate pesticide use to ensure a bountiful harvest of diverse crops that is needed for a healthy diet while, at the same time, making sure that pesticide uses do not have adverse effects on health?"[8(p725)]

On a global scale, estimates of annual use of pesticides are about 3 million metric tons; the United States alone accounts for about 1.2 billion pounds of this total.[8] According to the US Department of Agriculture,

> Pesticides are a vital input in today's agriculture, protecting food and fiber from damage by insects, weeds, diseases, nematodes, and rodents. US agriculture spends about 8 billion dollars annually on pesticides—about 70 percent of all pesticides sold in the country. It is estimated that each dollar invested in pesticide control returns approximately 4 dollars in crops saved. Nevertheless, pests still destroy nearly 13 percent of all potential food and fiber crops in the US Farmers' expenditures on pesticides are about 4–5 percent of total farm production costs.[9]

Sometimes the term *pesticide* is used interchangeably by the public with **insecticide**.[10] Nevertheless, these terms relate to distinct purposes. A pesticide is "any substance or mixture

Illicit Methamphetamine Laboratories

Methamphetamine, a central nervous system stimulant, is manufactured in illicit laboratories using over-the-counter ingredients. . . . Many of these ingredients are hazardous substances . . . that when released from active or abandoned methamphetamine laboratories can place first responders . . . at risk for serious injuries and death. . . .

Washington
In April 1996, an oven exploded as two persons were using acetone, hydrochloric acid, and sodium hydroxide to manufacture methamphetamine in an illicit apartment laboratory; one person sustained chemical burns and was taken to a hospital emergency department. The source of the burns was not revealed and, as a result, three hospital employees had nausea and vomited while treating the person. Three emergency medical technicians (EMTs) and two police officers exposed to emissions from the fire had eye and respiratory irritation. None of the injured first responders was wearing personal protective equipment (PPE) at the time of injury.

Oregon
In February 1999, a firefighter sustained chemical burns after exposure to hydrochloric acid and ephedrine during a fire at an illicit methamphetamine laboratory in a house in a residential neighborhood. Chemicals and other drug-manufacturing paraphernalia used to make methamphetamine were found after the fire was extinguished. The firefighter, who had worn turn-out gear [protective clothing] . . . as PPE at the time of injury, was decontaminated at the site, treated at a local hospital, and released.

Iowa
In March 1999, three police officers had respiratory irritation after exposure to anhydrous ammonia and ether emissions during a raid of an illicit residential methamphetamine laboratory. The officers were decontaminated at the site, treated at a local hospital, and released. They had not worn PPE at the time of injury.

Source: Adapted and reprinted from the Centers for Disease Control and Prevention. Public health consequences among first responders to emergency events associated with illicit methamphetamine laboratories—selected states, 1996–1999. *MMWR.* 2000;49:1021–1022.

of substances intended for preventing, destroying, repelling, or mitigating pests. Pests can be insects, rodents, weeds, and a host of other unwanted organisms. . . . Pesticides are usually divided on the basis of their target. The major classes are insecticides, herbicides, rodenticides, and fungicides."[11(p251)] In contrast with pesticides, insecticides are pesticide compounds that are used specifically to control insects. Table 7-3 presents definitions of terms that are related to the category of agents (i.e., pesticides) presented in this section.

Pesticides are applied by a number of methods including spraying from tractors and widespread broadcasting by aerial spraying, as shown in Figure 7-1.

Classes of Pesticides and Insecticides

Several categories of pesticides are in use at present; these include some types of inorganic chemicals; organic chemicals; and a variety of other substances including insecticidal soaps, contraceptives, insect growth regulators and hormones, as well as warfarin (an anticoagulant for control of rodents).

Four major classes of pesticides and insecticides are derived from organic chemicals: **organophosphates (OPs)**, organo-carbamates (also called carbamates), organochlorides (also known as **organochlorines**), and pyrethroids (from the class of pyrethrins).[12] Other chemicals not included in these classes are used as pesticides, such as chloropicrin (covered later in this chapter). Chloropicrin is an unclassified pesticide used as a soil fumigant.

Because they do not appear to persist in the environment, pesticides from the OP group are among those chosen most widely for agricultural purposes; yet, at the same time, OPs are among the most common sources of pesticide poisoning. Similarly, another group of so-called nonpersistent pesticides are the carbamates group, an example being aldicarb. Although pesticides of the OP class are implicated frequently in fatal poisoning incidents, carbamates are rarely a source of mortality from poisoning. Most of the pesticides from the third group, organochlorines, have been banned in the United States because of their propensity to remain in the environment.

TABLE 7-3 Definition of Pesticide and Related Terms

Term	Definition
Pesticide	Substances or mixture thereof intended for preventing, destroying, repelling, or mitigating any pest. Also, any substance or mixture intended for use as a plant regulator, defoliant, or desiccant.
Insecticide	A pesticide compound specifically used to kill or prevent the growth of insects.
Herbicide	A chemical pesticide designed to control or destroy plants, weeds, or grasses.
Fungicide	A pesticide that is used to control, deter, or destroy fungi.
Nematocide	A chemical agent that is destructive to nematodes.
Rodenticide	A chemical or agent used to destroy rats or other rodent pests, or to prevent them from damaging food, crops, etc.
Fumigant	A pesticide vaporized to kill pests. Used in buildings and greenhouses.

Source: Adapted and reprinted from US Environmental Protection Agency. Terms of Environment: Glossary. Available at: http://www.epa.gov/OCEPAterms/. Accessed March 31, 2010.

FIGURE 7-1 Helicopter spraying of Central Valley orchard crops during cold weather, when the trees are dormant, kills overwintering arthropod pests (such as scales and mites) and diseases. However, the organophosphate insecticides used as dormant sprays cause problems when drift occurs or when rainfall washes residues into rivers and streams.

Source: Reprinted from California Department of Pesticide Regulation. Dormant Spray Water Quality Initiative. Available at: http://www.cdpr.ca.gov/docs/emon/dormspray/. Accessed March 31, 2010.

The fourth group, pyrethrins, refers to an organic insecticide obtained from naturally occurring sources; often, pesticides derived from such natural sources are called botanicals. The insecticides from the pyrethrin group are useful for controlling insects and also have low toxicity for mammals.

Organophosphate Pesticides (Anticholinesterases)

In 1998, the EPA estimated that each year in the US the agricultural usage of organophosphates totaled 60 million pounds, which were spread on 38 million acres of cropland. An additional 17 million pounds were utilized for nonagricultural purposes.[13] (The use of OPs has declined during the 21st century in many states, as lower-risk alternatives have been implemented.) The agricultural uses of OPs are for control of insect pests on crops in fields, orchards, and vegetable plots. Nonagricultural uses include control of insects in homes, offices, and outdoors; for example, OP pesticides are used for mosquito and termite abatement. The popularity of OP pesticides arises from the facts that they are (1) inexpensive in comparison to alternatives; (2) can be used to control a wide range of insects, thus eliminating the need for multiple applications of different pesticides; and (3) have not been weakened by the resistance of insects. In addition, OPs tend not to persist in the environment.

Organophosphate pesticides are related to "nerve gases" such as sarin, soman, and tabun. In March 1995, the Aum Shinrikyo cult released sarin gas into the Tokyo subway system during the morning rush hour. As a result, 12 people died and 5,500 were injured.[14] In common with nerve gases, OP pesticides act on the nervous systems of insects and higher organisms by disrupting the transmission of nerve impulses. This effect occurs when OPs reduce the ability of the enzyme cholinesterase to regulate the neurotransmitter acetylcholine, which aids in cell-to-cell transfer of nerve impulses.[11]

Organophosphate poisoning can produce both acute and long-term effects. In the former case, the anticholinesterase activity happens soon after exposure and causes impairment of the neural impulse transfer mechanism. A group of immediate symptoms may occur: Nerves and muscles may become uncoordinated, producing respiratory paralysis and weakness; neurological symptoms may include seizures and loss of consciousness; cramping of the abdominal area may occur; and in extreme cases, death may ensue. The effects of long-term exposure may include a condition known as organophosphate-induced delayed polyneuropathy, which is manifested by numbness, loss of sensory abilities, and weakness. Clinicians believe that in most cases this delayed form of polyneuropathy is irreversible.

Examples of OP pesticides are diazinon, malathion, methyl parathion, and parathion. Pesticides from the organophosphate group appear in a wide variety of products: sprays, baits, indoor foggers and bombs, flea collars, pet shampoos, powders, animal dips, and granules. Some OP pesticides (e.g., malathion) are approved for direct application to food crops such as fruits (e.g., apples and grapes), row crops, and vegetables (e.g., tomatoes). A more extensive list of OP pesticides is provided in Table 7-4, with the trade names of some of the pesticides shown in brackets.

Despite the benefits that OP pesticides provide in the control of damage by insects to food crops and in the abatement of insect vectors, they also present several noteworthy hazards. Two of these hazards are the potential for harm to the persons who apply the pesticide and, more generally, the potential for harm to the entire population, particularly children. The extensive use of organophosphate pesticides worldwide increases the likelihood of pesticide poisoning, especially in the developing world, and thus is a major concern

TABLE 7-4 Partial List of Organophosphate Pesticides (Insecticides)

Acephate	Isofenphos+
Azinphos-methyl+	Isoxathion
Bensulide	Malathion
Cadusafos	Methamidophos+
Chlorethoxyfos	Methidathion+
Chlorfenvinphos	Methyl parathion+
Chlorpyrifos [Dursban]	Mevinphos+
Chlorthiophos+	Monocrotophos+
Coumaphos	Naled [Dibrom]
Dialifor+	Oxydemeton-methyl
Diazinon	Phorate+
Dichlorvos (DDVP)	Phosalone
Dicrotophos+	Phosmet [Imidan]
Dimethoate	Phosphamidon+
Dioxathion+	Phostebupirim
Disulfoton+	Pirimiphos-methyl
Ethion	Profenofos
Ethoprop	Propetamphos
Ethyl parathion+	Sulfotepp+
Fenamiphos+	Sulprofos
Fenitrothion	Temephos
Fenthion	Terbufos
Fonofos+	Tetrachlorvinphos
Isazophos	Trichlorfon

+ Indicates high toxicity.

Source: Adapted and reprinted from R Reigart, J Roberts, eds. *Recognition and Management of Pesticide Poisonings.* 5th ed. Washington, DC: US Environmental Protection Agency; 1999.

Metam Sodium Spill on the Upper Sacramento River

The upper Sacramento River is located in Northern California. This picturesque region, known for its natural beauty and abundant wildlife, attracts fishermen and vacationers from all over the world. On July 14, 1991, a massive spill of approximately 19,000 gallons of the fungicide metam sodium occurred when a freight train derailed on a section of the Southern Pacific tracks known as the Cantara Loop. (See Figure 7-2.) Seven derailed railroad tank cars cascaded directly into the river from an area on a trestle that was immediately above the river. One of them landed in the river at a point where the water was about one meter deep.[20,21]

The spill necessitated the evacuation of the nearby town of Dunsmuir. The effects of the spill were devastating to aquatic and terrestrial wildlife, resulting in a 36- to 45-mile long swath of destruction along the Sacramento River, which is a vital watershed for the state of California. A pea-green foam was reported to be coursing down the river, leaving in its poisonous wake numerous dead trout. Virtually all aquatic life was exterminated for almost 50 miles as the pesticide flowed downstream. Since 1991, extensive restoration of the affected areas has been under way.

In addition to eradicating aquatic life, the spilled pesticide seeped into shallow aquifers and released toxic gases into the air. Soon after the spill, eyewitnesses who were near Dunsmuir reported an obnoxious odor that made breathing difficult. A total of 705 persons sought medical assistance for health complaints that ranged from headache and eye irritations to nasal irritation and chest tightness.

From July 21 to July 22, 1991, inmates from the Shasta County jail and crew leaders were dispatched to pick up dead fish along the site of the spill. Among this group of 42 persons, 27 (64%) developed dermatitis on their lower extremities and some other sections of the body that came in contact with the river water. Nevertheless, according to the CDC, the pesticide was not identified definitely as the cause of the dermatitis cases, as the pesticide had degraded to very low concentrations by the time the workers contacted the river water.[22]

FIGURE 7-2 Metam sodium spill into the upper Sacramento River.

Source: © California Department of Fish and Game photo. Available at: http://www.fws.gov/contaminants/Documents/cantara_web.pdf. Accessed March 9, 2010.

for environmental health officials who work for public health departments and other environmental agencies.[15] Presently, diazinon is banned in the United States for use as a consumer product because of its toxicity to wildlife.

Methyl parathion is an example of an organophosphate pesticide that is used to control insects on crops. It is clas-

sified by the US EPA as a category I pesticide, which means that it is among the most toxic. A major incident of poisoning with methyl parathion occurred in Lorain County, Ohio, as a consequence of the pesticide being sprayed illegally for pest control in private residences over a period of years during the late 1980s and early 1990s until the practice was reported to authorities. Beginning in 1994, the EPA conducted an investigation that evaluated 254 area homes and 747 individuals. Results showed that residents in the exposed households reported that they were afflicted by a wide range of symptoms and that their pets died. Soon after their homes were sprayed, 49 residents were hospitalized and at least one died. Children were more likely to be affected than adults. EPA officials noted:

> Health care providers apparently did not consider pesticide poisoning when confronted with acute generic presentations, and although veterinarians may have diagnosed pesticide poisoning in pets, this information did not reach the public health system. . . . [A]cute and short-term organophosphate poisoning occurred but was not recognized in Lorain County during the years that methyl parathion was sprayed in private residences.[16(p1050)]

Carbamates

The pesticides in the class of carbamates are close relatives of the organophosphate pesticides. As is true of organophosphates, carbamates dissipate quickly from the environment as a result of breaking down into other substances. Farmers use carbamate-based pesticides as insecticides, fungicides, and herbicides. Some varieties are also in use around the home, an example being the carbamate insecticide carbyl (trade name Sevin), which is used to control garden pests (e.g., wasps, hornets, and snails) and is an ingredient in some products applied to furry pets to control ticks and fleas. Common types of the approximately 30 EPA-registered carbamates are aldicarb, fenoxycarb, and propoxur. The form of carbamates known as thiocarbamate is used mainly as an herbicide; the form known as dithiocarbamate is primarily for use as a fungicide. Metam sodium is a carbamate pesticide from the dithiocarbamate group. One of the pesticides used most frequently in the United States (with approximately 60 million pounds ap-

The Bhopal, India Incident

The Bhopal, India incident refers to history's most severe catastrophe that involved toxic chemicals. In this accident, methyl isocyanate (MIC) gases were released from a Union Carbide pesticide factory. Occurring on the night of December 2nd and early morning of December 3rd, 1984, this catastrophe resulted in the deaths of more than 3,800 residents (some estimates range as high as 7,500); in addition, an estimated 11,000 persons exposed to MIC were left with disabling conditions. Not confined to the acute effects of MIC release, the impact of the Bhopal incident remains today, with continuing adverse effects upon the health of those directly exposed as well as their children born after the disaster.

The Union Carbide factory was upwind of the city of Bhopal, which had a population of 900,000 at the time. Water that intruded accidentally into tank no. 610 (used for storing MIC) produced a chemical reaction that released nearly 40 tons of MIC into the atmosphere. Fumes from the plant floated over the unsuspecting city. Although workers became aware of the leak and reported it to plant authorities, action to control the toxic gas was delayed, allowing the escape of large quantities of MIC. Unfortunately, safety measures in place at the time (e.g., a siren to alert the community of dangers from the plant) were turned off or malfunctioning.

According to eyewitness reports, "Many died in their beds, others staggered from their homes, blinded and choking, to die in the street. Many more died later after reaching hospitals and emergency aid centres. The early acute effects were vomiting and burning sensations in the eyes, nose and throat, and most deaths have been attributed to respiratory failure. For some, the toxic gas caused such massive internal secretions that their lungs became clogged with fluids, while for others, spasmodic constriction of the bronchial tubes led to suffocation. Many of those who survived the first day were found to have impaired lung function. Further studies on survivors have also reported neurological symptoms including headaches, disturbed balance, depression, fatigue and irritability. [There also have been continuing reports of] [a]bnormalities and damage to the gastrointestinal, musculoskeletal, reproductive and immunological systems."

Source: US Environmental Protection Agency. Technology Transfer Network Air Toxics Website. Methyl Isocyanate. Available at: http://www.epa.gov/ttn/atw/hlthef/methylis.html. Accessed March 8, 2010; AcuSafe. Incidents: Bhopal, India (1984). Available at: http://www.acusafe.com/Incidents/Bhopal1984/incident-bhopal1984.html. Accessed March 8, 2010; and Greenpeace. Bhopal: the ongoing disaster 1984–2001. Available at: http://archive.greenpeace.org/toxics/html/content/bhopalbriefing.html. Accessed March 8, 2010.

plied annually), metam sodium is a common soil fumigant. (Refer to the text box for information on the 1991 chemical spill into the Sacramento River in the United States.)

Methyl isocyanate (MIC) is an intermediate chemical used for the manufacture of carbamate pesticides. Also, MIC is created as metam sodium breaks down. When acute exposure occurs, MIC is extremely toxic to life-forms (e.g., human beings, aquatic organisms, and plants). A notorious incident that involved the pesticide was the accidental release of MIC during a 1984 industrial accident in Bhopal, India, that killed more than 3,800 people. (Refer to the text box.)

Organochlorines

The third group of pesticides is derived from chlorinated hydrocarbons. *Chlorinated hydrocarbon* is

> a generic term given to compounds containing chlorine, carbon and hydrogen. The term can be used to describe organochlorine pesticides such as lindane and DDT, industrial chemicals such as polychlorinated biphenyls (PCB[s]), and chlorine waste products such as dioxins and furans. These compounds are persistent in the environment and most bioaccumulates [defined in Chapter 6] in the food chain. The human and environmental health risks of chlorinated hydrocarbons depend on the compound in question. As a general statement, exposure to chlorinated hydrocarbon[s] has been associated with suppression of the immune system and cancer.[17]

Organochlorines include

> a wide range of chemicals that contain carbon, chlorine and, sometimes, several other elements. A range of organochlorine compounds have been produced including many herbicides, insecticides, fungicides as well as industrial chemicals such as polychlorinated biphenyls (PCBs). The compounds are characteristically stable, fat-soluble and bioaccumulate. Organochlorines pose a range of adverse human health risks and some are carcinogens.[18]

Examples of organochlorine pesticides are:

- DDT
- Lindane
- Chlordane
- Mirex
- Hexachlorobenzene
- Methoxychlor

The organochlorine pesticide DDT (dichlorodiphenyltrichloroethane) is similar in chemical structure to DDE (dichlorodiphenyldichloroethylene) and DDD (dichlorodiphenyldichloroethane); frequently, both DDE and DDD are present as contaminants in DDT pesticides. DDE does not have commercial value; DDD was used in the past as a pesticide.[19] A metabolite of DDT, DDE is formed when DDT is ingested. For example, fish convert DDT to DDE when they consume DDT that is present in lower aquatic organisms.

In the United States, widespread use of organochlorine pesticides such as DDT began during the early 1940s and reached a maximum during the 1960s. Due to concerns about the possible adverse effects of DDT upon the health of humans and wildlife, application of DDT was prohibited in 1972 in the United States. (Refer to the text box.) Although most developed nations at present ban the use of DDT, some countries continue to use this pesticide.

DDT is not regarded as a highly toxic pesticide—a consideration that in the mid-20th century supported its use. For many years, DDT was employed worldwide to control insects and harmful mosquitoes that carry malaria. It was credited at one time for freeing a substantial segment of the world's population from the scourge of malaria and, consequently, with saving millions of persons from death due to malaria.

The downside of DDT is the fact that, in common with the organochlorines, it is a highly stable chemical that persists in the environment. This characteristic is associated with the phenomenon of bioaccumulation, the concentration of a chemical as it moves up the food chain. Amplification of the chemical's concentration may increase the likelihood of adverse health effects among animals at the upper end of the food chain. Specifically, DDT, which has the ability to become concentrated in the adipose (fatty) tissues of the body, has an estimated half-life of approximately 10 years; the term *half-life* indicates the time required for one half of the pesticide to be cleared from the body. So persistent and widespread is contamination of the environment with DDT, all living organisms on earth contain some levels of this pesticide. Nevertheless, it is noteworthy that average human body burdens of DDT have tended to decline with its decreasing use. US residents were reported to have the following average body fat concentrations of the pesticide for the years 1950, 1956, and 1980, respectively: 5 parts per million (ppm), 15.6 ppm, and 3 ppm.[23] However, levels of DDE, the DDT metabolite, have tended to remain constant, as people continue to ingest the DDE that is present in some species of fish and other DDE-containing foodstuffs.

DDT Ban Takes Effect (1972)

The general use of the pesticide DDT will no longer be legal in the United States after today, ending nearly three decades of application during which time the once-popular chemical was used to control insect pests on crop and forest lands, around homes and gardens, and for industrial and commercial purposes.

An end to the continued domestic usage of the pesticide was decreed on June 14, 1972, when William D. Ruckelshaus, Administrator of the Environmental Protection Agency, issued an order finally canceling nearly all remaining federal registrations of DDT products. Public health, quarantine, and a few minor crop uses were excepted, as well as export of the material.

The cancelation decision culminated three years of intensive governmental inquiries into the uses of DDT. As a result of this examination, Ruckelshaus said he was convinced that the continued massive use of DDT posed unacceptable risks to the environment and potential harm to human health.

DDT was developed as the first of the modern insecticides early in World War II. It was initially used with great effect to combat malaria, typhus, and the other insect-borne human diseases among both military and civilian populations.

A persistent, broad-spectrum compound often termed the "miracle pesticide," DDT came into wide agricultural and commercial usage in this country in the late 1940s. During the past 30 years, approximately 675,000 tons have been applied domestically. The peak year for use in the United States was 1959 when nearly 80 million pounds were applied. From that high point, usage declined steadily to about 13 million pounds in 1971, most of it applied to cotton.

The decline was attributed to a number of factors including increased insect resistance, development of more effective alternative pesticides, growing public and user concern over adverse environmental side effects—and governmental restriction on DDT use since 1969.

New DDT Report Confirms Data Supporting 1972 Ban, Finds Situation Improving

Residues of the pesticide DDT in the food supply, human tissues and in the environment have declined in recent years especially since the chemical was banned for major uses by EPA in 1972. . . . [T]he ban has contributed to the decline of DDT levels in fish. For example, one Federal study of Lake Michigan lake trout showed DDT levels decreased from 19.19 ppm in 1970 to 9.96 ppm in 1973. DDT levels in coho salmon declined from 11.82 ppm in 1969 to 4.48 . . . [ppm] in 1973. . . . DDT should still be considered a potential human cancer agent based on the results of animal studies. . . . DDT is stored in human fatty tissue, wildlife and fish; DDT is toxic to fish and birds and interferes with the reproduction of some species; DDT persists in soil and water for years.

Source: US Environmental Protection Agency. History: DDT Ban Takes Effect. Available at: http://www.epa.gov/history/topics/ddt/01.htm. Accessed March 8, 2010; and US Environmental Protection Agency. History: New DDT Report Confirms Data Supporting 1972 Ban, Finds Situation Improving. Available at: http://www.epa.gov/history/topics/ddt/03.htm. Accessed March 8, 2010.

In the developing world, people continue to consume foods that contain much higher levels of DDT and organochlorine pesticides than are permitted in the developed world. Exposure to high levels of DDT in developing countries is of particular concern for the health of children.

The various human health effects that have been linked to DDT include cancer, reproductive effects, impaired lactation, falling sperm counts, and impaired neurologic function. Among the forms of cancer associated with DDT in some studies are pancreatic cancer, non-Hodgkin's lymphoma, and breast cancer. DDT also causes nervous system abnormalities among pesticide workers; these symptoms include irritability, dizziness, and numbness. An extensive review of the literature suggested that "Other than the long-recognized neurologic toxicity associated with DDT poisoning, and laboratory abnormalities [e.g., abnormal results from blood tests] in DDT-exposed workers, human health effects of DDT exposure are not established."[24(p222)]

Pyrethrins

A pyrethrin is an insecticide derived from natural sources, namely certain varieties of chrysanthemum flowers.[25] Pesticides from this group have great ability to paralyze and kill flying insects, although some insects may recover because of their own defensive detoxifying enzymes. The paralyzing action of pyrethrins occurs through interference with the transmission of neural impulses via action on sodium channels.

Manufactured chemicals that have a composition similar to pyrethrins are called pyrethroids.[25] Although more than 1,000 types of pyrethroids have been synthesized, only a few are in use as insecticides in the United States. The most common pyrethroid is permethrin, with over 1 million pounds applied in the United States in 1997; other common pyrethroids are bifenthrin, cyfluthrin, cypermethrin, and telfluthrin.

Pyrethrin-based insecticides, having low concentrations of the active ingredient, are used inside the home in aerosol cans, insecticide bombs, insecticidal pet shampoos, treatments for lice applied directly to humans, and mosquito repellents. They degrade rapidly by the action of sunlight and are not very toxic when applied to animals, but are highly toxic to some beneficial insects (e.g., honeybees) as well as fish and other forms of aquatic life. People may inhale these insecticides as a result of spraying and may ingest them in foods. High levels of exposure to pyrethrin-based insecticides produce characteristic acute effects such as nausea, headache, dizziness, and neurologic symptoms. The following text box documents episodes of human illness due to exposure to pyrethrins and pyrethroids.

Herbicides/Defoliants

Examples of chemicals in the category of herbicides and defoliants are atrazine, paraquat, and Agent Orange (2,4-D [2,4-dichlorophenoxyacetic acid] and 2,4,5-T [2,4,5 trichlorophenoxyacetic acid]). Consider the first herbicide in the foregoing list, atrazine, which is one of the most widely used weed killers in the United States. When atrazine is applied as a weed killer on field crops such as corn, runoff from irrigation and rainfall may carry this herbicide into waterways. Some experts believe that atrazine has an estrogenic effect on frogs.[26] Estrogenic activity refers to the observation that a chemical has an effect that is similar to that of the female

Illnesses Associated with Use of Automatic Insecticide Dispenser Units—Selected States and United States, 1986–1999

To control indoor flying insects, restaurants and other businesses commonly use pyrethrin and pyrethroid insecticides sprayed from automatic dispensing units. Usually placed near entrances, these units are designed to kill flying insects in food service or work areas. On May 18, 1999, the Florida Department of Health (FDH) was notified by the Florida Department of Business and Professional Regulation (DBPR) that during May 12–17, three persons developed pesticide-related illnesses associated with improperly placed automatic insecticide dispensers. . . .

Cases 1–3

A 42-year-old cook working at a Florida restaurant developed a sore throat, dyspnea, headache, and dizziness on May 12, 1999, after a several-hour exposure to mist released from insecticide dispensers in the food preparation area. The insecticide dispensers had been installed on May 10, but it is unknown on what day the cook was first exposed. The cook removed the dispensers on May 12 and noted relief of his symptoms. However, the restaurant management reinstalled the dispensers on May 14, and on May 15, a 40-year-old male customer developed headache and shortness of breath within 1 hour of entering the restaurant. These symptoms lasted approximately 4 hours. On May 17, approximately 45 minutes after leaving this restaurant, a 47-year-old male customer experienced a sharp burning sensation in his left eye and noted swelling, redness, and irritation of the eyelid that persisted approximately 24 hours. The implicated pesticide dispenser was within 6 feet of the booth where this customer had been sitting, and it faced his left eye. This person reported his symptoms to DBPR on May 18. None of the three persons sought medical attention for their symptoms. The active ingredients released by these dispensers were pyrethrin and piperonyl butoxide.

Case 4

On August 20, 1995, a 17-year-old male restaurant employee in California was changing the cartridge of an automatic insecticide dispenser. When he closed the dispenser panel, the firing mechanism was activated and discharged a pyrethrin-containing mist into his right eye. The employee immediately experienced burning in the eye and promptly sought medical attention at the emergency department of a local hospital. He was diagnosed with chemical conjunctivitis and treated symptomatically.

Source: Adapted and reprinted from the Centers for Disease Control and Prevention. Illnesses associated with use of automatic insecticide dispenser units—selected states and United States, 1986–1999. *MMWR.* 2000;49:492–493.

sex hormone estrogen. One study suggested that there was an association between atrazine and prostate cancer among workers exposed at an atrazine manufacturing plant. The second herbicide, paraquat, is a standard herbicide used on many crops.[27] Some evidence indicates that paraquat, a highly toxic chemical, was applied in the past to marijuana plants; some marijuana in the United States showed paraquat contamination. The herbicide paraquat could cause lung damage when smoke from contaminated marijuana is inhaled.[28]

The third herbicide, Agent Orange, was applied by the US military as a defoliant in Vietnam during the Vietnam War of the 1960s and early 1970s to prevent the thick jungle foliage from concealing the enemy. During Operation Ranch Hand, which spanned the years from 1962 to 1971, approximately 19 million gallons of defoliants were sprayed on 3.6 million acres located in Vietnam and Laos.[29] Although the defoliants were mixtures of various herbicides, most contained the phenoxyacetic acid–based herbicides 2,4-D and 2,4,5-T. One of the most commonly used mixtures consisted of equal amounts of 2,4-D and 2,4,5-T. This herbicide mixture was shipped in drums marked with orange stripes; hence, it was given the name Agent Orange. Of particular concern was the fact that Agent Orange contained very small amounts of dioxins that originated from the manufacture of the herbicide.[29] (The health effects of dioxins will be covered later in this chapter.)

Around 1.5 million military personnel served during the time interval that the spraying with Agent Orange occurred. However, the exact number of persons exposed and the degree of their exposure to the herbicides can only be estimated. Returning veterans disclosed a number of unusual health outcomes that affected themselves (e.g., cancer and skin rashes) and their children (e.g., birth defects of various types). Some veterans attributed these occurrences to exposure to Agent Orange during the war.

Subsequently, a large number of epidemiologic studies have explored the health effects of veterans' exposures to Agent Orange. A report issued by the Institute of Medicine, an arm of the US National Academies, concluded that there was sufficient evidence that Agent Orange was associated with several forms of cancer (soft tissue sarcoma, non-Hodgkin's lymphoma, Hodgkin's disease, and chronic lymphocytic leukemia).[29] The linkage between Agent Orange and other health effects was reported to be less certain, although there have been some putative findings regarding this association. For example, another report from the Institute of Medicine stated that "there is limited suggestive/evidence of an association between exposure to the herbicides used in Vietnam or the contaminant dioxin and Type 2 diabetes."[30(p2)]

A list of herbicides is shown in Table 7-5. This list is provided for information only; the additional herbicides are not discussed in the text.

Other Health Effects of Pesticide Exposure

Pesticide exposures affect many classes of living beings, including agricultural workers, animals, and the general population. An English toxicologist concluded "that although we can be sure that pesticides pose no gross threat to health in the general population, subtle effects on more highly exposed subpopulations are, as yet, more difficult to rule out."[31(p219)]

Those most likely to experience the harmful effects of pesticides are people such as agricultural workers who are unwittingly exposed or misuse them. In addition, pesticides sometimes are used as a means of attempting suicide in agricultural areas.[31] Employees who have been exposed to pesticides in the workplace unknowingly may endanger their family members as well as themselves; workers' clothing may accumulate pesticides, which later may be carried into the workers' homes and contaminate unsuspecting family members.[32] Figure 7-3 demonstrates agricultural workers hoeing weeds around plants. Workers may come into contact with pesticides that have been applied to crops.

During the 1970s, in order to protect themselves from pesticides, some workers involved in spray applications donned the protective gear shown in Figure 7-4.

As noted previously, many products designed to control insect infestations on pets contain pesticides. The National

TABLE 7-5 Herbicides

Class	Example Pesticides
Phenoxyacetic acids	2,4-D; 2,4,5-T; silvex
Triazines	Atrazine, simazine
Bipyridyls	Diquat, paraquat
Amides	Propanil, diphenamide
Substituted ureas	Monuron, diuron
Carbamates	Pebulate, barban, CDEC
Arsenicals	DSMA, MSMA
Phthalamic acids	Dinoseb, naptalam
Benzoic acids	Dicamba; 2,3,6-TBA
Dinitroanilines	Trifluralin, nitralin
Others	Pichloram, bromacil

Source: Data reprinted from LR Shull and PR Cheeke. Effects of synthetic and natural toxicants on livestock. *Journal of Animal Science.* 1983;57(suppl 2):333

FIGURE 7-3 Agricultural workers hoeing weeds around plants. During the growing and processing stages of agriculture, workers may come into contact with pesticides that have been applied to plants.

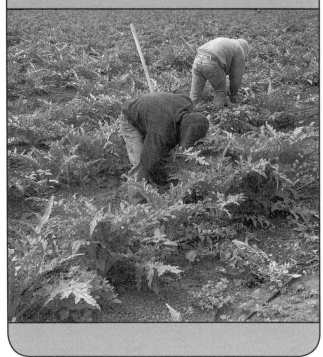

FIGURE 7-4 This individual was demonstrating the types of protective clothing worn by pesticide workers during the 1970s.

Source: Reprinted courtesy of the CDC Public Health Image Library. ID# 3912. Available at: http://phil.cdc.gov/Phil/detail.asp. Accessed March 27, 2010.

Resources Defense Council points out that it is likely that thousands of pets have been killed by pesticides intended to control fleas and ticks.[33] Even though these products have been labeled as safe for adults, they may pose hazards to children, whose developing bodies are more sensitive to toxic chemicals than are adults' bodies. Some children are exposed to pesticides applied to pets when the children play on the floor, put their pets' toys in their own mouths, and put their hands in their mouths after petting the animals.

The pesticides used in agriculture may have undesirable effects upon cattle and other livestock.[34] Exposure of livestock to pesticides may arise from contaminated feed, pesticides applied to fields, and agents used to control insect pests that plague food animals. The effects that animals may experience include acute and chronic toxicity. Pesticide residues also may build up in meat, poultry, and dairy products that subsequently are consumed by humans.

Another concern regarding pesticides is what may happen when they drift into schools and homes located near agricultural fields.[35] (Refer to the chloropicrin text box.) Pesticide drift may pose a greater hazard to children and sensitive subpopulations (e.g., pregnant women) than to healthy adults.

However, one California study reported no strong association between residential proximity to locations where pesticides were applied and fetal deaths.[36] Children appear to be more prone to pesticide poisoning than adults because children have large skin-surface to body-mass ratios.[37] Children also demonstrate personal hygiene deficiencies such as hand–mouth behaviors that could cause the ingestion of pesticides.

Biopesticides

In addition to chemical pesticides, other types include biopesticides, antimicrobials, and pest control devices. The text box

Illness Associated with Drift of Chloropicrin Soil Fumigant into a Residential Area—Kern County, California, 2003

Chloropicrin is the fourth most commonly used soil fumigant in California. Exposure to chloropicrin causes eye and respiratory tract irritation, vomiting, and diarrhea. . . . This report describes an investigation by the California Department of Pesticide Regulation (CDPR) and the Kern County Agriculture Commissioner (KCAC) into illnesses associated with the offsite drift of chloropicrin in Kern County. A total of 165 persons experienced symptoms consistent with chloropicrin exposure. The findings underscore health risks associated with fumigants and the usefulness of procedures adopted in California to ensure both prompt identification of exposure events and timely notification of the affected public.

On October 3, 2003, an agricultural pest control service began applying 100% chloropicrin at a concentration of 80 pounds/acre to 34 acres of fallow land in Kern County. Chloropicrin was injected 17–18 inches into the soil; a weighted board was used to compact the soil, treating 18 acres. That evening, residents living one quarter mile west of the application site experienced irritant symptoms. The Kern County Fire Department (KCFD) was contacted to investigate; however, darkness, distance from the treated field, and absence of chloropicrin odor prevented firefighters from identifying the source of the irritation. Records from a weather station approximately 7 miles southeast of the application site indicated low wind speeds and stable atmospheric conditions but also that the wind direction had changed that evening, blowing from the field toward the residential dwellings.

The next day, chloropicrin was applied to the remaining 16 acres. A 60-foot, chloropicrin-free buffer was maintained around the perimeter of the field because workers noted a persistent odor when they arrived. Residents one quarter mile west and south of the field complained about irritant symptoms that evening. Residents notified KCFD; several responding firefighters experienced eye irritation. The wind had changed again that evening and begun blowing from the field toward the residential dwellings. Suspecting a pesticide release, KCFD notified KCAC. The field was recompacted, and the odor ceased.

On October 6, KCAC notified CDPR about the incident. KCAC and CDPR conducted in-person interviews at 35 households located approximately one quarter mile west and south of the field and at a day care center; additional interviews were conducted on October 15. The 35 households and day care center had a total of 172 persons present during the exposure period. Representatives from each household and the day care center were interviewed by using a standardized questionnaire. . . . In addition, five workers involved with the fumigation were questioned informally, and KCFD records were reviewed to identify affected firefighters.

The investigation determined that 165 persons reported symptoms compatible with illness caused by chloropicrin; median age of the persons was 16 years (range: 3 months–63 years). Nearly all (99%) had irritant symptoms (e.g., eye or upper respiratory) . . . ; nine (5%) received medical evaluations. Seven had persistent respiratory symptoms when interviewed 11 days after the event. Follow-up medical care was limited because most of the affected persons lacked health insurance.

Source: Adapted and reprinted from the Centers for Disease Control and Prevention. Brief report: illness associated with drift of chloropicrin soil fumigant into a residential area—Kern County, California, 2003. *MMWR.* 2004;53:740.

provides additional information. (Instead of using pesticides, some farmers have been able to control pests by growing several types of crops in the same area at the same time, rotating crops, and applying compost; further discussion of this topic is beyond the scope of this text.)

DIOXINS

The term **dioxin** refers to "a family of chemical compounds that are unintentional byproducts of certain industrial, nonindustrial and natural processes, usually involving combustion."[38] The word *dioxin* usually means the chemical TCDD (2,3,7,8-tetrachlorodibenzo-*p*-dioxin),[39] which is the most toxic[40,41] and one of the most widely researched forms of dioxin. Researchers have observed that dioxins are among the most toxic chemicals ever used in experiments with laboratory animals.[39]

Other chemicals that are called "dioxin-like compounds" or simply "dioxins" come from three related chemical families: (1) chlorinated dibenzo-*p*-dioxins (CDDs), (2) chlorinated dibenzofurans (CDFs), and (3) certain polychlorinated biphenyls (PCBs).[42] A total of 419 compounds in the dioxin family are known to exist; however, scientists regard only about 30 of these as being the most poisonous.[40]

Both natural and human activities produce dioxins. Natural events such as forest fires and volcanic eruptions cause the emission of dioxins into the environment; dioxins that

Description of Biopesticides

Biopesticides are certain types of pesticides derived from such natural materials as animals, plants, bacteria, and certain minerals. For example, canola oil and baking soda have pesticidal applications and are considered biopesticides. . . .

- Microbial pesticides consist of a microorganism (e.g., a bacterium, fungus, virus or protozoan) as the active ingredient. [An example is Bacillus thuringiensis (Bt), which can kill inset larvae.]
- Plant-Incorporated-Protectants (PIPs) are pesticidal substances that plants produce from genetic material that has been added to the plant. For example, scientists can take the gene for the Bt pesticidal protein, and introduce the gene into the plant's own genetic material.
- Biochemical pesticides are naturally occurring substances that control pests by non-toxic mechanisms. . . . [Examples] include substances, such as insect sex pheromones, that interfere with mating, as well as various scented plant extracts that attract insect pests to traps.

Source: Adapted and reprinted from US Environmental Protection Agency. About pesticides: Types of pesticides. Available at: http://www.epa.gov/opp00001/about/types.htm. Accessed March 7, 2010.

the environment. (Refer to Table 7-2 for more information.) When they are released into the atmosphere from combustion, dioxins may drift over vast areas before settling on the earth's surface. They also may reach bodies of water as contaminants that unite with the sediments in the water. Aquatic organisms that feed on lake sediments may ingest these dioxins, which become ever more concentrated as they pass up the food chain to fish. The latter, in turn, may be consumed by organisms such as animals or man at the top of the food chain. Because dioxins are fat soluble, the process of bioconcentration may result in the accumulation of significant levels in animals' fatty tissues, the locus where dioxins tend to remain.

The health effects of exposure to dioxins depend on several factors: duration of exposure, frequency of exposure, when the exposure occurred, concentration of the agent, and route of entry into the body. Depending on these factors, the health effects of exposure to dioxins include:

- Chloracne
- Skin rashes
- Skin discoloration
- Growth of excessive body hair
- Liver damage
- Possible cancer risks
- Endocrine effects
- Reproductive and developmental effects

One of the most noteworthy health consequences of dioxin exposure at high concentrations is chloracne, a skin condition typified by a very severe and disfiguring type of acne.[42] Other dermal effects of high levels of exposure include patchy discoloration and increased growth of hair. Long-term exposure to dioxins has been associated with disruption of the immune, endocrine, reproductive, and nervous systems. Dioxins have been reported to cause cancer in laboratory animals.

There have been several documented examples of exposure of the population to potentially hazardous levels of dioxin. One is known as the Belgian PCB/dioxin incident, in which dioxin-contaminated chicken was distributed inadvertently to consumers in Belgium in 1999.[44] As a result of a processing accident, PCBs (that were secondarily contaminated with dioxins) became infused into a batch of recycled fats destined for use in animal fodder. The feeds, sold to more than 2,500 farms, apparently caused illnesses in the chickens but could not be documented as the cause of any illnesses in humans. Due to uncertainty about who consumed the tainted chickens and a long delay in discovering the contamination (until after the feeds had been distributed), the ultimate human health effects of this incident may be difficult to ascertain.[44] Two other dioxin exposure events occurred in Times Beach, Mis-

originate from these sources are called "natural background" dioxins.[42] With respect to human activities, incineration of industrial and municipal wastes produces dioxins, as does the burning of some fuels. Dioxins are produced when wood pulp is bleached in the paper manufacturing process and during the manufacture and application of some herbicides (e.g., dioxins were a contaminant in trace amounts in the herbicide Agent Orange). Burning of tobacco gives rise to minute amounts of dioxin in cigarette smoke.[43]

Dioxins, almost universal contaminants, are very stable chemicals that take many years to decompose. The World Health Organization refers to dioxins as members of the "dirty dozen club."[40] The club consists of persistent organic chemicals (POPs), so-named because of their tendency to remain in souri, and Seveso, Italy. (Refer to the following text boxes for more information.)

POLYCHLORINATED BIPHENYLS (PCBs)

Often, the group referred to as PCBs is presented as a single chemical. However, PCBs comprise an extensive class of organochlorines with 209 congeners (members of the same class), some of which are found more commonly in industrial chemicals than others.[45] Also, PCBs are classified as dioxin-like chemicals. Trade names for PCBs are Arochlor (formulated as nine common mixtures), Askarel, and Therminol.

Estimates indicate that from 1929 to 1977, about 700,000 tons of pure PCBs were manufactured in the United States.[46] PCBs won favor because of their chemical stability, low flammability, inexpensive cost, and insulating properties. Two of the common uses of PCBs were as an insulating fluid in transformers and capacitors and as a lubricant, although the use of PCBs for these purposes has been discontinued. Leakage of PCBs from aging transformers can contaminate the soil and environment. PCBs are known to be present at as many as 500 sites denoted on the 1,598 sites that the EPA has provided on the National Priorities List.[45] (*Note:* The National Priorities List was defined in Chapter 6.) Because of concerns about their environmental and health effects, the manufacture of PCBs was terminated in 1977.

One of the concerns voiced about PCBs is that they remain for long periods in the environment, for example, by binding to sediments. PCBs present in the environment tend to bioaccumulate in fish and other animals used for food and, in turn, impact human health. The ATSDR reports that human beings, their communities, and the environment will continue to face the effects of exposure to PCBs for many decades into the future.[47] This exposure will take place despite the slow, natural process of chemical degradation of PCBs and environmental cleanup efforts. Heavily contaminated US regions are the Hudson River in New York and the Lower Fox River in the Green Bay area of Wisconsin. For example, in New York, the Hudson Falls and Fort Edward General Electric Company plants discharged approximately 1.3 million pounds (600,000 kilograms) of PCBs into the Hudson River over a 30-year period that ended in 1977.[48] (See Figure 7-5 for a picture of the Hudson Falls plant.)

2,3,7,8-Tetrachlorodibenzo-p-dioxin Exposure to Humans—Seveso, Italy

At approximately noon on Saturday, July 10, 1976, an explosion occurred during the production of 2,4,5-trichlorophenol in a factory in Meda, about 25 km north of Milan, in the Lombardia region of Italy. A cloud of toxic material was released and included 2,3,7,8-tetrachlorodibenzo-p-dioxin (TCDD). Debris from this cloud fell south-southeast of the plant on an area of about 2.8 km^2 (700 acres), including parts of the towns of Seveso, Meda, Cesano Maderno, and Desio.

The size of the contaminated area was estimated primarily by measuring TCDD in the soil; additional criteria included the presence of dead animals (e.g., birds, rabbits, chickens) and detection of dermal lesions among persons in the area. The contaminated area was divided into three zones (A, B, and R) depending on the concentration of TCDD in the soil. . . . An additional zone, Zone S, outside the contaminated area was examined as a control zone. . . . Zone A, the most heavily contaminated section, was further divided into seven subzones, A1–A7, based on increasing distance from the factory.

The total amount of TCDD deposited in the contaminated area was initially estimated at about 165 g . . . ; subsequently, it has been estimated to be at least 1.3 kg. . . . Within 20 days of the explosion, the Italian authorities had evacuated the 211 families (735 persons) from the area later defined as Zone A and had taken immediate measures to minimize the risk of exposure to residents in nearby areas (primarily those in Zone B).

The Italian authorities were assisted by several national and international technical commissions in assessing adverse health effects. Residents of zones A, B, and R underwent extensive medical examinations from 1976 to 1985; chloracne, detected in a small segment of the population, was the only abnormal finding. . . . Only one potentially exposed person was measured for TCDD; she was a 55-year-old woman residing in a portion of Zone A (mean TCDD soil concentration of 185.4 Lgmg/m^2), who died from pancreatic adenocarcinoma 7 months after the explosion. Her TCDD whole-weight levels varied from 6 parts per trillion (ppt) in blood to 1840 ppt in adipose tissue. . . .

Source: Adapted and reprinted from the Centers for Disease Control and Prevention. International notes preliminary report: 2,3,7,8-tetrachlorodibenzo-p-dioxin exposure to humans—Seveso, Italy. *MMWR.* 1988;37:733–734.

PCBs have been shown conclusively to cause cancer in animals and are designated as probable human carcinogens.[49] Several mortality studies conducted among employees who had been exposed to PCBs suggested that malignant melanoma and liver, biliary tract, and intestinal cancers were associated with these substances. Effects of exposure to PCBs have been investigated in relation to the risk of breast cancer, although epidemiologic studies did not support this proposed association.[50]

PCBs also have been investigated with respect to their impact on the immune system, reproductive system, and children's intellectual development. PCB exposure may limit the development of immune responses to the Epstein-Barr virus and other viral and bacterial infections.[49] Exposure to PCBs is a possible risk factor for non-Hodgkin's lymphoma.[49] Findings suggest that PCBs cause menstrual disturbances and influence male fertility.[51] Prenatal PCB exposure has been linked to abnormal sperm morphology.[52] A number of studies indicate that prenatal exposure to PCBs is associated with children's lower performance on IQ tests.[53] One of the most strongly affected dimensions was performance tests of memory and attention.[54]

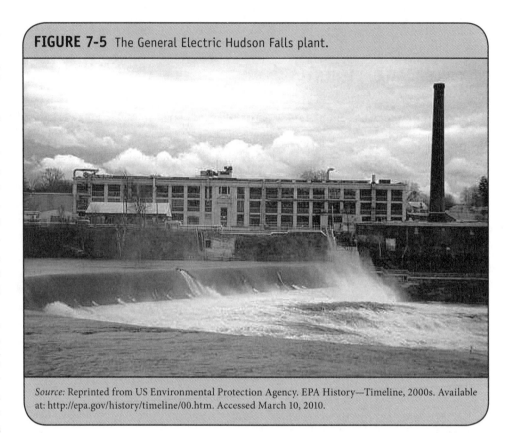

FIGURE 7-5 The General Electric Hudson Falls plant.

Source: Reprinted from US Environmental Protection Agency. EPA History—Timeline, 2000s. Available at: http://epa.gov/history/timeline/00.htm. Accessed March 10, 2010.

ORGANIC SOLVENTS

The term **solvent** refers to "a liquid substance capable of dissolving other substances; 'the solvent does not change in forming a solution.'"[55] How do people become exposed to solvents? There are several modes of exposure, including breathing their vapors directly, ingesting them in foods and water that have low levels of contamination, using foods and cosmetics packed in certain types of plastics, and sometimes by smoking cigarettes. Workers may be exposed chronically to solvents that are used by factories. When pregnant female workers are exposed to solvents, these substances are likely to cross the placental barrier and affect the developing fetus. Exposure to solvents among pregnant women has been linked to spontaneous abortions.[56]

Industrial facilities may release vapors from solvents into the surrounding neighborhoods where residents could inhale them. In addition to being emitted into the air from factories, solvents may enter the soil and groundwater through improper disposal or when they leach out of waste sites. Generally, most solvents do not persist in the environment (although there are some exceptions) because of their volatility. Also, research has not resolved fully the issue of their long-term environmental impacts. Only a few members of the solvent group are suspected carcinogens.[57] For example, the solvent benzene is a known carcinogen.

Following is an abbreviated list of solvents and a brief discussion of each one. The selection of compounds presented in this section is somewhat arbitrary, as there are thousands of such chemicals, many of which have both positive and negative impacts on the environment. Thus, this review cannot in any sense be considered comprehensive, but rather is generally representative of some of the issues that occur in the context of these chemicals. Examples of important solvents are the following:

- Tetrachloroethylene
- Trichloroethane
- Trichloroethylene (TCE)

- Toluene
- Acetone
- Benzene

Tetrachloroethylene (synonyms: perchloroethylene, PCE, perchlor, tetrachloroethene) is a synthetic, nonflammable solvent used in the dry cleaning industry and as a metal degreaser. This compound evaporates easily and has a distinctive odor.[58] Exposure to high levels causes neurologic effects and is capable of producing unconsciousness and death. The health effects of exposure to low levels have not been determined. Tetrachloroethylene exposure at very high levels caused liver and kidney cancer in studies of laboratory animals.[58] The International Agency for Research on Cancer (IARC) reported that there is

> sufficient evidence to designate PCE as carcinogenic in animals, with limited evidence in humans. With regard to occupational exposure through dry cleaning, PCE is considered to be possibly carcinogenic to humans. . . . The current epidemiologic evidence does not support a conclusion that occupational exposure to PCE is a risk factor for cancer of any specific site.[59(p473)]

Trichloroethane exists in two common forms: 1,1,1-trichloroethane and 1,1,2-trichloroethane. The form known as 1,1,1-trichloroethane (synonym: methylchloroform) is a solvent found in degreasing compounds and household cleaners that has had many other uses.[60] Depending upon the level of exposure, symptoms range from dizziness to loss of consciousness. Although not presently classified as a carcinogen, its manufacture has been discontinued since January 1, 2002, because of potential to harm the ozone layer.

The variant called 1,1,2-tricholorethane is a colorless, sweet-smelling solvent that has low flammability and is used as an intermediate chemical for the production of other chemicals.[61] Direct contact with the skin produces localized irritation. The compound breaks down very slowly after being released into the environment and is believed to persist indefinitely if it seeps into subsurface groundwater. To date, this compound has not been classified as a human carcinogen.

Trichloroethylene (TCE) is a grease-dissolving solvent that evaporates readily.[62] In addition to its use as a solvent, TCE is added to some cleaning agents, paint removers, and adhesives. In the environment, TCE may persist in underground water supplies for long periods. Low exposure levels produce neurologic effects such as dizziness and headaches. Inhalation or ingestion of large amounts of TCE can cause unconsciousness and death. The consumption of minute quantities of TCE present in public water supplies may lead to adverse health effects, although the consequences of long-term, low-level exposures have not been verified definitively. Research has suggested that TCE is a probable human carcinogen. In the chapter on water quality (Chapter 9), information on contamination of public drinking water supplies with TCE will be presented.

Toluene, used in the manufacture of nail polish, paints, and adhesives, is a clear, colorless liquid that has a characteristic odor.[63] Low to moderate degrees of exposure to toluene are known to cause reversible neurologic effects including anorexia, nausea, and confusion. Heavy exposures are capable of producing loss of consciousness and possibly death. Toluene is suspected of having adverse effects upon the renal system.

Acetone, a colorless liquid with a distinctive sweet odor, is used as an ingredient in nail polish, cleaners, and paints.[64] This highly volatile solvent is flammable and dissolves in water. Moderate levels of exposure to acetone can cause irritation of the eye (e.g., tearing) and the respiratory tract (e.g., nose, throat, and lungs). High levels are capable of causing headaches, vomiting, and loss of consciousness. Most volatile compounds have a threshold for irritating effects that is much higher than the human odor detection threshold. Habituation (desensitization) sometimes occurs among workers who are exposed repetitively; this phenomenon makes it difficult to establish appropriate exposure guidelines for volatile chemicals.[65] The EPA does not classify acetone as a carcinogen.

Benzene is a sweet-smelling, flammable, colorless liquid that evaporates rapidly.[66] Benzene is used as an intermediary chemical for the manufacture of plastics, resins, and synthetic fibers. It also is used as a solvent for waxes, paints, resins, oils, plastics, and rubber; it has been added as a component of fuels for motor vehicles.[67] Benzene occurs naturally in gasoline and crude oil, and as a component of cigarette smoke. The short-term effects of exposure to benzene vapors at moderate concentrations include depression of the central nervous system with effects similar to those of other solvents; very high concentrations of benzene vapors can be fatal.[68] In addition to damaging the blood and blood-forming organs, benzene is a known carcinogen that is causally related to the etiology of a form of leukemia called acute myelogenous leukemia.[69]

Muzaffer Aksoy, a Turkish hematologist, observed that many patients afflicted with leukemia were shoemakers.[70] At the time that he made this initial observation, benzene was used extensively in Turkey as a solvent in the manufacture of leather goods. Following this clinical observation, Aksoy conducted an epidemiologic study (from 1967 to 1974) of 28,500 employees involved with the manufacture of shoes, slippers, and handbags. In 1974, Aksoy reported a positive association between benzene exposure and leukemia on the basis of this epidemiologic research. His work led to the restriction in many countries of occupational benzene exposures, which now must be kept at negligible levels in the United States.

CHEMICALS USED IN THE MANUFACTURE OF PLASTICS

Included in the category of chemicals used in the manufacture of plastics are styrene and vinyl chloride. Chemicals called phthalates are used as plasticizers (a term that will be defined subsequently).

Styrene (styrene monomer) is a clear, colorless liquid that has an aromatic odor.[71] It is commercially important for the manufacture of polystyrene resins (used for many types of plastics, such as packaging, disposable drinking glasses, and building insulation). Short-term inhalation of styrene can produce central nervous system effects such as muscle weakness, and problems concentrating on tasks; irritation of the respiratory tract also can result. According to the IARC, styrene has been listed as possibly carcinogenic, although the evidence supporting this effect among humans and in animal studies is limited.

At room temperature, *vinyl chloride* (synonyms: chloroethene, chloroethylene, ethylene monochloride, monochloroethylene) is a colorless, flammable gas that has a distinctive sweet odor and is highly volatile.[72] When kept under pressure or at low temperatures, vinyl chloride becomes liquefied. In the United States, vinyl chloride is used mainly for the manufacture of polyvinyl chloride, which is an ingredient of a multitude of plastic products such as pipes, vinyl siding for houses, plastic coatings, and upholstery.

Depending upon the concentration, exposure to vinyl chloride can cause central nervous system effects, loss of consciousness, or death.[72] Workers who are exposed chronically to high levels of vinyl chloride may develop nerve and immune system damage, poor circulation in the hands and forearms, and damage to the bones at the tips of the fingers. The US Department of Health and Human Services classifies vinyl chloride as a human carcinogen. Numerous epidemiologic studies as well as case reports have verified that long-term chronic occupational exposure to vinyl chloride is associated with liver cancer (angiosarcoma of the liver).[73,74]

The term **plasticizer** denotes a substance that is added during the manufacture of a plastic to increase its durability as well as make it softer and more pliable. This section will focus on **phthalates** (e.g., diethyl phthalate [DEH]; di(2-ethylhexyl) phthalate [DEHP]; di-*n*-butyl phthalate [DDP]). Phthalates are a class of plasticizer that is used to increase the flexibility of plastics, such as plastic components for automobiles, packaging for foodstuffs, and toothbrushes; phthalates also are contained in polyvinyl chloride toys for infants.[75] In addition, phthalates are used as additives in cosmetics, aspirin, and insecticides. DBP is used in nail polish,[76] which is especially popular among women between the ages of 20 and 40 years. Many women of child-bearing age have significant concentrations of a DBP metabolite in their bodies. The importance of phthalates in causing adverse human health effects is unclear; the impact of DBP, in particular, on the health of unborn children is speculative.[77] DBP is thought to have

Bisphenol A (BPA)

BPA is a chemical used primarily in the production of polycarbonate plastics and resins. Polycarbonate plastics have many applications including food and drink packaging, e.g., water and infant bottles, compact discs, impact-resistant safety equipment, and medical devices.

- The primary source of exposure to BPA for most people is through the diet.
- BPA can leach into food from the protective internal epoxy resin lining of canned foods and from consumer products such as polycarbonate tableware, food storage containers, water bottles, and baby bottles.
- [People are concerned about BPA] because human exposure to BPA is widespread. Some animal studies report effects in fetuses and newborns exposed to BPA.
- More research is clearly needed to understand exactly how the findings relate to human health and development, but at this point we can't dismiss the possibility that the effects we're seeing in animals may occur in humans.

Source: Adapted and reprinted from National Institute of Environmental Health Sciences. National Toxicology Program. Bisphenol A (BPA). Available at: http://www.niehs.nih.gov/health/docs/bpa-factsheet.pdf. Accessed April 1, 2010.

an antiandrogenic effect (suppresses hormones related to the development of male sexual characteristics) in rats.

Phthalates are released rather easily from plastic products and can contaminate food wrapped in plastic packaging. When young children chew on toys made from polyvinyl chloride, some of the phthalate additives may be ingested and, conceivably, pose a health risk. In 2006, the European Union prohibited the use of several types of phthalates as additives to plastics in toys that can be placed in the mouth by toddlers younger than 3 years of age. The US in 2009 banned the use of phthalates for children's toys and child care products.[78]

The phthalate plasticizer DEHP is used in medical products formulated from polyvinyl chloride. Examples of such products are plastic bags used to contain intravenous solutions, blood products in plastic packaging, plastic tubing, and protective gloves. Concern has been raised over the possible toxic hazards associated with the use of polyvinyl products in the medical environment. Current information supports the view that the use of products that contain DEHP is generally safe, although some patients (e.g., children) may face the possibility of risks connected with DEHP.[79] The ATSDR asserts that "At the levels found in the environment, DEHP is not expected to cause harmful health effects in humans. Most of what we know about the health effects of DEHP comes from studies of rats and mice given high amounts of DEHP."[80]

Another chemical used in the manufacture of plastics is bisphenol A (BPA). The public has been concerned about BPA because its use is widespread and there have been some reports of animal studies that showed reproductive and developmental effects. Refer to the text box for more information.

CLEANING AND HOUSEHOLD PRODUCTS

The list of chemicals used commonly in household products is extensive. Table 7-6 provides some examples. Exposure to these products may be hazardous if they are used improperly or disposed of in an unsafe way. For example, care should be taken not to mix chlorine bleach and ammonia, because toxic chloramine gases will be released.

ENVIRONMENTAL ESTROGENS

Some organic chemicals (e.g., chlorinated hydrocarbon pesticides) are alleged to have estrogenic activity (defined previously). Sometimes DDT (and metabolites such as DDE) is referred to as an endocrine disruptor with respect to its ability to act as an antagonist to androgen, the male sex hormone. Another example comes from animal studies of the estrogenic pesticide methoxychlor, which has been shown to have negative consequences for fertility, pregnancy, and development.[81] It is possible that when estrogenic-like chemicals are present in

the environment, they may have abnormal influences on the reproductive systems of exposed humans and animals. In addition, these chemicals may act as cancer promoters by having an influence on the onset of female cancers that are thought to be caused by estrogenic activity. The following text box presents speculations regarding the possible role of estrogenic and other environmental chemicals in women's health.

Women's Health and the Environment

Women have a particular stake in environmental health research. Not only do they share many of the same diseases as men and children—in which the environment, along with genetic susceptibility, has an important role—but women also have particular environmental diseases related to their gender. . . . Women tend to carry more fat, in which substances introduced lower in the food chain may accumulate. . . .[a]

Breast Cancer and Exposure to Environmental Toxins
Controversy exists about the role of environmental toxins and breast cancer. Scientists agree that exposure to high doses of radiation before 30 years of age, such as being treated for Hodgkin's disease, places women at increased risk for breast cancer. Possible, but controversial, environmental risks for breast cancer include:

- passive smoking (second-hand smoke).
- PAHs (polycyclic aromatic hydrocarbons) produced by the burning of coal, oil, gas, garbage or other organic substances.
- certain organochlorine compounds, such as the polychlorinated biphenyls (PCBs) formerly used in consumer and industrial electronics.

Research has shown that human exposure to electromagnetic fields and DDT/DDE, a now-banned but previously widely used pesticide, are not associated with increased risk for breast cancer.[b]

Source: Adapted and reprinted from [a]Environment, Health and Safety Online. Women's Health and the Environment. Available at: http://www.ehso.com/ehshome/womenshealth2.htm. Accessed March 10, 2010; and [b]National Institutes of Health. National Institute of Environmental Health Sciences. Breast Cancer Fact Sheet. Available at: http://www.niehs.nih.gov/health/docs/breast-cancer-fs.pdf. Accessed March 31, 2010.

TABLE 7-6 Toxic Household Products

Product Name	Use(s)
Sodium hypochlorite	Chlorine bleach
Petroleum distillates	Metal polishes
Ammonia	Glass cleaner
Phenol and cresol	Disinfectants
Nitrobenzene	Furniture and floor polishes
Perchloroethylene or 1-1-1 trichloroethane	Solvents for use in dry cleaning fluids, spot removers, and carpet cleaners
Naphthalene or paradichlorobenzene	Mothballs, toilet bowl cleaners
Hydrochloric acid or sodium acid sulfate	Toilet bowl cleaners
Formaldehyde	Preservative in many household products; glue in particleboard and plywood furniture; spray starch
Formaldehyde, phenol, and pentachlorophenol	Spray starch

Source: Data are from Environmental Law Centre. Environment. Available at: http://www.elc.org.uk/pages/envirohome.htm. Accessed March 8, 2010.

CONCLUSION

Pesticides and other organic chemicals are indispensable to modern society; nevertheless, they have the potential to cause great harm. The average person is exposed to a multitude of chemicals—even a cup of coffee contains more than 1,000 chemicals. The ATSDR has compiled a list of 275 hazardous substances. Among the top 20 hazardous substances, nine are from chemical groupings such as PCBs, pesticides, and solvents. Throughout the world millions of tons of pesticides are used to control insects, weeds, and rodents. Organophosphate pesticides are used commonly for a number of reasons, including the fact that they tend not to persist in the environment; however, they can be hazardous when used inappropriately. Use of organochlorine pesticides such as DDT has been discontinued in many nations because of concerns about possible adverse health effects associated with the persistence of DDT in the environment. Although chemicals classified as solvents produce acute health effects, only a few of the chemicals in this group are documented carcinogens. In many cases, the long-term health effects of solvents are unknown. Continuing research is needed to ascertain the long-term health effects of pesticides and other organic chemicals.

Study Questions and Exercises

1. Define the following terms:
   a. Pesticide
   b. Insecticide
   c. Herbicide
   d. Pyrethroid

2. Describe the four major classes of pesticides. What are the advantages and disadvantages of each type?

3. What measures would you take to reduce the number of emergencies that involve hazardous substances? What are the three most common substances that produce personal injuries?

4. What was history's most severe incident that involved toxic chemicals? How could this accident have been prevented? Was the accident a one-time event, or are there continuing health problems?

5. What were some of the concerns that led to the banning of DDT in the United States and other developed countries? Do you believe that the hazards associated with DDT outweigh the pesticide's benefits?

6. Support or refute the following statement: Pyrethrin-based insecticides are unlikely to produce severe human health effects.

7. Describe Operation Ranch Hand, and state how Agent Orange received its name. Why is Agent Orange alleged to be a potential health hazard?

8. What type of agent is chloropicrin? Describe the hazards to the community associated with chloropicrin.

9. Name one of the most toxic groups of chemicals ever used in animal experiments. Describe the health effects of this family of chemicals.

10. Name three chemicals that the chapter identified as human carcinogens. Give some examples of accidents/incidents that involved these chemicals. What is being done to limit the human population's exposure to these chemicals?

REFERENCES

1. Gardella JR, Hill JA. Environmental toxins associated with recurrent pregnancy loss. *Semin Reprod Med.* 2000;18:407–424.

2. De Rosa CT. Restoring the foundation: tracking chemical exposures and human health. [Editorial] *Environ Health Perspect.* 2003;111:A374–A377.

3. National Center for Environmental Health. *Fourth National Report on Human Exposure to Environmental Chemicals.* Atlanta, GA: Centers for Disease Control and Prevention; 2009.

4. National Institute of Environmental Health Sciences. The New Environmental Health: Our chemical world, and our dilemma. NIH Publication #02-5081. Available at: http://www.niehs.nih.gov/health/scied/documents/NewEnviroHealth-FinalSm.pdf. Accessed March 6, 2010.

5. Carson R. *Silent Spring.* New York, NY: Houghton Mifflin Company; 1962.

6. National Center for Environmental Health. *Third National Report on Human Exposure to Environmental Chemicals.* NCEH Publication No.: 05-0725. Atlanta, GA: Centers for Disease Control and Prevention; 2005.

7. Casida JE, Quistad GB. Golden age of insecticide research: past, present, or future? *Ann Rev Entomol.* 1998;43:1–16.

8. Lockwood AH. Organophosphate pesticides and public policy. [Editorial] *Curr Opin Neurol.* 2002;15:725–729.

9. Kellogg RL, Nehring R, Grube A, et al. Environmental indicators of pesticide leaching and runoff from farm fields. Paper presented at: Conference on Agricultural Productivity: Data, Methods, and Measures; March 9–10, 2000; Washington, DC: United States Department of Agriculture, Natural Resources Conservation Service. Available at: http://www.nrcs.usda.gov/technical/NRI/pubs/eip_pap.html. Accessed March 31, 2010.

10. Reigart JR, Roberts JR. Pesticides in children. *Pediatr Clin North Am.* 2001;48:1185–1198.

11. Costa LG. Basic toxicology of pesticides. *Occup Med.* 1997;12(2):251–268.

12. Peter JV, Cherian AM. Organic insecticides. *Anaesth Intensive Care.* 2000;28:11–21.

13. US Environmental Protection Agency. Summary of organophosphate pesticide usage. Available at: http://www.epa.gov/oppfead1/trac/sumry5-1.htm. Accessed March 10, 2010.

14. The Japan Times Online. Mourners mark sarin attack 13 years on. March 21, 2008. Available at: http://search.japantimes.co.jp/cgi-bin/nn20080321a2.html. Accessed March 27, 2010.

15. Kwong TC. Organophosphate pesticides: biochemistry and clinical toxicology. *Ther Drug Monit.* 2002;24:144–149.

16. Rubin C, Esteban E, Kieszak S, et al. Assessment of human exposure and human health effects after indoor application of methyl parathion in Lorain County, Ohio, 1995–1996. *Environ Health Perspect.* 2002;110(suppl 6):1047–1051.

17. European Environment Agency. Chlorinated hydrocarbon. Available at: http://glossary.eea.europa.eu/EEAGlossary/C/chlorinated_hydrocarbon. Accessed March 7, 2010.

18. European Environment Agency. Organochlorines. Available at: http://glossary.eea.europa.eu/EEAGlossary/O/organochlorines. Accessed March 7, 2010.

19. Agency for Toxic Substances and Disease Registry (ATSDR). ToxFAQs for DDT, DDE, and DDD. Available at: http://www.atsdr.cdc.gov/tfacts35.html. Accessed February 16, 2010.

20. Gherman E. A toxic nightmare: the Dunsmuir metam sodium spill revisited. *Sonoma County Free Press.* July 1997. Available at: http://sonomacountyfreepress.com/reaction/a_toxic_nightmare.html. Accessed February 16, 2010.

21. US Fish and Wildlife Service. Restoring our resources: California's upper Sacramento River Cantara loop. Available at: http://www.fws.gov/contaminants/Documents/cantara_web.pdf. Accessed March 9, 2010.

22. Centers for Disease Control and Prevention. Dermatitis among workers cleaning the Sacramento River after a chemical spill—California, 1991. *MMWR.* 1991;40:825–827, 833.

23. Turusov V, Rakitsky V, Tomatis L. Dichlorodiphenyltrichloroethane (DDT): ubiquity, persistence, and risks. *Environ Health Perspect.* 2002;110:125–128.

24. Longnecker MP, Rogan WJ, Lucier G. The human health effects of DDT (dichlorodiphenyltrichloroethane) and PCBs (polychlorinated biphenyls) and an overview of organochlorines in public health. *Annu Rev Public Health.* 1997;18:211–244.

25. Agency for Toxic Substances and Disease Registry (ATSDR). ToxFAQs for pyrethrins and pyrethroids. Available at: http://www.atsdr.cdc.gov/tfacts155.html. Accessed February 16, 2010.

26. Natural Resources Defense Council. EPA won't restrict toxic herbicide atrazine, despite health threat. Available at: http://www.nrdc.org/health/pesticides/natrazine.asp. Accessed February 16, 2010.

27. US Environmental Protection Agency. Terms of environment: Glossary: P. Available at: http://www.epa.gov/OCEPAterms/pterms.html. Accessed February 16, 2010.

28. Centers for Disease Control and Prevention. Facts about paraquat. Available at: http://www.bt.cdc.gov/agent/paraquat/basics/facts.asp. Accessed February 16, 2010.

29. Frumkin H. Agent Orange and cancer: an overview for clinicians. *CA Cancer J Clin.* 2003;53:245–255.

30. National Academies, Institute of Medicine. *Veterans and Agent Orange: Herbicide/Dioxin Exposure and Type 2 Diabetes.* Washington, DC: National Academies Press; 2000.

31. Ray DE. Pesticide neurotoxicity in Europe: real risks and perceived risks. *Neurotoxicol.* 2000;21(1–2):219–221.

32. Hood E. Bringing home more than a paycheck: workers and pesticides. *Environ Health Perspect.* 2002;110:A765.

33. Wallinga D, Greer L. *Poisons on Pets: Health Hazards from Flea and Tick Products.* Natural Resources Defense Council; 2000. Available at: http://www.nrdc.org/health/effects/pets/pets.pdf. Accessed March 28, 2010.

34. Shull LR, Cheeke PR. Effects of synthetic and natural toxicants on livestock. *J Anim Sci.* 1983;57(suppl 2):330–354.

35. Ames RG. Pesticide impacts on communities and schools. *Int J Toxicol.* 2002;21:397–402.

36. Bell EM, Hertz-Picciotto I, Beaumont JJ. Case-cohort analysis of agricultural pesticide applications near maternal residence and selected causes of fetal death. *Am J Epidemiol.* 2001;154:702–710.

37. Sanborn MD, Cole D, Abelsohn A, et al. Identifying and managing adverse environmental health effects: 4. Pesticides. *CMAJ.* 2002;166:1431–1436.

38. DioxinFacts.org. Questions and answers: dioxins, furans, TCDD, PCBs. Available at: http://www.dioxinfacts.org/questions_answers. Accessed February 16, 2010.

39. Vanden Heuvel JP, Lucier G. Environmental toxicology of polychlorinated dibenzo-*p*-dioxins and polychlorinated dibenzofurans. *Environ Health Perspect.* 1993;100:189–200.

40. World Health Organization. Fact sheet no. 225: dioxins and their effects on human health. Available at: http://www.who.int/mediacentre/factsheets/fs225. Accessed February 16, 2010.

41. National Institutes of Health. National Institute of Environmental Health Sciences. Dioxins. Available at: http://www.niehs.nih.gov/health/topics/agents/dioxins. Accessed March 31, 2010.

42. US Food and Drug Administration (FDA). Food: Questions and answers about dioxins. Available at: http://www.fda.gov/Food/FoodSafety/FoodContaminantsAdulteration/Chemicalcontaminants/DioxinsPCBs/ucm077524.htm. Accessed March 31, 2010.

43. Agency for Toxic Substances and Disease Registry (ATSDR). Public health statement for chlorinated dibenzo-*p*-dioxins (CDDs). Available at: http://www.atsdr.cdc.gov/toxprofiles/phs104.html. Accessed March 28, 2010.

44. Bernard A, Fierens S. The Belgian PCB/dioxin incident: a critical review of health risks evaluations. *Int J Toxicol*. 2002;21:333–340.

45. Agency for Toxic Substances and Disease Registry (ATSDR). ToxFAQs for polychlorinated biphenyls (PCBs). Available at: http://www.atsdr.cdc.gov/tfacts17.html. Accessed February 16, 2010.

46. US Environmental Protection Agency. Office of Pollution Prevention and Toxics. Management of polychlorinated biphenyls in the United States. Available at: http://www.chem.unep.ch/pops/indxhtms/cspcb02.html. Accessed February 16, 2010.

47. Faroon OM, Keith S, Jones D, et al. Carcinogenic effects of polychlorinated biphenyls. *Toxicol Ind Health*. 2001;17:41–62.

48. US Environmental Protection Agency. EPA proposes comprehensive plan to clean up Hudson River PCBs. [EPA press release—December 6, 2000] Available at: http://www.epa.gov/history/topics/pcbs/02.htm. Accessed February 16, 2010.

49. US Environmental Protection Agency. Polychlorinated biphenyls (PCBs). Health effects of PCBs. Available at: http://www.epa.gov/epawaste/hazard/tsd/pcbs/pubs/effects.htm. Accessed March 7, 2010.

50. Negri E, Bosetti C, Fattore E, et al. Environmental exposure to polychlorinated biphenyls (PCBs) and breast cancer: a systematic review of the epidemiological evidence. *Eur J Cancer Prev*. 2003;12:509–516.

51. Faroon OM, Keith S, Jones D, et al. Effects of polychlorinated biphenyls on development and reproduction. *Toxicol Ind Health*. 2001;17:63–93.

52. Hsu PC, Huang W, Yao WJ, et al. Sperm changes in men exposed to polychlorinated biphenyls and dibenzofurans. *JAMA*. 2003;289:2943–2944.

53. Schantz SL, Widholm JJ, Rice DC. Effects of PCB exposure on neuropsychological function in children. *Environ Health Perspect*. 2003;111:357–376.

54. Jacobson JL, Jacobson SW. Intellectual impairment in children exposed to polychlorinated biphenyls in utero. *New Engl J Med*. 1996;335:783–789.

55. Hyperdictionary. Meaning of solvent. Available at: http://www.hyperdictionary.com/dictionary/solvent. Accessed February 16, 2010.

56. Lindbohm ML, Taskinen H, Sallmen M, et al. Spontaneous abortions among women exposed to organic solvents. *Am J Ind Med*. 1990;17:449–463.

57. Wernke MJ, Schell JD. Solvents and malignancy. *Clin Occup Environ Med*. 2004;4:513–527,vii.

58. Agency for Toxic Substances and Disease Registry (ATSDR). ToxFAQs for tetrachloroethylene (PERC). Available at: http://www.atsdr.cdc.gov/tfacts18.html. Accessed February 16, 2010.

59. Mundt KA, Birk T, Burch MT. Critical review of the epidemiological literature on occupational exposure to perchloroethylene and cancer. *Int Arch Occup Environ Health*. 2003;76:473–491.

60. Agency for Toxic Substances and Disease Registry (ATSDR). ToxFAQs for 1,1,1-trichloroethane. Available at: http://www.atsdr.cdc.gov/tfacts70.html. Accessed February 16, 2010.

61. Agency for Toxic Substances and Disease Registry (ATSDR). ToxFAQs for 1,1,2-trichloroethane. Available at: http://www.atsdr.cdc.gov/tfacts148.html. Accessed February 16, 2010.

62. Agency for Toxic Substances and Disease Registry (ATSDR). ToxFAQs for trichloroethylene (TCE). Available at: http://www.atsdr.cdc.gov/tfacts19.html. Accessed February 16, 2010.

63. Agency for Toxic Substances and Disease Registry (ATSDR). ToxFAQs for toluene. Available at: http://www.atsdr.cdc.gov/tfacts56.html. Accessed February 16, 2010.

64. Agency for Toxic Substances and Disease Registry (ATSDR). ToxFAQs for acetone. Available at: http://www.atsdr.cdc.gov/tfacts21.html. Accessed February 16, 2010.

65. Dalton P, Wysocki CJ, Brody MJ, et al. Perceived odor, irritation, and health symptoms following short-term exposure to acetone. *Am J Ind Med*. 1997;31:558–569.

66. Agency for Toxic Substances and Disease Registry (ATSDR). ToxFAQs for benzene. Available at: http://www.atsdr.cdc.gov/tfacts3.html. Accessed February 16, 2010.

67. US Environmental Protection Agency. Technology transfer network, air toxics website: benzene. Available at: http://www.epa.gov/ttnatw01/hlthef/benzene.html. Accessed February 16, 2010.

68. Canadian Centre for Occupational Health and Safety (CCOHS). OSH answers: health effects of benzene. Available at: http://www.ccohs.ca/oshanswers/chemicals/chem_profiles/benzene/health_ben.html. Accessed March 28, 2010.

69. Pyatt D. Benzene and hematopoietic malignancies. *Clin Occup Environ Med*. 2004;4:529–555, vii.

70. Yaris F, Dikici M, Akbulut T, et al. Story of benzene and leukemia: epidemiologic approach of Muzaffer Aksoy. *J Occup Health*. 2004;46:244–247.

71. Agency for Toxic Substances and Disease Registry (ATSDR). ToxFAQs for styrene. Available at http://www.atsdr.cdc.gov/tfacts53.html. Accessed February 16, 2010.

72. Agency for Toxic Substances and Disease Registry (ATSDR). Public health statement for vinyl chloride. July 2006. Available at: http://www.atsdr.cdc.gov/toxprofiles/phs20.html. Accessed February 16, 2010.

73. Bosetti C, La Vecchia C, Lipworth L, et al. Occupational exposure to vinyl chloride and cancer risk: a review of the epidemiologic literature. *Eur J Cancer Prev*. 2003;12:427–430.

74. National Institutes of Health. National Institute of Environmental Health Sciences, National Toxicology Program. Eleventh report on carcinogens. Substance profiles: vinyl chloride. Available at: http://ntp-server.niehs.nih.gov/ntp/roc/eleventh/profiles/s186viny.pdf. Accessed March 28, 2010.

75. Agency for Toxic Substances and Disease Registry (ATSDR). Public health statement for diethyl phthalate. June 1995. Available at: http://www.atsdr.cdc.gov/toxprofiles/phs73.html. Accessed February 16, 2010.

76. Agency for Toxic Substances and Disease Registry (ATSDR). ToxFAQs for Di-*n*-butyl phthalate. Available at: http://www.atsdr.cdc.gov/tfacts135.html. Accessed April 1, 2010.

77. Washam C. Baby ills from beauty aids? *Environ Health Perspect*. 2001;109:A202.

78. Brown P, KrennHrubec K. Issue Brief: Phthalates and children's products. Washington, DC: National Research Center for Women & Families; 2009.

79. Fanelli R, Zuccato E. Risks and benefits of PVC in medical applications. *Boll Chim Farm*. 2002;141:282–289.

80. Agency for Toxic Substances and Disease Registry (ATSDR). ToxFAQs for di(2-ethylhexyl) phthalate (DEHP). Available at: http://www.atsdr.cdc.gov/tfacts9.html. Accessed February 16, 2010.

81. Cummings AM. Methoxychlor as a model for environmental estrogens. *Crit Rev Toxicol*. 1997;27:367–379.

Ionizing and Nonionizing Radiation

INTRODUCTION

This chapter covers the topics of ionizing radiation and nonionizing radiation, including the similarities and differences between them as well as their sources and effects. The first half of the chapter will consider ionizing radiation, specifically an overview of the types of ionizing radiation, nomenclature used to describe its principal forms, and terms and methods related to its measurement. Then the chapter will review the major environmental sources of ionizing radiation and their possible health impacts. The second half of the chapter will cover the terminology used to describe the major categories of nonionizing radiation. The environmental sources of nonionizing radiation will be considered as well as its hypothesized health effects.

Let's begin with a few preliminary definitions. Generally speaking, radiation refers to energy that travels through space. The term **ionizing radiation** denotes radiation that "has enough energy to remove tightly bound electrons from atoms, thus creating ions. This is the type of radiation that people usually think of as 'radiation.' We take advantage of its properties to generate electric power, to kill cancer cells, and in many manufacturing processes."[1] Sources of ionizing radiation include those decaying radioactive materials that emit alpha and beta particles and gamma rays, medical procedures that employ radiopharmaceuticals and devices such as X-ray machines, and bodies in outer space that contribute to the earth's background radiation. (These types of radiation will be defined in more depth later in the chapter.)

In contrast to ionizing radiation, the term **nonionizing radiation** refers to "[r]adiation that has enough energy to move atoms in a molecule around or cause them to vibrate, but not enough to remove electrons. . . . Examples of this kind of radiation are sound waves, visible light, and microwaves."[1] Other examples include radio frequency energy (e.g., radiation from radio antennas), optical and ultraviolet radiation (e.g., from the sun), infrared (heat) radiation, and low-frequency radiation (e.g., radiation from electric power lines). Potential health effects of exposure to nonionizing radiation range from annoyance to acute symptoms such as pain and swelling to serious eye injury and long-term consequences such as cancer.

As shown in Figure 8-1, ionizing radiation and nonionizing radiation together make up the electromagnetic spectrum, which forms an energy continuum from the low-level energy fields associated with electric power lines to mid-level energy from radio stations to high levels of energy from medical X-rays. The highest levels of ultraviolet radiation demarcate the dichotomy between ionizing radiation and nonionizing radiation. The electromagnetic spectrum covers four major energy levels described in terms of their effects: nonthermal,

thermal, optical, and broken chemical bonds. We will begin with electromagnetic radiation on the right-hand side of the spectrum—ionizing radiation, which has sufficient energy to break chemical bonds.

OVERVIEW OF IONIZING RADIATION

Since Roentgen's discovery of X-rays in 1895, applications of radiation have proliferated in industry, biology, chemistry, medicine, and other fields such as nuclear weapons design. Exposure of human populations to ionizing radiation arises from two main sources, anthropogenic (man-made) and natural. Although many opportunities for the population's exposure to man-made ionizing radiation exist, natural ionizing radiation is responsible for most of the annual exposure and anthropogenic radiation for a minority of such exposure. Sources of natural ionizing radiation are cosmic rays, other forms of radiation that impinge upon earth from outer space, and radiation from geologic formations that contain radioactive elements (radioelements) such as uranium, from which radon gas is formed as a decay product. Also, radioelements are present naturally in the human body (an example is potassium-40). As noted previously, synthetic sources of ionizing radiation are medical X-rays and other procedures used in medicine (medical tests and therapies), consumer products, radioactive substances used in industry, nuclear power gen-erators, and radioactivity (e.g., radioactive fallout) from the production and detonation (primarily for testing purposes) of nuclear weapons. Consumer products that sometimes contain radioactive substances include:

- Radioluminescent paints and signs
- Mantles of camping lanterns
- Colorful ceramic glazes
- Potassium-based salt substitutes
- Dentures
- Tobacco products
- Ionization-type smoke detectors

With the increasingly numerous applications of radiation, a good understanding of the health effects of radiation exposure has developed. Quite early in the use of X-ray machines, health authorities and others observed the occurrence of radiation burns and radiation sickness among technicians. Other early observations included the recognition of health problems such as skin cancer and other cancers associated with ionizing radiation exposure. During the early 1900s, the radioactive element radium was used as a paint to create "glow-in-the-dark" watch and other instrument dials. The dials were hand-painted by workers who, before applying the paint, used mouth-tipping to create a point on the brushes that were coated with radium. After these workers began to develop a form of bone cancer known as "radium jaw," the practice of mouth-tipping was discontinued during the mid-1920s.[2] From these beginnings, the body of research information (from experimental and epidemiologic studies) regarding health effects of radiation exposure has become quite extensive, spanning a time period of more than a century.[3]

TYPES OF IONIZING RADIATION

Radiation and radioactivity are two important terms used in the context of ionizing radiation. The term **radiation** refers to "[e]nergy traveling through space. Some types of radiation associated with radioactivity are alpha and beta particles and gamma and X rays."[4] Radiation

FIGURE 8-1 Types of radiation in the electromagnetic spectrum: ionizing and nonionizing radiation.

Source: Reprinted from US Environmental Protection Agency. Radiation Protection: Understanding Radiation: Ionizing and Non-Ionizing Radiation. Available at: http://www.epa.gov/radiation/understand/ionize_nonionize.html. Accessed April 2, 2010.

also includes neutrons, which are uncharged. **Radioactivity** denotes "[t]he spontaneous emission of radiation from the nucleus of an unstable atom. As a result of this emission, the radioactive atom is converted, or decays, into an atom of a different element that might or might not be radioactive."[4] Radioactive decay is associated with the spontaneous disintegration of radioactive materials.

Related to the concept of radioactivity are the terms *isotope, nuclide, radioisotope*, and *radionuclide*. An **isotope** is "each of two or more forms of the same element that contain equal numbers of protons but different numbers of neutrons in their nuclei, and hence differ in atomic mass but not in chemical properties; in particular, a radioactive form of an element."[5] For example, carbon is an atom (atomic number 6), and two isotopes of carbon are carbon-12 and carbon-14. There are more than one dozen radioisotopes of uranium (atomic number 92) plus several nonradioactive isotopes. The term **nuclide** refers to a nucleus with a specific number of protons and neutrons and a specific energy state; it includes radioactive and nonradioactive atoms. A **radioisotope** is a natural or artificially produced isotope that is radioactive. For this reason, a radioisotope also is called a radioactive isotope. An example is the radioisotope of iodine, iodine-131 (^{131}I). A **radionuclide** is an atom that has an unstable nucleus; when a radionuclide decays, it can emit X- or gamma rays and/ or subatomic particles; ^{131}I also is a radionuclide as well as a radioisotope. Often radionuclides are described in terms of their half-life, meaning the time that it takes their level of radioactivity to decrease by one-half; the half-life of a radionuclide can range from a very brief time to millions of years. For example, ^{131}I has an eight-day half-life; the half-life of ^{227}U is 1.3 minutes and of ^{238}U, 4.47 billion years; stable elements (nonradioactive) have an infinite to near-infinite half-life.

Ionizing radiation consists of either particulate energy (e.g., highly energetic protons, neutrons, and α and β particles) or electromagnetic energy in the form of photons (e.g., γ rays and X-rays). Ionizing radiation is "radiation capable of producing ions or charged particles."[4] When ionization occurs, "[a]n orbital electron is stripped from a neutral atom, producing an ion pair (a negatively charged electron and a positively charged atom)."[4] Ionizing radiation may damage "living tissue in the human body. . . . The body attempts to repair the damage, but sometimes the damage is of a nature that cannot be repaired or it is too severe or widespread to be repaired. Also mistakes made in the natural repair process can lead to cancerous cells."[6]

The definitions of the terms **alpha particle, beta particle, gamma rays**, and **X-rays** are shown in the following text box.

Definitions: Alpha Particle, Beta Particle, Gamma Rays, and X-Rays

- *Alpha particle:* A subatomic particle made up of the nucleus of a helium atom that is ejected from a radioactive atom. It has low penetrating power and a short travel range. Alpha particles can be stopped by a piece of paper and, thus, generally will fail to penetrate the skin. However, alpha particles cannot be considered harmless. When introduced into the body (through diet, skin wounds, or inhalation of uranium-bearing ores and radioactive dusts), alpha particles irradiate the body's cells and may act as carcinogens or initiate other adverse health effects.

- *Beta particle:* An electron that is emitted from the nucleus of a radioactive atom. It has moderate penetrating power and a travel range of up to a few meters in air. Beta particles will penetrate only a fraction of an inch (up to 2 cm) of skin tissue. Again, internal exposure is a factor in producing potentially adverse effects.

- *Gamma rays, or gamma radiation:* These high-energy rays are part of the electromagnetic spectrum. Gamma rays, consisting of photons, are the most highly penetrating type of radiation; they are capable of passing through the body. When energy from photons interacts with bodily tissues, adverse effects such as cellular damage can result, even though the source of the photons is external to the body.

- *X-rays:* Penetrating electromagnetic radiation whose wavelengths are shorter than those of visible light. X-rays are used in medical diagnostic procedures because they are absorbed differentially by soft tissue and bone.

Source: Adapted and reprinted from Oak Ridge Institute for Science and Education, Radiation Emergency Assistance Center/ Training Site (REAC/TS). Guidance for Radiation Accident Management, Basics of Radiation: Definitions. Available at: http:// orise.orau.gov/reacts/guide/definitions.htm. Accessed April 2, 2010; and World Health Organization, International Agency for Research on Cancer. Ionizing Radiation, Part 1: X- and Gamma (γ)-Radiation, and Neutrons. *IARC Monographs.* 2000;75:36.

FIGURE 8-2 Measuring radiation levels with a Geiger counter.

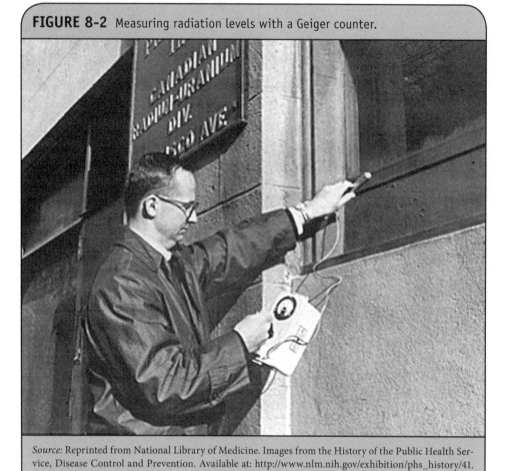

Source: Reprinted from National Library of Medicine. Images from the History of the Public Health Service, Disease Control and Prevention. Available at: http://www.nlm.nih.gov/exhibition/phs_history/41.html. Accessed April 2, 2010.

MEASUREMENT OF IONIZING RADIATION DOSE UNITS

One widely used device for measuring radiation is the Geiger counter, a hand-held device shown in Figure 8-2. The frequency of audible clicks that the device emits when gas in a detector tube is ionized is correlated with the intensity of radiation exposure. Also, a visual readout meter indicates the rate of exposure to radiation. The Geiger counter is best for detecting X-rays and β particles, so often other instruments are used for monitoring gamma rays and alpha particles. A device that is used most commonly in the occupational environment is a film badge, which is worn by workers who are potentially exposed to gamma radiation. The badge contains dental X-ray film that darkens in proportion to the degree of exposure to radiation.[7]

The unit of energy associated with emissions from a radioactive material (radionuclide) is the electron volt (eV). The units used for measurement of the amount of radioactivity, dosage, and exposure are shown in Table 8-1. The term **common units**, which refers to an earlier system of radiation measurement, is used often in the United States. The abbreviation **SI (System International) units**, which denotes the International System of Units, has been implemented more recently and has replaced the older system of common units. The terms shown in the table are discussed in the text.

Going across the top row of Table 8-1, we see the following terms: *radioactivity, absorbed dose, dose equivalent*, and *exposure*. Radioactivity was defined previously; the remaining terms are defined in Table 8-2.

TABLE 8-1 Ionizing Radiation Measurements

	Radioactivity	**Absorbed Dose**	**Dose Equivalent**	**Exposure**
Common Units	Curie (Ci)	Rad	Rem	Roentgen (R)
SI Units	Becquerel (Bq)	Gray (Gy)	Sievert (Sv)	Coulomb/kilogram (C/kg)

Source: Adapted and reprinted from Oak Ridge Institute for Science and Education. Guidance for Radiation Accident Management: Measurement. Available at: http://orise.orau.gov/reacts/guide/measure.htm. Accessed April 2, 2010.

TABLE 8-2 Radioactivity, Dose, and Exposure

Absorbed dose	"[T]he primary physical quantity of radiation dosimetry. It is defined as the radiation energy absorbed per unit mass of an organ or tissue and is used in studies of the damage to a particular organ or tissue."[a(p39)]
Dose equivalent (equivalent dose)	Obtained by weighting the absorbed dose in an organ or tissue by a radiation weighting factor that reflects the biological effectiveness of the charged particles that produce ionization within the tissue. Related to the concept of dose is *effective dose*, which measures the overall biological impact associated with radiation, by taking into account weighting factors and equivalent dose factors. Another aspect of dose is the *dose rate*, which is defined as "The dose delivered per unit time. It is usually expressed as rads per hour or in multiples or submultiples of this unit such as millirads per hour. The dose rate is commonly used to indicate the level of hazard from a radioactive source."[b]
Exposure	"A quantity used to indicate the amount of ionization in air produced by x- or gamma-ray radiation. The unit is the roentgen (R). For practical purposes, one roentgen is comparable to 1 rad or 1 rem for X and gamma radiation."[b] Exposure to ionizing radiation can come from an external source, which exposes (irradiates) the entire body or part of the body such as a targeted organ or tissue. Radiation of this type is called an *external radiation dose*. An *internal radiation dose* arises from a radioactive substance that has been deposited inside the body.[c]

Sources: Adapted from [a]World Health Organization, International Agency for Research on Cancer. Ionizing Radiation, Part 1: X- and Gamma (γ)-Radiation, and Neutrons. *IARC Monographs.* 2000;75:35–115; [b]Oak Ridge Institute for Science and Education. Guidance for Radiation Accident Management. Radiation Emergency Assistance Center/Training Site (REAC/TS). Basics of Radiation: Definitions. Available at: http://orise.orau.gov/reacts/guide/definitions.htm. Accessed April 2, 2010; [c]Health Physics Society. Radiation Dose Units. Available at: http://hps.org/publicinformation/ate/faqs/radiationdoses.html. Accessed March 11, 2010.

Returning to the first row in Table 8-1, we see the term *common units*. These units are the **curie**, rad, **rem**, and roentgen. The common units are defined in Table 8-3.

Table 8-1 contains the term *SI units*, which stands for the International System of Units. The SI units employ the terms *becquerel, gray,* and *sievert*. The definitions of the SI units and their equivalency in common units are shown in Table 8-4.

It is possible to express fractional units of radiation doses by using the following prefixes: milli (m) and micro (μ). In addition, the prefix kilo (k) is used. For example, when these prefixes are applied to a rad, an mrad is 1/1,000 of a rad; a μrad is 1/1,000,000 of a rad; a krad is 1,000 times one rad, or 1,000 rads. These prefixes may be applied to other measures of radiation (e.g., sievert and rem). Note that the amount of radioactivity (defined previously as curies or becquerels) present in a material does not depend on its weight or size but on the particular radioactive element or isotope. (See Figure 8-3.)

TABLE 8-3 Definitions of Common Units of Radiation

Curie (Ci)	A unit of measure used to describe the amount of radioactivity in a sample of material[a]; 1 Ci equals 3.7×10^{10} disintegrations per second.[b]
Rad	Radiation absorbed dose. The former unit of absorbed dose of ionizing radiation.[c]
Rem	Roentgen equivalent in man. A measure of radiation dose related to biological effect (i.e., the equivalent dose or effective dose).[a] A rem is a measure of dose deposited in body tissue, averaged over the mass of the tissue of interest. One rem is approximately the dose from any radiation corresponding to one roentgen of gamma radiation.[c]
Roentgen (R)	The unit of exposure from X- or gamma rays.[a]

Sources: Adapted and reprinted from [a]Oak Ridge Institute for Science and Education. Guidance for Radiation Accident Management. Radiation Emergency Assistance Center/Training Site (REAC/TS). Basics of Radiation: Definitions. Available at: http://orise.orau.gov/reacts/guide/definitions.htm. Accessed March 24, 2010; [b]Oak Ridge Institute for Science and Education. Guidance for Radiation Accident Management: Measurement. Available at: http://orise.orau.gov/reacts/guide/measure.htm. Accessed April 2, 2010; [c]Lawrence Berkeley National Laboratory. Nuclear Science Glossary, Appendix A Glossary of Nuclear Terms. Available at: http://www.lbl.gov/abc/wallchart/glossary/glossary.html. Accessed April 2, 2010.

TABLE 8-4 International System of Units (SI Units) and Their Equivalency in Common Units

Becquerel (Bq)	(Corresponds to radioactivity) The SI unit of activity, which is defined as one disintegration per second; 37 billion Bq = 1 curie; 1 Bq = 2.7×10^{-11} i.
Exposure	The SI unit of exposure is the coulomb per kilogram (C/kg). One R = 2.58×10^{-4} C/kg.
Gray (Gy)	(Corresponds to absorbed dose) The SI unit of absorbed dose; 1 gray = 100 rad; 1 rad = 0.01 Gy.
Sievert (Sv)	(Corresponds to dose equivalent) The SI unit of dose equivalent; 1 Sv = 100 rem; 1 rem = 0.01 Sv.

Source: Adapted and reprinted from Oak Ridge Institute for Science and Education, Radiation Emergency Assistance Center/Training Site (REAC/TS). Guidance for Radiation Accident Management, Basics of Radiation: Definitions. Available at: http://orise.orau.gov/reacts/guide/definitions.htm. Accessed March 24, 2010; and Oak Ridge Institute for Science and Education. Guidance for Radiation Accident Management, Radiation Emergency Assistance Center/Training Site (REAC/TS). Measurement. Available at: http://orise.orau.gov/reacts/guide/measure.htm. Accessed March 24, 2010.

FIGURE 8-3 Measurement: How much radiation is present?

The size or weight of a container or shipment does not indicate how much radioactivity is in it.

The amount of radioactivity in a quantity of material can be determined by noting how many curies of the material are present. This information should be found on labels and/or shipping papers.

More curies = a greater amount of radioactivity

A large amount of material can have a very small amount of radioactivity; a very small amount of material can have a lot of radioactivity.

For example, uranium-238 has 0.00015 curies of radioactivity per pound (0.15 millicuries), while cobalt-60 has nearly 518,000 curies per pound.

Source: Reprinted from Oak Ridge Institute for Science and Education. Guidance for Radiation Accident Management, Radiation Emergency Assistance Center/Training Site (REAC/TS). Measurement: Activity: How much is present? Available at: http://orise.orau.gov/reacts/guide/measure.htm. Accessed March 24, 2010.

TABLE 8-5 Nonstochastic Health Effects of Whole-Body Exposure for an Average Person and Time to Onset Following Acute Exposure

Exposure (rem)	Health Effect	Time to Onset
5–10	Changes in blood chemistry	
50	Nausea	Hours
55	Fatigue	
70	Vomiting	
75	Hair loss	2–3 weeks
90	Diarrhea	
100	Hemorrhage	
400	Possible death	Within 2 months
1,000	Destruction of intestinal lining	
	Internal bleeding	
	Death	1–2 weeks
2,000	Damage to central nervous system	
	Loss of consciousness	Minutes
	Death	Hours to days

Source: Reprinted from US Environmental Protection Agency. Radiation Protection: Understanding Radiation: Health Effects. Available at: http://www.epa.gov/radiation/understand/health_effects.html. Accessed March 11, 2010.

HEALTH EFFECTS OF EXPOSURE TO IONIZING RADIATION

The dose of radiation is associated with the amount of bodily tissue damage that may occur. Factors that govern the amount of exposure to radiation that a person receives (dose delivered) include:

- The total amount of time exposed to the radioactive source
- Distance from the radioactive source
- Degree of radioactivity (rate of energy emission) of a radioactive material

The amount of radiation dose that is absorbed—expressed as either grays or rads—may or may not be associated with acute health effects, depending upon individual susceptibility and amount of exposure as determined by the foregoing factors. The health effects of radiation exposure are described as nonstochastic and stochastic (acute) effects.[6]

Nonstochastic Effects

Table 8-5 shows the nonstochastic (acute) effects of varying levels of radiation exposure. Among the acute effects

of radiation exposure are tissue burns and radiation sickness (e.g., nausea, weakness, and loss of hair). At low levels, for example an exposure of 5 rads, radiation usually does not produce immediately detectable harm. The term **hormesis** refers to the belief that "[s]ome nonnutritional toxic substances also may impart beneficial or stimulatory effects at low doses, but at higher doses they produce adverse effects."[8(p15)] Consistent with the notion of hormesis, some scientists assert that low levels of radiation are beneficial to one's health. At high levels (e.g., an exposure of 350 to 400 rads or higher), ionizing radiation is capable of producing fatal injuries. The acute effects shown in Table 8-5 are cumulative, meaning that when a person experiences the health effect associated with an exposure at a higher level, the effects that occur at a lower level also will have been experienced. For example, subjects who experience hemorrhage at an exposure of 100 rems of radiation also will have had changes in blood chemistry.[6]

Stochastic Effects

Stochastic effects are those associated with low levels of exposure to radiation over long time periods. The term *stochastic* refers to an increased probability of the occurrence of an adverse health event. Among the effects linked potentially to low levels of exposure to radiation are carcinogenesis and genetic damage such as changes in DNA. These changes may be inherited by the progeny of exposed individuals who have experienced DNA damage. In some cases the damage to DNA is so severe that it is not transmitted (i.e., the germinal cells are incapable of viable cell division).

SOURCES OF ENVIRONMENTAL EXPOSURE TO IONIZING RADIATION

The human population is exposed to ionizing radiation from many sources. Ionizing radiation, produced from natural sources such as cosmic radiation (radiation from space) and uranium deposits, causes increases in background radiation

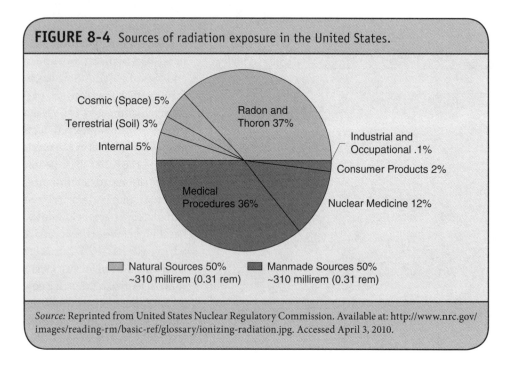

FIGURE 8-4 Sources of radiation exposure in the United States.

Cosmic (Space) 5%
Terrestrial (Soil) 3%
Internal 5%
Radon and Thoron 37%
Industrial and Occupational .1%
Consumer Products 2%
Medical Procedures 36%
Nuclear Medicine 12%

Natural Sources 50%
~310 millirem (0.31 rem)
Manmade Sources 50%
~310 millirem (0.31 rem)

Source: Reprinted from United States Nuclear Regulatory Commission. Available at: http://www.nrc.gov/images/reading-rm/basic-ref/glossary/ionizing-radiation.jpg. Accessed April 3, 2010.

levels in some geographic areas. A decay product of uranium, radioactive radon gas may seep into homes, thus exposing the residents. Although they are generally regarded as safe, nuclear power plants have been known to leak ionizing radiation into the environment under unusual conditions. Radioactive fallout from above-ground nuclear testing has exposed large populations to radiation. Still other exposure sources are decommissioned and abandoned nuclear weapons facilities and storage of nuclear wastes. Finally, medical X-rays and radiation diagnostic and therapy procedures produce exposures to ionizing radiation. Figure 8-4 shows the relative proportions of different radiation sources to which the US population is exposed.

Naturally Occurring Radiation

The estimated average annual exposure of the world's population to naturally occurring radiation is 2.4 mSv (0.0024 Sv 5 0.24 rem, or 240 mrem).[9] The sources of natural radiation include cosmic rays, terrestrial gamma rays, radionuclides that are present in the body, and radon gas. The relative distribution of the exposures from these sources is shown in Figure 8-5.

Uranium

A very common element in the earth's crust, uranium is present in soil and geologic formations almost universally. The uranium ores uraninite and pitchblende are found in large

amounts in North America, Africa, and Australia and in lesser amounts on other continents. Nearly all plants, animals, and aquifers contain tiny amounts of uranium. Coal used to fuel electrical generating plants has numerous impurities including radionuclides of uranium (plus thorium and radioactive decay products), which are not destroyed during burning and become concentrated in leftover ash. Fly ash that escapes from power plants into the environment can expose nearby residents to radioactivity from radionuclides; pollution control technology aids in removal of fly ash and radioactive particles from power plant emissions.

Estimates suggest that the bodies of typical nonoccupationally exposed persons who live in Europe and the United States contain about 22 µg of uranium. The three isotopes of uranium found in the natural environment are ^{234}U, ^{235}U, and ^{238}U, the last being the most common form. When ^{238}U that is present in the foundations of building sites and in building materials decays, it produces radon gas.

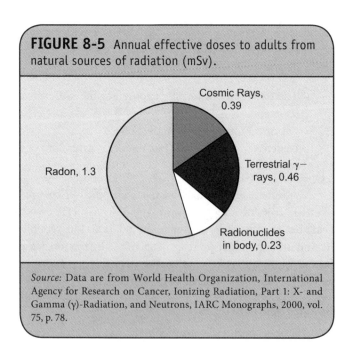

FIGURE 8-5 Annual effective doses to adults from natural sources of radiation (mSv).

Cosmic Rays, 0.39
Terrestrial γ−rays, 0.46
Radon, 1.3
Radionuclides in body, 0.23

Source: Data are from World Health Organization, International Agency for Research on Cancer, Ionizing Radiation, Part 1: X- and Gamma (γ)-Radiation, and Neutrons, IARC Monographs, 2000, vol. 75, p. 78.

Radon

An inert, colorless, and extremely toxic gas, radon is produced by the decay of radium and uranium. One of the radioactive decay products of uranium is radium-226 (^{226}Ra), which decays into radon-222 (^{222}Rn). Suspicions regarding the carcinogenic effect of radon were aroused by studies of miners who worked underground, where they were exposed to high levels of radon gas.[10] These miners had a lung cancer mortality rate that was five times that of the general population; concurrent cigarette smoking increased the risk of lung cancer. Classified as a Class A carcinogen (known human carcinogen) by the Environmental Protection Agency (EPA) and other agencies, radon gas causes no immediate symptoms but has been associated with long-term adverse health effects. Environmental radon produces one of the largest sources of human exposure to ionizing radiation and is thought to be one of the leading causes of lung cancer in the United States. Up to 20% of US lung cancer cases may be caused by radon despite evidence that cigarette smoking, asbestos exposure, and urban air pollution are the leading causes of lung cancer. Both lifetime risk of lung cancer and years of life lost show a dose–response increase with increasing radon exposure.[11] The induction period for lung cancer after radon exposure is believed to range from 5 to more than 20 years.

In addition to the association demonstrated between lung cancer and radon exposure among miners as well as among experimentally exposed laboratory animals, radon exposure that occurs in people's residences has been linked to lung cancer. An Iowa case-control study of lung cancer reported a positive association with cumulative radon exposure.[12] The area was selected for study because some Iowa homes—especially in the basement and on the first floor levels—have the highest indoor radon levels in the United States.

An estimated 15,000 to 22,000 lung cancer deaths are believed to be caused by radon in indoor air. According to EPA documents, approximately 50% of homes in some areas have high levels of radon gas. During the winter when windows are kept closed, radon levels increase. The EPA recommends that homeowners have their residences tested to verify that unsafe levels of radon gas are not present.

Another possible source of exposure to radon is drinking water. Waterborne radon may be released into the air, increasing the risk of lung cancer if inhaled; ingestion of water that contains radon may increase the risk of cancers in internal organs such as the stomach. The primary origins of waterborne radon are underground aquifers in some locales; not all water from underground sources contains radon, and surface water is generally free from radon contamination. Only a small percentage of the radon found in air originates from drinking water.

Extraterrestrial Radiation

Primary cosmic rays originate from outer space (e.g., the earth's galaxy and the sun) and interact with the earth's atmosphere to produce secondary cosmic rays.[9] Cosmic rays have the ability to penetrate and cross the human body easily. Radiation from the sun, called solar cosmic radiation, coincides with solar flares and sunspots on the surface of the sun. These solar events have the ability to increase ground-level radiation on the earth's surface. On February 23, 1956, the largest solar event observed to date caused the levels of neutron radiation to increase by a factor of 3,600% over the normal background radiation level.[9] Passengers and crew members of high-altitude aircraft receive higher exposures to the radiation from solar particle events than do persons who remain on the ground. However, a recent study of airline pilots failed to detect adverse health effects associated with exposures to ionizing radiation.[13]

Nuclear Facilities—Nuclear Accidents

Other potential sources for exposure of the population to ionizing radiation are nuclear facilities, which include weapons production plants, test sites, and nuclear power plants. Figure 8-6 illustrates the nuclear power plant on the Susquehanna River at Three Mile Island, Pennsylvania, which was the location of an accidental release of radiation into the environment on March 28, 1979.

The Three Mile Island accident involved a series of mechanical failures and mistakes that led to the accidental release of radiation into the environment when the core of the reactor experienced a partial meltdown. Following the incident, research studies suggested that the amount of human exposure to ionizing radiation was very low (less than 100 mrems).[14,15]

The association between exposure to ionizing radiation that occurred among residents who lived downwind of the nuclear reactor and health effects such as cancer remains a controversial issue. One study reported a modest association between postaccident cancer rates and proximity to the power plant. Although postaccident cancer rates increased during 1982 and 1983, and subsequently declined, plant emissions did not appear to account for the observed increase.[16] The major consequence of the Three Mile Island accident was that no new nuclear power plants have been built in the United States since 1979.[17] Despite the fact that the incident at Three Mile

FIGURE 8-6 Three Mile Island Nuclear Power Plant.

Source: Reprinted courtesy of the Centers for Disease Control and Prevention. Public Health Image Library, ID# 1194. Available at: http://phil.cdc.gov/Phil/details.asp. Accessed March 24, 2010.

Island has become a symbol for the antinuclear movement, the nuclear power industry argues that the containment of the meltdown reinforced the notion that the installed safety systems were effective.

In contrast to the Three Mile Island release, the nuclear power plant accident at Chernobyl, Ukraine, on April 26, 1986, was a major public health disaster that exposed a large portion of the European population to ionizing radiation. One consequence of the disaster was to call into question the safety of older nuclear reactors that use a similar design and are operating in Eastern Europe. Two explosions at the power plant and an associated fire required nine days to extinguish. One report stated that "a cloud of radioactivity rained down on western Europe as the fallout from the Chernobyl disaster spread with the wind. Plumes of radioactive waste covered the countryside, homes, people, land and food crops."[18(p16)]

Radioactive materials, primarily iodine and cesium, were deposited over wide swaths of Europe, including sections of the former Soviet Union, Sweden, Austria, Switzerland, and parts of Germany and northern Italy.[18] According to one account, "Half the reactor's caesium-137 and iodine-131 escaped and 3–5% of the remaining radioactive material escaped. . . . The accident killed 31 people; a further 209 suffered acute radiation sickness. About 185,000 people received radiation doses of over four times the internationally accepted limit; a much larger number received some increased radiation dose."[18(p16)] An exclusion zone with a 30-km radius around the reactor was created eventually. In some parts of the exclusion zone, ground radiation levels from the deposited ^{137}cesium were extremely high. In order to limit the spread of radioactivity from the damaged reactor, officials constructed a steel and concrete sarcophagus that encases the reactor. Noteworthy is the fact that the Chernobyl facility lacked an effective containment structure, which is not the case for US nuclear power reactors.

Carcinogenesis is one of the main health phenomena investigated as a consequence of the release of radioactivity from the Chernobyl power plant. Researchers have examined the occurrence of excess cases of cancer in neighboring sections of Europe that received radioactive fallout as well as those in close proximity to the reactor. A number of methodological issues cloud possible associations between cancer and exposure to radioactivity from Chernobyl. No method is available to distinguish between cancer (e.g., thyroid cancer and leukemia) that has resulted from the Chernobyl disaster and cancer that originates from other exposures. Exposures to natural background radiation and medical radiation among some European populations may exceed the radiation doses from the Chernobyl release. In addition, the residents of Europe generally were exposed to low doses of radiation. In summary, researchers have been unable to demonstrate any increase in rates of morbidity and mortality from cancer that can be assigned definitively to radioactivity from Chernobyl.[19] Another health effect of the Chernobyl accident could be the production of birth defects such as congenital anomalies. However, data from the EUROCAT epidemiologic surveillance of congenital anomalies have not suggested an increase in central nervous system anomalies or Down syndrome in Western Europe.[20]

Closer to the Chernobyl nuclear facility, however, there were marked increases in thyroid cancer as soon as 4 to 5 years after the accident. The Gomel region of Belarus in the former Soviet Union lies immediately to the north of Chernobyl. There was a sharp increase in the number of thyroid cancer cases among children in Gomel from 1 to 2 per year during 1986–1989 to 38 in 1991.[21] Subsequent research also demonstrated increases in the number of thyroid cancer cases in three radiation-affected countries (Belarus, Ukraine, and western parts of Russia). The number of such cases had totaled 5,000 by the year 2010, with 15,000 additional cases expected in the next 50 years among those exposed as children. Persons exposed as adults do not appear to demonstrate an increase in thyroid cancer rates.[22] Another outcome has been increases in the number of congenital abnormalities among children.[18]

In terms of cancer rates and proximity to other nuclear installations, studies with conflicting results have emerged. One study reported an excess of leukemia in a five-town area in Massachusetts in which one of the towns was the site of a commercial nuclear power plant. The excess cases were found mostly in adults and the elderly, but the authors believed that the results from this descriptive study were suggestive and warranted additional, more intensive follow-up investigations.[23] In contrast, no excess of cancer deaths was found among populations near the Rocky Flats nuclear weapons plant in Colorado[24] or California's San Onofre nuclear power plant (which has a formidable containment structure).[25] A systematic literature review concluded that although many studies of the health effects of community exposure to radiation were statistically sound, they did not provide adequate quantitative estimates of radiation dose that could be used to assess dose–response relationships.[26]

A major release of widespread radioactivity occurred in the Urals region of Russia.[27] In 1948, the former Soviet Union began production of its first atomic bomb at a plutonium separation plant near the city of Chelyabinsk. (Plutonium is a man-made element that is created by bombarding ^{238}U with neutrons; this heavy radioactive metal is used in nuclear reactors and for creating fissile materials in nuclear weapons.)[28] From 1949 to 1956, the plant discharged substantial amounts of nuclear waste into the nearby Techa River. An open depot for the storage of radioactive wastes contaminated Lake Karachay, which later evaporated and left residual radioactive dusts that affected the population downwind from the site. In 1957, a tank that stored nuclear wastes suffered a thermochemical explosion that spread radioactivity into the surrounding area. Exposed residents developed chronic radiation sickness, changes in blood parameters, and increased morbidity and mortality rates from leukemia and cancer. Refer to the text box for more information on nuclear accidents.

Nuclear Bomb Explosions

There are several types of nuclear bombs, including atom bombs and hydrogen bombs. Explosion of an atomic bomb is a fission reaction (splitting apart of uranium or plutonium atoms). In contrast, hydrogen bombs exploit the fusion reaction of hydrogen. The following text box describes the effects of a nuclear explosion.

Information presented in the text box indicates that persons near the site of a nuclear explosion would experience thermal burns and radiation-induced skin injuries. Figure 8-7 illustrates injuries to the skin caused by thermal burns and radiation burns (e.g., beta burns from beta radiation emitters). For a beta injury to occur, beta particle emitters (e.g., from the products of nuclear fission) must come into direct contact with skin and remain there for an extended time period. The injuries shown in Figure 8-7 resulted from the nuclear explosions that occurred in Japan during World War II.

Also as noted in the foregoing text box, one of the major by-products of the detonation of a nuclear weapon is radioactive fallout. When a nuclear weapon explodes above ground, it

Effects of a Nuclear Explosion

The effects of a nuclear weapon explosion are the blast (damage to or destruction of buildings and those in them), heat (destruction or injury by high temperatures or fire), intense light (damage to eyesight), and ionizing radiation (causing Acute Radiation Syndromes of different degrees of severity). A detonation similar in size to the bomb that was dropped on Hiroshima (15 kilotons) could result in a high-damage zone of a few kilometres radius where there would be few or no survivors. There would also be a significant number of injured people over a considerably larger area. However, the effects of nuclear explosion generated by the blast could be reduced somewhat by preparation in advance and prompt action during the event.

Detonating a nuclear weapon generates an intense and immediate pulse of radiation, and gives rise to longer lasting radioactive contamination. Objects close to the explosion can be made radioactive by neutrons from the explosion, but farther away objects become radioactive from fallout of radioactive debris generated by the weapon. The initial "prompt" radiation would directly affect everybody up to a few kilometres, whereas fallout can irradiate people over a much larger area in a number of ways. A radioactive cloud is spread by the wind, possibly over large distances. Rainfall can wash out some of the radioactive materials from the air and enhance fallout deposits onto surfaces where it has rained. Once this radioactive cloud deposits as particles on surfaces it can be picked up on clothing and other objects or inhaled or spread further. The radioactive fallout can also contaminate food and water supplies if it deposits on crops, animal feed, or in drinking water sources. The hazard from this fallout reduces with time but could last for many months or more.

Radioactive materials may be inhaled from the air or ingested in food causing internal radioactive contamination and damaging internal organs of the body. External exposure can be due to radioactive materials deposited on the ground, buildings, or even on our clothes or skin. If radioactive materials come into contact with the skin, they may cause radiation burns.

Persons near the site of detonation surviving the initial blast and thermal effects would be exposed to high levels of radiation and could develop symptoms of radiation sickness. Early symptoms of high radiation exposure include nausea, vomiting, diarrhea, fatigue, and headache. While thermal burns may appear within minutes, radiation induced skin injury and other early symptoms develop over days and weeks. Depending on the severity of exposure, victims may experience different symptoms and medical care will be needed. Following years or even some decades after exposures, an increased risk of cancer among the wider exposed population could be expected.

There will be considerable damage to the infrastructure of society. Communication systems may be severely disrupted and normal modes of transport may not be available. Consequently, there would be great difficulty in providing effective medical treatment to the large numbers of casualties.

Source: Adapted and reprinted with permission from World Health Organization Radiation and Environmental Health Unit. Health Protection Guidance in the Event of a Nuclear Weapons Explosion, WHO/RAD Information Sheet, February 2003. Available at: http://www.who.int/ionizing_radiation/en/WHORAD_InfoSheet_Nuclear_weapons21Feb.pdf. Accessed March 11, 2010.

produces large amounts of radioactive dusts that later become dispersed over the earth downwind from the burst. Some of the materials may even be injected into the upper atmosphere and, as they settle out, persist as residual hazards. A fission reaction may produce more than 300 radioactive products that have varying half-lives, ranging from a fraction of a second to many months or years. Integral to a nuclear explosion is the emission of neutrons that induce radioactivity in elements in the soil near the site of the explosion (ground zero). This radioactivity, which generally is confined to a limited area, decays gradually over time as beta and gamma radiation are released from the activated elements. Very fine particles (size range 10 nanometers to 20 micrometers) may be pushed up high into the atmosphere and can be dispersed worldwide. The heavier particles, such as vaporized water and soils, are incorporated into a radioactive cloud that settles over a wide geographic area of several hundred square miles, depending on wind and weather conditions. The initial level of radioactivity downwind and close to the explosion may be approximately 300 Gy per hour, the LD_{50} being a cumulative dose of 4.5 Gy. After the radioactivity from a nuclear weapon dissipates over several weeks, the nearby fallout zone becomes safe to enter, but crops and food animals taken from the area may be unsuitable to consume.

FIGURE 8-7 Upper left: Beta burn on the neck 1 month after exposure. Upper right: Beta burn one year after exposure. Lower left: Thermal (flash) burn—the patient's skin is burned in a pattern corresponding to the dark portions of a kimono worn at the time of the explosion. Lower right: Thermal (flash) burn—the skin under the areas of contact with clothing is burned and the protective effect of thicker layers of clothing can be seen on the shoulders and across the back.

Source: Adapted and reprinted from S Glasstone and PJ Dolan, eds. The Effects of Nuclear Weapons. 3rd ed. Washington, DC: US Department of Defense and the Energy Research and Development Administration; 1977:568, 569, 595, 597.

Among the components of fallout from weapons testing is radioactive iodine, which may become concentrated in the thyroid gland, potentially increasing the rate of thyroid cancer. There have been many studies of the health effects of fallout from aboveground atmospheric testing of nuclear weapons at the Nevada test site in the United States during 1951 to 1958. One cohort study followed young people who lived in proximity to the test site during infancy and childhood.[29] Three cohorts, similar in demographic and lifestyle characteristics, were selected. Two cohorts (exposure cohorts) were from Washington County, Utah, and Lincoln County, Nevada, both on the west side of the test site, close to the site, and in the pathway of the heaviest fallout. A third, unexposed, cohort (control cohort) was selected from Graham County,

Catalog of Nuclear Accidents

Since the 1940s, there have been numerous accidents that involved nuclear materials. In some instances, these accidents resulted in fatalities or exposed many people to ionizing radiation. Some of these accidents involved the manufacture of nuclear weapons, weapons testing, transport of nuclear devices, and accidents at electric power generating stations. Estimates indicate that more than 50 nuclear warheads and 10 nuclear reactors lie on the oceans' floors as a consequence of ships that have sunk and aircraft that have crashed or accidentally dropped nuclear bombs. A few examples follow:

- In the 1950s, several bomber aircraft accidentally dropped nuclear weapons or crashed with such weapons on board. In one incident on March 11, 1958, a B-47E en route to England dropped a nuclear weapon on Mars Bluff, South Carolina. The unarmed device landed on the property of Walter Gregg, destroying his house. Several of Gregg's family members were injured when the bomb's TNT-based trigger exploded on impact with the ground, causing a giant crater. Several nearby structures also were damaged.[a]
- On April 10, 1963, the nuclear submarine USS *Thresher* with its reactor core sank to the ocean floor in the vicinity of Boston, Massachusetts; all crew members perished.[b]
- During the 1970s, incidents included the sinking of a Soviet nuclear submarine, releases of radiation from nuclear power plants (e.g., Three Mile Island accident, discussed in text), and leakage of radioactive water from a nuclear fuel reprocessing plant.
- On April 26, 1986, the Chernobyl accident occurred (refer to text).
- On September 30, 1999, Japan's worst nuclear accident occurred when a tank located at a uranium reprocessing plant in Tokaimura exploded, killing two workers. The incident exposed reactor workers, rescue personnel, and community residents to excess levels of radiation.[c]
- On August 12, 2000, the Russian nuclear submarine *Kursk* sank in the Barents Sea.[d]

Sources: Data are from [a]*Columbia Star*. Atomic Bomb dropped on Florence, S.C., March 11, 1958. Available at: http://www.thecolumbiastar.com/news/2008-03-21/news/036.html. Accessed April 3, 2010; [b]Arlington National Cemetery. USS *Thresher* (SSN-593), 1961–1963. Available at: http://www.arlingtoncemetery.net/uss-thresher.htm. Accessed April 3, 2010; [c]R Toohey. The criticality accident at Tokaimura, Japan. *Health Phys.* 2002;82(suppl):S163; and *Guardian*. The wreck of the *Kursk* begins its journey home. Available at: http://www.guardian.co.uk/world/2001/oct/09/kursk.russia. Accessed April 3, 2010.

far to the south of the test site. At 12 to 15 years and 30 years after the heaviest fallout, there was a slight but nonsignificant increase in rates of thyroid cancer among the two exposure cohorts in comparison with the control cohort. Thus, it was concluded that living near the Nevada test site did not produce a statistically significant increase in thyroid neoplasms.

Studies of the long-term consequences of exposure to radiation from the atomic bombs dropped in Japan confirmed increases in the risk of breast cancer, especially if exposure occurred between the ages of 10 and 19 years.[30] Yet, some individuals seem to be resistant to the effects of radiation. Ms. Asa Takii, Japan's oldest person, who survived the Hiroshima atomic bomb blast, died in 1998 at the age of 114 years.[31] At the time of the detonation (August 6, 1945), Ms. Takii was hanging out the laundry to dry. She reported that she saw a flash and then her house caved in, trapping her for several days before she was rescued.[32]

Dirty Bombs

After the September 11, 2001, terrorist attacks in New York and Washington, DC, concern was raised over the possibility of additional incidents, particularly from a device known as a dirty bomb. A dirty bomb differs from an atomic bomb or other nuclear bomb in that the explosion, which disperses radioactive materials, is caused by conventional explosives and not by nuclear fission or fusion. In order to construct a dirty bomb, a terrorist would combine explosives with radioactive material from various sources and explode the bomb in a densely populated urban zone. Most likely, the effects of such an explosion would be confined to a small area. As a result, the most significant injuries caused by a dirty bomb would be from the explosives and explosion itself, rather than from radiation exposure. The main impact of the dirty bomb would probably be psychological by causing the population to panic.

Fact Sheet: Dirty Bombs

Basically, the principal type of dirty bomb, or Radiological Dispersal Device (RDD), combines a conventional explosive, such as dynamite, with radioactive material. In most instances, the conventional explosive itself would have more immediate lethality than the radioactive material. At the levels created by most probable sources, not enough radiation would be present in a dirty bomb to kill people or cause severe illness. For example, most radioactive material employed in hospitals for diagnosis or treatment of cancer is sufficiently benign that about 100,000 patients a day are released with this material in their bodies.

However, certain other radioactive materials, dispersed in the air, could contaminate up to several city blocks, creating fear and possibly panic and requiring potentially costly cleanup. Prompt, accurate, non-emotional public information might prevent the panic sought by terrorists.

A second type of RDD might involve a powerful radioactive source hidden in a public place, such as a trash receptacle in a busy train or subway station, where people passing close to the source might get a significant dose of radiation.

A dirty bomb is in no way similar to a nuclear weapon. The presumed purpose of its use would be therefore not as a Weapon of Mass Destruction but rather as a Weapon of Mass Disruption.

Source: Reprinted from United States Nuclear Regulatory Commission. Fact Sheet on Dirty Bombs. Available at: http://www.nrc.gov/reading-rm/doc-collections/fact-sheets/dirty-bombs.html. Accessed April 3, 2010.

The nuclear material, which would be dispersed, possibly could contaminate buildings and land for a period of time. However, the amount of radiation produced probably would not be sufficient to cause severe acute illnesses. Nevertheless, the long-term effects of radiation exposure might include increased incidence of cancers among persons exposed to the radiation. The cost of cleaning up after the explosion could also be extremely expensive, possibly amounting to millions of dollars.[33,34,35] The text box describes a dirty bomb, or **ra-**diological dispersal device (RDD), which has been the subject of much attention from the media.

MEDICAL USES OF IONIZING RADIATION

After accounting for the amount of radiation received from natural background sources, experts note that exposure of the population to ionizing radiation from medical procedures is the second largest source of exposure.[9] Approximately half of radiation exposure comes from natural background sources; about 40% of exposure has been attributed to medical exposure.[36] The risks of exposure to medically related ionizing radiation need to be balanced against the benefits that can be accrued from its helpful applications.

Medical devices that use radioactivity are essential for many common diagnostic and therapeutic regimens. These medical procedures include the use of X-ray machines, nuclear medicine, and radiation therapy. Not surprisingly, the number of procedures that employ radiation is substantially greater in developed countries than in less developed countries. In addition, people over the age of 40 in comparison with younger persons tend to be the recipients of a greater number of procedures that involve radiation. Radiation exposure during medical procedures does not affect only the patient; the medical staff who administer the procedures also may be exposed. Some members of the public may be exposed to radiation that emanates from patients who have undergone treatment. Nevertheless, the life-serving effects of nuclear medicine procedures appear to exceed greatly their risks to the public.

Medical X-rays and Fluoroscopy

The X-ray machine has been employed since the early 1900s for diagnosis and therapy in medicine and dentistry. A dental X-ray produces a typical effective dose of radioactivity of 2 to 3 mrems; a chest X-ray delivers 5 to 10 mrems. More recently, newer diagnostic procedures (e.g., computed tomography [CT]) have been developed that require exposure to relatively high doses of radiation. A CT scan of the abdomen exposes the subject to 1,000 mrems. In developed countries, technical developments such as the use of shielding have helped to minimize the amount of radiation exposure from X-ray machines.

Another diagnostic procedure known as fluoroscopy uses X-rays to generate real-time images of the interior of the body. Fluoroscopy has a number of important applications, such as angiography, biopsy, placement of drainage tubes, and use during orthopedic procedures. An example of a procedure that uses fluoroscopy involves the administration of barium for visualization of the colon. During the procedure, the patient receives a barium enema, which involves the placement of a solution that contains barium into the colon. The barium solution is a strong absorber of X-rays and helps to produce images that can be captured on film.[9]

Diagnostic Nuclear Medicine

In this application, health care personnel inject liquid radionuclides directly into the patient's body. Also, the patient may inhale gaseous radionuclides. Particular radionuclides have an affinity for specific target organs. After the nuclides are injected or inhaled, one may determine whether an organ is functioning properly or whether it is infused properly with blood. Among the uses of such techniques are diagnosis of cancer and tests of thyroid function. The most commonly used radionuclides include ^{123}iodine and ^{131}iodine (liquids) and ^{133}xenon (gas).

Radiation Therapy

The objective of radiation therapy is to kill cancerous cells in specific bodily sites, called the target volume. The three types of radiation therapy are teletherapy, brachytherapy, and nuclear therapy. In teletherapy, a beam of radiation originating from outside the patient is aimed at a lesion. Brachytherapy involves the placement of encapsulated radioactive material into a tumor. Nuclear therapy requires the oral ingestion or intravenous injection of radionuclides that travel to the site of a lesion in a target organ. A possible adverse side effect of radiation therapy is the increased risk of cancer developing outside the immediate area targeted for treatment. For example, radiation treatments for acne in the 1950s were linked to bone cancers.

NUCLEAR WASTE DISPOSAL

Nuclear wastes can present a significant public health hazard if not properly secured. In Goiânia, Brazil, during September 1987 local scavengers removed radioactive ^{137}cesium from a radiotherapy machine. An account of the incident follows in the text box.

NONIONIZING RADIATION

Nonionizing radiation is classified as the form of radiation on the left half of the electromagnetic spectrum shown in Figure 8-1, which portrays the following types of nonionizing radiation as we move up the energy spectrum: extremely low frequency (power line), radio (AM, FM, TV), microwave, infrared, visible light, and ultraviolet. The upper limit of ultraviolet radiation merges with the ionizing radiation portion of the electromagnetic spectrum.

The Goiânia Accident

In the Goiânia incident, authorities believe that scavengers dismantled a metal canister from a radiotherapy machine at an abandoned cancer clinic and left it in a junkyard. During the dismantling procedure the metal capsule that contained the caesium-137 source was ruptured. Over the next week, several hundred people in Goiânia were exposed to the caesium-137, but did not know it. Some children and adults, thinking the caesium powder was "pretty," even rubbed it over their bodies. Others inadvertently ate food that had been contaminated with the radioactive powder. After one week, a public health worker correctly diagnosed radiation syndrome when a sufferer visited a clinic. The Brazilian Nuclear Energy Commission sent in a team and they discovered that over 240 persons were contaminated with caesium-137, four of whom later died. The accident also contaminated homes and businesses and this required a major clean-up operation.

Source: Reprinted from International Atomic Energy Agency. IAEA Press Release 2002/09, Inadequate Control of World's Radioactive Sources. Available at: http://www.iaea.org/NewsCenter/PressReleases/2002/prn0209.shtml. Accessed April 3, 2010.

Radiation from the electromagnetic spectrum is measured in wavelengths and cycles per second (called hertz). Variations in the units assigned to hertz are as follows:

- Hertz (Hz)—cycles per second (e.g., 60 Hz)
- Kilohertz (KHz)—Hz times 1,000 (e.g., 100 KHz = 100,000 Hz)
- Megahertz (MHz)—Hz times 1 million (e.g., 50 MHz = 50 million Hz)
- Gigahertz (GHz)—Hz times 1 billion (e.g., 75 GHz = 75 billion Hz)

Energy at the low end of the electromagnetic spectrum has long wavelengths and low hertz; conversely, short wavelengths and high frequency characterize the energy at the upper end of the spectrum.[1] Here are some additional examples of nonionizing radiation:

- Extremely low frequency (ELF) radiation—ELF radiation has frequencies of 100 Hz or less and wavelengths of 100 million meters or longer. One source of ELF radiation is high tension power lines that run overhead; ELF radiation from power lines is in the range of 50 to 60 hertz. The frequency of alternating current electric power transmission in Europe and many countries is 50 Hz; in the United States, it is 60 Hz. When alternating currents pass through electric power transmission lines, sometimes they produce weak electromagnetic fields (EMFs).
- AM, FM, VHF-TV radio waves—These have frequencies between 1 million and 100 million hertz (1 MHz to 100 MHz) and wavelengths that range from 1 to 100 meters.
- Microwave radiation—Occurs in telecommunications equipment, radar, and ovens for heating food; frequencies are approximately 2.5 billion hertz (2.5 GHz) and wavelengths are approximately 1 hundredth of a meter long.
- Infrared radiation (IRA, IRB, IRC)—The source of heat in heat lamps used for keeping food warm.
- Visible light radiation.
- Ultraviolet radiation (UVA, UVB, UVC).

The human population is exposed ever more frequently to anthropogenic (man-made) sources of nonionizing radiation, such as radios and radio communications transmitters, cellular phones, medical equipment, microwave ovens, heat sealers, and radar transmitters. Even without the anthropogenic sources, nonionizing radiation impinges upon the human population from outer space and from the earth itself. According to one expert, "Environmental exposure to anthropogenic magnetic fields and radiation (EMFs) has steadily increased throughout this century. Today everyone is exposed to a complex mix of EMFs, both at home and at work, from the generation and transmission of electricity, from domestic appliances and industrial plant[s], and from telecommunications and broadcasting."[37(p185)]

Overview of Health Effects Associated with Nonionizing Radiation

The electromagnetic spectrum (nonionizing radiation) is subdivided into the nonthermal, thermal, and optical segments. The health effects of exposure to nonionizing radiation vary somewhat depending upon the segment of the spectrum considered and may be differentiated by their established and hypothesized short-term and long-term effects. Consider the

findings that have accumulated regarding specific types of nonionizing radiation (e.g., extremely low frequency radiation, radiofrequency radiation, and microwave radiation).

Extremely low frequency (ELF) radiation does not appear to produce many discernible short-term health effects. However, when we consider forms of nonionizing radiation that have higher frequency levels in comparison with ELF radiation (i.e., radiofrequency and microwave radiation), we find that the primary immediate health effect produced is heating of the body. Radiofrequency radiation produces effects on or near the skin's surface; in comparison, **microwave radiation** penetrates more deeply into the body, causing internal layers to heat up. Microwave radiation also can cause interference with implanted pacemakers. The fact that nonionizing radiation in the radiofrequency to microwave range produces heat makes this type of radiation useful for many applications such as heating food and in manufacturing processes, for example, those that use microwaves to power heat-sealing tools.

SOURCES OF EXPOSURE TO NONIONIZING RADIATION

Extremely Low Frequency (ELF) Radiation

Extremely low frequency (ELF) radiation is of the type in the range of 50 to 60 hertz that originates from electric power poles, wiring in the walls of buildings, and some electrical appliances. When associated with electric wiring and high-tension electrical lines, the source of ELF radiation is alternating electrical currents that flow through the circuits. Electricity that flows through transmission lines may produce electromagnetic fields (EMFs). For example, Figure 8-8 illustrates electric power lines that can produce extremely low frequency–associated EMFs. Because electrical power lines are designed to minimize power loss by keeping the energy inside the line, only very minute amounts of energy are released from the lines. Nevertheless, most communities prohibit construction of homes directly under high-tension lines because of concerns about health effects found in some epidemiologic studies. These findings have suggested that there are associations between EMFs from power lines and childhood cancers. The amount of ELF radiation emitted from the wiring and appliances inside homes is probably negligible.

Epidemiologic studies that have examined the health effects of exposure to ELF radiation have produced conflicting findings. Although many of the studies have reported negative findings, some research has reported low-level associations between ELF radiation exposure among persons who live near power lines and cancer (e.g., childhood leukemia and brain

FIGURE 8-8 High-tension power lines. Environmental health studies have examined their potential health effects.

cancers in children and adults). The International Agency for Research on Cancer considers EMFs emitted from ELF sources to be potentially carcinogenic.[38] The US EPA noted "that it can no longer categorically state that there is no effect from this radiation. Growing public concern about reported leukemia risk (especially in children), a possible connection with brain cancer, and potential interference with pacemakers has raised serious questions about the carcinogenicity of electromagnetic radiation."[39(p1447)]

Investigators have pursued the following three lines of research on possible linkages between cancer and EMFs from high-voltage power lines:[40]

- Associations between childhood cancer and residence near power lines
- Correlations between adult cancers and exposure to such radiation in occupations—an example being electrical contracting
- Associations between cancers among adults and exposure to power lines

The EMF and Breast Cancer on Long Island Study (EBCLIS) explored the possible relationship between breast cancer and women's exposure to EMFs.[41] During the course of this case-control study, researchers visited the Long Island, New York, homes of the study participants (576 breast cancer patients and 585 controls). EMF measurements in several areas of the houses (e.g., bedroom, front door, and the most lived-in room) were taken. These measurements were used to estimate the strengths of EMFs in the 60 Hz range. The EBCLIS study reported no association between the strength of EMF levels and risk of breast cancer.

Norwegian investigators performed a case-control study of women to determine whether exposure to electromagnetic fields such as those found at home and at work was associated with female breast cancer.[38] The study examined women who had residential exposure to EMFs from electric power lines located close to their homes and those who had occupational exposure to magnetic fields generated by 50 Hz currents. Rather than measuring residential exposure directly, researchers assessed exposure to EMFs on the basis of residence in a defined geographic corridor in proximity to a high-voltage power line. A total of 1,830 breast cancer cases and 3,658 controls participated in the study. The investigators reported a 60% increase in risk of breast cancer among women who had residential exposure to EMFs. Occupational exposure to EMFs was not related to breast cancer.

Another study, also conducted in Norway, assessed whether exposure to EMFs from high-voltage power lines was associated with increased incidence of hematological cancers in adults.[42] This research was a case-control study in which persons ($n = 1,063$) who resided in a corridor that had exposure to high-voltage power lines were matched with controls according to year of birth, sex, and municipality of residence. As there were only a few nonsignificant associations with some forms of hematological cancers (e.g., chronic lymphocytic leukemia), the researchers indicated that no firm conclusions could be drawn.

A nationwide cohort study of Finnish adults searched for an association between residence near high-voltage power lines and risk of cancer.[40] The study examined a cohort of 383,700 adult subjects who had lived for a period of 20 years within 500 meters of overhead power lines. The outcome variable was cancer of all sites as well as specific cancer diagnoses (e.g., stomach, colon, and nervous system). The researchers concluded that there was no association between ELF magnetic fields and adult cancers. The study's authors state, "The results of the present study suggest strongly that typical residential magnetic fields generated by high voltage power lines are not related to cancer in adults."[40(p1050)]

New Zealand researchers studied the relationship between EMF exposures and risk of childhood cancer.[43] Their case-control study examined 303 cases among children who ranged from newborns to 14 years of age. The cases were matched with an equivalent number of controls. Measurements of EMFs were taken in the children's bedrooms and the rooms in which they spent most of their time. Other EMF exposure sources that were considered were mothers' use of electric blankets and other electrical appliances during pregnancy. Similarly, children's use of such appliances also was evaluated. Risk of leukemia was one of the few outcomes associated significantly with EMF exposure, and the association was significant only for children who had the highest exposure levels. The investigators indicated that the findings should be interpreted with caution because of the small sample sizes employed in the investigation.

In summary, the research literature suggests that findings are inconsistent, not definitive, with respect to EMF exposure and cancer. "Overall, the few biological effects that may result from exposure to EMFs at levels normally encountered by members of the public have a tendency to be small in magnitude, short in duration and reversible. Effects may also be seen under very specific exposure and test conditions. This suggests that any risk to health would be small and possibly negligible."[37(p191)]

The long-term health effects ascribed to EMF exposure differ from the immediate effects and are open to debate or, at the very least, not well-understood. Jauchem and Merritt reported, "In general, the biological effect of EMF has been a controversial subject. Many highly speculative notions have become entrenched in the popular press; some unsubstantiated claims in the scientific literature are widely referenced and often misquoted in the lay literature."[44(p895)]

Radio Frequency Radiation

When an electric charge alternates (oscillates back and forth) very rapidly in a radio antenna, it produces radio waves, which move at the speed of light. The effect is similar to dropping a pebble into a smooth lake and causing ripples on the surface. The analogy breaks down in the sense that, in comparison with ripples on bodies of water, the electromagnetic waves oscillate at much higher frequencies; these waves also are referred to as electromagnetic radiation. **Radiofrequency (RF) radiation** covers the range of approximately 0.5 MHz to 300,000 MHz. (Refer to Table 8-6.) In comparison with ELF radiation, RF radiation produces higher amounts of energy. As a result, one who ventures too closely to a strong source of RF radiation may experience thermal effects such as heating.[45] Under certain circumstances, irreversible effects such as eye damage (cataracts) can occur.

Cancer is one health outcome that has been investigated in relationship to RF radiation. Several of these investigations have suggested that there may be an increased risk of some forms of cancer among persons who have had RF exposure; however, these findings are inconsistent.[46] "The evidence is weak in regard to its inconsistency, the weak design of the studies, the lack of detail on actual exposures, the limitations of the studies in their ability to deal with other likely factors, and in some studies there may be biases in the data used. Whereas the current epidemiologic evidence justifies further research to clarify the situation, there is no consistent evidence of any substantial effect on human cancer causation."[46(p166)]

TABLE 8-6 Examples of Frequencies in the Radio Range

Radiofrequency Radiation	Frequencies
AM radio	0.5 to 1.5 MHz
Amateur radio	3 to 30 MHz
FM, VHF-TV	50 to 150 MHz
UHF-TV	300 to 3,000 MHz
Microwave ovens	2,450 MHz
Radar, microwave communication	3,000 to 300,000 MHz or 3 to 300 GHz

Source: Data are from PA Valberg. Radio frequency radiation (RFR): the nature of exposure and carcinogenic potential. *Cancer Causes Control.* 1997;8:324.

Cell Phones

The cell phone is a very low-power apparatus that transmits in the radiofrequency range of 900 to 1,800 MHz. As of 2000, there were an estimated 92 million and 500 million cellular telephones in use in the United States and worldwide, respectively.[47] These numbers have risen dramatically: As of 2009, there were approximately 270 million subscribers (more than 85 percent of the population) in the United States.[48] During the same year, there were approximately 4.1 billion wireless telephone subscriptions worldwide.[49] The widespread popularity of cell phones means that even small adverse health effects could have substantial implications for population health.[50] Cell phone antenna banks are themselves a source of RF radiation. (See Figure 8-9.)

FIGURE 8-9 Cell phone antenna.

When communicating via a cell phone, the individual places the device close to his or her head. It has been suggested that RF radiation from cell phones can cause "hot-spots" inside the head.[45] The use of cell phones has raised the public's concern regarding several adverse effects, such as headaches, memory loss, sleep disturbance, nausea, dizziness, and forms of cancer such as brain tumors.[51] One legal case that reached national attention in the United States was a 1993 lawsuit filed in Florida by a man on behalf of his wife. The husband alleged that cell phone radiation caused his wife to die from a brain tumor. The case was subsequently dismissed when the court determined that the evidence was insufficient to show a causal link between cell phone use and brain tumors.[50] At present the hard evidence on the health effects of cell phone use is scant.[45]

In general, epidemiologic research findings do not support a clear relationship between use of cellular phones and morbidity and mortality. One study examined mortality differences between users of cellular phones, which usually require that the transmission antenna be held close to the head, and users of mobile telephones, which have an antenna that is located at a distance from the head. The age-specific mortality rates of the two types of telephone users were similar.[52] A case-control study of intracranial tumors of the nervous system did not substantiate a causal relationship between these forms of cancer and use of handheld cellular telephones.[47] Risk of intracranial tumors was not shown to increase with increasing use of cellular phones (e.g., more than 60 minutes per day for five years or more). Nevertheless, these and many other epidemiologic studies have not had an opportunity to examine health effects over a very long time period. A group of Swedish researchers conducted case-control studies on the relationship between certain types of brain tumors and use of mobile phones and cordless phones. The researchers found an association between the use of such phones and certain types of brain tumors (i.e., astrocytoma and acoustic neuroma). The highest risk level was found among subjects who had latency periods greater than 10 years.[53]

In summary, the National Toxicology Program has concluded that "[t]he weight of scientific evidence has not conclusively linked cell phones with any health problems. Additional research is needed."[48] The EPA stated, "Today, the only health problem known to be related to the use of cell phones is an increase in traffic accidents among voluble drivers. Nevertheless, the popular press tends to put a sensational spin on the idea that cell phones contribute to brain cancer, and anecdotal reports of headaches, skin numbing, and memory loss due to cell phone use have helped to heighten public fears."[50(pA475)]

Microwave Radiation

Microwave radiation, which is produced by radar, gained popularity during World War II because of its applications in devices used to track aircraft. This form of radiation also is used to heat foods. When the use of radar became more frequent, concerns about the health effects of radar exposure in occupational settings spurred an increase in the number of health research efforts. Over the years, the power emitted by radar devices has continued to increase, raising alarm about the possible health effects that might occur among exposed personnel. Standards now limit whole-body exposure to radar in occupational settings to 100 W/m^2.[54] (W/m^2 refers to watts per square meter—the amount of energy impacting the surface of the skin.) The exposure limit is believed to protect workers from ocular effects (lens opacities such as cataracts and clouding of the lenses of the eyes), one of the principal adverse health outcomes associated with microwave radiation exposure.

Ultraviolet Radiation (UVR)

Ultraviolet radiation (UVR) is a form of nonionizing radiation in the optical range. Sources of UVR include welders' arcs, lamps used for tanning beds, some flood lamps used in photography, halogen desk lamps, lightning, and electrical sparks. However, one of the most common sources of exposure to ultraviolet radiation is sunbathing, which is regarded as a popular and healthful pastime by many residents of sunny climes, for example, California and Florida. (Refer to Figure 8-10.) Evidence from epidemiologic research suggests strongly that sun exposure is associated with skin cancers of various forms.[55] (More information on skin cancer will be provided later in this section.) In the United States, areas located in lower geographic latitudes (e.g., New Orleans, Atlanta) that have higher levels of ambient UVR tend to have higher incidence rates for skin cancer than areas that fall in higher latitudes and have lower levels of UVR (e.g., Seattle,

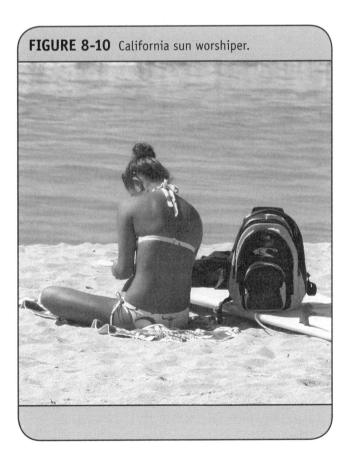

FIGURE 8-10 California sun worshiper.

The UV Index

The UV index provides a daily forecast of the expected risk of overexposure to the sun [see Table 8-7]. The index predicts UV intensity levels on a scale of 1 to 11+, where low indicates a minimal risk of overexposure and 11+ means an extreme risk. Calculated on a next-day basis for every ZIP code across the United States, the UV index takes into account clouds and other local conditions that affect the amount of UV radiation reaching the ground in different parts of the country.

TABLE 8-7 UV Index Value and Exposure Level

UV Index Number	Exposure Level
0 to 2	Low
3 to 5	Moderate
6 to 7	High
8 to 10	Very High
11+	Extreme

Source: Data from US Environmental Protection Agency. SunWise Program. UV Index. Available at: http://www.epa.gov/sunwise/uvindex.html. Accessed April 4, 2010; and US Environmental Protection Agency. SunWise Program. UV Index scale. Available at: http://www.epa.gov/sunwise/uviscale.html. Accessed April 4, 2010.

Minneapolis-St. Paul).[55] The thinning of the earth's ozone layer also may be responsible for increasing ambient levels of UVR.

UVR coming from the sun is subdivided into UVA, UVB, and UVC, depending upon the wavelength of the light. The wavelengths of these three forms are as follows: UVA—315 to 400 nanometers (nm); UVB—280 to 315 nm; and UVC—100 to 280 nm.[56] (Note that 1 nanometer equals 1 billionth of a meter.)

Many people enjoy some amount of sun exposure. However, as noted, excessive exposure can produce harmful consequences for one's health. To help protect exposed persons from excessive amounts of sunlight, the ultraviolet (UV) index provides a measure of the amount of UV exposure that one is likely to have on a given day. (Refer to the following text box.)

The health effects suspected of being associated with UVR include both dermal and ocular conditions. The former encompass temporary effects such as burns and longer-term consequences such as photoaging of the skin, nonmelanoma skin cancer (NMSC), and malignant melanoma (MM). The former encompass temporary effects such as burns and longer-term consequences such as photoaging of the skin. The latter (i.e., ocular effects) include acute temporary blinding, retinal damage, lens opacities and MM of the pigmented portion of the eye. Of the three forms of UVR, UVB is considered to be the most harmful to human health because it is the most effective in producing short-term and long-term adverse health effects.

Dermal Effects

The acute effects of UVR exposure upon the skin include erythema (skin reddening), inflammation, pain, swelling, tanning, photosensitization, phototoxicity, and photoallergic reactions. These reactions develop several hours after exposure. Among sensitive persons, intense sunlight exposure for short time periods may produce reddening of the skin (similar to a first-degree burn). Longer exposures to intense sunlight may result in more severe reactions such as swelling, blistering, and peeling of the skin. Thickening of the skin and tanning caused by changes in melanin are defensive responses that protect the skin from further injury.

Sunlight-associated photosensitivity refers to heightened sensitivity to sunlight; one of the causes of photosensitivity of the skin is previous exposure to sunlight, particularly the ultraviolet component. A sunlight-associated **photoallergy** is a type of dermatitis (intense itching rash) that is activated by sunlight, which sensitizes the skin to allergens. Sunlight-associated **phototoxicity** denotes a severe reaction to sunlight that occurs sometimes in conjunction with drugs (e.g., antibiotics and diuretics) that a person may be taking. A sunburned

area of skin that blisters, indicating that a second-degree burn has occurred, is one symptom of phototoxicity.

UVR exposure is linked to a number of long-term effects, which include photoaging, premalignant lesions, and malignant lesions such as skin cancer.[57] These effects may not appear for many years and tend to be cumulative. Persons who have spent a great deal of time outdoors over a period of years and who have not had adequate sun protection will be more likely to experience adverse effects from sunlight exposure than those who either tend to stay indoors or protect themselves with sun-blocking lotions and appropriate clothing. Photoaging of the skin is characterized by a leathery appearance and several important changes such as the occurrence of brown spots and loss of elasticity. The effects of photoaging are different from those of normal aging and can be observed when the areas of skin exposed to sunlight are compared with nonexposed areas in the same person. The exposed skin areas such as the faces of some elderly persons may have developed brown spots (hyperpigmentation), whereas nonexposed areas such as the legs appear smooth and without signs of hyperpigmentation.

Another adverse long-term health effect attributed to UVR exposure is skin cancer. The three types of skin cancer are squamous cell carcinoma (SCC), basal cell carcinoma (BCC), and malignant melanoma (MM). The two forms of nonmelanomatous skin cancer—SCC and BCC—account for about 40% of all cancers in the United States.[58] The occurrence of all three forms of skin cancer has shown an increasing trend.

Malignant melanoma is the most serious and potentially fatal form of skin cancer. In 1997, the incidence of malignant melanoma had risen to more than 40,000 cases annually and caused the deaths of more than 7,200 patients. Figure 8-11 presents data on the incidence and mortality from MM in the United States between the years 1988 and 1992. The highest incidence and mortality rates occurred among white men and women.

This most dangerous variety of skin cancer also is one of the most common types of cancer among young adults. Melanomas demonstrate well-known characteristics including lesions with irregular borders that may present with multiple colorations. (Refer to Figure 8-12.) The lesions, which may progress rapidly, often are vulnerable to injury and bleed easily. In many instances, the originating site of a malignant melanoma is a mole that demonstrates some of the foregoing characteristics. Men who develop MM are more likely than women to develop lesions on the head, neck, and trunk; women are more likely to develop MM on the lower limbs.[59]

The causes of malignant melanoma are not well understood. However, several risk factors have been established.

FIGURE 8-11 Incidence and mortality of melanoma of the skin, 1988–1992.

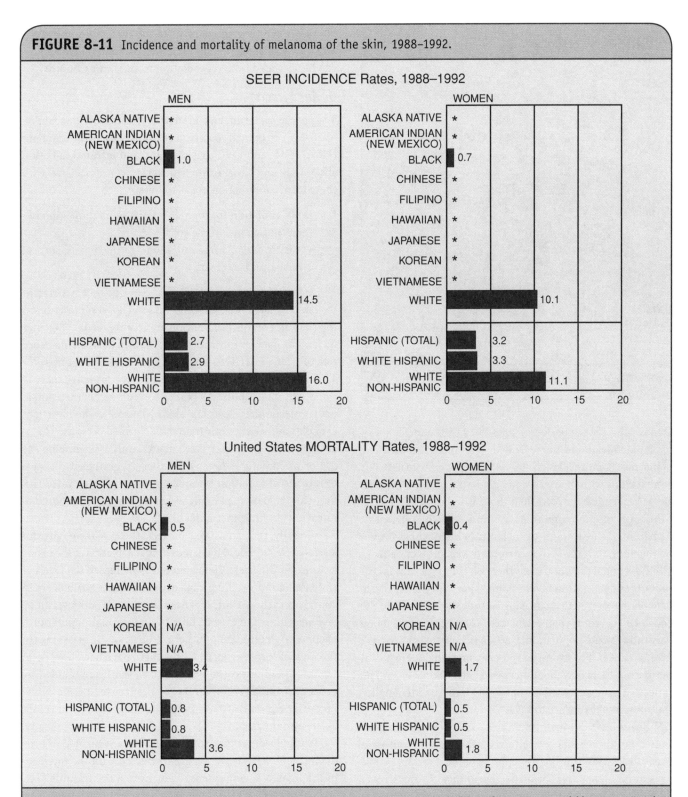

Figure Note: Rates are "average annual" per 100,000 population, age-adjusted to 1970 US standard; N/A = information not available; * = rate not calculated when fewer than 25 cases.

Source: Reprinted from National Cancer Institute, SEER Program. Racial/Ethnic Patterns of Cancer in the United States, 1988–1992: Melanoma, 1996, p. 85. NIH Pub. No. 96-4104. Bethesda, MD.

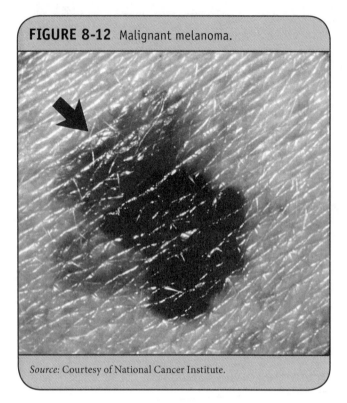

FIGURE 8-12 Malignant melanoma.

Source: Courtesy of National Cancer Institute.

One is age—for the period of 1988 to 1992, the incidence of malignant melanoma in the United States increased with age. White race is another risk factor for MM. People who have fair complexions with blue eyes and light hair (e.g., blond or red) are at higher risk for MM than those who have darker skin. MM is uncommon among Asians and African Americans. Apparently, the amount of melanin (which causes brown pigmentation) in the skin is correlated with protection from UVR. As noted previously, another risk factor for MM is latitude of residence. Among fair-skinned persons, the incidence of MM increases with decreasing latitude (living closer to the equator). The world's highest incidence of MM is found among Australia's white population. Certain occupations carry risk of skin cancer. For example, roofers who spend a great deal of time outdoors may incur increased risk of skin cancer. The reflective materials used in roofing surfaces tend to amplify the amount of exposure to UVR.

Spending too much time in the sun without adequate protection carries many health risks for the skin and eyes. Nevertheless, tanning booths remain a popular way for people to acquire a "healthy" bronzed appearance. In the United States, the indoor tanning industry generates over $1 billion in annual sales. Most tanning booth operators now use tanning machines that emit UVA primarily and have discontinued the once widely used UVB. Despite these modifications, the use of tanning booths is discouraged because of the risks of photoaging of the skin, damage to the eyes, and some of the forms of skin cancer. Phototoxic and photoallergic reactions can be activated by UVA radiation from tanning booths.

Ocular Effects

The optical spectrum and its adverse effects are shown in Figure 8-13. The optical spectrum encompasses ultraviolet light (UVA, UVB, and UVC), visible light, and infrared radiation (IRA, IRB, and IRC). Adverse ocular effects associated with these forms of radiation are as follows:

- UV radiation (particularly UVB radiation)—photokeratitis, a burn of the cornea
- Visible and infrared radiation—retinal burns, corneal burns, and cataracts

UV radiation has been identified as a possible risk factor for ocular melanoma, although the role of UV radiation in the causality of this form of cancer is controversial.[60] Ocular melanoma is a very rare cancer diagnosis that has an incidence rate of 0.5 to 1 per 100,000 per year in Western countries.[60] This very serious malignancy is the most common cancer of the eye among adults. As is true for cutaneous melanoma, ocular melanoma affects fair-skinned persons who have light eye color more frequently than dark-skinned persons.[61] Ocular melanoma must be treated aggressively by removing the eye or by radiation therapy. Further suggesting its linkage to ultraviolet radiation is the observation of an elevated risk for ocular melanoma among welders who may be exposed to ultraviolet light from arc welding.[60]

Usually, the ozone layer protects the eyes from harmful levels of UV radiation. It is believed that depletion of the ozone layer in the Southern Hemisphere has increased the levels of UVB radiation reaching the earth's surface, particularly in countries such as Chile.[62] These increased UVB levels may be harmful to the eyes of human and animal populations, particularly ruminants that graze outdoors in pastures. In the area of Punta Arenas, Chile, there have been anecdotal reports of domestic and wild animals that were blinded by the increasing levels of UVB radiation caused by the ozone hole over southern Chile; however, these reports have not been substantiated.

Sunlight and other sources of light are capable of producing acute effects, which are correlated with the intensity of the light. Viewing intense light from a light source (e.g., searchlights, lasers, welding arcs, and sunlight reflected by snow) may cause ocular injuries. As shown in Figure 8-13, intense visible light can burn the retina.

One of the most common causes of injury to the eyes from radiation in the ocular spectrum is UVR. Intense UVR

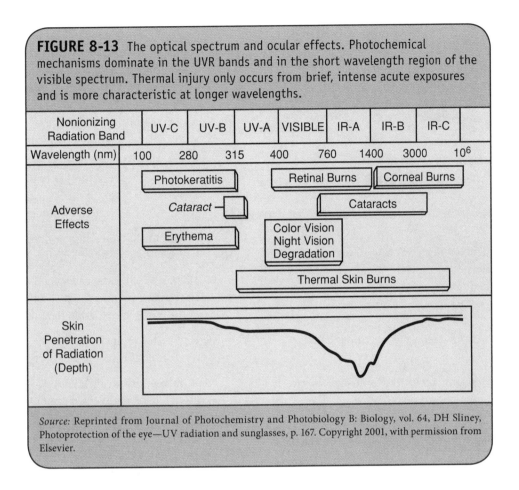

FIGURE 8-13 The optical spectrum and ocular effects. Photochemical mechanisms dominate in the UVR bands and in the short wavelength region of the visible spectrum. Thermal injury only occurs from brief, intense acute exposures and is more characteristic at longer wavelengths.

Nonionizing Radiation Band	UV-C	UV-B	UV-A	VISIBLE	IR-A	IR-B	IR-C	

| Wavelength (nm) | 100 | 280 | 315 | 400 | 760 | 1400 | 3000 | 10^6 |

Source: Reprinted from Journal of Photochemistry and Photobiology B: Biology, vol. 64, DH Sliney, Photoprotection of the eye—UV radiation and sunglasses, p. 167. Copyright 2001, with permission from Elsevier.

is hazardous to the cornea, lens, and sometimes the retina.[63] Acute UVB exposure can cause actinic keratitis, a condition also known as snow blindness.[62] Research studies have suggested that sunlight exposure may be associated with longer-term consequences such as cataracts (lens opacities), which are linked to age and cumulative amount of exposure to sunlight.[64] Ordinary, inexpensive sunglasses are effective in reducing the amount of ultraviolet radiation that reaches the eye.[65]

In summary, the health effects of UVR exposure are not all adverse. UVR in sunlight promotes vitamin D synthesis and reduction of seasonal affective disorder. Certain skin conditions (e.g., acne, psoriasis, and eczema) appear to be alleviated by UVR. Studies also suggest that UVR provides a protective effect against some internal cancers such as prostate cancer.[66]

CONCLUSION

Sharing the characteristic that they are components of the electromagnetic spectrum, ionizing and nonionizing radia-

tion differ in their levels of energy. Ionizing radiation is the kind of radiation that most people think of when they refer to radiation. This form of radiation has the capacity to remove electrons from atoms, whereas nonionizing radiation does not. Both ionizing and nonionizing radiation are integral for the functioning of modern society; for example, ionizing radiation is used in medical devices, electric power plants, and many other helpful applications, and nonionizing radiation is emitted by communication devices and many other sources. Although both forms of radiation present some documented hazards to the world's population, they also carry many benefits; it is necessary to balance their benefits against their potential harm. Protection of the population from radiation hazards can be accomplished through research that assesses the acute and long-term risks and hazards. Through well-conducted research studies, it may be possible to protect the health of the population, enjoy the benefits of radiation, and eliminate unnecessary alarm associated with any unsubstantiated claims about the adverse health effects of ionizing and nonionizing radiation.

Study Questions and Exercises

1. Define the following terms in your own words:
   a. Radiation
   b. Radioactivity
   c. Radioisotope
   d. Hertz
   e. Extremely low frequency radiation
   f. UV index

2. Describe the similarities and differences between ionizing and nonionizing radiation.

3. Define the term *stochastic*. How do the stochastic effects of ionizing radiation differ from the nonstochastic effects?

4. Match the term and its definition.

Becquerel	SI unit measure of amount of radioactivity present in a material
Coulomb	SI unit measure of amount of exposure to radioactivity
Curie	Common unit measure of amount of radioactivity present in a material
Gray	SI unit measure of absorbed dose of radiation
Rad	Common unit measure of absorbed dose of radiation
Rem	Common unit measure of radiation dose related to biological effect
Roentgen	Common unit measure of amount of exposure to radioactivity
Sievert	SI unit measure of radiation dose related to biological effect

5. Distinguish among α, β, and γ radiation. Explain how α radiation can be a health hazard.

6. Support or refute the statement that leakage from nuclear power plants is the greatest source of exposure of the human population to ionizing radiation.

7. How do the immediate effects of a nuclear explosion differ from the long-term effects?

8. Why might radar installations present a hazard to human health? Give two examples.

9. Define three types of ultraviolet radiation and discuss their health effects.

10. Discuss the risks and benefits to society associated with the use of devices that produce radiation (ionizing and nonionizing). What are the risks and benefits associated with radioisotopes?

11. Describe the ocular effects of nonionizing radiation in the optical spectrum.

12. What is meant by the term *dirty bomb*? What would be the main consequences of detonation of a dirty bomb in a large city?

REFERENCES

1. US Environmental Protection Agency. Radiation Protection: Understanding radiation: ionizing & non-ionizing radiation. Available at: http://www.epa.gov/radiation/understand/index.html. Accessed April 3, 2010.

2. Bistline RW. What have epidemiologic studies told us about radiation health effects? *Colo Med.* 1980;77(10):351–353.

3. Samet JM. Epidemiologic studies of ionizing radiation and cancer: past successes and future challenges. *Environ Health Perspect.* 1997:105(suppl 4):883–889.

4. Oak Ridge Institute for Science and Education. Guidance for Radiation Accident Management. Radiation Emergency Assistance Center/Training Site (REAC/TS). Basics of radiation: definitions. Available at: http://orise.orau.gov/reacts/guide/definitions.htm. Accessed March 11, 2010.

5. *The Oxford College Dictionary.* 2nd ed. New York: Spark Publishing, by arrangement with Oxford University Press, Inc.; 2007.

6. US Environmental Protection Agency. Radiation Protection: Health Effects. Available at: http://www.epa.gov/radiation/understand/health_effects.html. Accessed March 11, 2010.

7. Health Physics Society. Radiation Basics. Available at: http://www.hps.org/publicinformation/ate/faqs/radiation.html. Accessed April 2, 2010.

8. Eaton DL, Klaassen CD. Principles of toxicology. In: Klaassen CD, Watkins JB III, eds. *Casarett & Doull's Essentials of Toxicology.* New York, NY: McGraw-Hill; 2003.

9. World Health Organization, International Agency for Research on Cancer. Ionizing radiation, part 1: X- and gamma (γ)-radiation, and neutrons. *IARC Monographs.* 2000;75:35–115.

10. US Environmental Protection Agency. Ground water & drinking water. National primary drinking water regulations; radon-222; proposed rule. Available at: http://www.epa.gov/safewater/radon/radfr1.html. Accessed April 4, 2010.

11. Vonstille WT. Radon and cancer. *J Environ Health.* 1990;53:25–27.

12. Field RW, Steck DJ, Smith BJ, et al. The Iowa radon lung cancer study—phase I: residential radon gas exposure and lung cancer. *Sci Total Environ.* 2001;272:67–72.

13. Langner I, Blettner M, Gundestrup M, et al. Cosmic radiation and cancer mortality among airline pilots: results from a European cohort study (ESCAPE). *Radiat Environ Biophys.* 2004;42:247–256.

14. PBS Online. Frontline. Three Mile Island: the judge's ruling. Available at: http://www.pbs.org/wgbh/pages/frontline/shows/reaction/readings/tmi.html. Accessed April 4, 2010.

15. Warrick J. Study links Three Mile Island releases to higher cancer rates. Washingtonpost.com. February 24, 1997. Available at: http://www.washingtonpost.com/wp-srv/national/longterm/tmi/stories/study022497.htm. Accessed April 4, 2010.

16. Hatch M, Wallenstein S, Beyea J, et al. Cancer rates after the Three Mile Island nuclear accident and proximity of residence to the plant. *Am J Public Health.* 1991;81:719–724.

17. Stencel M. 20 years later: a nuclear nightmare in Pennsylvania. Washingtonpost.com. March 27, 1999. Available at: http://www.washingtonpost.com/wp-srv/national/longterm/tmi/tmi.htm. Accessed March 4, 2010.

18. Carlisle D. Bitter rain. *Nurs Times.* 1996;92(16):16–17.

19. Cardis E, Krewski D, Boniol M, et al. Estimates of the cancer burden in Europe from radioactive fallout from the Chernobyl accident. *Int J Cancer.* 2006;119:1224–1235.

20. Dolk H, Lechat MF. Health surveillance in Europe: lessons from EUROCAT and Chernobyl. *Int J Epidemiol.* 1993;22:363–368.

21. Kazakov VS, Demidchik EP, Astakhova LN. Thyroid cancer after Chernobyl [letter]. *Nature.* 1992;359:21.

22. Reiners C. Radioactivity and thyroid cancer. *Hormones.* 2009;8(3):185–191.

23. Clapp R, Cobb S, Chan C, et al. Leukemia near Massachusetts nuclear power plant [letter]. *Lancet.* 1987;2:1324–1325.

24. Johnson CJ. Cancer incidence in an area contaminated with radionuclides near a nuclear installation. *Ambio.* 1981;10:176–182.

25. Enstrom JE. Cancer mortality patterns around the San Onofre nuclear power plant, 1960–1978. *Am J Public Health.* 1983;73:83–91.

26. Shleien B, Ruttenber AJ, Sage M. Epidemiologic studies of cancer in populations near nuclear facilities. *Health Phys.* 1991;61:699–713.

27. Akleyev AV, Kossenko MM, Silkina LA, et al. Health effects of radiation incidents in the southern Urals. *Stem Cells.* 1995;13(suppl 1):58–68.

28. Natural Resources Defense Council. Glossary of environmental terms. Available at: http://www.nrdc.org/reference/glossary/p.asp. Accessed March 11, 2010.

29. Rallison ML, Lotz TM, Bishop M, et al. Cohort study of thyroid disease near the Nevada test site: a preliminary report. *Health Phys.* 1990;59:739–746.

30. Tokunaga M, Norman JE, Asano M, et al. Malignant breast tumors among atomic bomb survivors, Hiroshima and Nagasaki, 1950–1974. *J Natl Cancer Inst.* 1979;62:1347–1359.

31. Timelines of History. Today in history—July 31. Available at: http://www.timelines.ws/days/07_31.HTML. Accessed April 4, 2010.

32. Hiroshima Topics. Oldest A-bomb victim? Available at: http://www.chugoku-np.co.jp/weekly/1998/980731.html. Accessed March 11, 2010.

33. BBC News. Analysis: effects of a dirty bomb. June 11, 2002. Available at: http://news.bbc.co.uk/2/hi/health/2037769.stm. Accessed March 11, 2010.

34. Centers for Disease Control and Prevention. Radiation emergencies: frequently asked questions (FAQs) about dirty bombs. Available at: http://www.bt.cdc.gov/radiation/dirtybombs.asp. Accessed March 11, 2010.

35. United States Nuclear Regulatory Commission. Fact sheet on dirty bombs. Available at: http://www.nrc.gov/reading-rm/doc-collections/factsheets/dirty-bombs.html. Accessed April 4, 2010.

36. Jablon S, Bailar JC III. The contribution of ionizing radiation to cancer mortality in the United States. *Prev Med.* 1980;9:219–226.

37. Sienkiewicz Z. Biological effects of electromagnetic fields and radiation. *J Radiol Prot.* 1998;18:185–193.

38. Kliukiene J, Tynes T, Andersen A. Residential and occupational exposures to 50-Hz magnetic fields and breast cancer in women: a population-based study. *Am J Epidemiol.* 2004;159:852–861.

39. The hazards of extremely low frequency radiation. *Am J Public Health.* 1991;81:1447.

40. Verkasalo PK, Pukkala E, Kaprio J, et al. Magnetic fields of high voltage power lines and risk of cancer in Finnish adults: nationwide cohort study. *BMJ.* 1996;313:1047–1051.

41. Schoenfeld ER, O'Leary ES, Henderson K, et al. Electromagnetic fields and breast cancer on Long Island: a case-control study. *Am J Epidemiol.* 2003;158:47–58.

42. Tynes T, Haldorsen T. Residential and occupational exposure to 50 Hz magnetic fields and hematological cancers in Norway. *Cancer Causes Control.* 2003;14:715–720.

43. Dockerty JD, Elwood JM, Skegg DC, et al. Electromagnetic field exposures and childhood cancers in New Zealand. *Cancer Causes Control.* 1998;9:299–309.

44. Jauchem JR, Merritt JH. The epidemiology of exposure to electromagnetic fields: an overview of the recent literature. *J Clin Epidemiol.* 1991;44:895–906.

45. Verschaeve L, Maes A. Genetic, carcinogenic and teratogenic effects of radiofrequency fields. *Mutat Res.* 1998;410:141–165.

46. Elwood JM. A critical review of epidemiologic studies of radiofrequency exposure and human cancers. *Environ Health Perspect.* 1999;107(suppl 1):155–168.

47. Inskip PD, Tarone RE, Hatch EE, et al. Cellular-telephone use and brain tumors. *New Engl J Med.* 2001;344:79–86.

48. National Institute of Environmental Health Sciences, National Toxicology Program. Cell phone radiofrequency radiation studies. Available at:

http://www.niehs.nih.gov/health/docs/cell-phone-fact-sheet.pdf. Accessed April 4, 2010.

49. *Guardian.* Nice talking to you . . . mobile phone use passes milestone. Available at: http://www.guardian.co.uk/technology/2009/mar/03/mobile-phones1. Accessed April 4, 2010.

50. Forum: of mobile phones and morbidity. *Environ Health Perspect.* 1998;106:A474–A475.

51. Maier M, Blakemore C, Koivisto M. The health hazards of mobile phones. *BMJ.* 2000;320:1288–1289.

52. Rothman KJ, Loughlin JE, Funch DP, et al. Overall mortality of cellular telephone customers. *Epidemiol.* 1996;7:303–305.

53. Hardell L, Carlberg M. Mobile phones, cordless phones and the risk for brain tumours. *Int J Oncol.* 2009;35:5–17.

54. Osepchuk JM, Petersen RC. Historical review of RF exposure standards and the International Committee on Electromagnetic Safety (ICES). *Bioelectromagnetics.* 2003;suppl 6:S7–S16.

55. Armstrong BK, Kricker A. The epidemiology of UV induced skin cancer. *J Photochem Photobiol B.* 2001;63:8–18.

56. Tenkate TD. Ultraviolet radiation: human exposure and health risks. *J Environ Health.* 1998;61:9–15.

57. Urbach F. Ultraviolet radiation and skin cancer of humans. *J Photochem Photobiol B.* 1997;40:3–7.

58. Gilchrest BA, Eller MS, Geller AC, et al. The pathogenesis of melanoma induced by ultraviolet radiation. *New Engl J Med.* 1999;340:1341–1348.

59. Miller BA, Kolonel LN, Bernstein L, et al, eds. *Racial/Ethnic Patterns of Cancer in the United States, 1988–1992.* Bethesda, MD: National Cancer Institute; 1996. NIH Pub. No. 96-4104.

60. Guénel P, Laforest L, Cyr D, et al. Occupational risk factors, ultraviolet radiation, and ocular melanoma: a case-control study in France. *Cancer Causes Control.* 2001;12:451–459.

61. Neugut AI, Kizelnik-Freilich S, Ackerman C. Black-white differences in risk for cutaneous, ocular, and visceral melanomas. *Am J Public Health.* 1994;84:1828–1829.

62. Schein OD, Vicencio C, Muñoz B, et al. Ocular and dermatologic health effects of ultraviolet radiation exposure from the ozone hole in southern Chile. *Am J Public Health.* 1995;85:546–550.

63. Sliney DH. Photoprotection of the eye—UV radiation and sunglasses. *J Photochem Photobiol B: Biol.* 2001;64:166–175.

64. West SK, Duncan DD, Muñoz B, et al. Sunlight exposure and risk of lens opacities in a population-based study: the Salisbury Eye Evaluation Project. *JAMA.* 1998;280:714–718.

65. Rosenthal FS, Bakalian AE, Lou C, et al. The effect of sunglasses on ocular exposure to ultraviolet radiation. *Am J Public Health.* 1988;78:72–74.

66. Bodiwala D, Luscombe CJ, Liu S, et al. Prostate cancer risk and exposure to ultraviolet radiation: further support for the protective effect of sunlight. *Cancer Lett.* 2003;192:145–149.

PART III

Applications of Environmental Health

Water Quality

LEARNING OBJECTIVES

By the end of this chapter the reader will be able to:

- Describe sources of potable water
- Define what is meant by the hydrological cycle
- List hazardous substances that may be found in drinking water
- Describe how water is made safe for human consumption
- Discuss hazards to the aquatic environment (oceans, lakes, rivers) associated with environmental pollution

INTRODUCTION

This chapter covers the topics of water quality (e.g., freedom from waterborne diseases and hazards) and the water supply (e.g., sources and availability of water). Water quality represents a crucial topic for environmental health, because water is an essential element of life on earth. Residents of the United States and other developed countries take it for granted that they will be able to turn on a faucet and draw a refreshing glass of water that is free from dangerous contaminants and microbial agents. (Refer to Figure 9-1.) In contrast, a safe water supply is not always available in the less developed regions of the world, where waterborne diseases represent a significant public health threat.

Safe, high-quality drinking water is an essential aspect of public health. One of the most significant measures to protect the health of the public was the introduction of chlorination of drinking water. Since the early 20th century, drinking water chlorination has resulted in drastic reductions in waterborne infections (e.g., cholera and typhoid), in the United States.

FIGURE 9-1 A glass of pure water.

Source: Reprinted from US Environmental Protection Agency. Water on tap: What you need to know. Washington, DC: EPA Office of Water; 2003: back cover.

Vulnerable groups such as children, the elderly, and immunocompromised patients (e.g., those who are undergoing chemotherapy, taking steroids, or afflicted with HIV/AIDS) are at special risk of diseases caused by water contamination.[1,2] In the United States, water quality regulations are designed to protect the public from contaminated drinking water and from other forms of water pollution. Two major water quality regulations are the Safe Drinking Water Act and the Clean Water Act, both discussed previously in Chapter 4.

The US Environmental Protection Agency (EPA) notes some interesting facts about water: Although it is possible for a human being to live up to a month without food, that same individual can survive for only about a week without water.[3] The average requirement for human consumption of water per day is approximately 2.5 liters (about $2\frac{1}{2}$ quarts). This level is necessary to maintain health and includes water from all sources, including food sources. It is also noteworthy that approximately two-thirds of the human body is made up of water; this amount increases to about three-quarters for human brain tissue.

In the United States the average person uses about 100 gallons (about 400 liters) of water per day, and the average residence uses over 100,000 gallons (about 400,000 liters) during a typical year. From 50% to 70% of this household water is used for outdoor purposes such as watering lawns and washing cars. Figure 9-2 illustrates the relative percentage of different types of residential uses for water in a Southern California city in the United States. Because of its semiarid climate, this community uses more than half of its water for landscape maintenance; 5% is lost to system leaks.

In addition to its life-supporting role, water is required in immense quantities by agriculture and industry, such as new car manufacture, steel production, and production of canned foods. According to the EPA,[3] examples of the amounts of water required for industrial purposes are as follows:

- Manufacture of a new automobile and its four tires: 39,090 gallons (about 160,000 liters)
- Production of one barrel of beer: 1,500 gallons (about 6,000 liters)
- Production of one ton of steel: 62,600 gallons (about 250,000 liters)
- Processing one can of fruit or vegetables: 9.3 gallons (about 38 liters)

Despite the fact that water is a necessity of human life, about 20% of the world's population lacks safe drinking water. With the increasing world population, the problem of lack of access to safe drinking water is likely to worsen.[2] Although most developed nations treat industrial discharges and **sewage**, contamination of water supplies with chemicals such as arsenic and some microorganisms place public water supplies at risk. In the wealthier nations (e.g., Japan, Western European countries, and the United States), the public water supplies, although generally safe, may carry organic chemicals, lead, and arsenic, as well as bacteria, viruses, and parasites from fecal contamination.

The problem of water quality is especially acute for developing nations. In these countries up to 90% of the cities discharge their untreated sewage into rivers and streams. (Refer to Figure 9-3.) These surface waters in turn may be used for drinking and personal sanitation purposes. In the developing world, there are several large urban areas known as megacities, defined as cities with 10 million or more people. The unsanitary water supplies found in many of these densely populated areas foster the spread of gastrointestinal illnesses and serious infectious diseases that contribute greatly to the burden of morbidity and mortality in these regions.

FIGURE 9-2 Residential uses for water in a southern California community.

Showers, 9%
Clothes Washers, 11%
Toilets, 14%
Dish Washers, 1%
Baths, 1%
Leaks, 5%
Faucets, 8%
Landscape, 51%

Source: Data are from the Irvine Ranch Water District, Irvine, California.

FIGURE 9-3 A slum in Ecuador that was heavily affected by cholera due to its proximity to unsafe water sources.

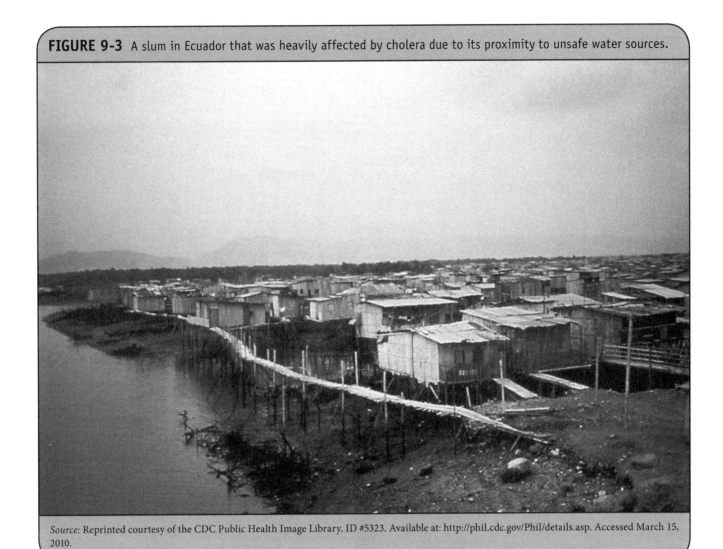

Source: Reprinted courtesy of the CDC Public Health Image Library. ID #5323. Available at: http://phil.cdc.gov/Phil/details.asp. Accessed March 15, 2010.

The lack of a safe water supply is compounded in some parts of the developing world by chronic water shortages. Regions that face a water shortfall include North Africa, the Middle East, and parts of sub-Saharan Africa. The residents of these areas are faced periodically with a chronic shortage of fresh water.

THE WATER SUPPLY

The two main sources of drinking water used by the human population are surface water and **groundwater**.[4] (Refer to the text box for definitions.) Surface waters are from rivers and lakes, as shown in Figure 9-4.

The second type of water available for human consumption is groundwater, which is stored naturally in underground aquifers. (See Exhibit 9-1 for a definition of the term **aquifer**.) Wastewater from human activities can find its way back into aquifers. In some regions of the world, communities treat wastewater and store it in percolation ponds so that it may recharge aquifers. Refer to Figure 9-5, which demonstrates that communities near the sea run the risk of saltwater intrusion into the aquifer when excessive amounts of water are withdrawn. Saltwater intrusion eventually may render the water unsuitable for human consumption.

The field of water science is known as hydrology. Some of the terms that relate to hydrology are *aquifer*, the **hydrological cycle, water scarcity**, and **water stress**. Some of these terms are discussed later in the chapter. (Refer to Exhibit 9-1 for a glossary of key hydrological terms.)

FIGURE 9-4 Examples of surface waters.

Water Definitions Used by Federal and State Water Authorities

Finished water—the water (e.g., drinking water) delivered to the distribution system after treatment, if any.

Groundwater—water that is contained in the interconnected pores in an aquifer.

Groundwater system—a system that uses water extracted from an aquifer (i.e., a well or spring) as its source.

Groundwater under the direct influence of surface water—as defined by the US Environmental Protection Agency (EPA), any water beneath the surface of the ground with substantial occurrence of insects or other macroorganisms, algae, or large-diameter pathogens (e.g, *Giardia intestinalis* or *Cryptosporidium*), or substantial and relatively rapid shifts in water characteristics (e.g., turbidity, temperature, conductivity, or PH) that closely correlate with climatologic or surface water conditions. Direct influence must be determined for individual sources in accordance with criteria established by the state [where the source is located].

Source water—untreated water (i.e., raw water) used to produce drinking water.

Surface water—all water on the surface (e.g., lakes, rivers, reservoirs, ponds, and oceans) as distinguished from subsurface or ground water.

Note: On December 16, 1998, the EPA's Interim Enhanced Surface Water Treatment Rule (IESWTR) appeared in the *Federal Register*. The purpose of the rule was to "[i]mprove control of microbial pathogens including specifically the protozoan *Cryptosporidium*, in drinking water"[a(p.69478)] as well as minimize risks associated with agents used to disinfect water. The control of *Cryptosporidium* applied both to surface waters and ground water under the influence of surface water. The IESWR mandated that "[s]tates are required to conduct sanitary surveys for all public water systems using surface water or ground water under the direct influence of surface water. . . Sanitary surveys are required no less frequently than every three years for community systems. . .."[a(p69484)] EPA standards for evaluation and processing of ground water under the influence of surface water are stricter than those applied to groundwater not under such influence.[b]

[a] Environmental Protection Agency. National Primary Drinking Water Regulations: Interim Enhanced Surface Water Treatment. *Federal Register*, Vol 63, No. 241, December 16, 1998, pp. 69478-69521.

[b] LO Gostin, Z Lazzarini, VS Neslund, MT Osterholm. Water quality laws and waterborne diseases: *Cryptosporidium* and other emerging pathogens. *Am J Public Health*. 2000;90:847-853.

Source: Adapted and reprinted from Centers for Disease Control and Prevention, Surveillance Summaries. Surveillance for waterborne disease and outbreaks associated with drinking water and water not intended for drinking—United States, 2005–2006. *MMWR*. 2008;57(SS-9):64–65.

FIGURE 9-5 Types of aquifers, wells, and groundwater flow.

Source: From Vital Water Graphics: Freshwater Resources, United Nations Environment Programme, © 2002 United Nations. Reprinted with the permission of the publisher. Available at: http://www.unep.org/dewa/assessments/ecosystems/water/vitalwater/a1.htm. Accessed April 5, 2010.

Exhibit 9-1

Glossary of Key Hydrological Terms

Aquifer: A layer or section of earth or rock that contains freshwater, known as groundwater (any water that is stored naturally underground or that flows through rock or soil, supplying springs and wells).[a]

Freshwater lakes: Most freshwater lakes are located at high latitudes, with nearly 50% of the world's lakes in Canada alone. Many lakes, especially those in arid regions, become salty through evaporation, which concentrates the inflowing salts. The Caspian Sea, the Dead Sea, and the Great Salt Lake are among the world's major salt lakes.[b]

Glaciers and icecaps: Glaciers and icecaps cover about 10% of the world's landmass. These are concentrated in Greenland and Antarctica and contain ~70% of the world's freshwater. Unfortunately, most of these resources are located far from human habitation and are not readily accessible for human use.

According to the United States Geological Survey (USGS), 96% of the world's frozen freshwater is at the South and North poles, with the remaining 4% spread over 550,000 km^2 of glaciers and mountainous icecaps measuring about 180,000 km^3. . . .[b]

Hydrological (water) cycle: The natural cycle by which water evaporates from oceans and other water bodies, accumulates as water vapor in clouds, and returns to oceans and other water bodies as precipitation.[a]

Nonrenewable water: Water in aquifers and other natural reservoirs that . . . [is] not recharged by the hydrological cycle or . . . [is] recharged so slowly that significant withdrawal for human use causes depletion. Fossil aquifers are in this category: They recharge so slowly over centuries that they are, in effect, a nonrenewable resource.[a]

Renewable water: Freshwater that is continuously replenished by the hydrological cycle for withdrawal within reasonable time limits, such as water in rivers, lakes, or reservoirs that fill from precipitation or from runoff. The renewability of a water source depends both on its natural rate of replenishment and the rate at which the water is withdrawn for human use.[a]

Reservoirs: Artificial lakes, produced by constructing physical barriers across flowing rivers, which allow the water to pool and be used for various purposes. The volume of water stored in reservoirs worldwide is estimated at 4,286 km^3. . . .[b]

Runoff: Water originating as precipitation on land that then runs off the land into rivers, streams, and lakes, eventually reaching the oceans, inland seas, or aquifers, unless it evaporates first. That portion of runoff that can be relied on year after year and easily used by human beings is known as stable runoff.[a]

Water withdrawal: Removal of freshwater for human use from any natural source or reservoir, such as a lake, river, or aquifer. If not consumed, the water may return to the environment and can be used again.[a]

Water scarcity: According to a growing consensus among hydrologists, a country faces water scarcity when its annual supply of renewable freshwater is less than 1,000 cubic meters per person. Such countries can expect to experience chronic and widespread shortages of water that hinder their development.[a]

Water stress: A country faces water stress when its annual supply of renewable freshwater is between 1,000 and 1,700 cubic meters per person. Such countries can expect to experience temporary or limited water shortages.[a]

Wetlands: Wetlands include swamps, bogs, marshes, mires, lagoons and floodplains. [In some cases, wetlands are associated with rivers.] According to the United Nations Environment Program, the earth's 10 largest wetlands are: West Siberian Lowlands, Amazon River, Hudson Bay Lowlands [in Canada], Pantanal [in mid-South America], Upper Nile River, Chari-Logone River [in Africa], Hudson Bay Lowlands in the South Pacific, Congo River, Upper Mackenzie River [in northwestern Canada], and North America prairie potholes [wetlands made up of shallow depressions in the northern Great Plains].

The total global area of wetlands is estimated at ~2,900,000 km^2. . . . Most wetlands range in depth from 0–2 metres. Estimating the average depth of permanent wetlands at about one metre, the global volume of wetlands could range between 2,300 km^3 and 2,900 km^3.[b]

Sources: [a]Reprinted from D Hinrichsen, B Robey, UD Upadhyay. Solutions for a Water-Short World. *Population Reports.* Series M, Number 14. Baltimore, Johns Hopkins University School of Public Health, Population Information Program, September 1998; [b]Adapted and reprinted from *Vital Water Graphics: Freshwater Resources,* United Nations Environment Programme, © 2002 United Nations. Reprinted with the permission of the publisher. Available at: http://www.unep.org/dewa/assessments/ecosystems/water/vitalwater/02.htm. Accessed April 5, 2010.

The Hydrological Cycle

The hydrological cycle is akin to a pumping system, driven by the sun, which moves freshwater from the oceans to landmasses and then returns it to the ocean.[5] This cycle describes the process by which the freshwater supply is continuously replenished. Refer to Figure 9-6.

The United Nations Environment Program provides the following description of the hydrological cycle:

> Water is transported in different forms within the hydrological cycle or "water cycle." . . . [E]ach year about 502,800 km^3 of water evaporates over the oceans and seas, 90% of which

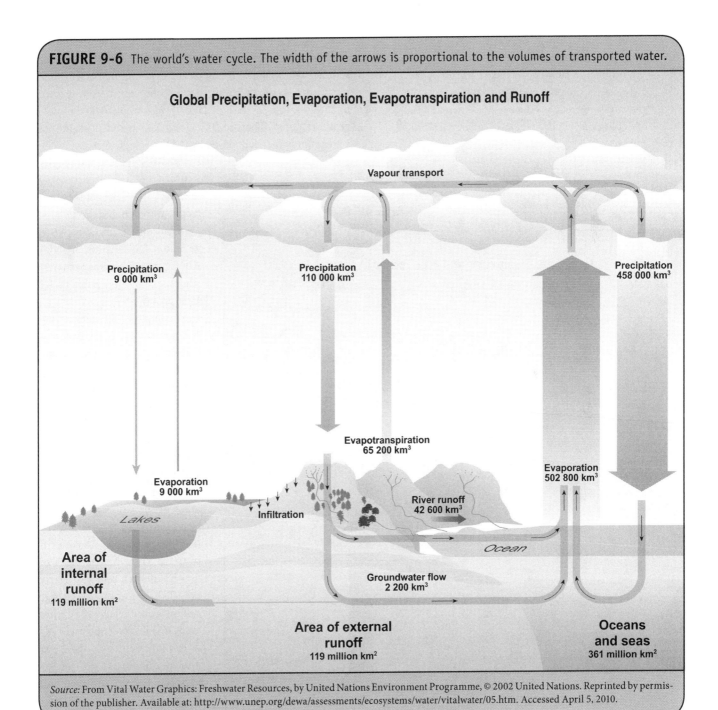

FIGURE 9-6 The world's water cycle. The width of the arrows is proportional to the volumes of transported water.

Global Precipitation, Evaporation, Evapotranspiration and Runoff

Vapour transport

Precipitation 9 000 km^3

Precipitation 110 000 km^3

Precipitation 458 000 km^3

Evapotranspiration 65 200 km^3

Evaporation 9 000 km^3

Infiltration

River runoff 42 600 km^3

Evaporation 502 800 km^3

Lakes

Ocean

Area of internal runoff 119 million km^2

Groundwater flow 2 200 km^3

Area of external runoff 119 million km^2

Oceans and seas 361 million km^2

Source: From Vital Water Graphics: Freshwater Resources, by United Nations Environment Programme, © 2002 United Nations. Reprinted by permission of the publisher. Available at: http://www.unep.org/dewa/assessments/ecosystems/water/vitalwater/05.htm. Accessed April 5, 2010.

(458,000 km³) returns directly to the oceans through precipitation, while the remainder (44,800 km³) falls over land. With evapo-transpiration totaling about 74,200 km³, the total volume in the terrestrial hydrological cycle is about 119,000 km³. About 35% of this, or 44,800 km³, is returned to the oceans as run-off from rivers, groundwater and glaciers. A considerable portion of river flow and groundwater percolation never reaches the ocean, having evaporated in internal runoff areas or inland basins lacking an outlet to the ocean. However, some groundwater that bypasses the river systems reaches the oceans. Annually the hydrological cycle circulates nearly 577,000 km³ of water. . . .[6]

Freshwater Resources

Figure 9-7 provides estimates of world freshwater reserves. No more water exists on earth than there was 2,000 years ago, but the human population has grown enormously since ancient times.[5]

Here are some facts about water availability[5]: Although about 70% of the earth's surface is covered by water, most of this water is unusable ocean water. Approximately 3% of all water is freshwater, of which the majority is unavailable for human use. This water is unavailable because nearly 75% of freshwater supplies are frozen in the polar ice caps and in glaciers. The remaining 1% of readily accessible water comes from surface freshwater; sources include lakes, rivers, and shallow underground aquifers. These readily accessible sources constitute the water supply that is renewed by the hydrological cycle.

Estimates suggest that only 0.01% of the world's total supply of water can be accessible for use by the human population.[5] This amount consists of about 12.5 to 14 billion cubic meters, or about 9,000 cubic meters for each person on earth. (One cubic meter is approximately 1,000 liters.) Unfortunately, the water supply is not distributed evenly across the world. This unequal distribution is exacerbated by the fact that there may be annual cycles of drought and flooding.

Figure 9-8 shows the earth's distribution of freshwater resources represented by glaciers, surface water, and other reserves. Many of the geographic areas of the world that receive heavy rainfall are located away from large population concentrations. The Amazon basin in South America receives nearly one-fifth of the global average rainfall runoff each year. Other areas that receive high amounts of rainfall are the Congo River and its tributaries on the African continent, and Asia and South America. The continent of North America has the larg-

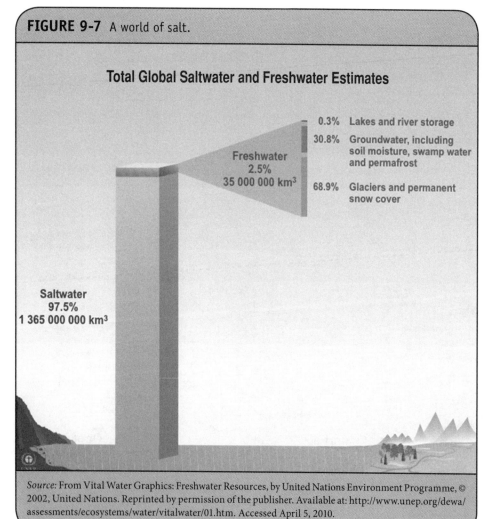

FIGURE 9-7 A world of salt.

Source: From Vital Water Graphics: Freshwater Resources, by United Nations Environment Programme, © 2002, United Nations. Reprinted by permission of the publisher. Available at: http://www.unep.org/dewa/assessments/ecosystems/water/vitalwater/01.htm. Accessed April 5, 2010.

est amount of freshwater available to the population. One extreme example of the unequal distribution of water resources is the water supplies of Kuwait versus Iceland. In the former country, the population has only about 75 cubic meters per person of available water; in the latter, almost one thousand times as much is available to the average person. Countries such as Mexico have an uneven distribution of rainwater; 90% of this country is chronically water short. In parts of Asia, such as India, the water supply is affected greatly by seasonal rains. Consequently, during the drier months very little water is available from rainfall.

Water Scarcity and Water Stress

In several areas of the world, the demand for water presently exceeds the available water supply as a result of water scarcity and water stress. (Refer to Exhibit 9-1 for definitions of water scarcity and water stress.) Ironically, two sections of the world that currently have severe water shortages also are experiencing some of the highest population growth rates in the world. These areas are Africa (sub-Saharan and North) and the Near East, regions that encompass 20 countries. In Saudi Arabia, for example, the supplies of so-called fossil groundwater that exist in aquifers are being rapidly depleted. As a means of supplanting diminishing groundwater sources, several Persian Gulf countries—Bahrain, Kuwait, Saudi Arabia, and the United Arab Emirates—now use desalinization as a method to convert sea water into freshwater.

Presently about 200 million people live in water-stressed countries. For ex-

ample, water shortages in China affect the northern part of the country, including the capital city, Beijing. Although the United States generally has adequate amounts of water, regional shortages occur from time to time. Some major aquifers in the Midwest are being overutilized and depleted. The western states (e.g., California), with rapidly expanding populations, periodically face water shortages during drought years.

The number of countries that will experience water scarcity is expected to increase as their populations continue to burgeon. Estimates suggest that by the year 2025, approximately 2.8 billion people will live in 48 countries that will experience water stress or water scarcity. These numbers will increase by the year 2050 to 54 countries with a combined population of 4 billion people. The world's population of approximately 6 billion is adding about 80 million members annually. This population increase represents a demand for

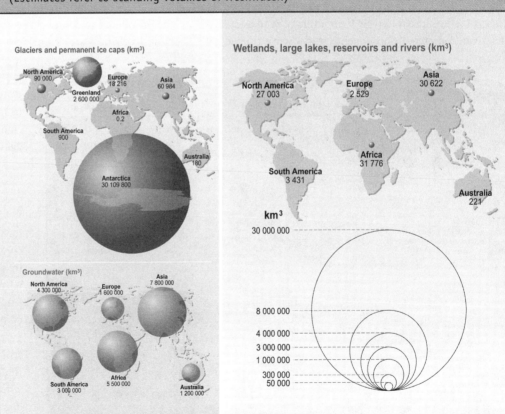

FIGURE 9-8 Global freshwater resources: quantity and distribution by region. (Estimates refer to standing volumes of freshwater.)

Source: From Vital Water Graphics: Freshwater Resources, by United Nations Environment Programme, © United Nations. Reprinted by permission of the publisher. Available at: http://www.unep.org/dewa/assessments/ecosystems/water/vitalwater/02.htm. Accessed April 5, 2010.

freshwater that is about that of the entire annual flow of Europe's Rhine River (64 billion cubic meters per year).

TREATMENT OF WATER FOR RESIDENTIAL CONSUMPTION

Water supplied to the public in the United States undergoes treatment in order to meet quality standards set by the EPA for safe levels of chemical contaminants and waterborne microorganisms. As noted previously, water sources include surface water (lakes and reservoirs) and water from aquifers. Processing of water takes place in water treatment plants, an example of which is shown in Figure 9-9. The four stages of water treatment in most plants are as follows: coagulation, sedimentation, filtration, and disinfection. These stages are presented in Figure 9-10.

As shown in Figure 9-11, after untreated water flows from a storage area into the plant, it first undergoes coagulation to remove suspended material. Aluminum sulfate is used as the coagulating agent. After the coagulating agent has been mixed with the water, the mixture is transferred to sedimentation tanks similar to the ones shown in Figure 9-12. The water then is filtered to remove smaller impurities. The filter is made of progressively finer layers of sand and a layer of activated charcoal. Subsequently, the water is treated with a disinfectant such as chlorine to destroy pathogens. (Refer to Figure 9-13.)

Fluoridation of Water

Some communities in the United States add fluoride to public drinking water in order to prevent tooth decay (dental caries). The rationale for this procedure came from the informal observations of dentists during the early 1900s, followed by epidemiologic studies.[7] Dr. Frederick McKay established a dental practice in 1901 in Colorado Springs, Colorado. (Refer to Figure 9-14.) He soon observed that many of his patients' teeth displayed stains, which he referred to as "mottled enamel" or "Colorado brown stain." McKay concluded that high levels of fluoride in the local drinking water probably were the cause of the stains, and also seemed to confer resistance against tooth decay.

Subsequently, dental researchers including Dr. H. Trendley Dean (during the 1930s) further investigated links between fluoride in drinking water and absence of dental caries. Dean used the term **fluorosis** to describe the dental condition in which teeth have been discolored by fluoride. In epidemiologic studies, Dean demonstrated an inverse relationship between the prevalence of dental caries and levels of naturally occurring drinking water fluoride levels. The optimal fluoride level was set at 0.7 to 1.2 parts per million (ppm) of drinking water. This level was thought to minimize the occurrence of fluorosis and confer protection against dental caries.

Water fluoridation as a means of preventing dental caries was tested in prospective field trials in four pairs of cities (one intervention and one control in each pair) beginning in 1945. For example, the intervention city Grand Rapids, Michigan, was paired with the control city Muskegon, Michigan. The field trials demonstrated a 50–70% reduction in the prevalence of dental caries with no apparent increase in dental fluorosis above what is seen in communities that have low levels of naturally occurring fluoride in their drinking water. Following these successful tri-

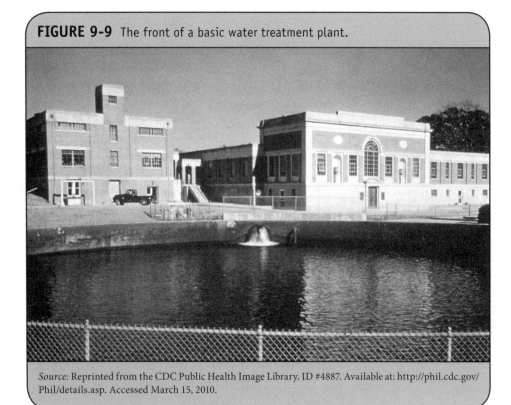

FIGURE 9-9 The front of a basic water treatment plant.

Source: Reprinted from the CDC Public Health Image Library. ID #4887. Available at: http://phil.cdc.gov/Phil/details.asp. Accessed March 15, 2010.

FIGURE 9-10 The stages of treatment at a water treatment plant.

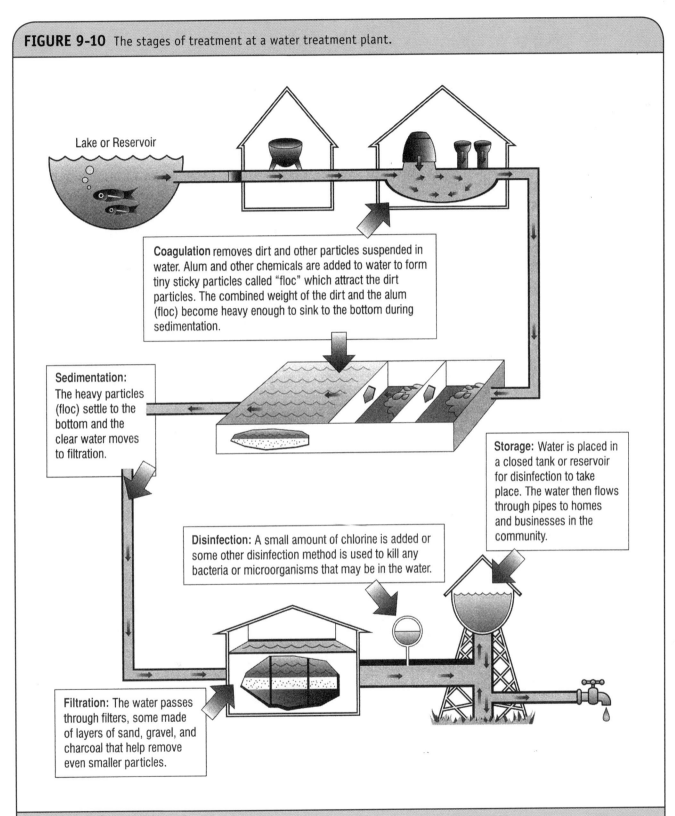

Lake or Reservoir

Coagulation removes dirt and other particles suspended in water. Alum and other chemicals are added to water to form tiny sticky particles called "floc" which attract the dirt particles. The combined weight of the dirt and the alum (floc) become heavy enough to sink to the bottom during sedimentation.

Sedimentation: The heavy particles (floc) settle to the bottom and the clear water moves to filtration.

Storage: Water is placed in a closed tank or reservoir for disinfection to take place. The water then flows through pipes to homes and businesses in the community.

Disinfection: A small amount of chlorine is added or some other disinfection method is used to kill any bacteria or microorganisms that may be in the water.

Filtration: The water passes through filters, some made of layers of sand, gravel, and charcoal that help remove even smaller particles.

Source: Reprinted from US Environmental Protection Agency. Water on tap: What you need to know. Washington, DC: EPA Office of Water; 2003: 8.

FIGURE 9-11 Storage tank for aluminum sulfate used to coagulate solids in water.

Source: Courtesy of Irvine Ranch Water District, Irvine, California.

FIGURE 9-12 Tanks used for additional skimming during secondary processing.

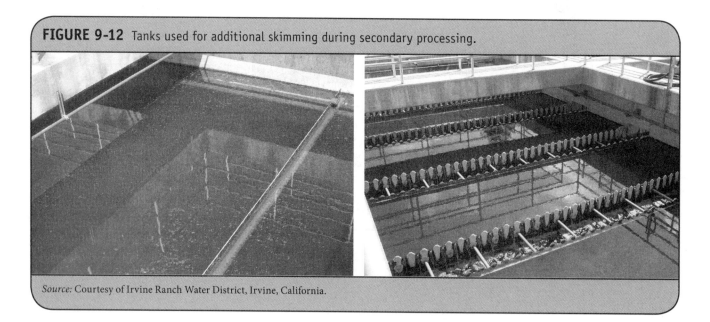

Source: Courtesy of Irvine Ranch Water District, Irvine, California.

FIGURE 9-13 On the top is a model of a sand and charcoal filter used in water processing. On the bottom is a chlorinator room for water disinfection.

Source: Courtesy of Irvine Ranch Water District, Irvine, California.

FIGURE 9-14 Dr. Frederick S. McKay, one of the pioneers in water fluoridation.

Source: Reprinted from the CDC Public Health Image Library. ID #4751. Available at: http://phil.cdc.gov/Phil/details.asp. Accessed April 5, 2010.

als, many communities in the United States added fluoride to public drinking water.

Treatment of Water from Aquifers

Aquifers are a common source of potable water in many communities. For high-quality water from aquifers, minimal aeration, filtration, and disinfection are necessary. In some cases, water drawn from aquifers is free from microorganisms, but undesirable for human consumption because of impurities and coloration that impair the esthetic qualities of this essential liquid. Such is the case of deep aquifers (present at 600 meters [2,000 feet]) found in some regions of the world (e.g., Southern California). This water can be made acceptable through a process of filtration that uses ultrafine filters, as shown in Figure 9-15. The figure shows pumps used to draw the water from the aquifer, banks of filters, and samples of water before and after filtration, in addition to the impurities that have been removed. In this example, the residual impurities removed through filtration are piped to the city's sanitary sewage processing plant.

DRINKING WATER CONTAMINATION

Many consumers in the United States are concerned about the safety of water supplied by municipal water plants. Some dramatic instances of waterborne diseases and the presence of lead and other heavy metals in water from the public water supply have been reported by the media. Despite these unusual instances of drinking water contamination, the public water supply generally is monitored carefully and must adhere to EPA safety standards. Nevertheless, consumers increasingly are adopting bottled water (shall we say "prestige water") as a substitute for tap water (refer to the following text box for a discussion of the relative merits of tap water versus bottled and vended water).

Potable water (drinking water) includes water from wells and runoff from the land's surface. Almost all water in its natural state is impure, because of common naturally occurring and anthropogenic sources of pollution. Naturally occurring sources of pollution arise from the diversity of aquatic animals

FIGURE 9-15 Water filtration system for water from aquifer (Parts A, B, and C).

A. Pump

B. Bank of filters

C. Samples of water before and after filtration

Source: Courtesy of Irvine Ranch Water District, Irvine, California.

Which Is Safer: Tap Water, Bottled Water, or Vended Water?

The growing public acceptance of bottled water may be the result of taste and health concerns. Also popular (particularly among Hispanic and Asian populations) is vended water. Here are some facts about the three types of water:

- Residents of communities that fluoridate water may be at increased risk of tooth decay should they drink bottled water exclusively, because bottled water usually is not fluoridated.
- Some bottled water may contain higher bacterial counts than tap water; all public drinking water sources are regulated by the EPA to ensure quality. The opened personal water bottles of school children have been reported to have fecal coliform contamination, possibly as a result of lapses in personal hygiene.
- Water purchased from water vending machines that are poorly maintained may be contaminated with coliform and other bacteria. Vended water comes from an approved source such as tap water; vending machines provide additional treatment to tap water by using carbon filtration and other methods.

Sources: JA Lalumandier, LW Ayers. Fluoride and bacterial content of bottled water vs tap water. *Arch Fam Med.* 2000;9:246–250; JA Oliphant, MC Ryan, A Chu. Bacterial water quality in the personal water bottles of elementary students. *Can J Public Health.* 2002;95:366–367; J Schillinger, S Du Vall Knorr. Drinking-water quality and issues associated with water vending machines in the city of Los Angeles. *J Environ Health.* 2004;66(6):25–31.

and plants that inhabit the bodies of water used eventually for human consumption. In addition to microbial organisms that live in water, fish, aquatic animals, and wildlife produce wastes that contaminate the water. Soils in contact with the water also harbor microorganisms. Decaying tree leaves and branches contribute organic materials. Natural rock and soil formations may introduce radionuclides, nitrogen compounds, and heavy metals such as arsenic, cadmium, chromium, lead, and selenium, as well as other chemicals.

Figure 9-16 demonstrates how man-made pollutants may enter the urban water supply. Water that courses across the surface of the land may incorporate various contaminants, which include the following[8,9]:

- Chemicals and nutrients (e.g., fertilizers and nitrates from agricultural lands)
- Rubber, heavy metals, and sodium (from roads)
- Petroleum by-products and organic chemicals (from dry cleaners, service stations, and leaking underground storage tanks)
- Chemicals used in the home (solvents, paints, used motor oil, lead, and copper)
- Heavy metals and toxic chemicals (from factories)
- Microbial pathogens (from human and animal wastes)

Runoff from urban streets is a growing contributor to water pollution, especially after periods of heavy rainfall. Pet wastes that are washed into storm drains can represent a hazard to human and animal health. As a result, many cities are attempting to curtail this source of water pollution through local ordinances. (See Figure 9-17.)

In summary, disease-causing agents that may be present in the water supply form four major groups. The first three groups represent agents that sometimes are excreted in feces: parasites (e.g., *Giardia, Cryptosporidia*), bacteria (e.g., *E. coli, Shigella*), and viruses (e.g., Norwalk virus, hepatitis viruses). The fourth group—chemicals (e.g., pesticides, heavy metals)—consists of pollutants that may enter the water from other sources.

Waterborne Diseases and Fecal Contamination

Waterborne diseases are conditions that are "transmitted through the ingestion of contaminated water and water acts as the passive carrier of the infectious agent."[10(p371)] Waterborne diseases are a source of ongoing concern to the residents of the developing world, where waterborne diarrheal conditions take a great toll in morbidity and mortality, and to tourists who travel in these areas. An example of a condition transmitted by water is gastroenteritis, defined as an "inflammation of the stomach and small and large intestines."[11] In addition to gastroenteritis, many serious diseases can be spread through the water supply. To some extent, these diseases also affect developed countries including the United States. The text box presents facts about the significance of waterborne diseases caused by bacterial agents.

Despite reassurances by officials about its safety, the public water supply in some areas of the United States occasion-

FIGURE 9-16 The urban water cycle: Man's impact on groundwater.

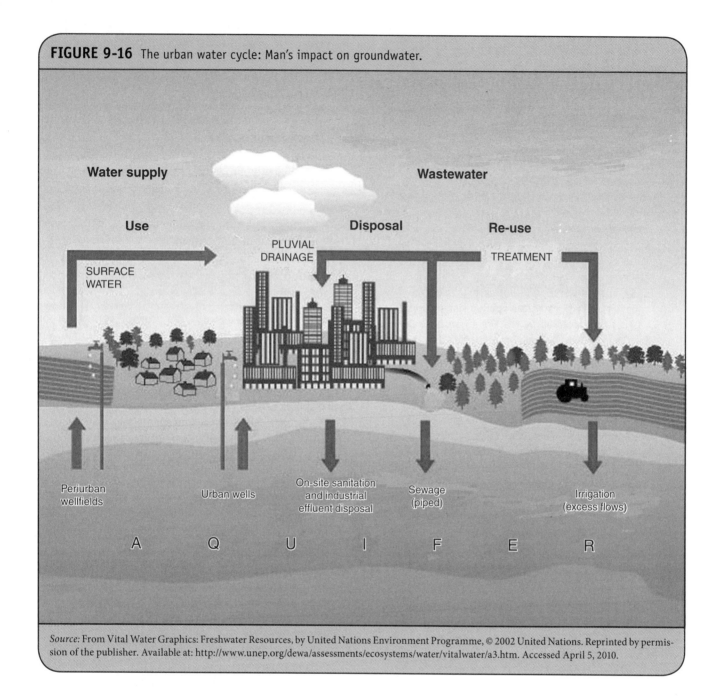

Source: From Vital Water Graphics: Freshwater Resources, by United Nations Environment Programme, © 2002 United Nations. Reprinted by permission of the publisher. Available at: http://www.unep.org/dewa/assessments/ecosystems/water/vitalwater/a3.htm. Accessed April 5, 2010.

ally may be responsible for transmitting serious waterborne diseases. When such transmission occurs via the public water supply, it is usually a consequence of a malfunctioning water-processing system (e.g., the 1993 cryptosporidiosis outbreak in Milwaukee, Wisconsin, discussed later in the chapter).

Many pathogens—bacterial, viral, and protozoan—are responsible for waterborne infections. Examples of waterborne diseases are cryptosporidiosis and giardiasis (both caused by protozoan agents), cholera (agent *Vibrio cholerae*), and

infection with *E. coli* O157:H7.[10] Other conditions that may be transmitted by water include infections caused by *Legionella pneumophila* and certain viruses (e.g., hepatitis A virus). Symptoms of waterborne diseases caused by bacteria include a form of severe diarrhea that can result in dehydration (as in cholera), fevers and abdominal distress of long duration (as in typhoid fever), and in some cases acute bloody diarrhea (as in *E. coli* O157:H7). The following is a list of some of the waterborne pathogens:

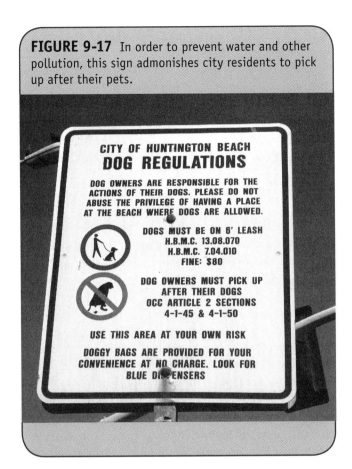

FIGURE 9-17 In order to prevent water and other pollution, this sign admonishes city residents to pick up after their pets.

- Enteric protozoal parasites
  - *Entamoeba histolytica*
  - *Giardia intestinalis*
  - *Cryptosporidium parvum*
  - *Cyclospora cayetanensis*
- Bacterial enteropathogens
  - *Salmonella*
  - *Shigella* (discussed in Chapter 11)
  - *Escherichia coli*
  - *Vibrio cholerae*
  - *Campylobacter* (discussed in Chapter 11)
- Viral pathogens
  - Enteroviruses
  - Adenoviruses
  - Noroviruses (formerly called Norwalk-like viruses)
- Other agents
  - *Dracunculus medinensis*
  - *Legionella pneumophila*

Enteric Protozoal Parasites

Cryptosporidiosis. The infectious agent that causes cryptosporidiosis is called *Cryptosporidium parvum*, a protozoal organism. The symptoms of cryptosporidiosis include watery

Preventing Bacterial Waterborne Diseases

Incidence Each year, an estimated 4 billion episodes of diarrhea result in an estimated 2 million deaths, mostly among children. Waterborne bacterial infections may account for as many as half of these episodes and deaths.

Sequelae Many deaths among infants and young children are due to dehydration, malnutrition, or other complications of waterborne bacterial infections.

Transmission Contaminated surface water sources and large, poorly functioning municipal water distribution systems contribute to transmission of waterborne bacterial diseases. Chlorination and safe water handling can eliminate the risk of waterborne bacterial diseases.

Risk Groups Over 2 billion persons living in poverty in the developing world are at high risk. Certain US groups (residents of periurban "colonias" and remote rural areas with poor water treatment and delivery systems) are also at risk.

Trends Despite global efforts, improvements in water and sanitation infrastructure have barely kept pace with population increases and migrations in the developing world.

Source: Adapted and reprinted from Centers for Disease Control and Prevention. Disease Listing: Preventing bacterial waterborne diseases. Available at: http://www.cdc.gov/ncidod/dbmd/diseaseinfo/waterbornediseases_t.htm. Accessed March 15, 2010.Preventing Bacterial Waterborne Diseases

TABLE 9-1 Cryptosporidiosis (Chronology)

1976	First human case diagnosed
1984	First well water outbreak
1987	First river water outbreak
1992	Multiple municipal water supply outbreaks
1993	Largest recorded waterborne outbreak in US history (Milwaukee, WI)
	Fresh-pressed apple cider outbreak (Central Maine)
1994	First outbreak in community with state-of-the-art water treatment (Las Vegas)

Source: Adapted and reprinted from the CDC Public Health Image Library. ID #109. NCID Content Provider. Available at: http://phil.cdc.gov/Phil/details.asp. Accessed March 15, 2010.

diarrhea, abdominal cramping, nausea, vomiting, and fever. The condition can be fatal among immunocompromised individuals.[12] Table 9-1 presents a chronology of cryptosporidiosis in the United States. The first human case was diagnosed in 1976. Since then, several outbreaks have been linked to drinking water sources including public drinking water supplies.

The complex life cycle of the different species of *Cryptosporidium* is shown in Figure 9-18. (Note that *Cryptosporidium parvum* is the species of *Cryptosporidium* that causes infections in humans.) *Cryptosporidium* oocysts, which are the infectious component for cryptosporidiosis, are excreted in the stools of infected persons.[13] Water used for recreation and drinking may be contaminated with sewage that contains the oocysts of *C. parvum*. Following ingestion by other human hosts, the oocysts (see Figure 9-19) reproduce. Resistant to chlorine treatment, infective oocysts may survive treatment by water treatment plants, even modern installations.

The most notorious waterborne outbreak of cryptosporidiosis in the United States occurred in southern Milwaukee in late March and early April 1993. More than 400,000 people were estimated to be affected during this major outbreak.[14] This number actually may undercount the number of affected persons, as the case definition was limited to watery diarrhea.[12]

The outbreak was linked to the Milwaukee Water Works (MWW), the supplier of water for the city of Milwaukee and nine surrounding municipalities in Milwaukee County. Investigators believed that *Cryptosporidium* oocysts (see Figure 9-19) from untreated Lake Michigan water were drawn into the water treatment plant. The usual water treatment processes (e.g., coagulation, filtration, and chlorination) were not adequate to remove the oocysts.

Two major rivers flow into the Milwaukee harbor. Along the rivers are slaughterhouses and effluents of human sewage. During a springtime period of heavy precipitation, the rivers may have transported oocysts into Lake Michigan, a source of water for the MWW. Between approximately March 21 and April 5, a marked increase in the turbidity of treated water was noted. On April 7 the MWW issued an advisory to customers to boil their water; subsequently, the MWW closed the plant temporarily on April 9. This massive outbreak in Milwaukee suggests the need to continuously monitor the quality of drinking water (especially for turbidity), to conduct **public health surveillance** of diarrheal illnesses caused by water, and to recognize the hazards that *Cryptosporidium* outbreaks pose for the public.

Contaminated water has been linked to most known outbreaks of cryptosporidiosis in the United States.[15] A study conducted in the San Francisco Bay area evaluated the risk of transmission of endemic cryptosporidiosis by drinking water. The study did not support the hypothesis that drinking water is a risk factor for cryptosporidiosis among the immunocompetent population. Cases of cryptosporidiosis identified by a surveillance system found that travel to another country was a strong and significant risk factor for cryptosporidiosis.

Other sources of *Cryptosporidium* infections are public swimming pools and water parks used by large numbers of diapered children. These settings have been implicated in outbreaks of cryptosporidiosis. It is known that very low doses of *C. parvum* are required for infection. The oocysts are resistant to chlorine treatment; therefore, bathers should avoid drinking water used in public swimming pools. Parents of diapered children should be educated regarding the supervision of their children so that swimming pools do not become contaminated with fecal material.[16]

Amebiasis.   Amebiasis is caused by the protozoal parasite *Entamoeba histolytica*, which produces cysts that are carried in human feces.[17] Transmission occurs via the ingestion of cysts that are contained in food and water that have been contaminated by feces. Both asymptomatic and symptomatic illnesses are associated with the organism. The latter include invasive intestinal amebiasis (e.g., dysentery, colitis, and appendicitis) and extraintestinal amebiasis (e.g., abscesses of the lungs and liver). When traveling to a less developed area of the world where sanitary conditions are wanting, tourists should avoid eating peeled fresh fruits and vegetables, unpasteurized milk and other dairy products, and food sold by street vendors.[18]

FIGURE 9-18 This illustration depicts the life cycle of different species of *Cryptosporidium*, the causal agents of cryptosporidiosis.

to 14 days, with approximately 7 days being typical. Symptoms of acute giardiasis include gastrointestinal effects such as diarrhea, nausea, and vomiting. A chronic form also can occur and may result in debilitation of the patient.

Cyclosporiasis (an emerging parasitic disease). In common with other protozoal parasites discussed in this section, the causative organism *Cyclospora cayetanensis* is transmitted via ingestion of food and water that have been contaminated with cysts (oocysts) from the organism. Foodborne outbreaks have involved fresh produce (e.g., snow peas and raspberries). During May through July 2007, a cluster of 29 cases of cyclosporiasis, reported in British Columbia, Canada, was linked to imported basil.[20] The protozoal parasite causes watery diarrhea and other symptoms of abdominal distress in addition to low-grade fever.

Bacterial Enteropathogens

Examples of microorganisms in this category are *Salmonella*, *Escherichia coli* O157:H7, and *Vibrio cholerae*. *Salmonella* bacteria are associated with a number of foodborne (see Chapter 11) and waterborne diseases. The variant (serogroup) of *Salmonella* called *Salmonella* serogroup Typhi (*S.* Typhi) causes typhoid fever, which is transmitted by fecal contaminated water and food (e.g., sold by street vendors). Typhoid fever is a very acute disease that causes fever, headache, and chills; in severe cases, it may produce confusion, delirium, and death.[21] According to the CDC about 400 typhoid fever cases occur

Giardiasis. The agent that is responsible for giardiasis is *Giardia intestinalis* (also known as *Giardia lamblia*), a protozoal organism.[19] (Refer to Figure 9-20.) *G. intestinalis* produces cysts that transmit the condition via contaminated food and water. The cysts have the ability to survive for long periods in cold water. The incubation period for giardiasis varies from 1

FIGURE 9-19 Oocysts of *Cryptosporidium parvum*. Oocysts are spheroidal objects, 4 to 6 microns (μm) in diameter.

Source: Reprinted courtesy of the CDC Public Health Image Library. ID #4384. Dr. Peter Drotman Content Provider. Available at: http://phil.cdc.gov/Phil/details.asp. Accessed April 5, 2010.

in the United States each year. Globally, typhoid fever causes approximately 21 million cases of disease and 200,000 deaths annually. Historically, there have been many examples of waterborne outbreaks: During 1973, an outbreak of 188 proved or presumptive cases occurred at a migrant labor camp in Dade County, Florida.[22] Another outbreak was reported in 1985 in Haifa, Israel, and involved 77 confirmed cases.[23]

The bacterium *E. coli* may be transmitted through contact with contaminated lakes and swimming pools and via ingestion of contaminated water. The same organism also may be transmitted by contaminated food, as discussed in Chapter 11. The following text box describes a waterborne outbreak of *E. coli*.

The bacterium that causes cholera is known as *Vibrio cholerae*. The inhabitants of developed countries such as the

United States (annual incidence 0 to 5 cases) have very low risk of contracting cholera, which primarily affects the developing world.[24] A continuing pandemic, lasting for four decades in Asia, Africa, and Latin America, has been a cause of epidemic diarrhea. The underlying factors responsible for cholera outbreaks are an inadequate infrastructure for processing water and migrations of large numbers of people to urban areas. Although cholera is a treatable condition, the disease has a case fatality rate of as high as 50% when untreated. The symptoms of cholera are vomiting and profuse watery diarrhea that can culminate in shock and death.

Viral Pathogens

Over 100 kinds of viruses are found in human stools and pose a potential for transmission by water.[25] "These viruses

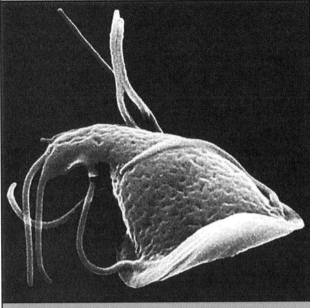

FIGURE 9-20 The protozoan parasite *Giardia lamblia*, causative agent for giardiasis.

Source: Reprinted courtesy of the CDC Public Health Image Library. ID #8698. Janice Haney Carr Content Provider. Available at: http://phil.cdc.gov/phil/details.asp. Accessed April 7, 2010.

A Waterborne Outbreak of *Escherichia coli* O157:H7

In the summer of 1998, a large outbreak of *Escherichia coli* O157:H7 infections occurred in Alpine, Wyoming. [There were] 157 ill persons; stool from 71 (45%) yielded *E. coli* O157:H7. In two cohort studies, illness was significantly associated with drinking municipal water. . . . The unchlorinated water supply had microbiologic evidence of fecal organisms and the potential for chronic contamination with surface water. Among persons exposed to water, the attack rate was significantly lower in town residents than in visitors (23% vs. 50%, p < 0.01) and decreased with increasing age. The lower attack rate among exposed residents, especially adults, is consistent with the acquisition of partial immunity following long-term exposure. Serologic data, although limited, may support this finding. Contamination of small, unprotected water systems may be an increasing public health risk.

Source: SJ Olsen, G Miller, T Brever, et al. A waterborne outbreak of *Escherichia coli* O157:H7 infections and hemolytic uremic syndrome: implications for rural water systems. *Emerg Infect Dis.* 2002;8:370–375. A Waterborne Outbreak of Escherichia coli O157:H7

are more resistant to environmental conditions and sewage treatment processes, including chlorination and UV radiation, than many of the sewage-associated bacteria."[25(p179)] Virus-associated conditions that may be spread through water are viral gastroenteritis and viral hepatitis. "The human enteric virus group, which includes Norwalk virus, rotavirus, hepatitis A virus, adenovirus, and enterovirus, is one of the leading causes of human illness."[25(p179)] The term *enteric* is defined as relating to the intestines. Disease outbreaks caused by enteric viruses have been associated with water and food that were contaminated by virus-laden human stools.

Two causes of viral gastroenteritis are noroviruses and adenoviruses. Infection with norovirus produces nausea, vomiting, and cramping. Norovirus-associated gastroenteritis usually has a brief duration (one to two days) but can produce severe and violent symptoms such as vomiting that happens without warning. Sometimes norovirus infection is labeled incorrectly as the stomach flu. However, this infection is unrelated to the influenza virus. Noroviruses can be carried in contaminated food and drink.[26]

The most common means for spreading adenoviruses is direct person-to-person contact. However, adenoviruses also are spread by waterborne transmission, although this mode is less common. Among the diseases that adenoviruses cause are respiratory illnesses, conjunctivitis, and gastroenteritis. Outbreaks of disease associated with fever and conjunctivitis, caused by adenoviruses, have been traced to waterborne transmission, particularly by human feces present in swimming pools and small lakes.[27] High concentrations of these viruses have been detected near the mouths of rivers in Southern California.[25]

Viral hepatitis A and viral hepatitis E (caused by the hepatitis A virus and the hepatitis E virus, respectively) can be spread via the fecal-oral route by contaminated food and water.[13,28,29] Hepatitis A outbreaks have been linked to the consumption of raw or incompletely cooked clams and other mollusks that were taken from contaminated bodies of water. Hepatitis E outbreaks have occurred in developing countries and have been associated with drinking-water contamination. In order to prevent hepatitis E infection, travelers who visit developing countries in South Asia and North Africa need to take care that their water supply is safe. Due to the presence of infectious agents and toxins in sewage, workers who come into contact with sewage are at increased risk in comparison to the general population of contracting infectious diseases, such as hepatitis C, caused by agents present in fecal matter.[30]

Other Agents

Guinea worm. Although there are several important waterborne diseases in this category, one that is noteworthy for the developing world is dracunculiasis (also called guinea worm disease).[31] As the result of an eradication campaign, the range for guinea worm is confined to rural sections of a small number of African countries. The causative organism is the nematode (a kind of roundworm) *Dracunculus medinensis*, which forms larvae that enter the water supply. The larvae infect small crustaceans in the water that are ingested in unfiltered water. In the abdominal cavity of the human host, the larvae mature into worms. Female worms that range in length from 3 to 6 feet (70 to 120 cm) then migrate to the surface of the skin of the feet where they produce painful blisters. The female worm then erupts from this lesion and, when the victim comes into contact with a body of water, releases larvae back into the water, thus perpetuating the cycle of infection. Refer to Figure 9-21 for an illustration of the clinical features of dracunculiasis as well as additional information.

Legionnaires' disease. Legionnaires' disease (legionellosis) is associated with infections by the bacterium *Legionella pneumophila*, which can produce lung infections that are a form of pneumonia.[13,32] The case-fatality rate for Legionnaires' disease is about 15%. *L. pneumophila* was first identified in 1977 after causing an outbreak of pneumonia that resulted in 34 deaths in 1976 at a meeting of the American Legion Convention—hence the name Legionnaires' disease. The symptoms of the disease include high fever, cough, chest pain and, in some cases, abdominal pain and diarrhea; a milder form of legionellosis with pneumonia absent is called Pontiac fever. More than 25,000 Legionnaires' disease cases (and over 4,000 deaths) occur annually.[32] Low levels of *L. pneumophila* are found in freshwater lakes, streams, and rivers. In the environment, some species of protozoa (e.g., some varieties of amoeba) serve as a host for *L. pneumophila*.[33] The organism can grow in domestic water systems, cooling systems, and stagnant water. Transmission of the bacterium can occur when water that is rich in *L. pneumophila* becomes aerosolized and is inhaled or ingested in such a way that it enters the respiratory system. The United States Department of Labor notes that "[c]ooling towers, evaporative condensers, and fluid coolers use a fan to move air through a recirculated water system. This allows a considerable amount of water vapor and sometimes droplets to be introduced into the surroundings, despite the presence of drift eliminators designed to limit droplet release. This water may be in the ideal temperature range for Legionnaires' disease bacteria (LDB) growth, 20°–50°C (68°–122°F)."[34] Figure 9-22 illustrates a cooling tower. Because the growth of *L. pneumophila* is possible in some types of cooling towers, proper maintenance of them is essential.

Chemicals in the Water Supply

As previously noted, chemicals enter the water supply from natural and anthropogenic sources. These substances may be present as contaminants in drinking water.

> A number of chemical contaminants have been identified in drinking water. These contaminants reach drinking water supplies from various sources, including municipal and industrial discharges, urban and rural runoff, natural geological formations, drinking water distribution materials and the drinking water treatment process. Chemical contaminants for which epidemiologic studies have reported associations include the following: aluminum, arsenic, disinfection by-products, fluoride, lead, pesticides and radon. Health effects reported have included various cancers, adverse reproductive outcomes, cardiovascular disease and neurological disease.[35(pS13)]

Pharmaceutical and personal care products (PPCPs) represent another source of water contamination. These chemicals may be either washed off or excreted from the body; examples of PPCPs that may end up in untreated sewage effluent, surface water, groundwater, and drinking water are analgesics, oral contraceptive agents, drugs for lowering cholesterol, and anticonvulsants.[36] In fact, the term *sewage epidemiology* describes a new field of monitoring excreted drugs in the sewer system to assess the level of illicit drug use in the community. Chapters 6 and 7 covered some of the hazards associated with metals, pesticides, and other chemicals. The following section will provide additional information about the effects of chemical contamination of drinking water.

Water Disinfection By-products (DBPs)

The chemicals used to disinfect water include chlorine, chloramines, chlorine dioxide, and ozone. These chemicals are associated with by-products of chlorination called DBPs.

FIGURE 9-21 Guinea worm disease and the use of filters.

A: Portable pipe filters are a convenient method for preventing Guinea worm disease. A young boy uses a portable pipe filter to prevent transmission of Guinea worm disease.

B: Traditional treatment of Guinea worm disease consists of wrapping the two- to three-foot-long worm around a small stick and extracting it: a slow, painful process that often takes weeks. The figure shows an emerging Guinea worm.

Photo credit: Emily Staub/TCC.

Photo credit: Elizabeth Wolfe.

C. President and Mrs. Carter examine a pipe filter.

D: Guinea worm disease incapacitates its victims so adults cannot work and children cannot play or attend school. Filters catch the microscopic water fleas that contain infective larvae. This woman is using such a cloth filter.

Photo credit: Annemarie Poyo.

Photo credit: Emily Staub/TCC.

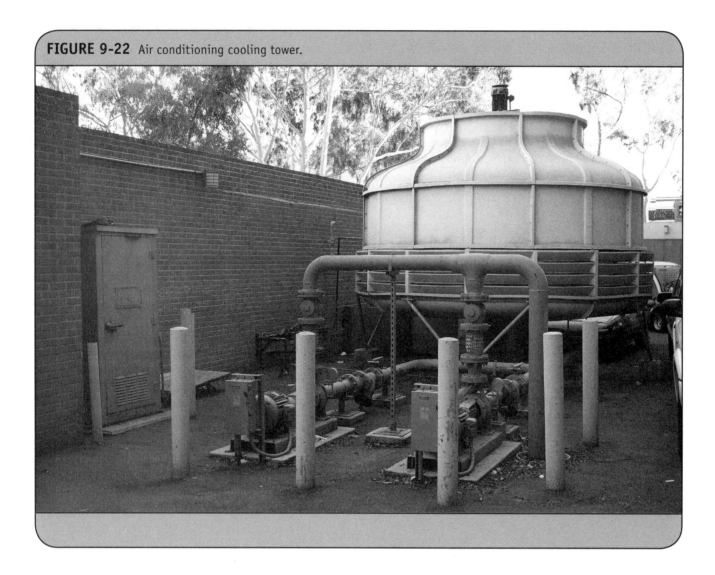

FIGURE 9-22 Air conditioning cooling tower.

For example, chlorine is associated with trihalomethanes (THMs), which are among the most common and widely measured DBPs.[37,38] Researchers have probed the relationship between DBPs and several forms of cancer (e.g., bladder and rectal cancer) as well as adverse reproductive outcomes. Several epidemiologic studies have investigated the association between chlorination of drinking water and risk of birth defects; two examples of supportive studies were those conducted by Aschengrau et al.[39] and Hwang et al.[37]

Aschengrau et al. reported an association between chlorine in drinking water and the frequency of late adverse pregnancy outcomes (e.g., congenital anomalies, stillbirths, and neonatal deaths).[39] Chlorinated surface water was associated with the frequency of stillbirths. The study involved approximately 1,200 cases of adverse pregnancy outcomes and a simi-

lar number of controls. Subjects were from the Brigham and Women's Hospital in Massachusetts.

Hwang et al. examined data from a cross-section of 285,631 Norwegian births in 1993–1998.[37] The results of this cross-sectional study suggested that consumption of chlorinated waters that contained large amounts of natural organic materials was related to increased risk of birth defects.

Nevertheless, at this stage, little is known about the potential adverse health effects of exposure to DBPs.[38] Many researchers who have addressed this topic have been confronted with methodological difficulties, especially with respect to exposure assessment. Typically, studies rely on approximate methods of exposure assessment that do not account for individual variability in patterns of water consumption (e.g., the amount of water consumed, whether water is consumed at work as well as at home, and use of bottled and filtered water).[40]

Solvent-Contaminated Drinking Water

Industrial chemicals may infiltrate the underground aquifers used for public water supplies. An example is contamination of water by a leaking underground solvent tank used by a semiconductor plant in Santa Clara County, California.[41,42] Although the tank held many different chemicals, the chemical solvent trichloroethane (discussed in Chapter 7) was present in the highest concentration. Unfortunately, the tank was located near a well used by the local water company. The leak was discovered in November 1981; by December 7 the levels of trichloroethane at the well were 1,700 parts per billion (ppb) and in mid-December reached 8,800 ppb. The level of 1,700 ppb exceeded by 8.5 times the level required by the state of California for remediation. Residents of an area affected by the contaminated water supply believed that an excessive number of spontaneous abortions and birth defects were occurring in their neighborhood. An investigation conducted in 1983 showed significant associations between exposure to the contaminated water and adverse pregnancy outcomes (congenital malformations and spontaneous abortions), but was unable to demonstrate a causal connection. A follow-up study suggested that the solvent leak was unlikely to have caused the increased numbers of adverse pregnancy outcomes.

BEACH AND COASTAL POLLUTION

The final topic in this chapter is pollution of ocean water. According to the Natural Resources Defense Council (NRDC), "Our vast oceans may seem indestructible, but pollution, ocean dumping of dredged material, sand and gravel mining, oil and gas development, shipping, habitat destruction and overfishing have taken a serious toll."[43]

Some estimates suggest that half of the world's coastal areas are endangered.[44] Figure 9-23 shows a number of human activities that lead to coastal degradation. These actions include draining of coastal ecosystems, dredging, solid waste disposal, construction of dams for flood control, discharge of wastes from farms and industries, and logging activities.

The approximately 1 billion people who live near coastal areas cause great stress on coastal ecosystems. Growth rates of populations near coastal regions are estimated to be twice the rate of worldwide population growth.[45] As the population mushrooms, coastal areas are threatened by overdevelopment, poor planning, and economic expansion. Each day the world's coastal regions are the recipients of billions of gallons of treated and untreated wastewater. During heavy rains urban runoff into the oceans degrades the quality of ocean water by adding microbial agents, nutrients, and chemical toxins. The problem of urban runoff is compounded by developments that result in the loss of **wetlands**, which act as natural water-filtering mechanisms. Excessive amounts of nutrients that enter the oceans may cause harmful blooms of algae, resulting in reduced levels of oxygen in the water (anoxic conditions). An anoxic ocean environment can bring about fish kills and damage other forms of ocean life.

Urban runoff and sewage contamination of the ocean expose swimmers to waterborne diseases—gastrointestinal, respiratory, skin, and eye infections. As a result of ocean water contamination, beach closings have become ever more frequent. (See Figure 9-24.)

The EPA conducts an ongoing survey of beaches through its BEACH Watch Program.[46] In 2002 the EPA surveyed a total of 2,823 beaches regarding advisories or closings and reported that about 25% had been issued an advisory or were closed. By far, the most frequent cause of beach closings was elevated bacteria levels. Figure 9-25 shows some of the reasons reported by the EPA for beach closings.

Storm water runoff is a leading cause of ocean pollution. Garbage that is discarded carelessly on the street may end up in the ocean or on beaches, as Figure 9-26 demonstrates. Following heavy rains, visitors to the beach are likely to find massive quantities of nonbiodegradable plastics (e.g., Styrofoam cups, rings from beverage six-packs, and plastic bags) that are littering the shoreline. In addition to being offensive, these materials endanger birds and fish. Motor vehicle oil and automotive chemicals that are dumped carelessly into storm drains also eventually pollute the ocean.

Petroleum Spills

Oil spills from tankers and off-shore drilling platforms can have a devastating impact on the shoreline, aquatic life, mammals, and birds. One of the worst oil spills in US history was caused by the tanker *Exxon Valdez*, described in the following text box and shown in Figure 9-27.

Oil platforms such as the one shown in Figure 9-28 have been associated with accidental releases of crude oil. January 28, 1969, was the date of an extensive oil spill off the coast of the city of Santa Barbara, California.[47] The spill originated from an offshore drilling rig known as platform Alpha, operated by the Union Oil Company. This episode, which lasted for 11 days and allowed 3 million gallons of oil to escape, caused an ecological catastrophe. The affected shoreline is an environmentally sensitive area noted for its pristine waters and abundant sea life. As a result of the spill, 3,600 ocean-feeding sea birds were killed. The carcasses of numerous poisoned seals and dolphins

FIGURE 9-23 Human actions leading to coastal degradation.

Cause of degradation	Estuaries	Intertidal Wetlands	Open Ocean
Drainage of coastal ecosystems for agriculture, deforestation, and mosquito control measures	●	◦	●
Dredging and channelisation for navigation and flood protection	●	●	·
Solid waste disposal, road construction, and commercial, industrial, or residential development	●	●	◦
Conversion for aquaculture	●	●	●
Construction of dykes, dams and seawalls for flood and storm control, water supply and irrigation	●	●	●
Discharge of pesticides, herbicides, domestic and industrial waste, agricultural runoff and sediment loads	●	●	●
Mining of wetlands for peat, coal, gravel, phospates, etc.	◦	·	◦
Logging and shifting cultivation	◦	●	·
Fire	◦	◦	·
Sedimentation of dams, deep channels and other structures	●	●	●
Hydrological alteration by canals, roads and other structures	●	●	●
Subsidence due to extraction of groundwater, oil, gas and other minerals	●	·	◦

● Common and major cause of degradation

◦ Present but not a major cause

· Absent or uncommon

Source: From Vital Water Graphics: Coastal and Marine, by United Nations Environment Programme, © 2002 United Nations. Reprinted by permission of the publisher. Available at: http://www.unep.org/dewa/assessments/ecosystems/water/vitalwater/38.htm. Accessed April 5, 2010.

FIGURE 9-24 Beach closing sign. With increasing levels of pollution in some areas, beach closings have become more frequent.

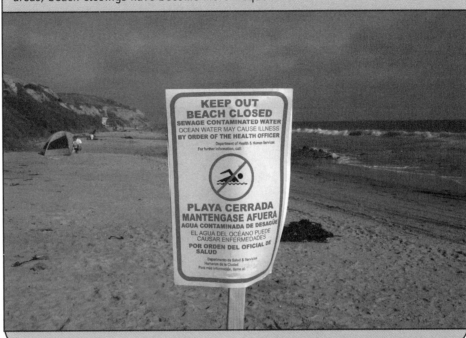

FIGURE 9-25 Sources of pollution that resulted in beach advisories and closings, 2002.

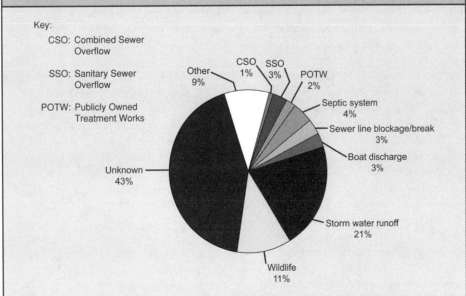

Key:
CSO: Combined Sewer Overflow

SSO: Sanitary Sewer Overflow

POTW: Publicly Owned Treatment Works

Other 9%
CSO 1%
SSO 3%
POTW 2%
Septic system 4%
Sewer line blockage/break 3%
Boat discharge 3%
Storm water runoff 21%
Wildlife 11%
Unknown 43%

Source: Reprinted from US Environmental Protection Agency, Office of Water. EPA's BEACH Watch Program: 2002 Swimming Season. EPA 823-F-03-007; 2003. Available at: http://www.epa.gov/waterscience/beaches/seasons/beachwatch2003-newformat.pdf. Accessed April 5, 2010.

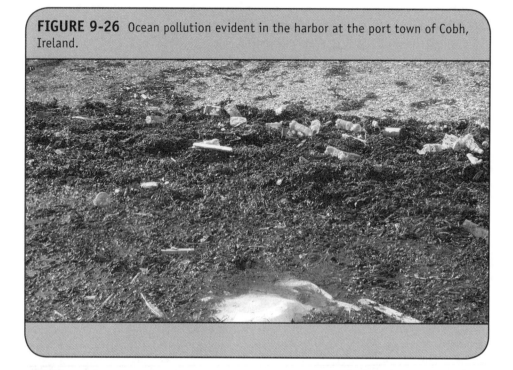

FIGURE 9-26 Ocean pollution evident in the harbor at the port town of Cobh, Ireland.

Exxon Valdez Oil Spill

On March 24, 1989, the tanker *Exxon Valdez*, en route from Valdez, Alaska, to Los Angeles, California, ran aground on Bligh Reef in Prince William Sound, Alaska. The vessel was traveling outside normal shipping lanes in an attempt to avoid ice. Within six hours of the grounding, the *Exxon Valdez* spilled approximately 10.9 million gallons of its 53 million gallon cargo of Prudhoe Bay Crude. Eight of the eleven tanks on board were damaged. The oil would eventually impact over 1,100 miles of non-continuous coastline in Alaska, making the *Exxon Valdez* the largest oil spill to date [as of 1992] in US waters.

The response to the *Exxon Valdez* involved more personnel and equipment over a longer period of time than did any other spill in US history. Logistical problems in providing fuel, meals, berthing, response equipment, waste management and other resources were one of the largest challenges to response management. At the height of the response, more than 11,000 personnel, 1,400 vessels and 85 aircraft were involved in the cleanup.

Concern over oil-related wildlife mortality was intense during the spill. The grounding occurred at the beginning of the bird migration season. The US Fish and Wildlife Service estimated that mortalities directly related to the spill range from 350,000 to 390,000 birds, especially common and thick-billed murres, assorted sea ducks, bald eagles, and pigeon guillemots, 3,500 to 5,500 sea otters and 200 harbor seals. In addition, killer whales may have been affected by the spill as their numbers in the area declined shortly after the spill. Of the 1,630 birds (over 36,000 dead birds were collected) and 357 sea otters that were trapped and treated by the International Bird Rescue Research Center (IBRRC)–run facilities (established in Homer, Kodiak, Seward and Valdez in response to this spill), the total survival rate was 50.7% for birds, and 62% for sea otters. These survival rates are considered very good for oil impacted animals.

Unlike birds, sea otters had to be anesthetized to be washed, which increases the risk to the animal, and increases the cost of rehabilitation. The sea otter rehabilitation program was complex, with a total of 29 veterinarians, and 9 veterinarian technicians scheduled to provide 24-hour care. The resulting cost of the sea otter rehabilitation program was at least $51,000 per sea otter. The highest percentages of sea otter fatalities (60%) were recorded in the first three weeks of the spill.

Source: Adapted and reprinted from National Oceanic and Atmospheric Administration. Oil Spill Case Histories, 1967–1991, Summaries of Significant US and International Spills. Report No. HMRAD 92-11. Seattle, Washington; 1992.

FIGURE 9-27 The Exxon Valdez oil spill. Upper left: Oil being removed (lightered) from the ship. Upper right: Exxon Valdez surrounded by a boom. Lower left: Biologist measuring depth of oil penetration. Lower right: Workers using high-pressure, hot-water washing to clean an oiled shoreline.

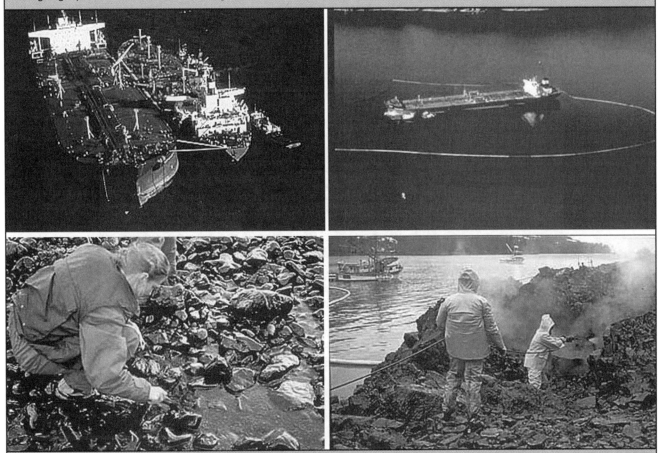

Source: Reprinted from National Oceanic and Atmospheric Administration, NOAA's Ocean Service, Office of Response and Restoration. Image Galleries: Exxon Valdez Oil Spill. Available at: http://response.restoration.noaa.gov/gallery_gallery_photo.php? Accessed April 5, 2010.

had to be removed from the beaches. This catastrophe was responsible for killing an untold number of fish and invertebrates and wreaked havoc on sensitive kelp forests.

In addition to the *Exxon Valdez* and Santa Barbara oil spills, there have been numerous other incidents. For example, the *Sea Empress* spilled approximately 72,000 tons of crude oil and 360 tons of heavy fuel oil when it ran aground at the entrance of Milford Haven harbor near Wales on February 15, 1996.[48] Nearby residents reported strong smells and complained of various symptoms that were associated with the spill. When contrasted with people living in control areas, residents in the exposed area indicated that they had higher rates of physical and psychological symptoms, which were consistent with the known toxicological effects of oil. The *Nakhodka* oil spill, which occurred on January 2, 1997, caused more than 6,000 tons of oil to be spilled into the Sea of Japan. Most of the oil drifted to the shoreline of the western portion of the island of Honshu, which is Japan's main island. Cleanup of the spill required the use of hand tools such as ladles and buckets because the area was inaccessible to machines. Local residents and those who were involved in the cleanup efforts experienced a number of acute symptoms of exposure, including low-back pain, headache, and effects on the eyes and skin.[49]

FIGURE 9-28 Oil platform off the California coast.

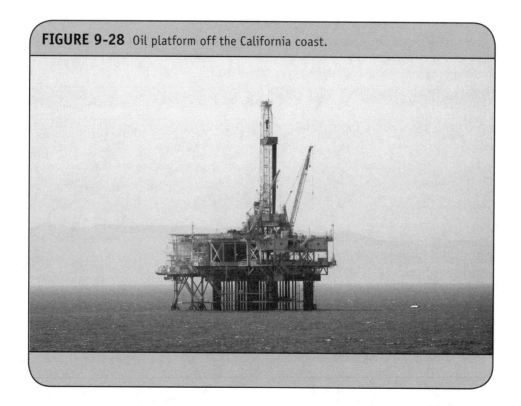

FIGURE 9-29 Deepwater Horizon fire.

Source: US Coast Guard, Visual Information Gallery. Deepwater Horizon fire. Available at: http://cgvi.uscg.mil/media/main.php?g2_itemId=836364. Accessed August 28, 2010.

The Deepwater Horizon Oil Spill, April 20 to July 15, 2010

The Deepwater Horizon oil spill was history's largest accidental marine oil spill. Although initial reports suggested that only about 1,000 barrels of oil per day were spewing from 5,000 feet beneath the water surface of the Gulf of Mexico, subsequent estimates increased periodically as the full scale of the catastrophe became known. The official estimate eventually grew to 60,000 barrels per day, 12 times the first estimate. By the time the wellhead had been capped, nearly 5 million barrels of oil are believed to have contaminated the gulf.

This catastrophe eclipsed all previous marine oil spills that occurred in the United States and anywhere else in the world. The second largest marine release of oil in history also occurred in the gulf during 1979 in the Bay of Campeche from the Mexican oil rig Ixtoc 1. Estimates placed the total from this spill at 3.3 million barrels. The largest (nonmarine) oil spill in history was the 36 billion gallons released by retreating Iraqi soldiers in Kuwait in 1991.

On the night of April 20, 2010, an explosion (caused by methane gas) followed by a conflagration devastated the Deepwater Horizon oil platform, which eventually sank into the deep water. The drilling rig, owned and operated by Transocean Ltd. under contract with the BP Oil Company, was located approximately 50 miles southeast of Venice, LA, and was staffed by a crew of 126 at the time. Most of the crew members were able to evacuate by lifeboats. Tragically, the explosion and fire injured 17 crew members, four of them critically. An additional 11 workers, assumed to have perished at sea, remained unaccounted for despite an extensive three-day search by the US Coast Guard.

The wellhead is located about one mile below the surface of the water, a factor that presented a major technological challenge to efforts to stem the flow gushing deep beneath the surface. Various measures attempted to stop the leak: using undersea robots to repair a blowout preventer on the wellhead, attempting to cap the well, and pumping drilling mud into the well (a technique known as "top kill"). Nevertheless, massive quantities of oil continued to spew nearly unabated for 86 days until the wellhead was finally capped on July 15 and the flow stanched. After this apparently successful effort to cap the well, additional efforts to implement a permanent solution followed. These measures included drilling relief wells that would facilitate sealing off the leakage completely.

Oil slicks from the gushing well covered thousands of square miles of gulf waters. As oil moved toward landfall, it eventually impacted the coastal areas of Louisiana and the neighboring states of Mississippi, Alabama, and Florida. Crude oil worked its way into the ecologically sensitive marshes at the mouth of the Mississippi River.

Efforts to mitigate the effects of the spilled oil included direct recovery from the wellhead, use of chemical dispersants, construction of sand berms that would prevent oil from reaching the bayous, emplacement of thousands of feet of floating containment booms, deployment of skimmer ships, and burning of crude oil that had accumulated on the water's surface. Estimates indicate that these actions resulted in the containment of 74% of the oil. As of August, 2010, the remaining one-quarter was either floating on or beneath the surface or had washed ashore. Natural forces buried some of this oil in the sand; cleanup workers collected visible remains such as tar balls.

The spill had immediate and devastating consequences for the local economy in oil-affected areas. In addition to discouraging tourism, a mainstay of the region, the catastrophe severely curtailed the fishing industry. Government authorities prohibited fishing at the mouth of the Mississippi River and nearby affected areas. Seafood could no longer be harvested from waters that had supported generations of fishermen by providing a bounty of shrimp, crabs, oysters, and fish.

Although the long-term environmental consequences of the spill will not be known for many decades, its immediate effects became apparent within a few days. Oil worked its way into sensitive Louisiana marshes that support the brown pelican (the state bird) and numerous aquatic organisms that form an essential component of survival of the coastal ecosystem. Oil-soaked pelicans and other oiled birds floundered on the beach. Tar balls and "oil mousse" fouled the coasts. Deep underwater plumes, some more than 20 miles long, clouded the normally pristine gulf waters.

The thousands of gallons of dispersants applied to the floating crude oil were potentially toxic to marine life forms. In fact, one of the dispersants used extensively in the gulf was no longer approved for use in Britain, because of the chemical's suspected adverse effects.

Species of marine life impacted by the spill included birds, dolphins, blue crabs, and turtles. Particularly at risk were Kemp's ridley turtles, which are endemic to the gulf coast. Their numbers had crashed during the Ixtoc 1 spill and, in recent years, had rebounded slightly. An unanswered question is whether crude oil that might have soiled the turtles' coastal nesting areas will cause their extinction. Dissolved oil near the site of the spill endangers the ecosystems of deepwater gulf reefs, known to support a variety of corals, crustaceans, fish, and other marine creatures. Another environmental concern has been how to dispose safely of the immense quantity of oil-saturated debris produced by the spill and gathered by clean-up personnel, who themselves were exposed to toxins from the spill.

Source: Data from *The New York Times*. Available at: http://www.nytimes.com. Accessed 8/15/2010; and The White House Blog, New report: 74% of oil in Deepwater Horizon oil spill has been contained or mitigated. Available at: http://www.whitehouse.gov. Accessed 8/10/2010.

The process of extracting oil from petroleum fields has caused significant environmental damage in some areas of the world. The tropical forest areas of the Ecuadorian Amazon hold large oil reserves. As a result of drilling and extraction activities, billions of gallons of untreated wastes and oil have been dumped into the environment in this region. To prevent further damage to this ecologically sensitive area, controls will be needed to stem the flow of pollutants.[50]

On April 20, 2010, an explosion at the Deepwater Horizon oil platform and the resulting damage to the wellhead caused the largest marine oil spill in history up to that time. The catastrophe released 5 million barrels of oil into the Gulf of Mexico, from a location that is about 50 miles south of the Louisiana coastline. Information about the spill is provided in a text box. Figure 9-29 illustrates fire-fighting efforts at the site. A report of the effects of the oil spill is available from the Institute of Medicine.[51]

CONCLUSION

Water is an essential element of life on earth—a human being can survive for only about one week without water. As the global population expands and increasing industrialization creates ever-growing demands for water, supplies of this vital commodity have become endangered. Several areas of the world currently face chronic shortages and water stress; often these are the same areas that are experiencing skyrocketing population growth.

Surface water and groundwater are used as the sources of potable water in the majority of the countries of the world. These sources are vulnerable to contamination from human activities such as sewage disposal, large-scale farms, manufacturing facilities, and urban runoff. Standard water processing methods are unable to remove many toxic chemicals and some pathological microbes. In the developing world, where adequate water processing methods are not in place, water-borne infections are a major cause of morbidity and mortality. The world's oceans, which seem to be vast and invulnerable to pollution, are rapidly degrading, especially in the coastal areas. The 21st century will need to become the era for implementing pollution abatement measures in order to protect a finite and increasingly endangered resource—water.

The cost of water to the consumer varies greatly across the globe and depends on local supply availability and demand. In some countries, bottled water accounts for 10 percent or more of drinking water supplies because water is unavailable or unsafe. Melting of the world's glaciers, which in some regions replenish vitally needed surface water, ultimately may cause further exacerbation of water shortages when the glaciers disappear completely. For an excellent overview of water availability, see the issue of *National Geographic* devoted to water.[52]

Study Questions and Exercises

1. Define the following terms:
   a. Surface water
   b. Groundwater
   c. Hydrology
   d. Hydrological cycle

2. Describe the principal reserves for water. Which areas of the world have adequate supplies and which are facing a chronic shortage?

3. How is the majority of water used in the average household? What are some ways in which households might conserve water and prevent waste of water?

4. Why has bottled water garnered favor in recent years? To what extent is bottled water safer than tap water? What safeguards are in place to protect the quality of bottled water?

5. Explain the four stages of water treatment. How is it possible for waterborne pathogens such as *Cryptosporidium* to contaminate water that has been treated in modern treatment plants?

6. Describe three waterborne diseases and suggest methods for their prevention.

7. What historical observations led to the fluoridation of water? Take a position for or against the fluoridation of water.

8. What are some examples of toxic chemicals that may enter the public water supply? Describe some of the health effects that are attributed to toxic chemicals present in drinking water.

9. Defend or refute the hypothetical statement that the world's oceans, because of their vast size, are invulnerable to pollution from microbial agents and toxic chemicals.

10. Find an article in your local newspaper or other media source regarding local efforts by citizens to clean up the beach at a nearby lake or ocean. What steps can individuals take to prevent water pollution?

REFERENCES

1. US Environmental Protection Agency, Office of Water. Drinking water and health: what you need to know! EPA 816-K-99-001. 1999. Available at: http://www.epa.gov/safewater/dwh/dw-health.pdf. Accessed April 5, 2010.

2. Tibbetts J. Water world 2000. *Environ Health Perspect.* 2000;108:A69–A73.

3. US Environmental Protection Agency. Safe Drinking Water Act 30th anniversary water facts. EPA 816-F-04-036. 2004. Available at: http://www.epa.gov/safewater/sdwa/pdfs/fs_30ann_waterfacts_web.pdf. Accessed April 5, 2010.

4. Holt MS. Sources of chemical contaminants and routes into the freshwater environment. *Food Chem Toxicol.* 2000;38(1 suppl):S21–S27.

5. Hinrichsen D, Robey B, Upadhyay UD. Solutions for a water-short world. *Population Reports.* Baltimore: Johns Hopkins University School of Public Health, Population Information Program; 1998. Series M, No. 14.

6. United Nations Environment Programme. Vital water graphics: freshwater resources. Available at: http://www.unep.org/dewa/assessments/ecosystems/water/vitalwater/05.htm. Accessed April 5, 2010.

7. Centers for Disease Control and Prevention. Achievements in public health, 1900–1999: fluoridation of drinking water to prevent dental caries. *MMWR.* 1999;48:933–940.

8. Tong ST, Chen W. Modeling the relationship between land use and surface water quality. *J Environ Manage.* 2002;66:377–393.

9. US Environmental Protection Agency. *Water on Tap: What You Need to Know.* Washington, DC: EPA Office of Water; 2003.

10. Leclerc H, Schwartzbrod L, Dei-Cas E. Microbial agents associated with waterborne diseases. *Crit Rev Microbiol.* 2002;28:371–409.

11. Centers for Disease Control and Prevention. Viral gastroenteritis. Available at: http://www.cdc.gov/ncidod/dvrd/revb/gastro/faq.htm. Accessed April 5, 2010.

12. MacKenzie WR, Hoxie NJ, Proctor ME, et al. A massive outbreak in Milwaukee of *Cryptosporidium* infection transmitted through the public water supply. *N Engl J Med.* 1994;331:161–167.

13. Heymann DL, ed. *Control of Communicable Diseases Manual.* 19th ed. Washington, DC: American Public Health Association; 2008.

14. Dillingham RA, Lima AA, Guerrant RL. Cryptosporidiosis: epidemiology and impact. *Microbes Infect.* 2002;4:1059–1066.

15. Khalakdina A, Vugia DJ, Nadle J, et al. Is drinking water a risk factor for endemic cryptosporidiosis? A case-control study in the immunocompetent general population of the San Francisco Bay Area. *BMC Public Health.* 2003;3:11.

16. Carpenter C, Fayer R, Trout J, et al. Chlorine disinfection of recreational water for *Cryptosporidium parvum. Emerg Infect Dis.* 1999;5:579–584.

17. Centers for Disease Control and Prevention. Parasites and health: amebiasis. Available at: http://www.dpd.cdc.gov/dpdx/HTML/Frames/A-F/Amebiasis/body_Amebiasis_page1.htm. Accessed April 5, 2010.

18. Centers for Disease Control and Prevention. Parasitic disease information. Fact sheet: amebiasis. Available at: http://www.cdc.gov/ncidod/dpd/parasites/amebiasis/factsht_amebiasis.htm. Accessed April 5, 2010.

19. Centers for Disease Control and Prevention. Parasites and health: giardiasis. Available at: http://www.dpd.cdc.gov/dpdx/HTML/Frames/G-L/Giardiasis/body_Giardiasis_page1.htm. Accessed April 5, 2010.

20. Shah L, MacDougall L, Ellis A, et al. Challenges of investigating community outbreaks of cyclosporiasis, British Columbia, Canada. *Emerg Infect Dis.* 2009;15:1286–1288.

21. Centers for Disease Control and Prevention. Disease listing: typhoid fever. Available at: http://www.cdc.gov/ncidod/dbmd/diseaseinfo/typhoidfever_t.htm. Accessed February 22, 2010.

22. Hoffman TA, Ruiz CJ, Counts GW, et al. Waterborne typhoid fever in Dade County, Florida. Clinical and therapeutic evaluation of 105 bacteremic patients. *Am J Med.* 1975;59:481–487.

23. Finkelstein R, Markel A, Putterman C, et al. Waterborne typhoid fever in Haifa, Israel: clinical, microbiologic and therapeutic aspects of a major outbreak. *Am J Med Sci.* 1988;296:27–32.

24. Centers for Disease Control and Prevention, National Center for Zoonotic, Vector-Borne, and Enteric Diseases. Cholera: Technical information. Available at: http://www.cdc.gov/nczved/divisions/dfbmd/diseases/cholera/technical.html. Accessed April 6, 2010.

25. Jiang S, Noble R, Chu W. Human adenoviruses and coliphages in urban runoff-impacted coastal waters of Southern California. *Appl Environ Microbiol.* 2001;67:179–184.

26. Centers for Disease Control and Prevention. Norovirus: food handlers. Available at: http://www.cdc.gov/ncidod/dvrd/revb/gastro/norovirus-foodhandlers.htm. Accessed April 6, 2010.

27. Centers for Disease Control and Prevention. National Center for Immunization and Respiratory Diseases, Division of Viral Diseases. Adenoviruses. Available at: http://www.cdc.gov/ncidod/dvrd/revb/respiratory/eadfeat.htm. Accessed April 7, 2010.

28. Centers for Disease Control and Prevention. Hepatitis A information for the public. Available at: http://www.cdc.gov/hepatitis/A/index.htm. Accessed April 7, 2010.

29. Centers for Disease Control and Prevention. Information for the public: Hepatitis E. Available at: http://www.cdc.gov/hepatitis/E/index.htm. Accessed April 7, 2010.

30. Brautbar N, Navizadeh N. Sewer workers: occupational risk for hepatitis C—report of two cases and review of literature. *Arch Environ Health.* 1999;54:328–330.

31. Centers for Disease Control and Prevention. Public information fact sheet. Parasites and health: dracunculiasis. Available at: http://www.dpd.cdc.gov/dpdx/HTML/Frames/A-F/Dracunculiasis/body_Dracunculiasis_page1.htm. Accessed April 7, 2010.

32. US Department of Labor. Occupational Safety and Health Administration. Legionnaires' disease. Available at: http://www.osha.gov/dts/osta/otm/legionnaires/disease_rec.html. Accessed April 7, 2010.

33. Cirillo JD, Falkow S, Tompkins LS. Growth of *Legionella pneumophila* in *Acanthamoeba castellanii* enhances invasion. *Infect Immun.* 1994;62:3254–3261.

34. US Department of Labor. Occupational Safety and Health Administration. Legionnaires' disease: Cooling towers, evaporative condensers, and fluid coolers. Available at: http://www.osha.gov/dts/osta/otm/legionnaires/cool_evap.html. Accessed April 7, 2010.

35. Calderon RL. The epidemiology of chemical contaminants of drinking water. *Food Chem Toxicol.* 2000;38(1 suppl):S13–S20.

36. Potera C. Drugged drinking water. *Environ Health Perspect.* 2000;108:A446.

37. Hwang B-F, Magnus P, Jaakkola JK. Risk of specific birth defects in relation to chlorination and the amount of natural organic matter in the water supply. *Am J Epidemiol.* 2002;156:374–382.

38. Nieuwenhuijsen MJ, Toledano MB, Eaton NE, et al. Chlorination disinfection byproducts in water and their association with adverse reproductive outcomes: a review. *Occup Environ Med.* 2000;57:73–85.

39. Aschengrau A, Zierler S, Cohen A. Quality of community drinking water and the occurrence of late adverse pregnancy outcomes. *Arch Environ Health.* 1993;48:105–113.

40. Zender R, Bachand AM, Reif JS. Exposure to tap water during pregnancy. *J Expo Anal Environ Epidemiol.* 2001;11:224–230.

41. Deane M, Swan SH, Harris JA, et al. Adverse pregnancy outcomes in relation to water contamination, Santa Clara County, California, 1980–1981. *Am J Epidemiol.* 1989;129:894–904.

42. Wrensch M, Swan S, Lipscomb J, et al. Pregnancy outcomes in women potentially exposed to solvent-contaminated drinking water in San Jose, California. *Am J Epidemiol.* 1990;131:283–300.

43. Natural Resources Defense Council. An environmental agenda for the 109th Congress. 2005. Available at: http://www.nrdc.org/legislation/109congressinx.asp. Accessed February 22, 2010.

44. United Nations Environment Programme. Vital water graphics: coastal and marine. Available at: http://www.unep.org/dewa/assessments/ecosystems/water/vitalwater/38.htm. Accessed April 5, 2010.

45. Hendrickson SE, Wong T, Allen P, et al. Marine swimming-related illness: implications for monitoring and environmental policy. *Environ Health Perspect*. 2001;109:645–650.

46. US Environmental Protection Agency, Office of Water. EPA's BEACH Watch Program: 2002 swimming season. EPA 823-F-03-007. 2003. Available at: http://www.epa.gov/waterscience/beaches/seasons/beachwatch2003-newformat.pdf. Accessed April 7, 2010.

47. Clarke KC, Hemphill JJ. The Santa Barbara oil spill: a retrospective. In: Danta D, ed. *Yearbook of the Association of Pacific Coast Geographers*. Honolulu, Hawaii: University of Hawaii Press; 2002:157–162.

48. Lyons RA, Temple JM, Evans D, et al. Acute health effects of the *Sea Empress* oil spill. *J Epidemiol Community Health*. 1999;53:306–310.

49. Morita A, Kusaka Y, Deguchi Y, et al. Acute health problems among the people engaged in the cleanup of the *Nakhodka* oil spill. *Environ Res*. 1999;81:185–194.

50. San Sebastián M, Armstrong B, Stephens C. Outcomes of pregnancy among women living in the proximity of oil fields in the Amazon basin of Ecuador. *Int J Occup Environ Health*. 2002;8:312–319.

51. Institute of Medicine. *Assessing the Effects of the Gulf of Mexico Oil Spill on Human Health*. Washington, D.C.: The National Academies Press; 2010.

52. *National Geographic*. Water: Our Thirsty World. April 2010;217(4).

Air Quality

INTRODUCTION

This chapter covers the sources and causes of air pollution, the components of air pollution (e.g., gases and particles), and some of the health and environmental effects that have been linked to air pollution, including greenhouse gases and global warming. As so eloquently stated by the Natural Resources Defense Council, "No element of the natural world is more essential to life than air, and no environmental task more critical than keeping it clean."[1]

The causes of poor outdoor air quality and smog include the automobile and industrial processes that involve combustion of fossil fuels. The products of fossil fuel consumption are sulfur dioxide, particles, ground-level ozone, nitrogen oxides, carbon monoxide, and lead. In the developed world many nations have formulated air quality standards in order to protect public health. Nevertheless, many European cities do not meet World Health Organization (WHO) air quality standards for at least one pollutant, and in the United States, about a quarter of the population lives in areas that do not meet US air qual-

ity standards, which are similar to WHO standards.[2] Refer to Figure 10-1 for an example of air quality in New York City on a smoggy day; air pollution obscures famous landmarks such as the Brooklyn Bridge. Recently, air quality has improved considerably in most of the United States.

The potential damaging effects of air pollution are numerous: adverse human health effects (e.g., lung damage) and adverse environmental effects (e.g., acid rain and global warming). Most people who live in urban areas have experienced, at one time or another, the effects of outdoor air pollution. Symptoms can include burning eyes, aching lungs, difficulty breathing, wheezing, coughing, headache, and other symptoms such as an irritated throat and nose.[3,4] In recent years the United States and many other developed countries have made significant progress in improving air quality as a result of measures such as catalytic converters in automobiles, control of emissions from factories, and use of less-polluting fuels. However, in the large cities of many developing nations, for example, Beijing, China, and Mexico City, Mexico, air quality has continued to degrade.

Often people refer to air pollution as **smog**. Originally, smog referred to smoke plus fog. Also, smog denotes

> A mixture of pollutants, principally ground-level ozone [discussed later in this chapter], produced by chemical reactions in the air involving smog-forming chemicals. [These chemicals can arise from both anthropogenic (due to human activities) and natural sources.] A major portion of smog-formers come from burning of petroleum-based fuels such as gasoline. Major smog

FIGURE 10-1 Smog in New York City.

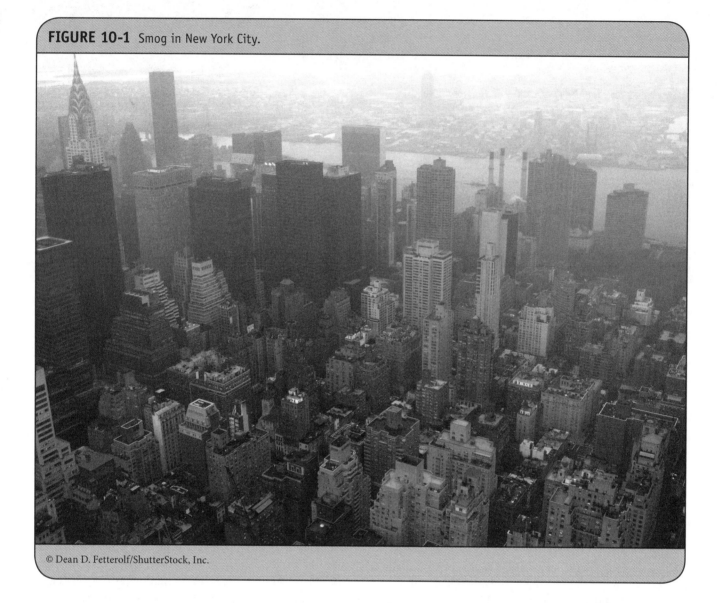

© Dean D. Fetterolf/ShutterStock, Inc.

occurrences are often linked to heavy motor vehicle traffic, sunshine, high temperatures, and calm winds or temperature inversion (weather condition in which warm air is trapped close to the ground instead of rising).[5]

The term **smog complex** refers to "eye irritation, irritation of the respiratory tract, chest pains, cough, shortness of breath, nausea and headache" associated with smog.[3] In our homes, at work, and in other enclosed spaces, we may be exposed to secondhand cigarette smoke, allergens, potentially toxic molds, and hazardous chemicals.

High levels of air pollution can endanger our health and can kill people as well, especially when reactive gases are discharged into the atmosphere and when vulnerable

persons are exposed. Health effects associated with air pollution include some forms of cancer such as lung cancer and skin cancer (from possible depletion of the ozone layer), damage to vital tissues and organs such as the nervous system, and impairment of lung and breathing function. There have been numerous occasions of air pollution–caused mortality. For example, in Chapter 7 it was noted that during a release of toxic air pollutants in Bhopal, India, large numbers of people were killed by toxic fumes released into the environment. A second incident happened in London, England, where a 1952 great "smog disaster" killed several thousand people.[6] Similar examples will be cited later in this chapter.

Air pollution damages the environment and causes property damage. It reduces visibility in national parks such as the

FIGURE 10-2 Haze above northern India as seen from a satellite.

Source: Reprinted from MODIS Rapid Response System—Image Gallery. Available at: http://rapidfire.sci.gsfc.nasa.gov/gallery/?2004352-1217/India. A2004352.0520.2km.jpg. Accessed April 15, 2010.

Grand Canyon in the United States and can even interfere with aviation. Environmental damage linked to air pollution includes harm to forests, lakes and other bodies of water, wildlife, and buildings. Visit many large cities of the world and you will see that their structures often are blackened from many years of exposure to smog and smoke. These types of environmental damage are not geographically limited in scope; air pollution is a global problem. One example is shown in Figure 10-2, which portrays haze across northern India in a picture taken from a satellite above the earth. Satellites and other technologies make it possible to view similar clouds of air pollution over many parts of the earth.

The problem of urban air pollution is continuing to grow more acute in the developing world, where populations are expanding rapidly and fast-paced industrialization is coupled with increasing use of motor vehicles. In the developing areas, the use of fossil fuels has contributed to worsening air pollution. In some megacities—Beijing, Delhi, Jakarta, and Mexico City—the air quality is becoming as bad as it was in London during the 1950s.[2]

NOTORIOUS AIR POLLUTION EPISODES IN HISTORY

Major lethal air pollution episodes include those in the Meuse Valley in Belgium (1930); Donora, Pennsylvania (1948); and London, England (1952).[3]

Meuse Valley, Belgium

One of the earliest modern episodes of hazardous air pollution occurred during the first week of December 1930, in the Meuse Valley in Belgium. The Meuse Valley is located near Liege, Belgium, which at the time had a high concentration of steel industry operations (e.g., foundries, mills, coke ovens, and smelters). During an infamous episode of severe air pollution, sulfur dioxide, sulfuric acid mists, and fluoride gases rose to extremely high levels. This noxious mixture was thought to be associated with the deaths of more than 60 persons during the last two days of the incident. The resulting mortality was more than 10 times the normal mortality rate.[7] Most of the fatalities occurred among the elderly who had preexisting heart and lung diseases.[3]

Donora, Pennsylvania

During the time interval from approximately October 27 to October 30, 1948, an environmental air pollution disaster occurred in Donora, Pennsylvania, a small town located on the Monongahela River about 30 miles south of Pittsburgh. The disaster was associated with an air inversion (defined later in the chapter) in the valley in which the town was located. In this very severe episode of air pollution, fog combined with particulate matter and industrial and other contaminants. The sources of the contaminants were iron and steel mills, coal-fired home stoves, factories that burned coal, coke ovens, and metal works. This episode caused some form of illness among approximately half of the town's 14,000 residents; about 400 of them were hospitalized, and 20 died before the smog finally lifted at the end of October.[7,8] Figures 10-3 and 10-4, respectively, show how the town was obscured by air pollution on various days around the time of the smog episode and the locations of people who died.

Although the episode of late October affected a wide cross-section of age groups, those who were aged 55 years

FIGURE 10-3 Views of Donora, Pennsylvania, taken at about the time of the 1948 smog episode.

Source: Adapted and reprinted from the US National Library of Medicine, National Institutes of Health, Images from the History of Medicine. Available at: http://www.nlm.nih.gov. Accessed August 28, 2010.

FIGURE 10-4 A sketch of Donora made by Charles Shinn for the US Public Health Service in 1949. The circle indicates the locations of more than half of the deaths that occurred during the killer smog.

Zone where 12 of 20 deaths occurred

Source: Data from D Davis, When Smoke Ran Like Water: Tales of Environmental Deception and the Battle Against Pollution. New York, NY: Basic Books; 2002. Sketch by Charles Shinn. Adapted and reprinted from the US National Library of Medicine, National Institutes of Health, Images from the History of Medicine. Available at: http:/www.nlm.nih.gov. Accessed August 28, 2010.

and older tended to be the most severely affected. During the incident, persons who were stricken reported respiratory symptoms (cough, sore throat, difficulty breathing) and gastrointestinal symptoms (nausea and vomiting). Previous histories of heart disease and lung disease were contributing factors to the adverse outcomes of smog exposure.[3]

The Lethal London Fog of 1952

During December 5 through December 9, 1952, a very severe episode of air pollution settled on London, England. Traditionally, London had been known for its foggy climate coupled with smoke caused by the use of coal and other fossil fuels to heat homes, run power plants, and operate factories. At least 1 million coal stoves spewed forth choking sulfurous smoke. As a result, so-called "pea-souper" fogs were well-known to the residents of the English metropolis. The consequence of the

particularly lethal fog that occurred in December 1952 was a reported excess of 3,000 deaths above normal. Many environmental health experts consider the London fog of 1952 to be a landmark for the study of the health effects of air pollution and a catalyst that has led to research in this field.[7]

The foregoing examples (in the Meuse Valley, Donora, and London) illustrate the growing accumulation of evidence regarding associations between acute episodes of air pollution and increased mortality, evidence that spurred air pollution research and galvanized public health officials.

SOURCES AND CAUSES OF AIR POLLUTION

What is meant by the term **air pollution**? First consider perfectly clean air—which is not found in the natural environment, even in the most remote locations such as up in the mountains far away from human activities. In the laboratory, it is possible to produce clean air artificially by using filtration and other methods. After removing contaminants, we would find that the largest components (by weight) are nitrogen (76%), oxygen (23%), argon (1%), carbon dioxide (0.03%), plus a variety of other gases in lesser amounts and water vapor depending upon the relative humidity.[9]

The normal ambient air—air that we breathe—might be thought of as a kind of soup composed of particles and vapors that arise from natural and anthropogenic sources. Each liter of air may contain thousands of invisible suspended particles and also hundreds of invisible vapors; because these constituents are invisible, we are unaware of their presence.[9] Air pollution refers to the presence, in various degrees, of those substances (e.g., suspended particles and vapors) not found in perfectly clean air.

Numerous sources emit pollutants; these sources can be dichotomized into natural and anthropogenic sources. The former include volcanic ash, dusts, and organic materials carried by the wind. The latter are subdivided roughly into stationary sources (e.g., power plants, oil refineries) and mobile sources (e.g., on-road vehicles, off-road vehicles, and nonroad vehicles).

The types of pollutants may be classified as either primary or secondary. Primary air pollutants (discussed later in the chapter) are those emitted directly by sources of pollution. Examples are ozone, nitrogen dioxide, and carbon monoxide. Secondary air pollutants are those generated from atmospheric chemical reactions among primary pollutants.[9] An example would be the production of smog (discussed subsequently).

Naturally Occurring Air Pollution

Several natural events produce air pollutants, especially particulate matter. These phenomena include wind storms that spread dust clouds, salt evaporation along the earth's coasts, and production of materials that have a biologic origin (e.g., mold spores, pollen, and organic material from plants and animals).[10] In some areas of the world, raging forest fires emit huge amounts of smoke and ash into the atmosphere. The smoke trails can be seen by satellites hovering above the earth. In some cases, forest fires are truly natural events, such as when caused by lightning strikes. In other cases they are man-made events, for example, when caused by human carelessness, arson, or efforts to clear vegetation from the land.

Volcanic eruptions are another natural source of air pollution. Examples are the dust clouds produced by the eruptions of El Chichon near Mexico City; Galunggung in West Java, Indonesia; and Mount Pinatubo, in the Philippines. In the US state of Washington, the 1980 Mount Saint Helens

eruption spewed forth tons of fine ash that descended upon a wide geographic area. (Refer to Figure 10-5.) Volcanic dusts often contain free crystalline silica, which is a toxic mineral.[11] The acute effects of exposure to volcanic dusts are irritation of the eyes and upper respiratory tract. Repeated exposure is thought to be a risk factor for the lung disease **pneumoconiosis**, especially when fine particles (less than 10 micrometers in diameter) are inhaled. However, a five-year longitudinal follow-up study of loggers who were exposed to ash from Mount Saint Helens indicated that the risks of lung diseases such as chronic bronchitis and pneumoconiosis are minimal when exposure is initially high and then tapers off over time.[11]

Anthropogenic Sources of Air Pollution

As noted previously, anthropogenic sources of air pollution include stationary sources and mobile sources.

Stationary Sources of Air Pollution

Stationary sources include electric generating plants (see Figure 10-6), factories and manufacturing complexes, oil refineries (see Figure 10-7), chemical plants, and incinerators.

Mobile Sources of Air Pollution

Mobile sources include on-road vehicles (e.g., cars, trucks, buses), off-road vehicles (e.g., dune buggies, snowmobiles), and nonroad vehicles (e.g., airplanes, ships, trains).[3,12] According to the US Environmental Protection Agency (EPA), motor vehicles produce nearly half of two major causes of smog—volatile organic compounds (VOCs) and nitrogen oxides (NO_x)—almost 75% of carbon monoxide, and more than half of emissions of toxic air pollutants.[13]

- *On-road vehicles*—The contribution of motor vehicles to air pollution is likely to continue as the number of drivers on the road increases, although technical improvements have reduced emissions from passenger vehicles. (Refer to Figure 10-8 for a view of a crowded freeway during rush hour in Southern California.) The number of miles traveled each year on US highways increased by 178% between 1970 and 2005.[13] During the current century, vehicle miles increase by about 2% to 3% annually. In the United States, most drivers commute to work alone despite the availability of car pool lanes in many locations. Many geographically dispersed regions of the United States do not have convenient public transportation systems in place. This situation contrasts with developed European countries and Japan, two areas of the world that have excellent

FIGURE 10-5 Eruption of Mount Saint Helens on May 18, 1980.

Source: Reprinted from the Centers for Disease Control and Prevention. Public Health Image Library. ID #4726. Available at: http://phil.cdc.gov/Phil/details.asp. Accessed March 22, 2010.

FIGURE 10-6 Electric power plant—example of a stationary source of air pollution.

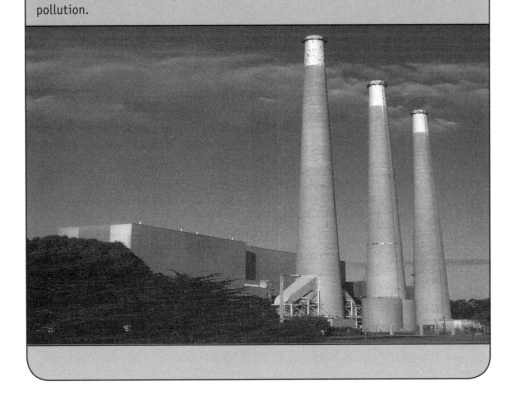

FIGURE 10-7 Stationary source of air pollution: oil refinery.

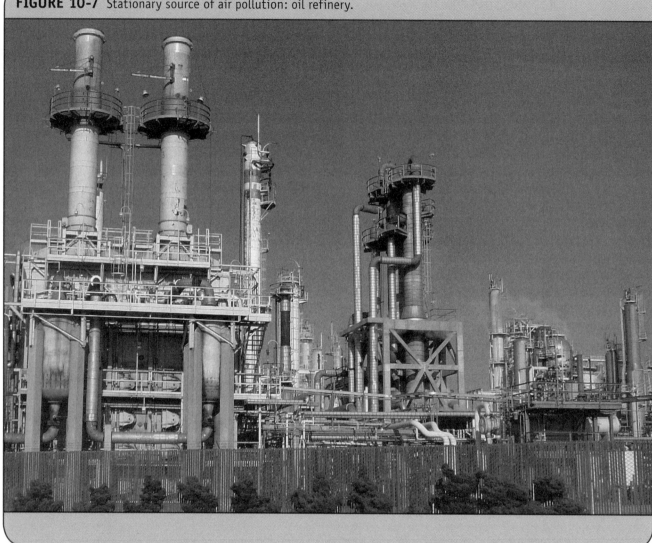

public transportation systems, which make the use of cars unnecessary or, at least, less frequent. Also contributing greatly to the air pollution problem are buses and trucks, which can cause more pollution (e.g., particle emissions) than automobiles.

- Modern automobiles produce much less pollution than automobiles did in the 1970s. Improvements include low-sulfur fuels, emission control technology, removal of lead from gasoline, and use of alternative fuels. Other innovations to reduce air pollution include electrically powered and hybrid vehicles.
- *Off-road vehicles*—Although their use is less frequent than that of on-road vehicles, off-road vehicles such as

dune buggies and snowmobiles can add to air pollution in the areas where they are used. For example, they may be a cause of air pollution in national parks and wilderness areas where their use is permitted.

- *Nonroad vehicles*—Trains, airplanes, and ships also contribute to the burden of air pollution.

COMPONENTS OF AIR POLLUTION

How do scientists classify air contaminants? According to Phalen, "One classification segregates air contaminants into the broad categories of infectious agents, allergens, chemical irritants, and chemical toxicants (biologic and nonbiologic).

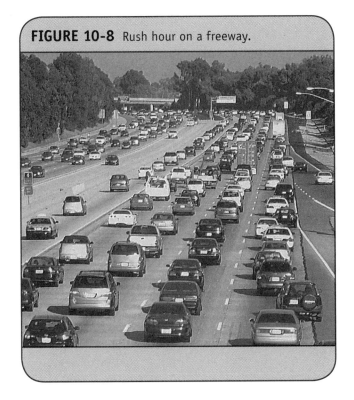

FIGURE 10-8 Rush hour on a freeway.

Another classification segregates air contaminants into particles, gases, and vapors. . . ."[9(p2)]

Pollution is composed of a number of components.[14] What we see as air pollution (for example, in Figure 10-13) is actually a mix of contaminants, particularly in the case of smog. Note also that there may be substances present that are not visible to the human eye. As a result of chemical reactions (described in the section on temperature inversion) that take place in the presence of certain atmospheric conditions, some of the contaminants become visible. Among the constituents of air pollution (although these vary from one location to another depending upon the types of fuels in use) are sulfur oxides, particulate matter, oxidants (including ozone), carbon monoxide, **hydrocarbons**, nitrogen oxides, lead, and some other heavy metals.[15]

The term **criteria air pollutants** is used to describe "A group of very common air pollutants regulated by EPA on the basis of criteria (information on health and/or environmental effects of pollution)."[5] Criteria air pollutants are present everywhere in the United States.[16] Criteria air pollutants are ozone, nitrogen oxides, carbon monoxide, sulfur dioxide, particulate matter, and lead.[16] In addition, several other pollutants are relevant to air quality: volatile organic compounds and smog (a mixture of pollutants). Table 10-1 presents a summary of the names of common air pollutants, sources, health effects,

and environmental effects. The following discussion presents a detailed examination of these pollutants, with the exception of lead and smog (defined previously). Lead, once a universal component of gasoline, has been phased out or is being phased out in most areas of the world; nevertheless, lead remains an important environmental contaminant that arises from many sources in addition to air pollution. Refer to Chapter 6 (Toxic Metals and Elements) for coverage of lead.

Ozone is a gas that is one of the molecular forms of oxygen. The ordinary oxygen gas found in air is a molecule made up of two oxygen atoms bonded together (O_2). Ozone (O_3) consists of three oxygen atoms bonded together into a molecule.[5] Occurring in nature, ozone has the sharp smell associated with sparks from electrical equipment. Ozone is a main component of photochemical smog. Found near ground level, ozone in smog stems from a series of chemical reactions among the products of combustion of fossil fuels (including gasoline) in combination with various chemicals found in products such as solvents and paints.

Previously, in Chapter 8, we considered the role of ozone in protecting the earth from ultraviolet light as well as the influence of human activities on the environment that are hypothesized to have reduced the ozone layer. The health effects attributed to ground-level ozone include respiratory difficulties such as reduced lung function, exacerbation of allergic respiratory disease, local irritation of the eyes and respiratory tract, and reduction of the ability to fight off colds and related respiratory infections. Besides reducing visibility, environmental effects include damage to forests and plants and oxidation effects that cause damage to certain kinds of fabric and rubber.

Nitrogen oxides (NO_x) refer to gases made up of a single molecule of nitrogen combined with varying numbers of molecules of oxygen. Nitrogen oxides are "produced from burning fuels, including gasoline and coal, and react with volatile organic compounds to form smog. Nitrogen oxides are also major components of acid rain."[5]

Although clean air is mostly nitrogen, some forms of nitrogen are considered to be major environmental pollutants.[17] Although the primary source of nitrogen pollution is fertilizer used in agriculture, approximately 25% of nitrogen generation (in the form of NO_x or NO_2—nitrogen dioxide) is the product of combustion of fossil fuels, for example, gasoline used in automobiles, as well as other fuels such as natural gas, diesel oil, and coal. Air pollution scientists attribute urban ozone, acid rain, and oxygen depletion of coastal waters to NO_x. Travelers to London and European cities can observe readily the damage to ancient marble-faced buildings, stone structures, and public monuments that has resulted from the

TABLE 10-1 Overview of Common Air Pollutants

Name of Pollutant	Symbol	Example of Source	Health Effects	Environmental Effects	Property Damage
Ozone (**criteria pollutant**)	O_3	Variety of oxygen formed by chemical reaction of pollutants	Breathing impairment; eye irritation	Can damage plants and trees; contributes to smog	Affects rubber, fabrics
Nitrogen dioxide, nitrogen oxides (**criteria pollutant**)	NO_2 NO_x	Combustion of gasoline and fossil fuels; cars	Damage to lungs and respiratory system; aggravates asthma	Contributes to acid rain, which damages trees and lakes	Acids produced can eat away stones used in buildings and monuments
Carbon monoxide (**criteria pollutant**)	CO	Combustion of gasoline and fossil fuels; cars	Reduction in oxygen-carrying capacity of the blood	Contributes to the formation of smog	—
Particulate matter (**criteria pollutant**)	PM_{10} $PM_{2.5}$	Burning of wood and diesel fuels	Respiratory irritation; lung and heart effects	Causes haze	Discolors buildings, furniture, and clothing
Sulfur dioxide (**criteria pollutant**)	SO_2	Burning of fossil fuels	Breathing problems; lung damage; aggravates asthma	Contributes to acid rain, which can damage trees and lakes	Acids produced can eat away stones used in buildings and monuments
Lead (**criteria pollutant**)	Pb	Leaded gasoline, paint, batteries; lead smelters	Damages brain/CNS, immune system, and kidneys	Can harm plants and animals; causes losses in biodiversity	Persists in environment; accumulates in soil, sediments
Smog		Mixture of pollutants, esp. ozone; originates from petroleum-based fuels	Irritation of respiratory system, eyes	Reduces visibility	—
Volatile organic compounds (VOCs)		Burning fuels; released from certain chemicals (e.g., solvents)	Acute effects similar to those of smog; possible carcinogen	Can damage plants	—

Source: Adapted from US Environmental Protection Agency. What are the six common air pollutants? Available at: http://www.epa.gov/air/urbanair/. Accessed May 5, 2010; and US Environmental Protection Agency. National Risk Management Research Laboratory. EPA 625/R-02/009. Appendix B: Glossary of terms. Available at: http://www.epa.gov/nrmrl/pubs/625r02009/html/appendixb.html. Accessed April 14, 2010.

acids in air pollution. With respect to human health, NO_2 and NO_x are potentially harmful to the respiratory system.

Carbon monoxide (CO) is defined as "A colorless, odorless, poisonous gas, produced by the incomplete burning of solid, liquid, and gaseous fuels. Appliances fueled with natural gas, liquified petroleum (LP gas), oil, kerosene, coal, or wood may produce CO. Burning charcoal produces CO and car exhaust contains CO."[5] Exposure to high levels of CO can result in death or serious health consequences. Indoor use

of unventilated charcoal barbecues and inappropriate use of ovens (powered by natural gas) for space heating have been associated with fatalities. Smokers are exposed routinely to carbon monoxide from tobacco smoke, although this level of exposure is not sufficient to cause death. Carbon monoxide levels can become dangerous in poorly ventilated mines. On January 2, 2006, an explosion at the Sago coal mine in West Virginia was linked to the deaths of 12 of 13 miners who were trapped deep underground. The sole immediate survivor demonstrated symptoms of severe carbon monoxide poisoning for which treatment was rendered in a hyperbaric chamber. High levels of toxic carbon monoxide impeded rescue efforts at a Montcoal, West Virginia, mine, where an explosion on April 5, 2010, killed 29 miners.

Inhaled carbon monoxide aggravates coronary heart disease, as well as circulatory, lung, and respiratory diseases, due to reduced oxygen-carrying capacity of the blood and increased demand on the heart and lungs. Carbon monoxide has 210 times more affinity for binding with hemoglobin in the blood than oxygen does. The combination of carbon monoxide and hemoglobin is called **carboxyhemoglobin**. High levels of carboxyhemoglobin limit the oxygen-carrying capacity of blood.[18] Patients who suffer from carbon monoxide poisoning can experience a range of symptoms, such as visual disturbances and impairment of mental and physical functioning.

Aerosol particles, also known as **particulate matter (PM)**, include dust, soot, and other finely divided solid and liquid materials that are suspended in and move with the air.[5,9] The sources of particles include diesel exhaust from trucks and buses; smoke from incineration of garbage, wastes from crops, and slash burning; industrial activities; and effluents from wood-burning fireplaces. Particulate matter, which has been linked to lung damage, bronchitis, and early mortality, also causes environmental degradation through the deposition of soot on vehicles, clothing, and buildings. Such pollutants are known to irritate the eye, nose, and throat.

Particulate air pollution is a worldwide problem, producing—in some cases—what we observe as visible haze. Using the standard of 50 micrograms of suspended particles per cubic meter of air ($\mu g/m^3$), one can compare various regions with respect to pollution. In developed regions (e.g., Western Europe and North America), levels of suspended particulate matter typically do not exceed 50 $\mu g/m^3$. Cities in many Central and Eastern European countries often have double this level and exceed 100 $\mu g/m^3$; similarly high levels of particulate air pollution are found in many developing countries.[19]

Particulate matter refers generically to a mixture of particles that can vary in size.[14] Let's consider as a reference point the thickness of a human hair (about 100 micrometers in diameter) and compare it with two particle sizes that are used as air pollution standards: PM_{10} and $PM_{2.5}$. Particles classified as PM_{10} are larger than 2.5 micrometers in diameter and range up to 10 micrometers in diameter. The $PM_{2.5}$ pollutants include the class of particles that are called ultrafine (diameter of 0.01 to 0.1 micrometers) and fine (diameter of 0.1 to 2.5 micrometers). Both are criteria air pollutants, as

noted previously. The general health effects of particulate matter include respiratory system irritation, lung damage, and development of bronchitis. (More information on the health effects associated with PM is presented later in this chapter.)

In comparison with the larger particles, the invisible particles of diameter 2.5 micrometers ($PM_{2.5}$) or smaller have been of greater concern recently. $PM_{2.5}$ particles have the capability to bypass the body's normal defenses and can be inhaled deeply into the lungs where they are deposited; if they do not dissolve, the body's natural clearance mechanisms are unable to remove them efficiently. (Refer to the lung diagram in the section on lung anatomy: Figure 10-15). Some of the fine particles may contain liquid acid condensates and toxic heavy metals. Some researchers have claimed that $PM_{2.5}$ is associated with approximately 60,000 smog-related deaths annually in the United States[20]; not all agree that the figure is this large.

Large amounts of PM were released following the collapse of the World Trade Center in New York City after the terrorist attacks on September 11, 2001. Examples of materials that could have been incorporated in the dusts include asbestos, fiberglass, and crystalline mineral components of concrete and wallboard. The Centers for Disease Control and Prevention (CDC) has developed a registry of persons (e.g., nearby residents, workers, schoolchildren, and first responders) who were most highly exposed to the dusts, smoke, and other airborne materials.[21] These individuals will be followed over time to assess whether there have been any adverse health effects associated with their exposures.

Sulfur dioxide (SO_2) is a gas produced by burning sulfur contaminants in fuel, for example, coal. Power plants that use high-sulfur coal or do not have effective emission controls are a source of SO_2. Some industrial processes, including production of paper and smelting of metals, also produce sulfur dioxide, which can form sulfuric acid (H_2SO_4), a strong acid. Thus, SO_2 can play an important role in the production of acid rain.[5] Health effects associated with sulfur dioxide include bronchoconstriction (as in asthma attacks) and production of excess mucus, which can produce coughing.

Volatile organic compounds (VOCs) refer to a class of chemicals that contain carbon (C), the basic chemical element found in living beings. Essentially all carbon-containing chemicals belong to the group that is called organic. Volatile chemicals evaporate and thus escape into the air easily.[5] Not classified as criteria air pollutants, VOCs are the product of combustion of fuel (e.g., diesel fuel, gasoline, coal, and natural gas). Products used frequently in the workplace and at home release VOCs; examples are paints and lacquers, some types

FIGURE 10-9 Acid rain formation.

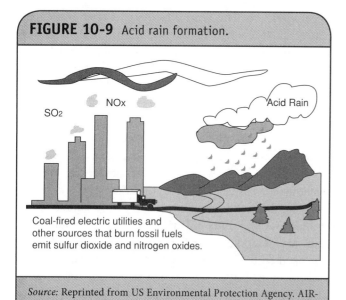

SO₂   NOx   Acid Rain

Coal-fired electric utilities and
other sources that burn fossil fuels
emit sulfur dioxide and nitrogen oxides.

Source: Reprinted from US Environmental Protection Agency. AIR-Trends 1995 Summary: Acid Rain. Available at: http://www.epa.gov/air/airtrends/aqtrnd95/acidrain.html. Accessed March 22, 2010.

of glues, construction materials, and solvents such as benzene and toluene. One of the most significant sources of VOCs is automobiles. VOCs interact with other pollutants to form smog. The impact of VOCs on human health can be serious (e.g., cancers at various bodily sites). Some VOCs are known to be injurious to plants.

Acid Rain

The term **acid rain** refers to the precipitation of acidic compounds formed when components of air pollution (e.g., SO_2 and NO_x) interact with other components in the air such as water, oxygen, and oxidants.[22] Emissions of SO_2 and NO_x are produced by installations such as electric utility plants. (Refer to Figure 10-9.) Eventually the acid rain settles on the earth, creating abnormally high levels of acidity that are potentially damaging to the environment, wildlife, and human health. For example, acid rain is believed to harm forests and certain species of fish, and to contribute to the deterioration of structures. (Refer to Figure 10-10.)

FIGURE 10-10 Deterioration of the exterior of a building in Dublin, Ireland. Air pollution, solar radiation, moisture, and cold–heat cycling are contributing causes.

Temperature Inversion

The term **temperature inversion** refers to an atmospheric condition during which a warm layer of air stalls above a layer of cool air that is closer to the surface of the earth, as shown in Figure 10-11. A temperature inversion is the reverse of the usual situation in which the air closer to the surface of the earth is warmer than the air in the upper atmosphere. Solar radiation causes the earth's surface to become heated and warms the air near the surface. The usual temperature gradient (hot air below and cool above) allows convection of warm air from the earth's surface into the upper atmosphere, thus removing pollutants from the breathing zones of people. During a temperature inversion, pollutants (e.g., smog, smog-forming chemicals, and VOCs) can build up

when they are trapped close to the earth's surface. Continuing release of smog-forming pollutants from motor vehicles and other sources during an inversion exacerbates air pollution. A temperature inversion layer as seen from an airplane is shown in Figure 10-12.

Temperature inversions contribute to the creation of smog, which is aggravated in cities such as Los Angeles that have unfavorable topographical characteristics and prevailing winds. In the Los Angeles Basin, under certain conditions, coastal on-shore winds push pollutants farther inland, away from their sources; these pollutants are stopped by nearby mountains, creating higher levels of air pollution than existed along the coast. This concentration of pollutants then may be trapped under an inversion layer; a series of chemical reactions among the pollutants produces smog. Figure 10-13 shows smog caused by an inversion layer in the Inland Empire region of Southern California. You can see that, even on this relatively clear day during spring, air pollution obscures a nearby mountain. The type of smog shown in Figure 10-13 also is called photochemical smog, which is caused by the interaction of NO_x with VOCs. Ozone near the earth's surface is another major constituent of smog.

Diesel Exhaust

Widespread exposure to diesel exhaust occurs in the general community and in the workplace. A meta-analysis reviewed studies of the possible etiologic role of occupational exposure to diesel exhaust in the induction of lung cancer. The authors reported that across the group of research reports, the pooled risk of lung cancer among workers exposed to diesel exhaust was statistically significantly elevated after controlling for smoking.[23] As a result of its association with elevated risk of lung cancer, public health experts have named diesel exhaust as a probable carcinogen.[24] For example, epidemiologic evidence suggests that in comparison with nonexposed groups, two categories of workers (truck drivers and railroad crews) exposed directly to diesel exhaust have lung cancer incidence rates that are 20% to 40% higher.[25] The level of exposure to diesel exhaust among both types of transportation workers is roughly equivalent.[26] One study reported that some groups of miners were exposed to diesel exhaust levels above recommended standards.[24]

Diesel exhaust, a complex mixture of particles and gases, includes the element carbon, condensed hydrocarbon gases, and **polycyclic aromatic hydrocarbons (PAHs)**, the latter suspected of being carcinogens.[24] Other constituents are hundreds of organic and inorganic compounds, some of which are regarded as toxic air pollutants.[25] Most of the particles in diesel exhaust are very fine and capable of being inhaled deeply

FIGURE 10-11 Diagram of temperature inversion.

Cooler

Cool

Warm

Warm air rising

Altitude

Temperature

Cooler

Warm

Cool

Rising warm air inhibited by inversion

Altitude

Temperature

Source: Reprinted from US Environmental Protection Agency. Air Pollution Control Orientation Course. Control Emission Technologies—Transport & Dispersion of Air Pollutants. Available at: http://www.epa.gov/air/oaqps/eog/course422/ce1.html. Accessed March 22, 2010.

FIGURE 10-12 Inversion layer as seen from an airplane.

FIGURE 10-13 Air pollution in southern California on a spring day.

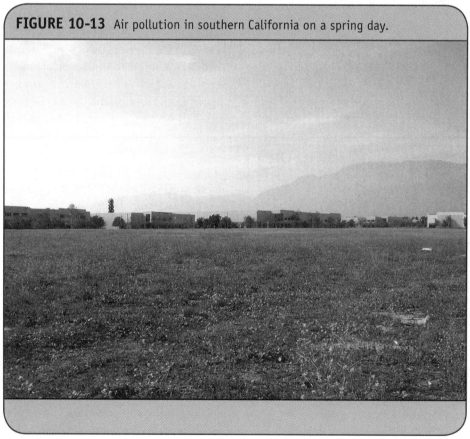

into the lungs where they may have a carcinogenic effect. For this reason, lung cancer has been a particular focus of research on the effects of diesel exhaust, which is also thought to contribute to airway inflammation, allergies, and asthma.

When the cost of fuel for vehicles is high and as oil shortages persist, the use of diesel engines will tend to grow in popularity because of their greater energy efficiency and endurance.[25] Even though there have been improvements in diesel engine design that reduce NO and particulate emissions, these newer engines continue to emit higher levels of carcinogenic and toxic substances than do conventional gasoline engines that have catalytic converters.[25] Many of the diesel-driven vehicles (e.g., buses and trucks) in use in the United States are 15 years old or older, indicating that these vehicles do not have the advantages of the latest emissions reduction technology.

Likely to be more vulnerable to the effects of diesel exhaust exposure than adults are children, whose defenses to ward off disease are not as well developed as those of adults. Children who ride in school buses powered by diesel engines are exposed to diesel exhaust. Residents (both children and adults) of urban areas may be exposed to diesel exhaust from motor vehicle traffic. For example, adolescent residents of upper Manhattan in New York City were reported to receive frequent exposures to diesel exhaust from vehicles that travel on city streets.[27] The role that these exposures play in exacerbation of lung disorders needs to be explored more fully.

Despite the supportive findings regarding the potentially carcinogenic role of diesel exhaust exposures, this topic of research remains highly controversial.[28] Some researchers remain skeptical about whether, in fact, a risk to human health exists from exposures to diesel exhaust. Researchers have questioned the validity of data and methods used in risk assessments of diesel exhaust exposure. For example, some of the studies of truck drivers have not controlled adequately for smoking status and the level of diesel exhaust exposure.[29]

AIR QUALITY STANDARDS

This section presents information on the Air Quality Index and National Ambient Air Quality Standards (NAAQS).

The Air Quality Index

The **Air Quality Index** is used to provide the public with an indication of air quality in a local area:

> The AQI is an index for reporting daily air quality. It tells you how clean or polluted your air is, and what associated health effects might be a concern for you. The AQI focuses on health ef-

fects you may experience within a few hours or days after breathing polluted air. EPA calculates the AQI for five major air pollutants regulated by the Clean Air Act: ground-level ozone, particle pollution (also known as particulate matter), carbon monoxide, sulfur dioxide, and nitrogen dioxide. For each of these pollutants, EPA has established national air quality standards to protect public health. . . .

Air Quality Index (AQI) Values	Levels of Health Concern	Colors
When the AQI is in this range:	*...air quality conditions are:*	*...as symbolized by this color:*
0 to 50	Good	Green
51 to 100	Moderate	Yellow
101 to 150	Unhealthy for sensitive groups	Orange
151 to 200	Unhealthy	Red
201 to 300	Very unhealthy	Purple
301 to 500	Hazardous	Maroon

Each category corresponds to a different level of health concern. The six levels of health concern and what they mean are:

- "Good" AQI is 0–50. Air quality is considered satisfactory, and air pollution poses little or no risk.
- "Moderate" AQI is 51–100. Air quality is acceptable; however, for some pollutants there may be a moderate health concern for a very small number of people. For example, people who are unusually sensitive to ozone may experience respiratory symptoms.
- "Unhealthy for Sensitive Groups" AQI is 101–150. Although general public is not likely to be affected at this AQI range, people with lung disease, older adults, and children are at a greater risk from exposure to ozone, and persons with heart and lung disease, older adults, and children are at greater risk from the presence of particles in the air.
- "Unhealthy" AQI is 151–200. Everyone may begin to experience some adverse health effects, and members of the sensitive groups may experience more serious effects.

- "Very Unhealthy" AQI is 201–300. This would trigger a health alert signifying that everyone may experience more serious health effects.
- "Hazardous" AQI is greater than 300. This would trigger a health warning . . . of emergency conditions. The entire population is more likely to be affected.[30]

National Ambient Air Quality Standards

Federal standards for air pollution are called the National Ambient Air Quality Standards (NAAQS). The EPA reviews the scientific literature at five-year intervals and decides whether to revise each standard. Current standards (as of 2010) are presented in the following text box.

HEALTH EFFECTS OF AIR POLLUTION

The aesthetic impacts of air pollution include reduction in the quality of our lives by obscuring the natural environment, by damaging property, and, in some cases, by being malodorous. This section will focus on the human health effects of air pollution and will present information on methods for the measurement of air pollution in the laboratory.

Measurement of Air Pollution in Experimental Studies

Improvements in air quality in the United States have reduced the levels of pollutants in the air substantially. Consequently, increasingly sensitive techniques are needed to define the current health effects of air pollution. Examples of these sensitive techniques are shown in Figure 10-14, which illustrates scientific devices used in air pollution health effects studies, primarily with small animals. Air purifiers are used to create artificially purified air that has known levels of contaminants. Laser particle analyzers are used to quantify precisely the amount of particulate matter in a sample of air. Exposure chambers administer precise amounts of pollutants under controlled conditions to small mammals. Through the use of devices such as these, air pollution researchers are able to measure exposure to air pollution much more definitively than is possible through studies conducted in the ambient environment.

Human Health Effects

Among human populations, air pollution is associated with short-term (acute) and long-term effects.[6] The former can include irritation of the eyes, nose, and throat; aching lungs; bronchitis and pneumonia; wheezing; coughing; nausea; and headaches. Examples of long-term effects are heart disease, chronic obstructive pulmonary disease, and lung cancer.

Population subgroups differ in their susceptibility to air pollution. Vulnerable groups who are at increased risk of being affected by air pollution include the elderly, persons afflicted with chronic diseases, and growing children. Persons who have low educational attainment or diabetes or who are African American appear to be more susceptible to the adverse affects of air pollution and might be particularly likely to benefit from air pollution emissions controls.[31] On the other hand, another viewpoint is that introduction of emission controls could pose an economic burden for small businesses that employ minority groups that have low incomes.

As they grow and develop, children who live in some areas of the world are exposed to air pollution numerous times over the course of their lives. A meaningful question for researchers pertains to the effects of the cumulative impact of air pollution on children over long time periods.[32] According to one estimate, air pollution in cities of the developing world produces about 50 million cases per year of chronic cough among children who are younger than 14 years of age.[19]

National Ambient Air Quality Standards

The Clean Air Act, which was last amended in 1990, requires EPA to set National Ambient Air Quality Standards for pollutants considered harmful to public health and the environment. The Clean Air Act established two types of national air quality standards. *Primary standards* set limits to protect public health, including the health of "sensitive" populations such as asthmatics, children, and the elderly. *Secondary standards* set limits to protect public welfare, including protection against decreased visibility, damage to animals, crops, vegetation, and buildings.

The EPA Office of Air Quality Planning and Standards (OAQPS) has set National Ambient Air Quality Standards for six principal pollutants, which are called "criteria" pollutants. They are listed in Table 10-2. Units of measure for the standards are parts per million (ppm) by volume, milligrams per cubic meter of air (mg/m^3), and micrograms per cubic meter of air ($\mu g/m^3$).

TABLE 10-2 National Ambient Air Quality Standards

Pollutant	Primary Standards		Secondary Standards	
	Level	Averaging Times	Level	Averaging Time
Carbon Monoxide	9 ppm (10 mg/m^3)	8-hour[a]	None	
	35 ppm (40 mg/m^3)	1-hour[a]		
Lead	1.5 μg/m^3	Quarterly Average	Same as Primary	
Nitrogen Dioxide	53 ppb (0.053 ppm)	Annual (Arithmetic Average)	Same as Primary	
	100 ppb	1-hour	None	
Particulate Matter (PM$_{10}$)	150 ug/m^3	24-hour[b]	Same as Primary	
Particulate Matter (PM$_{2.5}$)	15.0 μg/m^3	Annual[c] (Arithmetic Average)	Same as Primary	
	35 ug/m^3	24-hour[d]	Same as Primary	
Ozone	0.075 ppm (2008 std)	8-hour[e]	Same as Primary	
	0.12 ppm	1-hour[f]	Same as Primary	
Sulfur Oxides	0.03 ppm	Annual (Arithmetic Average)	0.5 ppm	3-hour[a]
	0.14 ppm	24-hour[a]		
	75 ppb	1-hour	None	

[a]Not to be exceeded more than once per year.

[b]Not to be exceeded more than once per year on average over 3 years.

[c]To attain this standard, the 3-year average of the weighted annual mean PM$_{2.5}$ concentrations from single or multiple community-oriented monitors must not exceed 15.0 μg/m^3.

[d]To attain this standard, the 3-year average of the 98th percentile of 24-hour concentrations at each population-oriented monitor within an area must not exceed 35 μg/m^3.

[e]To attain this standard, the 3-year average of the fourth-highest daily maximum 8-hour average ozone concentrations measured at each monitor within an area over each year must not exceed 0.075 ppm.

[f](a) EPA revoked the 1-hour ozone standard in all areas, although some areas have continuing obligations under that standard.

(b) The standard is attained when the expected number of days per calendar year with maximum hourly average concentrations above 0.12 ppm is ≤ 1.

Source: Adapted and reprinted from US Environmental Protection Agency. Air and Radiation. National Ambient Air Quality Standards (NAAQS). Available at: http://www.epa.gov/air/criteria.html. Accessed August 25, 2010.

Three of the major health effects are airway sensitivity disorders (e.g., asthma), lung cancer, and heart attacks.[14] In addition, heavy episodes of air pollution have been correlated with increased mortality rates. The specific effects of air pollution are related to total exposure—duration of exposure (for example, how long one lives in a smoggy environment) and the type and concentration of the pollutant. Also a consideration in health effects are environmental and temporal factors—temperature, climate, and timing of exposure.[3]

Anatomy of the Lung and Impact of Air Pollution on the Body

This section will describe how components of air pollution enter the human lung and how they impact the body. (Refer to Figure 10-15.) During respiration, air is drawn in through the nose and mouth. The air then passes through the windpipe into the right and left lungs, which have three and two lobes, respectively. Each lobe is supplied with bronchial tubes that branch several times and terminate in bronchioles and alveoli. The lobes of the lungs, bronchioles, and alveoli are shown in Figure 10-15, part A. Figure 10-15, parts B and D, illustrate the structure of the bronchial tubes, bronchioles, and alveoli; exchange of oxygen between inhaled air and the circulatory system takes place in the alveoli. Figure 10-15, part C (left side), shows the complete structure of a right lung that was taken from a dog.

Consider one of the major components of air pollution—smog. According to animal studies, smog has the capacity

FIGURE 10-14 Devices employed in experimental studies of air pollution. The exposure chambers are used with small animals: (A) Laser particle analyzer. (B) Exposure chamber. (C) Air purifier. (D) Exposure chamber. (E) Exposure chamber.

A

B

C

D

E

Source: Courtesy of Dr. Robert Phalen, Air Pollution Lab, University of California, Irvine.

to damage the cellular structure of airways (e.g., windpipe, bronchial tubes) to the lungs. In response to ozone exposure, the exposed airways sometimes manifest swelling and inflammation. People who are exposed to smog may experience breathing difficulties and may develop acute or chronic cough.

Other conditions that are believed to be associated with the irritating effects of smog are chronic obstructive pulmonary disease and, among sensitive persons, exacerbation of asthma. Also suspected of being associated with smog and other forms of air pollution are some types of cancer.

FIGURE 10-15 Lung anatomy: (A) Diagram of the lungs. (B) Human tracheobronchial tree. (C) Right lung and left tracheobronchial tree. (D) The bronchial tree dissected showing (respectively) bronchial tubes, bronchioles, and alveoli.

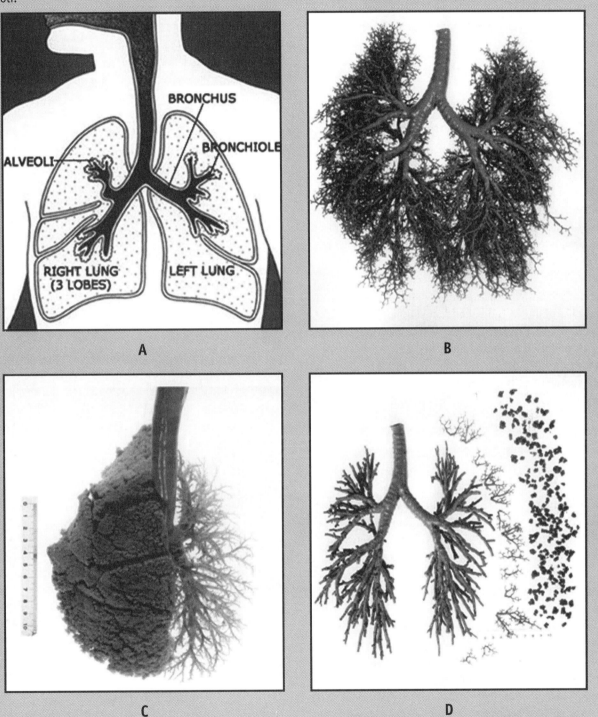

Source: (A) Reprinted from the Centers for Disease Control and Prevention. Basic information about lung cancer. Available at: http://www.cdc.gov/cancer/lung/basic_info. Accessed May 5, 2010. (B, C, and D) Dr. Robert Phalen, Air Pollution Laboratory, University of California, Irvine.

Epidemiologic Studies of Air Pollution Health Effects

This section covers the following outcomes that have been studied in relation to air pollution: mortality, coronary heart disease, chronic obstructive pulmonary disease, asthma, and lung cancer.

Mortality

Air pollution levels, which in many urban areas (e.g., Mexico City) are alarmingly high, are related to human mortality. According to one report, the estimated number of cases of mortality associated with outdoor air pollution worldwide ranges from 200,000 to 570,000 per year, or about 0.4% to 1.1% of annual deaths.[19] Dockery et al. demonstrated statistically significant associations between air pollution and mortality in a prospective study of 8,111 adults who resided in six US cities.[33] In a study conducted among the predominantly Mormon residents of Utah Valley in central Utah, elevated concentrations of particles (PM_{10}) were associated with increased mortality, particularly from respiratory and cardiovascular causes.[34] Other epidemiologic studies conducted in large urban areas such as New York City have investigated associations between rising air pollution levels and mortality.

One type of epidemiologic study has examined the relationship between daily mortality and air pollution levels. The historically significant extreme air pollution episodes noted previously (e.g., the London fog in 1952) appeared to provide at least anecdotal evidence of the correlation of increased mortality with the times that air pollution levels rose to very high levels. Ito et al. examined London data for the period 1965 through 1972 for levels of air pollution classified according to type of pollutant.[35] Statistically significant associations were found between air pollution variables and mortality.

Another study that reported a correlation between increases in total daily mortality and increased air pollution (SO_2 and smoke shade) was conducted in New York City.[36] Daily mortality was related to particulate air pollution in St. Louis, Missouri, and the counties in eastern Tennessee.[37] Researchers estimated the daily mortality rate associated with gaseous air pollution and particulate air pollution—inhalable particles (PM_{10}) and fine particles ($PM_{2.5}$). For each 100 micrograms per cubic meter increase in PM_{10}, the total mortality was reported to increase by 16% in St. Louis, Missouri, and by 17% in the eastern Tennessee counties. Weaker associations were reported for $PM_{2.5}$; associations between mortality and gaseous pollutants (e.g., SO_2, NO_2, and O_3) were not statistically significant. Another study conducted by Dominici et al. found that daily variations in PM_{10} and daily variations in mortality were positively associated. Cardiovascular and respiratory mortality were more closely related to particulate pollution than were other forms of mortality.[38]

Coronary Heart Disease (CHD)

Individuals who have preexisting heart or lung disease may be at particular risk for the fatal or aggravating effects of air pollution. People who are afflicted with ischemic heart disease combined with arrhythmias or congestive heart failure may have heightened sensitivity to pollutants from motor vehicle emissions.[39] Cigarette smoking and air pollution may act synergistically to aggravate lung diseases such as emphysema.[15] Extreme temperatures may add to this synergistic effect.

Carbon monoxide arises from cigarette smoke, automobile exhaust, and certain types of occupational exposures. An investigation into the possible association between angina pectoris and heavy freeway traffic found no direct association between myocardial infarction and ambient carbon monoxide. It was hypothesized that there was an indirect association between exposure to carbon monoxide in the ambient air and acute myocardial infarction through smoking, which is associated with elevated blood carbon monoxide levels.[40]

The air of one large metropolitan city exposed pedestrians and persons who worked outdoors to carbon monoxide levels that ranged from 10 to 50 ppm; there were even higher levels in poorly ventilated areas of the city.[41] The recommended standard for carbon monoxide in occupational settings is a maximum of 50 ppm. Pedestrians and workers who have heart problems may be at increased risk of aggravation of their conditions when exposed to high levels of ambient carbon monoxide in the urban environment.

Chronic Obstructive Pulmonary Disease (COPD)

A major investigation, the Tucson Epidemiological Study of Airways Obstructive Diseases, has tracked the etiology and natural history of COPD.[42] (Chapter 13 defines and provides more information on COPD.) Based on a multistage stratified cluster sample of white households in the Tucson, Arizona, area, it has generated many important findings, including the effects of passive smoking on children.[43]

Asthma

One of the most frequent chronic conditions in the United States, **asthma** has shown an increasing prevalence since 1980.[44-46] This increase has happened even as air pollution has declined steadily. Currently asthma is regarded as a key public health problem that confronts the United States.[45] Residents of inner-city areas (notably children) seem to be more affected by the condition than are persons who live in other areas.[47] The growing problem of childhood asthma is significant to public health because of the burden of morbidity and suffering that this condition contributes to the lives of children and their parents. Interestingly, in the United States, the prevalence of childhood asthma varies by socioeconomic status and racial and ethnic group. African American children who live in low income areas have the highest asthma prevalence and morbidity in comparison with other ethnic and racial groups.[48] Indoor air quality and genetic factors may be relevant to the occurrence of this significant respiratory disease. Some facts regarding asthma are the following:

> Asthma is a chronic respiratory illness often associated with familial, allergenic, socioeconomic, psychological, and environmental factors. . . . Although recent reports suggest asthma-related mortality has been declining since 1996, a disparity remains between rates for non-Hispanic whites and those for non-Hispanic blacks and other racial/ethnic populations. . . . Non-Hispanic blacks experience higher rates than non-Hispanic whites for ED [emergency department] visits, hospitalizations, and deaths; these trends are not explained entirely by higher asthma prevalence among non-Hispanic blacks. . . . Other racial/ethnic populations experience higher asthma mortality and hospitalization rates than non-Hispanic whites while also reporting lower asthma prevalence and fewer outpatient and ED visits.[46(p147)]

Symptoms of asthma—difficulty breathing and tightness of the chest—are a response to muscle contractions that constrict the trachea, lungs, and other parts of the airway. Excess mucus secretion also contributes to breathing difficulties. Asthma is believed to have a complex etiology that involves both genetic and environmental factors.[49] Among the triggers for asthma attacks are allergens, pollutants, and viral infections; examples of sources of allergens are vermin (i.e., cockroaches and rodents), dust mites, mold, and household pets (i.e., dogs and cats).[50] Other potential triggers are **environmental tobacco smoke**, cold air, exercise, stress, and aspirin.

Air pollution has been studied as a possible factor in asthma occurrence. Exploration of this association presents methodologic difficulties due to the facts that air pollution contains a complex mixture of substances and asthma has a complex, heterogeneous etiology.[51] Examples of components of air pollution studied in relation to asthma include particles, molds, nitrogen dioxide, ozone, and pollen.

Epidemiologic studies have reported an association between high concentrations of air pollution and asthma prevalence.[52] Among schoolchildren in Japan, incidence rates of asthma were associated with air pollution components such as particles (PM_{10}) and nitrogen dioxide.[52] A Los Angeles study of asthma among African American children found that particles and molds were related to respiratory symptom occurrence.[53]

Lung Cancer

Although air pollution is a suspected cause of lung cancer, researchers have had difficulty in establishing a definitive association because of problems in measuring the effects of low-level exposures and problems in measuring air pollution itself. An example of research on air pollution's health effects is that conducted by Henderson et al.[54] Census tracts in Los Angeles were aggregated into 14 study areas that represented homogeneous air pollution profiles. The study reported a correlation between the geographic distribution of lung cancer cases and the general location of emission sources for hydrocarbons.

One of the components of air pollution that may be implicated in lung cancer mortality is fine particulate matter. Pope et al. conducted an analysis of a data set that contained information on risk factors, air pollution levels, and mortality from approximately 500,000 adults who resided in metropolitan areas throughout the United States.[55] These individuals were part of a large, ongoing, prospective study called the Cancer Prevention II study, which was conducted by the American Cancer Society. The investigators concluded that exposure to fine particulate matter over extended time periods was a risk factor for both lung cancer and cardiopulmonary mortality.

In large population studies, the effects of air pollution exposure may be impossible to disentangle from the effects of other exposures, for example, tobacco smoke. A retrospective study conducted in Erie County, New York, found that air pollution alone was not associated with lung cancer.[56] However, the same study reported that the risk of lung cancer increased among heavy smokers who had extensive exposure to air pollution.

A Swedish study reported that air pollution from vehicle exhaust emissions may be important for increasing the risk of lung cancer.[57] According to the Swedish group, one of the components of vehicle emissions that may increase risk of lung cancer is NO_2.

INDOOR AIR QUALITY

Indoor air that is of poor quality can be a significant factor in the etiology of lung disease and exacerbation of existing conditions such as asthma and bronchitis. A report authored by four leading health and governmental organizations states:

> Studies from the United States and Europe show that persons in industrialized nations spend more than 90 percent of their time indoors. . . . For infants, the elderly, persons with chronic diseases, and most residents of any age, the proportion is probably higher. In addition, the concentrations of many pollutants indoors exceed those outdoors. The locations of highest concern are those involving prolonged, continuing exposure—that is, the home, school, and workplace.[58(p1)]

The indoor environment provides many opportunities for exposure to potentially irritating and harmful substances. Examples are aerosolized chemicals, fumes from gas appliances, components of building materials, and secondhand smoke from tobacco products. Adverse health outcomes that have been linked to indoor pollution include respiratory diseases such as asthma, Legionnaires' disease, the sick building syndrome, hypersensitivity pneumonitis, and multiple chemical sensitivity.[59]

Indoor Air Quality in the Home

Sources of indoor air pollution in the home are shown in Figure 10-16. Residential indoor air pollution poses risks for respiratory illness of various types.[60] For example, certain environmental characteristics tend to be found in the dwellings of inner-city children who have asthma; these characteristics include the presence of cockroaches, persistent dampness, wall-to-wall carpeting in children's bedrooms, exposure to environmental tobacco smoke, infestations with rodents, and pets that have fur.[47] Other factors that influence the quality of indoor air are effluents from gas stoves and the use of construction materials that contain formaldehyde.[60] Dust mites, molds, and bacteria, all of which are linked with asthma, also may be identified in indoor air.[61] Evidence suggests that children who become sensitized to allergenic indoor air pollutants such as molds and animal fur may incur an increased risk for the development of asthma.[61] Dwellings that have damp, odiferous interiors may be conducive to the growth of fungi, dust mites, and bacterial pathogens, all of which, in turn, tend to be related to respiratory symptoms.[62]

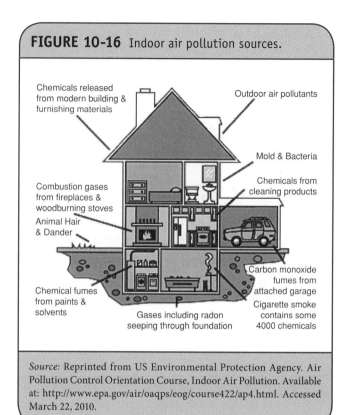

FIGURE 10-16 Indoor air pollution sources.

Chemicals released from modern building & furnishing materials

Outdoor air pollutants

Mold & Bacteria

Chemicals from cleaning products

Combustion gases from fireplaces & woodburning stoves

Animal Hair & Dander

Carbon monoxide fumes from attached garage

Chemical fumes from paints & solvents

Gases including radon seeping through foundation

Cigarette smoke contains some 4000 chemicals

Source: Reprinted from US Environmental Protection Agency. Air Pollution Control Orientation Course, Indoor Air Pollution. Available at: http://www.epa.gov/air/oaqps/eog/course422/ap4.html. Accessed March 22, 2010.

Indoor Use of Biomass Fuels

A frequent cause of indoor air pollution in developing countries is the use of unventilated indoor cooking stoves that burn biomass fuels (wood, animal dung, or cuttings from crops). (Refer to Figure 10-17.)

Approximately half the global population uses biomass fuels for cooking and heating; in some areas of the world (e.g., South Asia and sub-Saharan Africa), this figure reaches 80%. Often biomass fuels are combusted in crude stoves or pits that have been dug into the floor. Due to inefficient combustion and the lack of ventilation in household areas used for cooking, the house fills up with smoke. As a result, the persons who occupy the dwelling may be exposed to substantial amounts of pollutants: PM_{10}, carbon monoxide, nitrous oxides, sulfur compounds, and polycyclic aromatic hydrocarbons (PAHs). Some estimates indicate that the level of indoor air pollutants in such homes exceeds US EPA standards by several orders of magnitude. As shown in Figure 10-17, women who are responsible for cooking receive the largest doses of indoor air pollution, as do their infants who may be strapped to the women's backs. Other household residents who may be at risk of the adverse effects of indoor air pollution are the elderly, who spend more time indoors than do other family mem-

FIGURE 10-17 Woman cooking with an indoor stove.

Source: Photo by Nigel Bruce. Reprinted with permission from J Van Hise Heart, The Air That They Breathe, UC Berkeley Public Health, Berkeley, CA: School of Public Health, Spring 2003, p. 5, © 2003 The Regents of the University of California.

bers. A study conducted in India reported that elderly men and women who live in homes that use biomass fuels have a higher prevalence of asthma than elderly persons who live in homes that use cleaner fuels.[49]

Sick Building Syndrome and Building-Related Illness

Sick building syndrome (SBS) is another example of a condition ascribed to indoor air pollution.[63,64] SBS

> is used to describe situations in which building occupants experience acute health and comfort effects that appear to be linked to time spent in a building, but no specific illness or cause can be identified. The complaints may be localized in a particular room or zone, or may be widespread throughout the building. In contrast, the term "building related illness" (BRI) is used when symptoms of diagnosable illness are identified and can be attributed directly to airborne building contaminants.[65]

SBS is a temporary phenomenon that is relieved when affected persons are no longer inside the building. Symptoms of SBS can include headache, respiratory tract irritation, dry skin, and fatigue; the cause of the symptoms of SBS is unknown. In comparison, **building-related illness (BRI)** describes symptoms of diagnosable illnesses that can be linked to specific pollutants; examples are Legionnaires' disease and hypersensitivity pneumonitis. Possible causes of SBS are inadequate building ventilation, chemical contaminants, and biological contaminants.[65]

A condition that bears similarity to sick building syndrome is multiple chemical sensitivity. The onset of multiple chemical sensitivity is described as the development of sensitivity at about the same time to several chemicals, which are present in the ambient environment at low levels. The onset of the condition occurs in many cases following exposure to indoor air that has quality problems.[59] Also hypothesized as being related to low-quality indoor air is hypersensitivity pneumonitis, an illness "characterized by flu-like symptoms that include fever, chills, fatigue, cough, chest tightness, and shortness of breath."[59(p402)] Causal factors associated with the illness include exposure to molds, fungi, and bacteria found in indoor air.

Secondhand Smoke

Figure 10-18 demonstrates the lungs of two smokers—the lungs on the left are those of a smoker who had quit briefly before succumbing to a heart attack. The lungs shown on the right are those of a smoker who quit for several years. Note that the long-term quitter's lungs show horizontal striping, which corresponds to remaining deposits of carbon from cigarette smoke. The smoker who had quit for only a short period of time had lungs with more extensive deposits of carbon.

The harmful effects of smoking upon smokers have been well known for some time. Some of these harmful effects are

FIGURE 10-18 A: Dorsal view of the lungs of a male heavy smoker who quit 18 months prior to a fatal heart attack at 71 years of age. B: The lungs of a smoker who had quit smoking for a number of years.

A

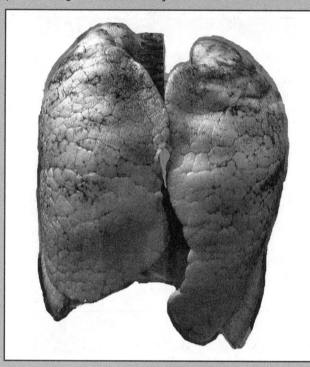

B

Source: Courtesy of Dr. Robert Phalen, Air Pollution Lab, University of California, Irvine.

lung conditions such as emphysema and chronic obstructive pulmonary disease, heart disease, as well as lung cancer and cancers at other bodily sites. More recently the effects of exposure to environmental tobacco smoke (ETS) have become recognized more clearly. Exposure to ETS is also called "secondhand smoking," "passive smoking," or "involuntary smoking."[58]

The term **passive smoking**, also known as exposure to sidestream cigarette smoke, refers to the involuntary breathing of cigarette smoke by nonsmokers in an environment where there are cigarette smokers present. In restaurants, waiting rooms, international airliners, and other enclosed areas where there are cigarette smokers, nonsmokers may be unwillingly (and, perhaps, unwittingly) exposed to a potential health hazard. The effects of chronic exposure to cigarette smoke in the work environment were examined in a cross-sectional study of 5,210 cigarette smokers and nonsmokers. Nonsmokers who did not work in a smoking environment were compared with nonsmokers who worked in a smoking environment as well as with smokers. Exposure to smoke in

the work environment among the nonsmokers was associated with a statistically significant reduction in pulmonary function test measurements in comparison with the nonsmokers in the smoke-free environment.[66] A 1992 report from the US Environmental Protection Agency concluded that environmental tobacco smoke is a human lung carcinogen responsible for approximately 3,000 lung cancer deaths annually among US nonsmokers.[67] The nonsmoking spouses of smokers are at greater risk of dying than are the nonsmoking spouses of nonsmokers. Eleven studies conducted in the United States have shown an average 19% increase in risk of death among nonsmoking spouses of smokers.[68] Among children, passive smoking is associated with bronchitis, pneumonia, fluid in the middle ear, asthma incidence, and aggravation of existing asthma.

Research on passive smoking presents several methodologic difficulties. Relatively small increases in risk of death from passive smoking are difficult to demonstrate, given the use of questionnaires to quantify smoking by spouses, the long- and short-term variability in exposures to cigarette smoke from sources other than the spouse (e.g., those at work, restaurants, and entertainment venues), and the long latency period between exposure to cigarette smoke and onset of disease. Additional research will be required to improve methods, such as the use of biologic markers, for assessing exposure to cigarette smoke.

Many states (e.g., California, Massachusetts) in the United States have banned smoking in locations such as restaurants where nonsmokers (both customers and employees) may be exposed to secondhand smoke. Smoking is no longer permitted on domestic airlines in the United States. Many foreign countries have begun to introduce smoking bans in public areas including restaurants; an example is Ireland. These steps will help to protect the public's health by reducing exposure to secondhand cigarette smoke.

GLOBAL CLIMATE CHANGE AND GLOBAL WARMING

According to one source, the term **global warming** is defined as follows:

> An increase in the near surface temperature of the Earth. Global warming has occurred in

the distant past as the result of natural influences, but the term is most often used to refer to the warming predicted to occur as a result of increased emissions of greenhouse gases. Scientists generally agree that the Earth's surface has warmed by about 1 degree Fahrenheit in the past 140 years.[69]

The use of fossil fuels, including coal and petroleum-based fuels, causes the release of gases, including **carbon dioxide**, methane, chlorofluorocarbon gases, and nitrous oxide. Chlorofluorocarbon gases used in air conditioners have been linked to the depletion of the ozone layer. Reduction of ozone levels in the upper atmosphere produces increased levels of ultraviolet radiation, normally absorbed by stratospheric ozone. The result could be an increased incidence of skin cancers and cataracts.

Gases that arise from natural sources and anthropogenic activities such as the burning of fossil fuels may accumulate in the atmosphere. Sometimes these gases are referred to as **greenhouse gases**, owing to the fact that in sufficient concentrations in the atmosphere, they may have the effect of trapping heat and causing the earth's temperature to rise. This principle is illustrated in Figure 10-19.

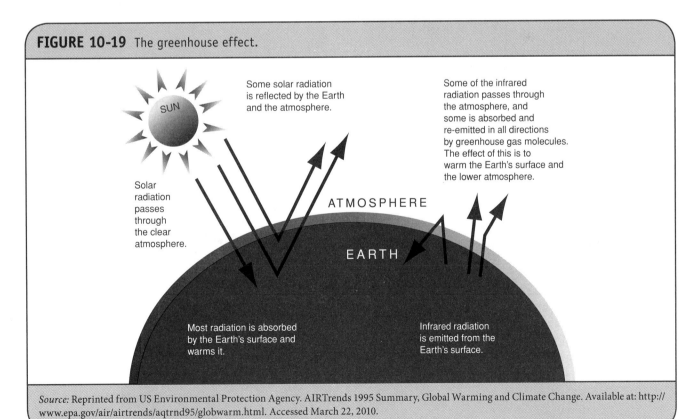

FIGURE 10-19 The greenhouse effect.

Source: Reprinted from US Environmental Protection Agency. AIRTrends 1995 Summary, Global Warming and Climate Change. Available at: http://www.epa.gov/air/airtrends/aqtrnd95/globwarm.html. Accessed March 22, 2010.

Have the earth's surface temperatures actually increased during the past century? According to the National Oceanic and Atmospheric Administration, the answer is "yes," with some qualifications.[70] Since the end of the 19th century, temperatures at the surface of the earth have increased generally by about 0.74 degrees Celsius, and for the past 50 years the linear trend of increase is about 0.13 degrees Celsius, although some areas (e.g., the southeastern United States and sections of the North Atlantic) have cooled. Temperatures in North America and Eurasia have shown the greatest warming trend. Figure 10-20 portrays global temperature anomalies during the period 1880 to 2001 (anomalies refer to departures from the long-term average temperature during the same time period). The trends shown by the data in Figure 10-20 suggest that global temperatures have been increasing since early in the 20th century. The scientific community has concluded with "virtual certainty" that anthropogenic activities have increased the levels of greenhouse gases such as CO_2. Increases in greenhouse gases tend to cause warming of the planet. Unknown at present is how much and how quickly warming will happen.[71]

A key issue is whether the increases in global temperature that have been observed during the past century represent natural temperature variability or are the effect of greenhouse gases. Analyses of temperature changes over the past millennium have used data from tree rings and ice cores. These analyses indicate that the recent large temperature increases during the late 20th century are most likely due to anthropogenic activities that have increased levels of greenhouse gases in the atmosphere.[72]

FIGURE 10-20 Jan–Dec global surface mean temperature anomalies.

Source: Reprinted from US Department of Commerce, National Climatic Data Center, NOAA Satellite and Information Service. Available at: http://www.ncdc.noaa.gov/oa/climate/globtemp.html. Accessed April 13, 2010.

FIGURE 10-21 Brazilian deforestation of the state of Rondonia. These images from the Moderate Resolution Imaging Spectroradiometer on NASA's Terra satellite were obtained in 2000 (left) and 2009 (right). The two images show the effects of increasing deforestation, which appears as a fishbone pattern that merges into large, cleared areas. During the past 30 years, approximately 68,000 square kilometers of Rondonia's original 208,000 square kilometers of forested areas have been cleared.

2000

2009

Source: Reprinted from NASA's Earth Observatory. Amazon Deforestation. Available at: http://earthobservatory.nasa.gov/Features/WorldOfChange/deforestation.php. Accessed May 5, 2010.

Deforestation

Contributing to the greenhouse effect is deforestation, which decreases the capacity of trees and the forest ecosystem to reduce the amount of CO_2 in the atmosphere. When deforestation occurs, biodiversity is reduced, resulting in the loss of plants that someday might yield valuable medicines and other products. Deforestation often is the result of burning huge swaths of land, further adding to air pollution.

Extensive areas of the world have been affected by deforestation including the Brazilian Amazon jungle, the largest tropical forest in the world (31% of the world's total). Figure 10-21 provides earlier and later satellite images that show the progress of deforestation during a 9-year period.

Deforestation is not limited to the Amazon region; vast sections of the United States also have suffered from the widespread removal of trees. Forests, which take up about 33% of the land mass in the United States, contribute clean air, water, habitat for animals, recreational opportunities, and valuable lumber. One of the areas that have been affected is the US Pacific Northwest. In this region, logging of old-growth forests by the method of clear-cutting has caused habitat fragmentation, whereby continuously forested areas are segmented into smaller parcels that are separated by nonforested zones. The net result is the destruction of habitat needed for the survival of animals that must leave the protective cover of the forest and traverse nonforested segments in order to seek food and water. (Refer to Figure 10-22 for an example of clear-cutting.)

FIGURE 10-22 Deforestation caused by clear-cutting practices in the United States.

Potential Impacts of Global Warming

The potential consequences of global warming include disturbances in the native habitats of plant and animal species. Another possible end result could be the production of an environment that is conducive to the growth of vector-borne diseases, growth of organisms in the ocean that cause foodborne seafood poisoning, and exacerbation of the effects of air pollution. Global warming, which has been linked to extreme climatic conditions such as heat waves, droughts, and monsoons, may cause disruption of the food supply and dwindling of food resources, especially in developing areas. Refer to Figure 10-23 for an overview of the potential health effects associated with climate variability and change. Potential health effects shown in the figure range from temperature-related illnesses and deaths to vector- and rodentborne diseases. Moderating influences involve nonclimatic factors such as population growth, changes in the standard of living, and improvements in health care and the public health infrastructure. Adaptation measures are steps that can be taken to lessen the possibility of adverse health outcomes linked to climate change. Examples of these measures are increasing the protection of populations via public health programs such as immunizations as well as the use of protective technologies (e.g., air conditioning and water treatment).[73]

Changes in the Distribution of Endemic Diseases

As global mean temperatures increase, changes in the ecological system favor the growth of some disease-causing agents (e.g., bacteria and fungi) and disease-carrying vectors. The increases in the prevalence and incidence of emerging and reemerging infectious diseases have been attributed to some degree to climate changes that are occurring in some regions of the world.[74] For example, as the temperature increases, the range of arthropods such as the *Aedes aegypti* mosquito can expand farther north. Normally, freezing temperatures during winter kill off this species of mosquito, which can carry viruses that cause diseases such as dengue fever and yellow

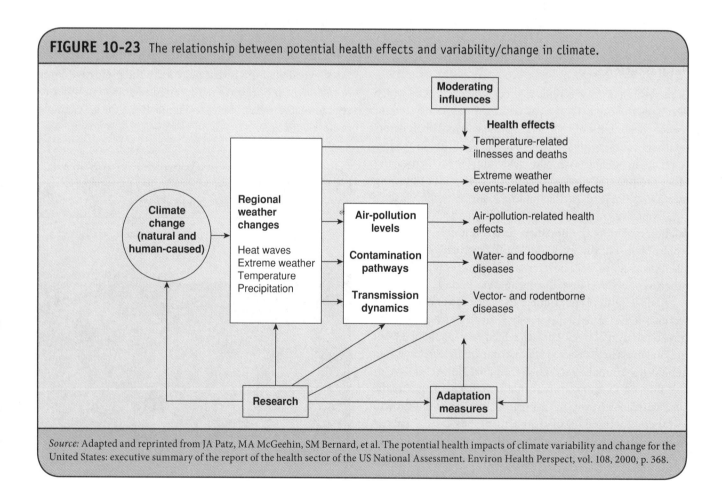

FIGURE 10-23 The relationship between potential health effects and variability/change in climate.

Source: Adapted and reprinted from JA Patz, MA McGeehin, SM Bernard, et al. The potential health impacts of climate variability and change for the United States: executive summary of the report of the health sector of the US National Assessment. Environ Health Perspect, vol. 108, 2000, p. 368.

fever. Also, extreme weather conditions such as heavy rainfall provide breeding grounds that contribute to the growth of mosquito populations.

Some Canadian experts believe that global warming might cause higher temperatures and longer summers that enable disease vectors to expand northward.[75] Another consequence could be that a warmer climate in Canada would permit the establishment of formerly exotic zoonoses (defined in Chapter 5). As a result, Canadians would be at increased risk of contracting vector-borne diseases such as arboviral encephalitis, rickettsial diseases, and Lyme arthritis. Increased temperatures might contribute to the contamination of food sources derived from animals due to *Salmonella* and *E. coli* O157:H7. If summers become longer and winters milder, rodents and small mammal species that are reservoirs for zoonotic diseases might be able to breed and survive for longer time periods. Consequently, the human population would be at increased risk of zoonotic diseases such as hantavirus infection and plague.

Retreating Glaciers and Rising Oceans

Evidence of a changing global climate is the retreat of glaciers in high mountain areas worldwide. High-altitude areas on earth that are showing the retreat of perennial snow and glaciers are Glacier National Park in Montana (United States), Mount Kilimanjaro in Africa, and the Alps in Europe.[76] Regions such as these could be completely devoid of glaciers in 20 to 25 years. Figure 10-24 demonstrates how the Cascade Glacier in the Washington Cascade Mountains has receded from 1928 to 2000.

Another apparent effect of global warming has been for the average height of the world's oceans to rise gradually as

Is Sea Level Rising?

Global mean sea level has been rising at an average rate of 1.7 mm/year (plus or minus 0.5 mm) over the past 100 years, which is significantly larger than the rate averaged over the last several thousand years. Depending on which greenhouse gas scenario is used (high or low) projected sea-level rise is projected to be anywhere from 0.18 (low greenhouse gas increase) to 0.59 meters for the highest greenhouse gas increase scenario.

Source: Reprinted from National Oceanic and Atmospheric Administration. Global Warming Frequently Asked Questions: Is sea level rising? Available at: http://www.ncdc.noaa.gov/oa/climate/globalwarming.html#Q9. Accessed March 22, 2010.

water stored in frozen sources melts. Refer to the following text box.

Particularly at risk of flooding due to a rise in the level of the sea are low-lying areas (especially low-lying coastal cities), deltas, and coral atolls.[77] Rising sea levels will cause intrusion of salt water and erosion of coastal areas. Countries that would be most affected are Vietnam, Egypt, Bangladesh, and low-lying island nations. According to a mid-range scenario in which the level of the ocean rises by 16 inches (40 cm) by the year 2080, as many as 200 million people would be affected

---

FIGURE 10-24 South Cascade Glacier in the Washington Cascade Mountains, in 1928, 1979, and 2000.

Source: Images courtesy of the National Snow and Ice Data Center. Reprinted from E Yohe, Sizing Up the Earth's Glaciers, 2004, National Aeronautics and Space Administration, Earth Observatory. Available at: http://earthobservatory.nasa.gov/Study/GLIMS. Accessed April 13, 2010.

by surges in the ocean level. An even greater increase in sea level by 1 meter would affect additional millions of people in China, Bangladesh, Egypt, and Indonesia.

Extreme Climatic Conditions

Evidence suggests that global warming is associated with extreme climatic conditions including heat waves and severe rain storms.

> Small changes in global mean temperatures can produce relatively large changes in the frequency of extreme temperatures. . . . Higher average ambient air temperatures are likely to induce more vigorous cycles of evaporation and precipitation. Indeed, a trend of increasing climate variability and extreme precipitation events has been observed over the past century, and recent models strongly correlate this trend with anthropogenic production of greenhouse gases.[78(p2283)]

From 1979 to 1995 (the most recent period for which data are available), the United States experienced a total of 6,615 heat-related deaths that were distributed as follows: heat due to weather conditions (2,792); heat due to man-made factors (327); and unspecified heat-related cause (3,496).[79] The major risk factors for heat-related death include excessive physical exertion during high temperatures, alcohol consumption, being overweight, using certain medications, and age. (Refer to Figure 10-25.)

Among significant episodes of heat-related mortality, two of particular note occurred: in Chicago, Illinois (US), and in France. The July 12 to July 16, 1995, heat wave in Chicago caused the daily high temperatures to rise to the range of 93°F to 104°F; the city had a record high temperature of 119°F on July 13. The resulting high temperatures were responsible for 465 deaths that were certified as heat-related during the period of the heat wave.[80]

During August 2003, a blistering heat wave descended on France, causing a death toll of almost 15,000.[81] Many of the deaths occurred among the elderly after temperatures reached the low 100s Fahrenheit (low 40s Celsius) in a country where it is uncommon to use air conditioning. One account indicated that "Morgues and funeral parlours coped with an overflow of

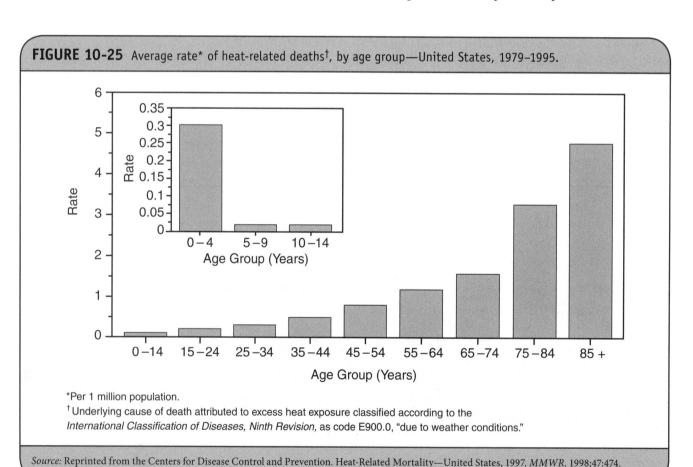

FIGURE 10-25 Average rate* of heat-related deaths†, by age group—United States, 1979–1995.

*Per 1 million population.
†Underlying cause of death attributed to excess heat exposure classified according to the *International Classification of Diseases, Ninth Revision,* as code E900.0, "due to weather conditions."

Source: Reprinted from the Centers for Disease Control and Prevention. Heat-Related Mortality—United States, 1997. *MMWR.* 1998;47:474.

victims. Refrigerated storerooms were set up; and temporary workers hired to collect bodies from private homes and hotels. Grave diggers worked overtime."[82(p411)]

CONTROLLING AIR POLLUTION AND GLOBAL WARMING

The United States holds the distinction of producing 23% of the earth's emissions of greenhouse gases.[83] The major source of air pollution in the United States is combustion of fossil fuels, particularly by coal-fired electric generating plants and internal combustion engines. With only about 4% of the world's population, the United States is the leading source of carbon dioxide pollution.[84] In addition, the world's developing nations are increasing their contribution of greenhouse gases as these countries add to their populations and increase their levels of industrialization. A number of steps

have been proposed to reduce the emissions of harmful air pollution: technological controls, the Kyoto Protocol, and energy conservation.

Using Technology to Control Particulate Matter

Several mechanical devices that are used to reduce industrial emissions of particulate matter are scrubbers, filters, and electrostatic precipitators. Scrubbers are machines that transfer particles in gases to a collecting liquid. An electrostatic precipitator (see Figure 10-26) confers negative or positive electrical charges to particles that are present in gases and collects them on a surface that has the opposite charge.[85]

The Kyoto Protocol

The Kyoto Protocol is an international and legally binding compact that was initiated in Kyoto, Japan, in 1997.[86,87] The purpose of the protocol is to reduce emissions of greenhouse gases that are believed to be the cause of recent climate changes. The protocol requires developed countries to reduce their emissions by targeted amounts. For example, the United States would be required to cut emissions by 7% and European countries (Switzerland, Central and Eastern Europe, and the European Union) by 8%. In order for the Kyoto Protocol to come into effect, it needed to be ratified by a sufficient number of industrialized countries that in combination produce at least 55% of the world's total CO_2 emissions. For some time, implementation of the Kyoto Protocol was stalled because an adequate number of countries, including the United States, had failed to ratify it. By February 2005, 141 nations including Russia had ratified the protocol, meaning that it could be implemented. The Kyoto Protocol went into force on February 16, 2005.[87] The United States, the world's largest producer of CO_2, has not

FIGURE 10-26 Conventional electrostatic precipitator.

Transformer - Rectifier Sets

Rappers

Collection Plates

Clean Gas Out

Flue Gas In

Discharge Electrodes

Hoppers

Source: Adapted and reprinted from US Environmental Protection Agency. Basic Concepts in Environmental Sciences, Module 6: Air Pollutants and Control Techniques—Particulate Matter. Available at: http://www.epa.gov/apti/bces/module6/matter/control/control.htm#precipit. Accessed April 13, 2010.

ratified the protocol; Australia is the only other developed country that has not signed the agreement.

From December 7 to December 18, 2009, delegates from 192 countries assembled in Copenhagen, Denmark, to attempt to reach a new international agreement for counteracting global warming.[88–90] Development of a new agreement known as the Copenhagen Accord was spearheaded by the United States, China, and a small group of other countries. Participants in the Copenhagen climate talks asserted that climate change is a major contemporary environmental challenge that should be addressed by curbing greenhouse gases. Delegates proposed that any increase in global temperature between the years 2010 and 2050 should be kept below 2 degrees Celsius. The agreement was not legally binding and was opposed by many countries, especially in the developing world, because of the monetary costs that would be involved. At the conclusion of the conference, talks became deadlocked. Nevertheless, this international conference ultimately may have the positive effect of increasing the world's awareness of control of greenhouse gases and related issues.

Energy Conservation

From a global perspective, the Kyoto Protocol, the Copenhagen Accord, and similar agreements should be helpful in reducing the emission of greenhouse gases. In addition, a number of other steps can be taken to reduce the emission of greenhouse gases and prevent global warming[83,84]:

- Increase the efficiency of older power plants.
- Develop more renewable and alternative energy sources (e.g., wind turbines and solar panels).
- Use energy-efficient designs in home construction and electrical appliances; try to reduce dependence on such appliances.
- Increase the fuel efficiency of motor vehicles as in the use of hybrid gas-electric and other high-mileage designs.
- Increase the use of public transportation.

CONCLUSION

Clean air is an essential element for the survival of life on earth. Air that is polluted can endanger our health and cause damage to trees, wildlife, and property. Sources of air pollution can be subdivided into natural and anthropogenic sources. Natural pollution arises from volcanoes, dust storms, and fires. Anthropogenic sources arise from stationary and mobile sources. The former include factories, oil refineries, and incinerators; examples of the latter are various types of vehicles used on air, water, and land. The health effects of air pollution include increased mortality rates and lung and cardiovascular diseases. As a result of growing emissions of greenhouse gases associated with the consumption of fossil fuels, the phenomenon of global warming is believed to be causing extreme climatic changes and rises in the average sea level. Air pollution and global warming can be reduced through the use of more efficient energy technologies, by limiting population growth, and by conserving energy. Many developed countries have expended significant efforts toward reduction of air pollution. Although these efforts have helped to produce cleaner air, additional steps need to be taken.

Study Questions and Exercises

1. Define the following terms in your own words:
   a. Smog
   b. Air pollution
   c. Criteria air pollutants
   d. Normal ambient air

2. Give examples of how air pollution endangers human health. Include in your discussion a review of the short-term and long-term health effects of air pollution.

3. How does air pollution impact the environment? In what ways can the pollutants NO_x and SO_2 damage structures and monuments over long periods of time?

4. Define the following sources of air pollution and give examples:
   a. Stationary
   b. Mobile
   c. Natural
   d. Anthropogenic

5. Describe how ground-level ozone can be harmful to our health while ozone in the upper stratosphere plays an important role in protecting our health.

6. Explain the adverse health effects attributed to carbon monoxide. Which population groups are likely to be most vulnerable to the effects of carbon monoxide exposure?

7. Define what is meant by a temperature inversion. Explain how temperature inversions contribute to the creation of smog.

8. Explain why environmental health experts are concerned about the possible adverse consequences of exposure to diesel exhaust. Describe one major adverse health effect that has been attributed to diesel exhaust. Name the risk groups that are most affected by exposure to diesel exhaust.

9. Refer to the diagram that shows the anatomy of the human respiratory system (Figure 10-15, part A, page 261). Which parts of the respiratory system are most likely to be affected by fine particulate matter?

10. Define the term *Air Quality Index*. How does the Air Quality Index aid in protecting the health of the population?

11. Epidemiologic analyses have demonstrated a correlation between an increase in total daily mortality and an increase in air pollution. Give examples of historically significant fatal air pollution episodes that were characterized by extreme increases in air pollution and accompanying increases in mortality.

12. Explain the difference between sick building syndrome and building-related illness. Describe the sources of indoor air pollution that can affect human health adversely.

13. Define what is meant by greenhouse gases and describe how they contribute to the greenhouse effect.

14. Describe three methods for the control of greenhouse gases. Which method, if any, is likely to be most effective?

15. Define the term *global warming* and present arguments for and against the proposition that global warming has occurred during the past century. What environmental outcomes have been attributed to global warming?

REFERENCES

1. Natural Resources Defense Council. An Environmental Agenda for the 109th Congress. Available at: http://www.nrdc.org/legislation/109congressinx.asp. Accessed April 14, 2010.

2. World Health Resources Institute. Rising energy use: Health effects of air pollution. Available at: http://www.wri.org/publication/content/8463. Accessed April 13, 2010.

3. South Coast Air Quality Management District (AQMD). Smog and health. Available at: http://www.aqmd.gov/smog/historical/smog_and_health.htm. Accessed April 13, 2010.

4. US Environmental Protection Agency. The plain English guide to the Clean Air Act: why should you be concerned about air pollution? Available at: http://www.epa.gov/air/caa/peg/concern.html. Accessed April 14, 2010.

5. US Environmental Protection Agency. National Risk Management Research Laboratory. EPA 625/R-02/009. Appendix B: Glossary of Terms. Available at: http://www.epa.gov/nrmrl/pubs/625r02009/html/appendixb.html. Accessed April 14, 2010.

6. Lawrence Berkeley National Laboratory. How can air pollution hurt my health? Available at: http://www.lbl.gov/Education/ELSI/Frames/pollution-health-effects-f.html. Accessed April 14, 2010.

7. Bell ML, Davis DL. Reassessment of the lethal London fog of 1952: novel indicators of acute and chronic consequences of acute exposure to air pollution. *Environ Health Perspect.* 2001;109(suppl. 3):389–394.

8. Helfand WH, Lazarus J, Theerman P. Donora, Pennsylvania: an environmental disaster of the 20th century. *Am J Public Health.* 2001;91:553–554.

9. Phalen RF. *The Particulate Air Pollution Controversy: A Case Study and Lessons Learned.* Boston, MA: Kluwer Academic Publishers; 2002.

10. Health Effects Institute. Understanding the health effects of components of the particulate matter mix: progress and next steps. Boston, MA: Health Effects Institute; 2002.

11. Centers for Disease Control and Prevention. Epidemiologic notes and reports cytotoxicity of volcanic ash: assessing the risk for pneumoconiosis. *MMWR.* 1986;35:265–267.

12. California Environmental Protection Agency, Air Resources Board. Glossary of air pollution terms. Available at: http://www.arb.ca.gov/html/gloss.htm. Accessed April 14, 2010.

13. US Environmental Protection Agency. The plain English guide to the Clean Air Act: Cars, trucks, buses, and "nonroad" equipment. Available at: http://epa.gov/air/caa/peg/carstrucks.html. Accessed April 14, 2010.

14. US Department of Health and Human Services. Statement by Dr. Kenneth Olden on health effects of air pollution. September 3, 2002. Available at: http://www.os.dhhs.gov/asl/testify/t020903.html. Accessed February 22, 2010.

15. Mitchell RS, Judson FN, Moulding TS, et al. Health effects of urban air pollution. *JAMA.* 1979;242:1163–1168.

16. US Environmental Protection Agency. Air & Radiation. What are the six common air pollutants? Available at: http://www.epa.gov/air/urbanair/. Accessed April 14, 2010.

17. Kaiser J. The other global pollutant: nitrogen proves tough to curb. *Science.* 2001;294(5545):1268–1269.

18. AllRefer.com. Hemoglobin derivatives. Available at: http://health.allrefer.com/health/hemoglobin-derivatives-info.html. Accessed April 15, 2010.

19. World Resources Institute. Urban air: health effects of particulates, sulfur dioxide, and ozone. Available at: http://pubs.wri.org/publication/content/8335. Accessed April 15, 2010.

20. Novel technologies measure ultrafine air pollution in the L.A. Basin. *J Environ Health.* 2004;66(8):51.

21. Centers for Disease Control and Prevention. Potential exposures to airborne and settled surface dust in residential areas of Lower Manhattan following the collapse of the World Trade Center—New York City, November 4–December 11, 2001. *MMWR.* 2003;52:131–136.

22. US Environmental Protection Agency. AIRTrends 1995 summary: acid rain. Available at: http://www.epa.gov/air/airtrends/aqtrnd95/acidrain.html. Accessed February 22, 2010.

23. Lipsett M, Campleman S. Occupational exposure to diesel exhaust and lung cancer: a meta-analysis. *Am J Public Health.* 1999;89:1009–1017.

24. Cohen HJ, Borak J, Hall T. Exposure of miners to diesel exhaust particulates in underground nonmetal mines. *AIHA J.* 2002;63:651–658.

25. Kagawa J. Health effects of diesel exhaust emissions—a mixture of air pollutants of worldwide concern. *Toxicol.* 2002;181–182:349–353.

26. Liukonen LR, Grogan JL, Myers W. Diesel particulate matter exposure to railroad train crews. *AIHA J.* 2002;63:610–616.

27. Northridge ME, Yankura J, Kinney PL, et al. Diesel exhaust exposure among adolescents in Harlem: a community-driven study. *Am J Public Health.* 1999;89:998–1002.

28. Stayner L. Protecting public health in the face of uncertain risks: the example of diesel exhaust [editorial]. *Am J Public Health.* 1999;89:991–993.

29. Steenland K. Lung cancer and diesel exhaust: a review. *Am J Ind Med.* 1986;10:177–189.

30. US Environmental Protection Agency. AIRNow: Air Quality Index (AQI)—A guide to air quality and your health. Available at: http://www.airnow.gov/index.cfm?action=aqibasics.aqi. Accessed April 15, 2010.

31. Levy JI, Greco SL, Spengler JD. The importance of population susceptibility for air pollution risk assessment: a case study of power plants near Washington, DC. *Environ Health Perspect.* 2002;110:1253–1260.

32. Health and Clean Air. Saving the children. *Health & Clean Air Newsletter.* Spring 2003. Available at: http://www.healthandcleanair.org/newsletters/spring2003.html. Accessed April 15, 2010.

33. Dockery DW, Pope CA III, Xu X, et al. An association between air pollution and mortality in six U.S. cities. *New Engl J Med.* 1993;329:1753–1759.

34. Pope CA III. Adverse health effects of air pollutants in a nonsmoking population. *Toxicol.* 1996;111:149–155.

35. Ito K, Thurston GD, Hayes C, et al. Associations of London, England, daily mortality with particulate matter, sulfur dioxide, and acidic aerosol pollution. *Arch Environ Health.* 1993;48:213–220.

36. Schimmel H, Greenberg L. A study of the relation of pollution to mortality: New York City, 1963–1968. *J Air Pollut Control Assoc.* 1972;22:607–616.

37. Dockery DW, Schwartz J, Spengler JD. Air pollution and daily mortality: associations with particulates and acid aerosols. *Environ Res.* 1992;59:362–373.

38. Dominici F, McDermott A, Zeger SL, et al. National maps of the effects of particulate matter on mortality: exploring geographical variation. *Environ Health Perspect.* 2003;111:39–43.

39. Mann JK, Tager IB, Lurmann F, et al. Air pollution and hospital admissions for ischemic heart disease in persons with congestive heart failure or arrhythmia. *Environ Health Perspect.* 2002;110:1247–1252.

40. Kuller LH, Radford EP, Swift DP, et al. Carbon monoxide and heart attacks. *Arch Environ Health.* 1975;30:477–482.

41. Wright GR, Jewizyk S, Onrot J, et al. Carbon monoxide in the urban atmosphere. *Arch Environ Health.* 1975;30:123–129.

42. Lebowitz MD, Holberg CJ, Knudson RJ, Burrows B. Longitudinal study of pulmonary function development in childhood, adolescence, and early adulthood. *Am Rev Respir Dis.* 1987;136:69–75.

43. Lebowitz MD. The relationship of socio-economic factors to the prevalence of obstructive lung diseases and other chronic conditions. *J Chronic Dis.* 1977;30:599–611.

44. Mannino DM, Homa DM, Pertowski CA, et al. Surveillance for asthma—United States, 1960–1995. *MMWR Surveill Summ.* 1998;47:1–28.

45. Mannino DM, Homa DM, Akinbami LJ, et al. Surveillance for asthma—United States, 1980–1999. *MMWR Surveill Summ.* 2002;51:1–13.

46. Rhodes L, Bailey CM, Moorman JE, et al. Asthma prevalence and control characteristics by race/ethnicity—United States, 2002. *MMWR.* 2004;53:145–148.

47. Crain EF, Walter M, O'Connor GT, et al. Home and allergic characteristics of children with asthma in seven U.S. urban communities and design of an environmental intervention: the Inner-City Asthma Study. *Environ Health Perspect.* 2002;110:939–945.

48. Klinnert MD, Price MR, Liu AH, et al. Unraveling the ecology of risks for early childhood asthma among ethnically diverse families in the Southwest. *Am J Public Health.* 2002;92:792–798.

49. Mishra V. Effect of indoor air pollution from biomass combustion on prevalence of asthma in the elderly. *Environ Health Perspect.* 2003;111:71–77.

50. National Institutes of Health. Of Air and Asthma: Air Pollution's Effects. Bethesda, MD: National Institutes of Health (NIH); 2008.

51. Delfino RJ. Epidemiologic evidence for asthma and exposure to air toxics: linkages between occupational, indoor, and community air pollution research. *Environ Health Perspect.* 2002;110(suppl 4):573–589.

52. Shima M, Nitta Y, Ando M, et al. Effects of air pollution on the prevalence and incidence of asthma in children. *Arch Environ Health.* 2002;57:529–535.

53. Ostro B, Lipsett M, Mann J, et al. Air pollution and exacerbation of asthma in African-American children in Los Angeles. *Epidemiol.* 2001;12:200–208.

54. Henderson BE, Gordon RJ, Menck H, et al. Lung cancer and air pollution in south-central Los Angeles County. *Am J Epidemiol.* 1975;101:477–488.

55. Pope CA III, Burnett RT, Thun MJ, et al. Lung cancer, cardiopulmonary mortality, and long-term exposure to fine particulate air pollution. *JAMA.* 2002;287:1132–1141.

56. Vena JE. Air pollution as a risk factor in lung cancer. *Am J Epidemiol.* 1982;116:42–56.

57. Nyberg F, Gustavsson P, Jarup L, et al. Urban air pollution and lung cancer in Stockholm. *Epidemiol.* 2000;11:487–495.

58. The American Lung Association (ALA), the Environmental Protection Agency (EPA), the Consumer Product Safety Commission (CPSC), and the American Medical Association (AMA). *Indoor Air Pollution: An Introduction for Health Professionals.* Washington, DC: US Government Printing Office; 1994. Publication 1994-523-217/81322.

59. Oliver LC, Shackleton BW. The indoor air we breathe: a public health problem of the '90s. *Public Health Rep.* 1998;113:398–409.

60. Lebowitz MD, Holberg CJ, Boyer B, Hayes C. Respiratory symptoms and peak flow associated with indoor and outdoor air pollutants in the southwest. *J Air Pollut Control Assoc.* 1985;35:1154–1158.

61. Vojta PJ, Friedman W, Marker DA, et al. First national survey of lead and allergens in housing: survey design and methods for the allergen and endotoxin components. *Environ Health Perspect.* 2002;110:527–532.

62. Engvall K, Norrby C, Norbäck D. Asthma symptoms in relation to building dampness and odour in older multifamily houses in Stockholm. *Int J Tuberc Lung Dis.* 2001;5:468–477.

63. Jaakkola JJK, Tuomaala P, Seppänen O. Air recirculation and sick building syndrome: a blinded crossover trial. *Am J Public Health.* 1994;84:422–428.

64. Mendell MJ, Fine L. Building ventilation and symptoms—where do we go from here? *Am J Public Health.* 1994;84:346–348.

65. US Environmental Protection Agency. Indoor air facts no. 4 (revised): sick building syndrome. Available at: http://www.epa.gov/iaq/pubs/sbs.html. Accessed February 22, 2010.

66. White JR, Froeb HF. Small-airways dysfunction in nonsmokers chronically exposed to tobacco smoke. *New Engl J Med.* 1980;302:720–723.

67. US Environmental Protection Agency. *Respiratory Health Effects of Passive Smoking: Lung Cancer and Other Disorders.* Washington, DC: EPA; 1992. EPA publication 600/6-90/006F.

68. Boyle P. The hazards of passive—and active—smoking. *N Engl J Med.* 1993;328:1708–1709.

69. National Aeronautics and Space Administration. Earth Observatory glossary. Available at: http://earthobservatory.nasa.gov/Glossary/?mode=alpha&seg=f&segend=h. Accessed April 5, 2010.

70. National Oceanic and Atmospheric Administration. Global warming frequently asked questions: is the climate warming? Available at: http://www.ncdc.noaa.gov/oa/climate/globalwarming.html. Accessed April 15, 2010.

71. Centers for Disease Control and Prevention. Climate change—science: state of knowledge. Available at: http://www.epa.gov/climatechange/science/stateofknowledge.html. Accessed April 17, 2010.

72. Crowley TJ. Causes of climate change over the past 1000 years. *Science.* 2000;289:270–277.

73. Patz JA, McGeehin MA, Bernard SM, et al. The potential health impacts of climate variability and change for the United States: executive summary of the report of the health sector of the U.S. National Assessment. *Environ Health Perspect.* 2000;108:367–376.

74. McMichael AJ, Patz J, Kovats RS. Impacts of global environmental change on future health and health care in tropical countries. *Br Med Bull.* 1998;54:475–488.

75. Charron DF. Potential impacts of global warming and climate change on the epidemiology of zoonotic diseases in Canada. *Can J Public Health.* 2002;93:334–335.

76. Yohe E. Sizing up the Earth's glaciers. 2004. Available at: http://earthobservatory.nasa.gov/Features/GLIMS/. Accessed April 15, 2010.

77. Patz JA, Kovats RS. Hotspots in climate change and human health. *BMJ.* 2002;325:1094–1098.

78. Patz JA, Khaliq M. Global climate change and health: challenges for future practitioners. *JAMA.* 2002;287:2283–2284.

79. Centers for Disease Control and Prevention. Heat-related mortality—United States, 1997. *MMWR.* 1998;47:473–476.

80. Centers for Disease Control and Prevention. Heat-related mortality—Chicago, July 1995. *MMWR.* 1995;44:577–579.

81. CBSNEWS.com. France ups heat toll. September 25, 2003. Available at: http://www.cbsnews.com/stories/2003/08/29/world/main570810.shtml. Accessed April 15, 2010.

82. Dorozynski A. Heat wave triggers political conflict as French death rates rise. *BMJ.* 2003;327:411.

83. A wake-up call for environmental health. *Lancet.* 2003;362:587.

84. Natural Resources Defense Council. Global warming basics. Available at: http://www.nrdc.org/globalWarming/f101.asp. Accessed April 15, 2010.

85. US Environmental Protection Agency. Basic concepts in environmental sciences. Module 6: air pollutants and control techniques—particulate matter-control techniques. Available at: http://www.epa.gov/apti/bces/module6/matter/control/control.htm. Accessed April 15, 2010.

86. About.com. Environmental Issues. What is the Kyoto Protocol? Available at: http://environment.about.com/od/kyotoprotocol/i/kyotoprotocol.htm. Accessed April 15, 2010.

87. The Woods Hole Research Center. The Kyoto Protocol. Available at: http://www.whrc.org/resources/online_publications/warming_earth/kyoto.htm. Accessed April 17, 2010.

88. The New York Times. Copenhagen Climate Talks. Updated Dec. 18, 2009. Available at: http://topics.nytimes.com/top/reference/timestopics/subjects/u/united_nations_framework_convention_on_climate_change/index.html. Accessed April 20, 2010.

89. The Guardian. Climate change talks yield small chance of global treaty. Available at: http://www.guardian.co.uk/environment/2010/apr/11/climate-change-talks-deal-treaty. Accessed April 20, 2010.

90. World Business Council for Sustainable Development. Climate: Is the Copenhagen Accord already dead? Available at: http://www.wbcsd.org/plugins/DocSearch/details.asp?type=DocDet&ObjectId=Mzc0NzE. Accessed April 20, 2010.

CHAPTER **11**

Food Safety

LEARNING OBJECTIVES

By the end of this chapter the reader will be able to:

- State three measures for preventing foodborne illness
- Discuss 10 microbiological agents that are implicated in foodborne illness
- Explain the significance of foodborne illness for the world's population
- List five categories of contaminants in the food supply
- Describe one major regulation for protecting the safety of food from carcinogens

INTRODUCTION

The focus of this chapter is on food safety, including foodborne diseases, foodborne infections, and foodborne outbreaks. The term **foodborne diseases** (which includes **foodborne intoxications** and **foodborne infections**) refers to "illnesses acquired by consumption of contaminated food; they are frequently and inaccurately referred to as food poisoning."[1(p239)] A **foodborne outbreak** indicates "the occurrence of a similar illness among two or more people which an investigation linked to consumption of a common meal or food items, except for botulism (one case is an outbreak)."[2(p4)]

The problem of foodborne illness is well known to the general public, due to the media's frequent coverage of outbreaks. For example, your local newspaper will occasionally print stories about foodborne illness outbreaks that happen in restaurants in your community; even the major restaurant chains are not immune to such incidents. Another example comes from media reports of dramatic foodborne illness outbreaks on cruise ships; often these outbreaks devastate the

vacations of passengers who must terminate their cruises prematurely. Other foodborne outbreaks are associated with foreign travel; at one time or another, many travelers to foreign countries have experienced illnesses caused by unsanitary or improperly prepared meals. Travelers to exotic locales may acquire foodborne pathogens—uncommon in their usual place of residence—that challenge health care providers who are unfamiliar with the resulting diseases.[3]

Foodborne illness can be both acute and long term. In this chapter, we will learn that some of the causes of acute foodborne illness are microbiologic agents and toxic chemicals such as pesticides and heavy metals. In addition, other contaminants that may be present in food are suspected of affecting human health adversely; these contaminants include food additives, antibiotics used to promote growth in animals used for food, and low levels of potential carcinogens. Sources of food contamination are pollutants in water used to process foods, chemicals used by the agricultural industry, and even pollutants found in the air. The role that food contaminants play in causing ill-defined gastrointestinal and other diseases is suspect, yet unclear. Many cases of such illness probably go unreported, so their scope is unknown. A pressing question is whether, and to what extent, human exposure to low levels of toxic contaminants in foods increases the risk of adverse health effects or is entirely benign.

In addition to providing information about causes of foodborne illness, the chapter also will cover foodborne disease prevention, methods for food safety inspection, and enforcement of government regulations. One of the important responsibilities of local and federal government agencies is to ensure the quality of foodstuffs. This goal is supported by

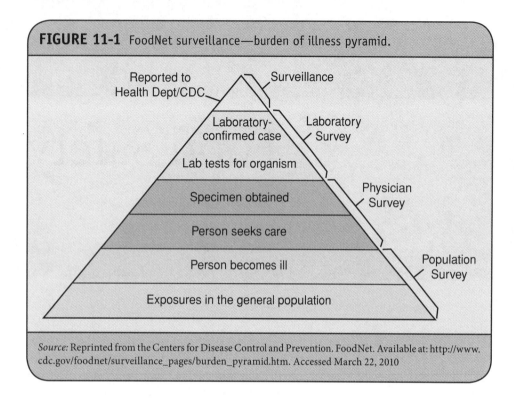

FIGURE 11-1 FoodNet surveillance—burden of illness pyramid.

Reported to Health Dept/CDC

Surveillance

Laboratory-confirmed case

Laboratory Survey

Lab tests for organism

Specimen obtained

Physician Survey

Person seeks care

Person becomes ill

Population Survey

Exposures in the general population

Source: Reprinted from the Centers for Disease Control and Prevention. FoodNet. Available at: http://www.cdc.gov/foodnet/surveillance_pages/burden_pyramid.htm. Accessed March 22, 2010

foodborne illness in the United States has tended to remain stable over time, with recent declines in some conditions (e.g., *E. coli* O157 infection) and the need to sustain these declines.

Surveillance of Foodborne Illness

In the United States, the CDC maintains responsibility at the federal level for surveillance of foodborne illness. For many types of foodborne diseases, only a small proportion may be reported by so-called passive surveillance systems, which rely on the reporting of cases of foodborne illness by clinical laboratories to state health departments and ultimately to the CDC.[7] In contrast, the CDC Foodborne Diseases Active Surveillance Network (FoodNet) is an active system whereby public health officials maintain frequent direct contact with clinical laboratory directors to identify new cases of foodborne illness. The focus of the FoodNet program is diarrheal illnesses caused by emerging infectious disease agents; foodborne diseases are monitored in several US sites, which are part of the CDC's Emerging Infections Program. Examples of the foodborne diseases that are monitored are those caused by parasites such as *Cyclospora* and *Cryptosporidium* (see Chapter 9) and bacterial agents such as *Campylobacter*, *E. coli* O157:H7, *Listeria monocytogenes*, *Salmonella*, *Shigella*, and *Vibrio*. Infections with *Vibrio parahaemolyticus* and *Vibrio vulnificus* often are associated with consumption of undercooked oysters taken from waters that have been contaminated by these bacteria. The other conditions are described later in the chapter.

The CDC has developed a model, called the burden of illness pyramid, for describing how reporting of foodborne disease takes place. Figure 11-1 illustrates the burden of illness pyramid.

> This illustration [of the burden of illness pyramid] shows the chain of events that must occur for an episode of illness in the population to be registered in surveillance. At the bottom of the pyramid, 1) some of the general population is ex-

cadres of government-employed environmental health workers who inspect the food supply and investigate foodborne illness outbreaks. The chapter will conclude with a review of new trends in production of foods and possible implications for human health.

THE GLOBAL BURDEN OF FOODBORNE ILLNESS

From the global perspective, foodborne illness is a major cause of morbidity (and occasionally mortality). Illnesses transmitted by foods can cause adverse birth outcomes, chronic illnesses, and disabilities (e.g., miscarriages, neurologic sequelae from meningitis, and kidney failure). Within the past few years, the incidence of foodborne illnesses has increased in industrialized nations.[4] This increase has been attributed to changes in agricultural and food processing methods, globalization in food distribution, and other social and behavioral changes among the human population.

According to the US Centers for Disease Control and Prevention (CDC), foodborne illness continues to be a public health problem of great importance for the United States.[5] Some estimates suggest that foodborne illnesses (reported and unreported) affect almost one-quarter of the population each year in the United States. Other estimates indicate that foodborne illnesses cause 9,000 deaths annually with an economic cost of $5 billion.[6] In recent years, the incidence of

TABLE 11-1 Number and Percentage of Reported Foodborne Disease Outbreaks and Outbreak-Associated Illnesses, by Etiology—United States, 2006

Etiology	No. of Outbreaks	No. of Illnesses
Bacterial	295	7,241
Chemical	66	267
Parasitic	12	147
Viral	511	14,855
Single etiology	884	22,510
Multiple etiologies	23	794
Unknown etiology	363	4,330
Total 2006	1,270	27,634

Totals include confirmed and suspected etiology

Source: Adapted from the Centers for Disease Control and Prevention. Surveillance for foodborne disease outbreaks—United States, 2006. *MMWR.* 2009;58:611.

posed to an organism; 2) some exposed persons become ill; 3) the illness is sufficiently troubling that some persons seek care; 4) a specimen is obtained from some persons and submitted to a clinical laboratory; 5) a laboratory appropriately tests the specimen; 6) the laboratory identifies the causative organism and thereby confirms the case; 7) the laboratory-confirmed case is reported to a local or state health department.

FoodNet conducts laboratory surveys, physician surveys, and population surveys to collect information about each of these steps.[8]

Table 11-1 tallies the number of outbreaks that occurred in 2006 by cause; during 2006 a total of 1,270 outbreaks and 27,634 illnesses were reported.

Figure 11-2 shows data reported from 1990 to 2002 on combined foodborne disease outbreaks for the causes shown

FIGURE 11-2 Foodborne-disease outbreaks reported to the CDC January 1, 1990, through March 15, 2002.

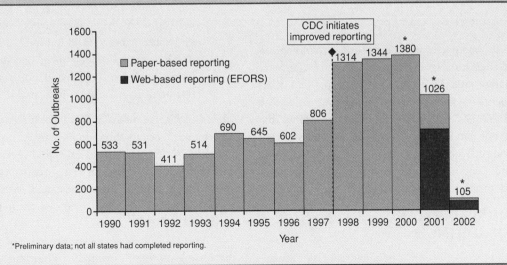

*Preliminary data; not all states had completed reporting.

Source: Adapted and reprinted from the Centers for Disease Control and Prevention. Surveillance for Foodborne-Disease Outbreaks—United States, 1998-2002. Surveillance Summaries, November 10, 2006. *MMWR.* 2006;55(No. SS-10):8.

> **TABLE 11-2** Contaminants That May Be Present in Food
>
> - Pathogenic microbial agents
>   - Examples: bacteria, worms, protozoa, fungi, viruses, prions, and (in certain cases) toxins from such organisms
> - Chemically related foodborne hazards
>   - Marine toxins, mushroom toxins
>   - Heavy metals
>   - Pesticides, herbicides, and fungicides
>   - Preservatives and additives
> - Residues of medicines administered to food animals
>   - Antibiotics, growth-promoting hormones
> - Foreign objects and other physical contaminants
>   - Natural components: bones, shells, seeds
>   - Other: glass and metal fragments, stones
> - Radioactive materials
> - Materials used in packaging
>   - Residues of plastics
>   - Waxes
> - Miscellaneous contaminants
>   - Debris from insects (insect parts, ova) and from rodents (fecal material, fur)
>   - Cleaning agents used in the food processing environment

in Table 11-1. Although some major bacterial foodborne illnesses caused by agents such as *Campylobacter* and *Listeria* have shown a sustained decline over time, others caused by *Vibrio* have not (2009 data). These trends suggest that continued efforts will be required to reduce further the incidence of some types of foodborne illness.

CATEGORIES OF FOOD HAZARDS

The "big three" categories of food hazards are biological, physical, and chemical.[9] In addition, nutritional hazards are those associated with the presence of nutrients and other food constituents in excessive or deficient amounts that lead to disease. Table 11-2 provides a list of contaminants that may be present in food. Physical hazards encompass foreign objects in food such as stones, glass, metal (e.g., bullets), and pieces of wood. Food hazards may be introduced when foods are harvested, processed, shipped, or stored.

COMMON MICROBIAL AGENTS OF FOODBORNE ILLNESS

The media and the CDC publish frequent reports of disease outbreaks caused by microbial agents. Some microbial pathogens (e.g., *Salmonella*) are more common agents of foodborne illness than are others (e.g., *Clostridium botulinum*). In ad-

dition, a type of microbial agent referred to as an emerging foodborne disease pathogen increasingly is causing foodborne infections. Emerging foodborne disease pathogens are a subset of agents from the general category of emerging infectious disease agents, which cause emerging infections. These infections, which include cholera, Rift Valley fever, and Lyme disease, "have newly appeared in the population, or have existed but are rapidly increasing in incidence or geographic range. . . ."[10(p7)] Emerging foodborne disease pathogens include *E. coli* O157:H7, *Campylobacter jejuni*, and *Listeria monocytogenes*. As they increase in frequency and scope, emerging foodborne diseases are a major concern of environmental health workers across the globe.

Chapter 5 focused mainly on zoonotic emerging infectious diseases. Some of these same emerging infectious disease pathogens represent hazards to the food supply. The rise in newly recognized pathogens has altered the epidemiology of foodborne illness by increasing the occurrence and sequaelae of emerging foodborne diseases.[3] Some of the microbial agents that cause foodborne illness have adapted to changes in food production, causing their reemergence and the development of new pathogens.[11] Another factor that has contributed to the rise of these pathogens is globalization of the food supply, as explained in an editorial in the *New England Journal of Medicine*:

> The surge in livestock production around the world, including most parts of Asia, has resulted in unprecedentedly large populations of closely confined animals, particularly pigs and chickens. . . . Today, large hog-raising operations, with tens of thousands of animals on a single farm, are common throughout parts of Asia, North and South America, and Europe. . . . A number of infectious agents tend to be associated with an increasing intensity of production and concentration of animals in limited spaces.[12(p1280)]

The editorial also indicates that these infectious agents "pose a potentially serious threat to human health."[12(p1280)] Other potential hazards arise from fruits and vegetables that originate in developing countries and are consumed in developed countries. In addition, the processes (e.g., cooking, treatment, and pasteurization) designed to deactivate pathogens "can and do fail."[12(p1281)]

Table 11-3 provides an abbreviated list of microbial agents responsible for foodborne illness. The agents form three general classes (bacteria, parasites, and viruses) plus a fourth class called "other." Some also are classified as agents of emerging foodborne disease. Excluded from this section are parasitic protozoal organisms, which were discussed in Chapter 9. Microbes vary greatly in the dose that is required to produce human illness.[11] In some instances the ingestion of only a single virus particle can cause disease; in others only a few organisms (viruses, bacteria, or parasites) need be consumed.

BACTERIAL AGENTS

The pathogens *Salmonella*, *Clostridium botulinum*, *Staphylococcus aureus*, and *Clostridium perfringens* are bacteria—unicellular organisms that have characteristic shapes, such as rod shaped (in some instances a slender, curved rod), spherical (cocci), or spiral. Bacteria can be moving (motile)—propelled by flagella or projections from cells—or nonmoving (nonmotile).

Bacteria may be classified as *gram-positive* or *gram-negative*, terms that refer to Gram's method, which is a staining technique for classifying bacteria. Using this methodology, technicians stain bacteria with a dye known as gentian violet; then they expose the bacteria to Gram's solution (a mixture of iodine, potassium iodide, and water) and other chemicals. After washing, bacteria that retain the gentian violet are gram-positive and those that do not retain it are gram-negative.

Foodborne infections should be differentiated from foodborne intoxications. Foodborne infections are induced by infectious agents such as some bacteria (e.g., *Salmonella*) that cause foodborne illness directly; symptoms of such infection are variable and may include nausea, diarrhea, vomiting, headaches, and abdominal pain. Foodborne intoxications result from other agents that do not cause infections directly but produce spores or toxins as they multiply in the food; these toxins then can affect the nervous system (neurotoxins) or the digestive system. An example of such a bacterial agent is *Staphylococcus aureus*.

Salmonella

Known as the genus *Salmonella*, this organism embodies approximately 2,000 serotypes that can cause human illness.[13] Used to identify subspecies of bacteria, the process of serotyping involves determining whether bacterial isolates react with the blood serum from animals that have formed antibodies against specific types of bacteria. Bacteria that react with specific sera are called members of that serotype.

The causative agents for the foodborne infection salmonellosis, *Salmonella* are described as rod-shaped, motile, gram-negative, and non-sporeforming bacteria. Figure 11-3 shows an image of *Salmonella* bacteria. (Note that some serotypes of *Salmonella* are nonmotile.)

The two most common serotypes in the United States are *Salmonella* serotype Enteritidis and *Salmonella* serotype Typhimurium, although the numbers of isolates of these serotypes have declined since 1996.[14] In 2006, a total of 34% of laboratory-confirmed cases of salmonellosis were caused by these two serotypes.[15] Four serotypes (Enteritidis, Typhimurium, Newport, and Heidelberg) accounted for 45% of isolates. A variety of *Salmonella* called *S.* Typhi causes typhoid fever. (This disease, which can be transmitted by contaminated food and water, was discussed in Chapter 9.)

Salmonellosis is ranked among the most frequent types

TABLE 11-3 Abbreviated Listing of Foodborne Pathogens and Diseases

Type of Organism	Name of Disease
Bacteria: Pathogenic Bacteria	
Salmonella	Salmonellosis
Clostridium botulinum	Botulism
Clostridium perfringens	*Clostridium perfringens* food intoxication
Staphylococcus aureus	Staphylococcal food intoxication
Campylobacter jejuni	Vibrionic enteritis
Shigella	Shigellosis
Listeria monocytogenes	Listeriosis
Bacteria: Enterovirulent *Eschericia Coli* Group (EEC Group)	
Escherichia coli O157:H7 enterohemorrhagic (EHEC) serotype	*E. coli* O157:H7 infection
Parasites: Worms	
Trichinella spiralis	Trichinellosis, trichinosis
Taenia solium, Taenia saginata	Taeniasis, cysticercosis (*T. solium*)
Viruses	
Norovirus (formerly called Norwalk virus group)	Epidemic viral gastroenteropathy
Other Pathogenic Agents	
Prions	Bovine spongiform encephalopathy (BSE), commonly referred to as mad cow disease

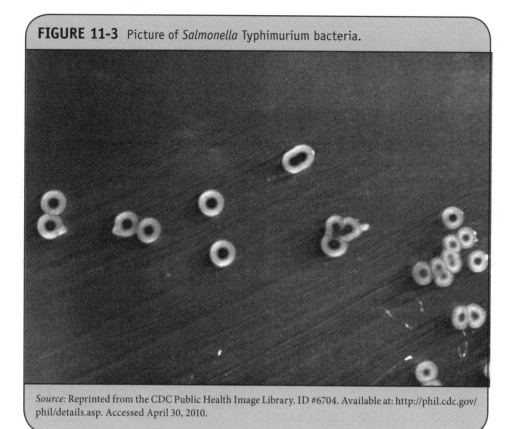

FIGURE 11-3 Picture of *Salmonella* Typhimurium bacteria.

Source: Reprinted from the CDC Public Health Image Library. ID #6704. Available at: http://phil.cdc.gov/phil/details.asp. Accessed April 30, 2010.

of foodborne illness in the United States.[14] Approximately 2 to 4 million cases of salmonellosis (reported and nonreported) are estimated to occur each year in the United States; about 500 deaths each year are caused by *Salmonella* infections. The number of cases of salmonellosis (excluding typhoid fever) reported each year ranges between 40,000 and 50,000.[16] Until the late 1980s, the United States and other developed countries experienced a rising incidence of salmonellosis. Since then, the rates of this condition have tended to stabilize in the United States. The number of *S.* Enteritidis isolates taken from human specimens has tended to increase relative to the other three common isolates. Refer to Figure 11-4 for numbers of reported cases of salmonellosis in comparison with cases of shigellosis (covered later in the chapter). Figure 11-4 also shows the rates of four common serotypes of *Salmonella*.

Salmonella are known to occur widely in wild and domestic animal reservoirs.[1] Animals that are used for human consumption—poultry, swine, cattle—may harbor *Salmonella*. Pet animals such as cats, dogs, and turtles also can be reservoirs for *Salmonella*. Some animals and birds are chronic carriers of the bacteria. *Salmonella* bacteria may be

transferred to environmental surfaces at work and at home (e.g., the kitchen) from raw meats, poultry, and seafood; from animal feces; and from contaminated water and soil. Symptoms and characteristics of *Salmonella* infections are shown in the text box.

Salmonella infections have been associated with diverse scenarios. Here are five examples of the many documented foodborne disease outbreaks caused by *Salmonella*:

1. Consumption of raw, unpasteurized milk was initially implicated in the cases of two children hospitalized with *Salmonella* infection. Subsequent investigations identified a total of 62 affected persons. The outbreak was linked to a dairy farm that served food and had a petting zoo. The farm legally sold raw milk and products made with raw milk.[17]

2. Eating cantaloupe imported from Mexico was associated with multistate outbreaks of *Salmonella* infections. The outbreaks affected more than 100 persons in 12 US states and Canada. Traceback investigations revealed that sanitary conditions at Mexican farms where the cantaloupes

FIGURE 11-4 Salmonellosis and shigellosis. Number of reported cases, by year—United States, 1977–2007, shown on the top. *Salmonella*, serotype isolates rates in the United States per 100,000 population, 1970–2006, shown on the bottom.

(a)

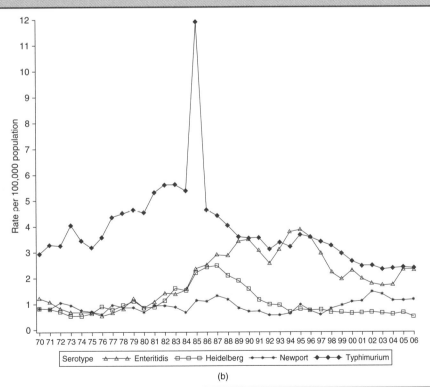

(b)

Source: Reprinted from the Centers for Disease Control and Prevention. Summary of Notifiable Diseases—United States, 2007. Published July 9, 2009 for *MMWR* 2007;56(No. 53):68; and the Centers for Disease Control and Prevention. Salmonella Surveillance: Annual Summary, 2006. Atlanta, GA: US Department of Health and Human Services, CDC, 2008:85.

Salmonellosis (*Salmonella* spp.)

Nature of disease: The acute symptoms of salmonellosis are nausea, vomiting, abdominal cramps, diarrhea, fever, and headache. Chronic consequences include arthritic symptoms that may follow 3–4 weeks after onset of acute symptoms. The onset time is 6–48 hours.

Infective dose: As few as 15–20 cells can cause infection; occurrence of infection depends upon age and health of host, and strain differences among the members of the genus.

Duration of symptoms: Acute symptoms may last for 1 to 2 days or may be prolonged, again depending on host factors, ingested dose, and strain characteristics.

Diagnosis of human illness: Serological identification of culture isolated from stool.

Associated foods: These include raw meats, poultry, eggs and egg shells, milk and dairy products, fish, shrimp, frog legs, yeast, coconut, sauces and salad dressing, cake mixes, cream-filled desserts and toppings, dried gelatin, peanut butter, cocoa, and chocolate. Various *Salmonella* species have long been isolated from the outside of egg shells.

Target populations: All age groups are susceptible, but symptoms are most severe in the elderly, infants, and the infirm. AIDS patients suffer salmonellosis frequently (estimated 20-fold more than general population) and suffer from recurrent episodes.

Source: Adapted and reprinted from US Food and Drug Administration. Center for Food Safety and Applied Nutrition, Bad Bug Book—*Salmonella* spp. Available at: http://www.fda.gov/Food/FoodSafety/FoodborneIllness/FoodborneIllnessFoodbornePathogensNaturalToxins/BadBugBook/ucm069966.htm. Accessed April 30, 2010.

originated could have been responsible (e.g., possible sewage-contaminated irrigation water and poor hygienic practices of workers).[18]

3. During winter of 1995–1996, ingestion of contaminated alfalfa sprouts was linked to 133 cases of salmonellosis in Oregon and British Columbia. Investigations suggested that the source of the *Salmonella* bacteria was contaminated alfalfa seeds.[19]

4. A multistate outbreak of *Salmonella* serotype Agona infections affected more than 200 persons in 11 states during April through May 1998. The outbreak was linked to Toasted Oats cereal that had been contaminated with this serotype of *Salmonella* bacteria.[13]

5. During 1985, the CDC became aware of the largest number of culture-confirmed cases of *Salmonella* ever reported for a single outbreak—5,770 by April 16, 1985.[20] This large number of cases was responsible for the increase shown in Figure 11-4. The cause of the incident was pasteurized milk, which ordinarily would be free from *Salmonella*. Apparently, the pasteurization process was inadequate, or the milk became contaminated after pasteurization.

Several of the strains of *Salmonella* have developed antibiotic resistance, making their treatment more difficult. The development of antimicrobial-resistant *Salmonella* has been tied to the administration of antibiotics to animals consumed for food; these resistant forms of *Salmonella* are capable of being transmitted to the human population.[21] For example, during the first four months of the year 2002, the CDC reported the characteristics of 47 cases of antibiotic-resistant *Salmonella* infections that occurred in five US states. These cases were caused by a serotype of *Salmonella* called *Salmonella* serotype Newport. The source of many of these cases was raw or undercooked ground beef.[22]

Clostridium botulinum

Clostridium botulinum causes the foodborne disease botulism, a form of foodborne intoxication. *C. botulinum* grows in an anaerobic (oxygen-free) environment and produces a potent toxin (a neurotoxin) that affects the nervous system.[23] The organism is rod shaped, as shown in Figure 11-5.

The organism forms spores that are resistant to heat; the spores are able to survive in foods that have been incorrectly or minimally processed. However, the organism can be eradicated by heating at a temperature of 80°C (176°F) for 10 or more minutes. When present in foods, the toxin produces a very severe disease that has a high mortality rate, particularly if not treated promptly. The disease has a low incidence in the United States; about 10 to 30 outbreaks occur each year. The form of the disease called infant botulism has been linked to consumption of honey by infants.

FIGURE 11-5 A photomicrograph of *Clostridium botulinum* bacteria.

Source: Reprinted from the CDC Public Health Image Library. ID #2107. Available at: http://phil.cdc.gov/phil/details.asp. Accessed April 30, 2010.

Other facts regarding botulism are listed in the following text box.

Exhibit 11-1 presents two case studies of botulism that were reported by the CDC.

Clostridium perfringens

Clostridium perfringens causes perfringens food poisoning, a common source of foodborne illness in the United States.[26] The CDC estimates that about 10,000 cases occur each year. *C. perfringens* is anaerobic, rod shaped, and forms spores. The organism occurs commonly in the environment (e.g., in soil and sediments), especially in those areas contaminated with feces; *C. perfringens* is a frequent resident of the intestines of humans and animals. The following text box contains some facts regarding *C. perfringens*.[26]

Here is an example of an outbreak: In 1993, *C. perfringens* caused illness outbreaks after diners consumed St. Patrick's Day meals of corned beef in Ohio and Virginia. The Ohio incident sickened at least 156 persons. The Virginia outbreak caused 115 persons to become ill. In both situations, the causative factor was *C. perfringens* intoxication, apparently from consuming meat that had been kept at improper holding temperatures, which allowed the spores and bacteria to proliferate.[27]

Clostridium botulinum

- Symptoms: A very small amount (a few nanograms) [or billionths of a gram] of toxin can cause illness. Onset of symptoms in foodborne botulism is usually 18 to 36 hours after ingestion of the food containing the toxin, although cases have varied from 4 hours to 8 days. Early signs of intoxication consist of marked lassitude, weakness and vertigo, usually followed by double vision and progressive difficulty in speaking and swallowing. Difficulty in breathing, weakness of other muscles, abdominal distention, and constipation may also be common symptoms.
- Associated Foods: The types of foods involved in botulism vary according to food preservation and eating habits in different regions. Any food that is conducive to outgrowth and toxin production, that when processed allows spore survival, and is not subsequently heated before consumption can be associated with botulism. Almost any type of food that is not very acidic (pH above 4.6) can support growth and toxin production by *C. botulinum*. Botulinal toxin has been demonstrated in a considerable variety of foods, such as canned corn, peppers, green beans, soups, beets, asparagus, mushrooms, ripe olives, spinach, tuna fish, chicken and chicken livers and liver pate, and luncheon meats, ham, sausage, stuffed eggplant, lobster, and smoked and salted fish.

BIOHAZARD

Source: Adapted and reprinted from US Food and Drug Administration. Center for Food Safety and Applied Nutrition, Bad Bug Book—*Clostridium botulinum*. Available at: http://www.fda.gov/Food/FoodSafety/FoodborneIllness/FoodborneIllnessFoodbornePathogensNaturalToxins/BadBugBook/ucm070000.htm. Accessed April 26, 2010.

Exhibit 11-1

CASE STUDY:
Botulism

1. On June 30, 1994, a 47-year-old resident of Oklahoma was admitted to an Arkansas hospital with subacute onset of progressive dizziness, blurred vision, slurred speech, difficulty swallowing, and nausea. . . . He developed respiratory compromise and required mechanical ventilation. The patient was hospitalized for 49 days, including 42 days on mechanical ventilation, before being discharged. The patient had reported that, during the 24 hours before onset of symptoms, he had eaten home-canned green beans and a stew containing roast beef and potatoes. Although analysis of the leftover green beans was negative for botulism toxin, type A toxin was detected in the stew. The stew had been cooked, covered with a heavy lid, and left on the stove for 3 days before being eaten without reheating.[24(pp200–201)]
2. On November 23, 1997, a previously healthy 68-year-old man became nauseated, vomited, and complained of abdominal pain. During the next 2 days, he developed diplopia, dysarthria, and respiratory impairment, necessitating hospitalization and mechanical ventilation. Possible botulism was diagnosed, and . . . antibotulinum toxin was administered. . . . A food history revealed no exposures to home-canned products; however, the patient had eaten pickled eggs that he had prepared 7 days before onset of illness; gastrointestinal symptoms began 12 hours after ingestion. The patient recovered after prolonged supportive care. The pickled eggs were prepared using a recipe that consisted of hard-boiled eggs, commercially prepared beets and hot peppers, and vinegar. The intact hard-boiled eggs were peeled and punctured with toothpicks then combined with the other ingredients in a glass jar that closed with a metal screw-on lid. The mixture was stored at room temperature and occasionally was exposed to sunlight. Cultures revealed *Clostridium botulinum* type B, and type B toxin was detected in samples of the pickled egg mixture. . . .[25(pp778–779)]

Source: The Centers for Disease Control and Prevention. Foodborne botulism from eating home-pickled eggs—Illinois, 1997. *MMWR.* 2000;49:778–780; the Centers for Disease Control and Prevention. Foodborne botulism—Oklahoma, 1994. *MMWR.* 1995;44:200–202.

Staphylococcus aureus

Staphylococcus aureus is a spherically shaped bacterium that causes a foodborne intoxication with rapid onset.[28] Figure 11-6 illustrates a grape-like cluster of *S. aureus* bacteria. During growth in foods, *S. aureus* elaborates a toxin that is extremely resistant to cooking at high temperatures. The organism can thrive in an environment that has heavy concentrations of salt or sugar (ham is a frequent vehicle for foodborne *S. aureus* poisoning); most other bacteria are unable to tolerate such an environment. Frequently, *S. aureus*–associated foodborne

Clostridium perfringens (C. perfringens)

- Onset and Symptoms: The common form of perfringens poisoning is characterized by intense abdominal cramps and diarrhea which begin 8–22 hours after consumption of foods containing large numbers of those *C. perfringens* bacteria capable of producing the food poisoning toxin. The illness is usually over within 24 hours but less severe symptoms may persist in some individuals for 1 or 2 weeks.
- Associated Foods: In most instances, the actual cause of poisoning by *C. perfringens* is temperature abuse of prepared foods. Small numbers of the organisms are often present after cooking and multiply to food poisoning levels during cool down and storage of prepared foods. Meats, meat products, and gravy are the foods most frequently implicated.

Source: Adapted and reprinted from US Food and Drug Administration. Center for Food Safety and Applied Nutrition, Bad Bug Book—*Clostridium perfringens.* Available at: http://www.fda.gov/Food/FoodSafety/FoodborneIllness/FoodborneIllnessFoodbornePathogensNaturalToxins/BadBugBook/ucm070483.htm. Accessed April 26, 2010.

FIGURE 11-6 Scanning electron micrograph of *Staphylococcus aureus* bacteria.

Source: Reprinted from the Centers for Disease Control and Prevention. Methicillin-resistant *Staphylococcus aureus* infections in correctional facilities—Georgia, California, and Texas, 2001–2003. *MMWR*. 2003;52:992.

Staphylococcal Food Poisoning

- Symptoms: The onset of symptoms in staphylococcal food poisoning is usually rapid and in many cases acute, depending on individual susceptibility to the toxin, the amount of contaminated food eaten, the amount of toxin in the food ingested, and the general health of the victim. The most common symptoms are nausea, vomiting, retching, abdominal cramping, and prostration.
- Foods Incriminated: Meat and meat products; poultry and egg products; salads such as egg, tuna, chicken, potato, and macaroni; bakery products such as cream-filled pastries, cream pies, and chocolate eclairs; sandwich fillings; and milk and dairy products. Foods that require considerable handling during preparation and that are kept at slightly elevated temperatures after preparation are frequently involved in staphylococcal food poisoning.
- Reservoir: Staphylococci exist in air, dust, sewage, water, milk, and food or on food equipment, environmental surfaces, humans, and animals. Humans and animals are the primary reservoirs. Staphylococci are present in the nasal passages and throats and on the hair and skin of 50 percent or more of healthy individuals. [They may exist in great numbers in skin lesions and lacerations.]

Source: Adapted and reprinted from US Food and Drug Administration. Center for Food Safety and Applied Nutrition, *Bad Bug Book—Staphylococcus aureus*. Available at: http://www.fda.gov/Food/FoodSafety/FoodborneIllness/FoodborneIllnessFoodbornePathogensNaturalToxins/BadBugBook/ucm070015.htm. Accessed April 26, 2010.

outbreaks are linked to foods that have not been stored in a safe temperature range (below 45°F [7.2°C] and above 140°F [60°C]).

Some of the additional characteristics of staphylococcal food poisoning are listed in the following text box.

The CDC reported the occurrence of an *S. aureus*–associated foodborne outbreak in 1997. Refer to the case study in Exhibit 11-2.

Escherichia coli O157:H7 (*E. coli* O157:H7)

E. coli O157:H7 is one of four classes of *E. coli* that are designated enterovirulent, meaning that they cause inflammation of the intestines and the stomach. The disease caused by *E. coli* O157:H7 is called hemorrhagic colitis, because one of the dramatic symptoms of the illness produced by the toxin from *E. coli* O157:H7 is bloody diarrhea. For the same reason, *E.*

coli O157:H7 is referred to as an enterohemorrhagic (EHEC) strain of *E. coli*. Figure 11-7 shows an electron micrograph of *E. coli* bacteria.

Nonpathogenic strains of *E. coli* reside harmlessly in the intestinal tracts of animals and humans and are part of the normal bacterial flora. Apparently, they retard the growth of pathogenic bacteria and synthesize vitamins. However, a few strains of *E. coli* are pathogenic, an example being the rare strain *E. coli* O157:H7.

Exhibit 11-2

CASE STUDY:
S. aureus Food Outbreak Associated with Ham

On September 27, 1997, a community hospital in northeastern Florida notified the St. Johns County Health Department about several persons who were treated in the emergency department because of gastrointestinal illnesses suspected of being associated with a common meal. Self-administered questionnaires were distributed to the 125 attendees to document food histories, illnesses, and symptoms. A case was defined as nausea and/or vomiting in a person who attended the party or consumed food served at the party and who became ill within 8 hours after eating. Leftover food was collected and submitted for laboratory analysis. Food preparers were interviewed about the purchase and preparation of food served at the party.

Of the approximately 125 persons who attended the party, 98 completed and returned questionnaires. Of these, 31 persons attended the event but ate nothing, and none of them became ill; they were excluded from further analysis. A total of 18 (19%) persons had illnesses meeting the case definition, including 17 party attendees and one person who ate food brought home from the party. Ill persons reported nausea (94%), vomiting (89%), diarrhea (72%), weakness (67%), sweating (61%), chills (44%), fatigue (39%), myalgia (28%), headache (11%), and fever (11%). Onset of illness occurred at a mean of 3.4 hours after eating (range: 1–7 hours); symptoms lasted a median of 24 hours (range: 2–72 hours). Seven persons sought medical treatment, and two of those were hospitalized overnight.

Illness was strongly associated with eating ham. Of the 18 ill persons, 17 (94%) had eaten ham. The ill person who had not attended the party had eaten only leftover ham. None of the other foods served at the party were significantly associated with illness. One sample of leftover cooked ham and one sample of leftover rice pilaf were analyzed and were positive for staphylococcal enterotoxin type A. Samples of stool or vomitus were not obtained from any ill persons, and cultures from nares or skin were not obtained from the food preparers.

On September 25, a food preparer had purchased a 16-pound precooked packaged ham, baked it at home at 400°F (204°C) for 1.5 hours, and transported it to her workplace, a large institutional kitchen, where she sliced the ham while it was hot on a commercial slicer. The food preparer reported having no cuts, sores, or infected wounds on her hands. She reported that she routinely cleaned the slicer in place rather than dismantling it and cleaning it according to recommended procedures and that she did not use an approved sanitizer. All 16 pounds of sliced ham had been placed in a 14-inch by 12-inch by 3-inch plastic container that was covered with foil and stored in a walk-in cooler for 6 hours, then transported back to the preparer's home and refrigerated overnight. The ham was served cold at the party the next day. The rice pilaf was prepared the day of the party by a different person.[29(pp1189–1190)]

Source: The Centers for Disease Control and Prevention. Outbreak of Staphylococcal food poisoning associated with precooked ham—Florida, 1997. *MMWR.* 1997;46:1189–1191.

The agent *E. coli* O157:H7 gained notoriety when it was associated with consumption of undercooked hamburger meat at a fast-food restaurant.[3] The organism, found in the intestines of healthy cattle, may invade meat during the slaughter process.[30] Outbreaks have occurred among visitors to petting farms.[31] In the United States, this organism—which causes both bloody and nonbloody diarrhea—has been linked to approximately 73,000 cases and 61 deaths annually.[32] Among children, infection with *E. coli* O157:H7 is the leading cause of hemolytic uremic syndrome (HUS), which produces such adverse consequences as acute kidney failure, end-stage renal disease, and hypertension. Young children are particularly vulnerable to HUS caused by *E. coli* O157:H7.[33] Refer to Table 11-4 for a chronology of the *E. coli* O157:H7 pathogen, and refer to the following text box for the characteristics of *E. coli* O157:H7–associated foodborne illness.

Among the foodborne illness outbreaks associated with *E. coli* O157:H7 is an incident that affected the patrons of a hamburger chain and impacted four western states. Refer to Exhibit 11-3.

Shigella

Shigella bacteria, which are highly infectious, are the cause of shigellosis (bacillary dysentery); an example of this agent

FIGURE 11-7 A cluster of *E. coli* bacteria.

Source: Reprinted from US Department of Agriculture, Agricultural Research Service. News & Events, Image Gallery, Image Number K11077-2. Photo by Eric Erbe, Colorization by Christopher Pooley. Available at: http://www.ars.usda.gov/is/graphics/photos/mar04/k11077-2.htm. Accessed May 6, 2010.

is *Shigella sonnei*. The bacteria can be transmitted via the fecal-oral route through contaminated water and foods that are handled in an unsanitary manner. In the United States, approximately 300,000 cases of shigellosis occur each year; the percentage of these cases that is caused by food is unknown. However, fewer than 10% of foodborne disease outbreaks in the United States are believed to be caused by *Shigella*.[34] Other facts regarding *Shigella* are presented in the following text box.

TABLE 11-4 *E. coli* O157:H7 (chronology)

1982	First recognized as a pathogen
1985	Associated with hemolytic uremic syndrome
1990	Outbreak from drinking water
1991	Outbreak from apple cider
1993	Multistate outbreak from fast-food hamburgers
1995	Outbreak from fresh produce
1996	Outbreak in Japan Multistate outbreak from unpasteurized apple juice

Source: Adapted and reprinted from the Centers for Disease Control and Prevention. Public Health Image Library, ID #107. Available at: http://phil.cdc.gov/Phil/details.asp. Accessed May 1, 2010.

Characteristics of *E. coli* O157:H7–Associated Foodborne Illness

- Symptoms: The illness is characterized by severe cramping (abdominal pain) and diarrhea which is initially watery but becomes grossly bloody. Occasionally vomiting occurs. Fever is either low-grade or absent. The illness is usually self-limited and lasts for an average of 8 days. Some individuals exhibit watery diarrhea only. . . .
- Associated Foods: Undercooked or raw hamburger (ground beef) has been implicated in many of the documented outbreaks; however, *E. coli* O157:H7 outbreaks have implicated alfalfa sprouts, unpasteurized fruit juices, dry-cured salami, lettuce, game meat, and cheese curds. Raw milk was the vehicle in a school outbreak in Canada.

Source: Adapted and reprinted from US Food and Drug Administration. Center for Food Safety and Applied Nutrition, Bad Bug Book—*Escherichia coli* O157:H7. Available at: http://www.fda.gov/Food/FoodSafety/FoodborneIllness/FoodborneIllnessFoodbornePathogensNaturalToxins/BadBugBook/ucm071284.htm. Accessed April 26, 2010.

Exhibit 11-3

CASE STUDY:
Multistate *E. coli* O157:H7 Outbreaks

From November 15, 1992, through February 28, 1993, more than 500 laboratory-confirmed infections with *E. coli* O157:H7 and four associated deaths occurred in four states—Washington, Idaho, California, and Nevada.

On January 13, 1993, a physician reported to the Washington Department of Health a cluster of children with hemolytic uremic syndrome (HUS) and an increase in emergency room visits for bloody diarrhea. During January 16–17, a case-control study comparing 16 of the first cases of bloody diarrhea or postdiarrheal HUS identified with age- and neighborhood-matched controls implicated eating at chain A restaurants during the week before symptom onset. On January 18, a multistate recall of unused hamburger patties from chain A restaurants was initiated.

As a result of publicity and case-finding efforts, during January–February 1993, 602 patients with bloody diarrhea or HUS were reported to the state health department. A total of 477 persons had illnesses meeting the case definition of culture-confirmed *E. coli* O157:H7 infection or postdiarrheal HUS. Of the 477 persons, 52 (11%) had close contact with a person with confirmed *E. coli* O157:H7 infection during the week preceding onset of symptoms. Of the remaining 425 persons, 372 (88%) reported eating in a chain A restaurant during the 9 days preceding onset of symptoms. Of the 338 patients who recalled what they ate in a chain A restaurant, 312 (92%) reported eating a regular-sized hamburger patty. Onsets of illness peaked from January 17 through January 20. Of the 477 patients, 144 (30%) were hospitalized; 30 developed HUS, and three died. The median age of patients was 7.5 years (range: 0–74 years). [During approximately the same time period, additional cases occurred in Idaho, California, and Nevada. These cases also were linked to the chain A restaurants.]

During the outbreak, chain A restaurants in Washington linked with cases primarily were serving regular-sized hamburger patties produced on November 19, 1992; some of the same meat was used in "jumbo" patties produced on November 20, 1992. The outbreak strain of *E. coli* O157:H7 was isolated from 11 lots of patties produced on those two dates; these lots had been distributed to restaurants in all states where illness occurred. Approximately 272,672 (20%) of the implicated patties were recovered by the recall.

A meat traceback by a CDC team identified five slaughter plants in the United States and one in Canada as the likely sources of carcasses used in the contaminated lots of meat and identified potential control points for reducing the likelihood of contamination. The animals slaughtered in domestic slaughter plants were traced to farms and auctions in six western states. No one slaughter plant or farm was identified as the source.

Source: Adapted and reprinted from the Centers for Disease Control and Prevention. Update: multistate outbreak of *Escherichia coli* O157:H7 infections from hamburgers—western United States, 1992–1993. *MMWR.* 1993;42:258–259, 261.

Shigella

- Symptoms: Abdominal pain; cramps; diarrhea; fever; vomiting; blood, pus, or mucus in stools. The onset time for shigellosis ranges from 12 to 50 hours. Infections are associated with mucosal ulceration, rectal bleeding, drastic dehydration; fatality may be as high as 10% to 15% with some strains.
- Associated Foods: Salads (potato, tuna, shrimp, macaroni, and chicken), raw vegetables, milk and dairy products, and poultry.
- Risk Groups: Infants, the elderly, and the infirm are susceptible to the severest symptoms of disease, but all humans are susceptible to some degree. Shigellosis is a very common malady suffered by individuals with acquired immune deficiency syndrome (AIDS).

Source: Adapted and reprinted from US Food and Drug Administration. Center for Food Safety and Applied Nutrition, Bad Bug Book—*Shigella* spp. Available at: http://www.fda.gov/Food/FoodSafety/FoodborneIllness/FoodborneIllnessFoodbornePathogensNaturalToxins/BadBugBook/ucm070563.htm. Accessed April 26, 2010.

FIGURE 11-8 Relative rates of laboratory-confirmed infections with *Campylobacter*, STEC* O157, *Listeria*, *Salmonella*, and *Vibrio* compared with 1996-1998 rates, by year—Foodborne Diseases Active Surveillance Network, United States, 1996–2007.[†]

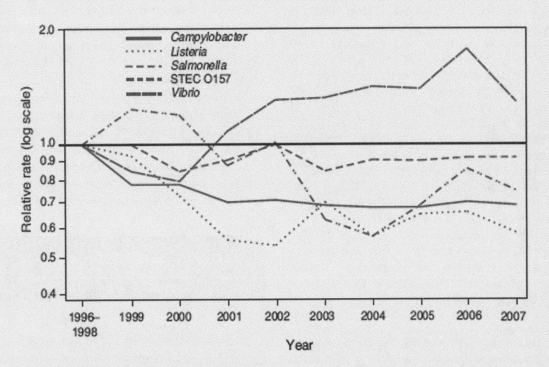

* Shiga toxin-producing *Escherichia coli*.
[†] The position of each line indicates the relative change in the incidence of that pathogen compared with 1996–1998. The actual incidences of these infections can differ.

Source: Reprinted from the Centers for Disease Control and Prevention. Preliminary FoodNet data on the incidence of infection with pathogens transmitted commonly through food—10 states, 2007. *MMWR*. 2008;57:368.

Campylobacter jejuni

Campylobacter jejuni is responsible for an illness known as campylobacteriosis. Among the bacterial causes of foodborne infections, *C. jejuni* is among the most commonly reported agents. About 2.1 to 2.4 million cases of campylobacteriosis occur each year in the United States.[35] Shown in Figure 11-8 are data on the relative rates of laboratory-confirmed infections with *Campylobacter*, Shiga toxin-producing *Escherichia coli* (STEC) O157, *Listeria*, *Salmonella*, and *Vibrio* reported by the CDC's FoodNet program.

Some of the characteristics of foodborne campylobacteriosis are listed in the text box titled "*Campylobacter jejuni*."

Among the *C. jejuni*–associated outbreaks reported by the CDC was the occurrence of 75 cases of illness in December 2002 related to consumption of unpasteurized milk in Wisconsin.[36] The unpasteurized milk was distributed by a retail dairy farm store. Unpasteurized milk can serve as a vehicle for *C. jejuni* and several other pathogens. The CDC noted that

> The facility that supplied milk to patients was a Grade A organic dairy farm with 36 dairy cows. The farm also had a retail store in which milk and other food products were available. In addition, farm operators provided unpasteurized milk samples at community events and to per-

Campylobacter jejuni

- Symptoms: *C. jejuni* infection causes diarrhea, which may be watery or sticky and can contain blood. Other symptoms often present are fever, abdominal pain, nausea, headache and muscle pain. The illness usually occurs 2–5 days after ingestion of the contaminated food or water. Illness generally lasts 7–10 days, but relapses are not uncommon (about 25% of cases). Most infections are self-limiting and are not treated with antibiotics.
- Associated Foods: *C. jejuni* frequently contaminates raw chicken. Surveys show that 20 to 100% of retail chickens are contaminated. This is not overly surprising since many healthy chickens carry these bacteria in their intestinal tracts. Raw milk is also a source of infections. The bacteria are often carried by healthy cattle and by flies on farms. Non-chlorinated water may also be a source of infections. However, properly cooking chicken, pasteurizing milk, and chlorinating drinking water will kill the bacteria.

Source: Adapted and reprinted from US Food and Drug Administration. Center for Food Safety and Applied Nutrition, Bad Bug Book—*Campylobacter jejuni*. Available at: http://www.fda.gov/Food/FoodSafety/FoodborneIllness/FoodborneIllnessFoodbornePathogensNaturalToxins/BadBugBook/ucm070024.htm. Accessed April 30, 2010.

sons who toured the farm, including children from childcare facilities. Because unpasteurized milk cannot be sold legally to consumers in Wisconsin, the dairy distributed unpasteurized milk through a cow-leasing program. Customers paid an initial fee to lease part of a cow. Farm operators milked the cows and stored the milk from all leased cows together in a bulk tank. Either customers picked up milk at the farm or farm operators had it delivered. On December 8, investigators obtained a milk sample from the farm's bulk milk tank, and cultures of the milk samples grew *C. jejuni* with a PFGE pattern that matched the outbreak strain. Farm operators

were ordered to divert all milk to a processor for pasteurization.[36(p548)]

Listeria monocytogenes

The illness listeriosis is caused by the bacterium *Listeria monocytogenes*, which has been found in some domestic mammals and several species of birds. The bacterium occurs widely in plant-related materials such as vegetables that may have been contaminated with sewage used as a fertilizer.[37] These vegetables may be consumed raw or after minimal processing. In the United States, *L. monocytogenes* is associated with about 2,500 cases of illness and 500 fatalities per year.[38] The characteristics of listeriosis are listed in the following text box.

A decline in the incidence of listeriosis has occurred in recent years, although sporadic outbreaks have been reported.[38] A 2002 outbreak in eight northeastern US states was respon-

Listeria monocytogenes

- Symptoms: Septicemia, meningitis (or meningoencephalitis), encephalitis, and intrauterine or cervical infections in pregnant women, which may result in spontaneous abortion (2nd/3rd trimester) or stillbirth. The onset of the aforementioned disorders is usually preceded by influenza-like symptoms including persistent fever. Gastrointestinal symptoms such as nausea, vomiting, and diarrhea may precede more serious forms of listeriosis or may be the only symptoms expressed.
- Associated Foods: *L. monocytogenes* has been associated with such foods as raw milk, supposedly pasteurized fluid milk, cheeses (particularly soft-ripened varieties), ice cream, raw vegetables, fermented raw-meat sausages, raw and cooked poultry, raw meats (all types), and raw and smoked fish. Its ability to grow at temperatures as low as 3°C permits multiplication in refrigerated foods.

Source: Adapted and reprinted from US Food and Drug Administration. Center for Food Safety and Applied Nutrition, Bad Bug Book—*Listeria monocytogenes*. Available at: http://www.fda.gov/Food/FoodSafety/FoodborneIllness/FoodborneIllnessFoodbornePathogensNaturalToxins/BadBugBook/ucm070064.htm. Accessed April 30, 2010.

sible for 46 confirmed cases, 7 fatalities, and 3 stillbirths or miscarriages.[39] The multistate outbreak was associated with eating sliceable turkey deli meat.

WORMS

Trichinella

Trichinosis is a foodborne disease associated with eating meat that contains a nematode (also called a roundworm) from the genus *Trichinella*.[40,41] The classic agent of trichinosis is *Trichinella spiralis*, which can be found in many carnivorous and omnivorous animals (e.g., pigs, bears, walruses, rodents, and cougars). The disease may be transmitted from animals such as these to humans when meat that contains the cysts of *T. spiralis* has not been cooked adequately. For example, outbreaks have been associated with eating pork from local farms and from consumption of grizzly bear meat.[42]

Formerly trichinosis was common in the United States, because garbage that contained raw meat was used routinely as feed for swine. Trichinosis outbreaks have been prevented following the elimination of this practice. Consumers can protect themselves further by cooking pork and wild game products adequately; also, freezing kills the worms of *T. spiralis*.

Infection with *T. spiralis* can be asymptomatic, as in the instance of light infections, or can include gastrointestinal effects in more severe infections. After about one week, when the organism migrates into muscle tissues, symptoms can range from fever and facial edema to life-threatening effects upon the heart and central nervous system.

The life cycle of *Trichinella* is shown in Figure 11-9. Following ingestion of meat that contains cysts, the larvae are released due to the action of stomach acids on the cysts. The larvae subsequently may invade the small intestine and develop into adult worms. The female adult worms release larvae that can migrate into muscle tissue and become encysted. The human host is a dead-end host, meaning that the disease cannot be spread to other humans.

Tapeworms

Taeniasis is a parasitic disease caused by tapeworms.[43] One form is caused by the beef tapeworm (*Taenia saginata*) and the other by the pork tapeworm (*Taenia solium*). These organisms may induce human illness

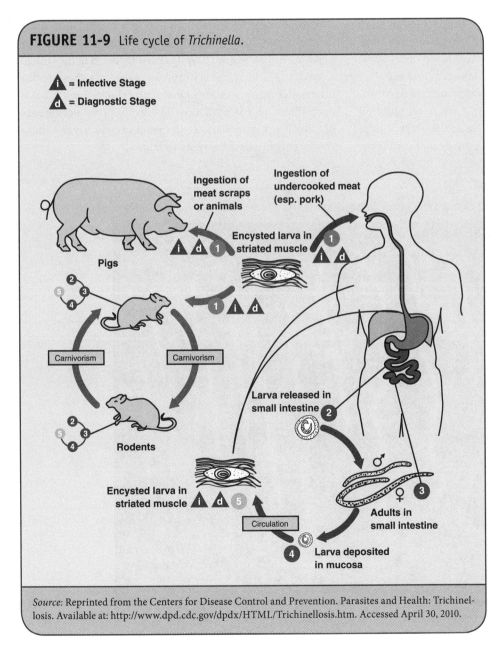

FIGURE 11-9 Life cycle of *Trichinella*.

Source: Reprinted from the Centers for Disease Control and Prevention. Parasites and Health: Trichinellosis. Available at: http://www.dpd.cdc.gov/dpdx/HTML/Trichinellosis.htm. Accessed April 30, 2010.

following the consumption of raw or undercooked infected beef or pork. Usually the symptoms of taeniasis are limited to mild abdominal distress; one of the main symptoms is the passage of the proglottids (the section of the worm that contains eggs) of *T. saginata* and *T. solium* in stools. *T. solium* can cause a serious condition termed cysticercosis, in which the organism migrates to muscle or brain tissue and forms cysts. The worms of *T. saginata*, which reside in human intestines, can be quite long. (See Figure 11-10.)

VIRAL AGENTS

Hepatitis A Virus (HAV)

Chapter 9 indicated that HAV can be transmitted by both contaminated food and water. Foods that are associated commonly with HAV outbreaks include fruits, sandwiches made with cold cuts, dairy products, vegetables, and shellfish.[44] A common mode for contamination of foods is by HAV-infected workers in food processing plants and restaurants. Of the 23,000 cases of hepatitis A reported in the United States annually, about 7% are believed to be food- or waterborne.

One instance of a large hepatitis A outbreak occurred from February to March 1997; this incident caused 213 cases in Michigan and 29 cases in Maine, and seemed to be linked to sporadic cases in several other states.[45] The source of the outbreak was frozen strawberries fed to schoolchildren in schools that had purchased the contaminated product from the same commercial processor. Other examples of hepatitis A outbreaks include those linked to sandwich shops and to national hamburger chains.

Hepatitis A outbreaks that involved almost 1,000 cases occurred in Tennessee, North Carolina, Georgia, and Pennsylvania from September to November 2003.[46] The outbreak in Pennsylvania was associated with a single restaurant and was responsible for more than 600 infected persons and 3 deaths. This outbreak was the largest episode of foodborne hepatitis A that, to date, ever has been reported in the United States. The Pennsylvania outbreak, as well as those in the other three states, was associated with green onions that had been imported from Mexico. This widespread occurrence of hepatitis A demonstrates the need to cook green onions thoroughly instead of serving them raw.

FIGURE 11-10 Adult tape worm (*Taenia saginata*).

Source: Reprinted from the CDC Public Health Image Library, ID #5260. Available at: http://phil.cdc.gov/Phil/details.asp. Accessed May 1, 2010.

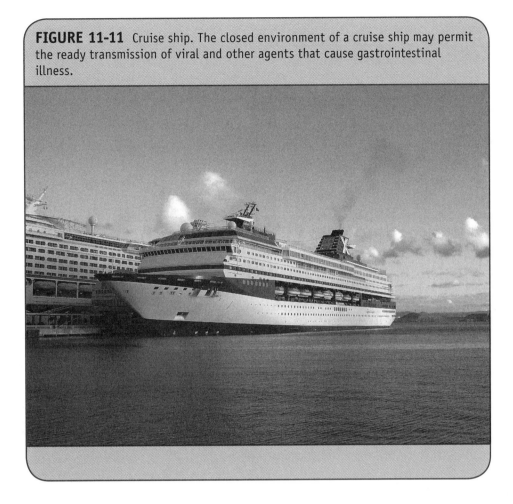

FIGURE 11-11 Cruise ship. The closed environment of a cruise ship may permit the ready transmission of viral and other agents that cause gastrointestinal illness.

Norovirus

Chapter 9 presented the topic of noroviruses, particularly with respect to waterborne norovirus infections. This virus is transmitted easily within closed environments such as cruise ships.[47] (See Figure 11-11.) Some cases may be brought on board by passengers who fall ill just before embarking on a cruise. It is also possible that crew members and shipboard environmental contamination can act as disease reservoirs.[48]

Outbreaks of gastrointestinal illness have been responsible for sickening hundreds of passengers on cruise ships.[49] The culprit for many outbreaks is believed to be a virus similar to the Norwalk virus, which is also called the winter vomiting virus. During one month in fall 2002, the toll was estimated to be 1,400 infected passengers and crew members on 10 ships. One outbreak that occurred on the *Amsterdam* (operated by Holland America) afflicted 163 passengers and 18 crew members out of 1,905 primarily elderly persons who went on the cruise. Illness symptoms consisted of vomiting and diarrhea as well as associated dehydration and abdominal cramps. These symptoms lasted from one to two days.

Just as the occurrence of gastrointestinal illness has continued to be reported throughout the United States, the CDC expects to continue to see increases in the number of reported gastrointestinal illness cases on some cruises.[50] Annually, about 6.8 million passengers in North America took cruises during the late 1990s. During the six-year period from 1993 to 1998, the number of passengers who embarked on cruises from the United States increased by 50%.[51] The number of North American cruise passengers increased by 11% from 2003 to 2004 (a record year with nearly 9 million passengers) and by 9% between 2004 and 2005.

US government regulations state:

> Cruise vessels sailing to U.S. ports are required to notify the CDC of all reported gastrointestinal illnesses that have been reported to the ships'

Outbreaks on Cruise Ships

Sundream (Sun Cruises, UK): January 20 to February 3, 2003. This vessel reported 95 of 1,085 passengers (8.8%) and 12 of 403 crew (3.0%) with gastrointestinal illness. The vessel made one US port of call in St. Thomas, US Virgin Islands on January 31, and then proceeded onto [*sic*] Venezuela. A UK public health laboratory confirmed gastrointestinal illness from the ill passengers and crews' stool samples. The *Sundream* crew conducted extensive cleaning and disinfection of the vessel.

Olympia Voyager (Royal Olympic Cruises, Greece): January 15 to February 3, 2003. This vessel reported 35 of 756 passengers (4.6%) and 5 of 356 crew (1.4%) ill with gastrointestinal illness. The cruise began in Port Everglades Florida and concluded in Houston, Texas. Extensive cleaning and disinfection was initiated [*sic*] during the first week of the cruise as the initial cases were identified. No new cases were identified the second week.

Carnival Spirit (Carnival Cruise Lines): January 27 to February 4, 2003. *Carnival Spirit* reported 102 of 2143 passengers (4.8%) and 10 of 902 crew (1.0%) were ill with a gastrointestinal illness. This vessel sails a 7-day cruise from Miami. Stool specimens were collected and submitted to [the] CDC for analysis. Clinical presentation of the illness [was] consistent with a noroviral outbreak. *Carnival Spirit* crew [conducted] extensive cleaning and disinfection aboard the vessel and additional staff will board in Miami on February 4th to assist.

Sun Princess (Princess Cruise Lines): January 25 to February 9, 2003. On January 28, the VSP was notified that 267 of 2029 passengers (13.1%) and 29 of 877 crew (3.3%) reported ill with a gastrointestinal illness. The cruise sails from Los Angeles to Hawaii, and return[s] to Los Angeles. On February 4th, Princess Cruises made the decision to terminate the 15 day cruise in Hawaii and not continue with the remaining five days transit from Hawaii to Los Angeles. This measure [was] taken to protect the health and safety of both passengers and crew by adopting every precaution possible to avoid the risk of any further transfer of this illness. All passengers [were] flown home.

Cruise ship travelers are reminded that simple hygienic practices, such as frequent and thorough hand washing and avoiding contact with other passengers when ill, are important measures to prevent the spread of disease.

Source: Reprinted from the Centers for Disease Control and Prevention, Vessel Sanitation Program. Investigation update on the *Carnival Legend*— February 4, 2003. Available at: http://www.cdc.gov/nceh/vsp/surv/outbreak/2003/update_feb4.htm. Accessed March 22, 2010.

medical staff. This report must be filed 24 hours prior to arrival at a U.S. port, from a foreign port. If the number of ill passengers or crewmembers reaches 2%, the vessel is required to file a special report. The CDC continues to closely monitor illness reports on a daily basis. An "outbreak" of gastrointestinal illness is defined as having 3% or more of either passengers or crew reported with a gastrointestinal illness.[50]

The CDC operates the Vessel Sanitation Program (VSP), which aims to keep the risks of diarrheal disease outbreaks among passengers at a minimum. A component of the VSP program is twice-yearly inspections of cruise ships that enter US waters; these inspections are not announced in advance.[51] Refer to the text box for a description of outbreaks that occurred on four cruise ships: *Sundream, Olympia Voyager, Carnival Spirit*, and *Sun Princess*.

OTHER AGENTS

Prions

Prions are hypothesized to be a modification of a normal protein; the modified protein is called a prion protein, which is a pathogenic agent that can damage the central nervous system of cattle. Infections with prions are regarded as the cause of **bovine spongiform encephalopathy (BSE)**, a neurologic disease in cattle.[52] The course of BSE (also known as mad cow disease) is progressive, ultimately fatal, and is potentially transmissible among cattle; an extensive outbreak among cattle occurred in the United Kingdom beginning in 1986. At the conclusion of 2008, the number of BSE cases in cattle exceeded 184,500 in the UK. Since the outbreak in the UK, cases also have been reported in 20 European countries as well as Japan, Israel, Canada, and the United States.

In North America (Canada and the United States), a total of 21 cases of BSE were reported between 1993 and early

Exhibit 11-4

CASE STUDY:

Bovine Spongiform Encephalopathy in a Dairy Cow—Washington State, 2003

On December 23, 2003, the US Department of Agriculture (USDA) made a preliminary diagnosis of bovine spongiform encephalopathy (BSE) in a single "downer" (i.e., nonambulatory disabled) dairy cow in Washington state. . . . The BSE-positive cow was aged 6.5 years when it was slaughtered on December 9. Before slaughter, the cow was nonambulatory; its condition was attributed to complications from calving. The animal was examined by a USDA Food Safety and Inspection Service (FSIS) veterinary medical officer both before and after slaughter. After examination, the carcass was released for use as food for human consumption. Tissues (e.g., brain, spinal cord, and small intestine) considered to be at high risk for the transmission of the BSE agent were removed from the cow during slaughter and sent for inedible rendering (often used for nonruminant animal feed). Because the cow was nonambulatory at slaughter, brain tissue samples were taken by USDA's Animal and Plant Health Inspection Service (APHIS) as part of its targeted surveillance for BSE. On December 23, a presumptive diagnosis of BSE was made, and the herd to which this cow belonged was placed under a state hold order.

On December 24, FSIS recalled beef from cattle slaughtered in the same plant on the same day as the BSE-positive cow. Some of the beef subject to the recall had been shipped to several establishments, which processed it further. Meat products manufactured from the recalled meat were distributed primarily to locations in Oregon and Washington, with smaller quantities distributed to locations in California, Idaho, Montana, and Nevada. FSIS continues to verify the distribution and control of all recalled products.

APHIS, in collaboration with CFIA, traced the birth of the BSE-positive cow to a farm in Alberta, Canada. On January 6, USDA and CFIA announced that DNA evidence had confirmed this traceback to Canada with a high degree of certainty. This line of investigation indicates that the BSE-positive cow was one of 82 animals from a Canadian herd cleared for shipment to the United States; 81 of the cattle listed on the Canadian animal health certificate entered the United States on September 4, 2001, through Oroville, Washington.

Source: Adapted and reprinted from the Centers for Disease Control and Prevention. Bovine spongiform encephalopathy in a dairy cow—Washington State, 2003. *MMWR.* 2004;52:1280–1281.

FIGURE 11-12 A: BSE-affected cow, showing incoordination and difficulty standing. B: Brain tissue from a BSE-affected cow with vacuoles, or microscopic holes.

Source: Reprinted from the CDC Public Health Image Library, ID #5438 and #5435, US Dept. of Agriculture, Animal and Plant Health Inspection Service, APHIS content provider. Photo credit (A): Dr. Art Davis, (B): Dr. Al Jenny. Available at: http://phil.cdc.gov/Phil/details.asp. Accessed March 24, 2010.

TABLE 11-5 Foodborne Chemical Hazards

Etiologic agent	Incubation period	Clinical syndrome
1. Marine toxins		
a. Ciguatoxin	1–48 hrs, usually 2–8 hrs	Usually gastrointestinal symptoms followed by neurologic symptoms (including paresthesia of lips, tongue, throat, or extremities) and reversal of hot and cold sensation
b. Scombroid toxin (histamine)	1 min–3 hrs, usually <1 hr	Flushing, dizziness, burning of mouth and throat, headache, gastrointestinal symptoms, urticaria, and generalized pruritus
c. Paralytic or neurotoxic shellfish poison	30 mins–3 hrs	Paresthesia of lips, mouth or face, and extremities; intestinal symptoms or weakness, including respiratory difficulty
d. Puffer fish, tetrodotoxin	10 mins–3 hrs, usually 10–45 mins	Paresthesia of lips, tongue, face, or extremities, often following numbness; loss of proprioception or "floating" sensations
2. Heavy metals a. Antimony b. Cadmium c. Copper d. Iron e. Tin f. Zinc	5 mins–8 hrs, usually <1 hr	Vomiting, often metallic taste
3. Monosodium glutamate (MSG)	3 mins–2 hrs, usually <1 hr	Burning sensation in chest, neck, abdomen, or extremities; sensation of lightness and pressure over face or heavy feeling in chest
4. Mushroom toxins		
a. Shorter-acting toxins:	≤ 2 hrs	Usually vomiting and diarrhea, other symptoms differ with toxin:
Muscimol		Confusion, visual disturbance
Muscarine		Salivation, diaphoresis
Psilocybin		Hallucinations
Coprinus artrementaris		Disulfiram-like reaction
Ibotenic acid		Confusion, visual disturbance
b. Longer-acting toxin (e.g., Amanita spp.)	6–24 hrs	Diarrhea and abdominal cramps for 24 hrs followed by hepatic and renal failure

Source: Adapted and reprinted from NH Bean, JS Goulding, C Lao, et al. Surveillance for foodborne disease outbreaks—United States, 1988–1992. In: *CDC Surveillance Summaries, MMWR.* 1996;45(SS-5):63–65.

2010. The majority of these cases (18) occurred in Canada; the most recent case was reported during the month of February 2010. On December 23, 2003, the first known case of BSE was reported in the United States. An account of that case is presented in Exhibit 11-4. As of February 2010, a total of three cases (one from a cow born in Canada) were reported in the United States.

BSE appears to be spread among cattle by feeds that contain rendered cattle products. Figure 11-12 shows a cow that has BSE and brain tissue affected by BSE. A crucial issue is whether the agent that causes BSE in cattle can be transmitted to humans. Epidemiologic and laboratory evidence suggest an association between BSE in cattle in the UK and a new human prion disease in humans. According to *Control of*

Communicable Diseases Manual, 19th edition, "Variant CJD . . . has been linked causally to bovine spongiform encephalopathy, with human cases thought due to dietary exposure to BSE-contaminated tissues."[1(p217)] The form of the disease in humans is a type of dementia called **variant Creutzfeldt-Jakob disease (vCJD)**.

CHEMICALLY RELATED FOODBORNE HAZARDS

Referring back to Table 11-2, you will see that in addition to microbial agents, other types of agents represent foodborne hazards. These include toxins, heavy metals, pesticides, herbicides, and fungicides; veterinary medicines in meat; and additives used for various purposes. Rocourt et al. point out that "Exposure to chemicals in food can result in acute and chronic toxic effects ranging from mild and reversible to serious and life threatening. These effects may include cancer, birth defects and damage to the nervous system, the reproductive system and the immune system."[2(p2)] Table 11-5 presents selected examples of chemical hazards as well as their associated incubation periods and clinical symptoms.

Toxins

Naturally occurring toxins, such as those from seafood and mushrooms, may be associated with foodborne illness. Other naturally occurring toxins (not covered in detail in this textbook) include oxalic acid found in rhubarb and other plant leaves, nitrites and nitrates found in beets and other vegetables, and aflatoxin (a type of mycotoxin) produced by molds that grow on peanuts and some grains.

Marine Toxins

In the United States, the annual number of reported cases of poisoning from marine toxins is estimated to be 30, although the actual number of cases may be much higher, as not all

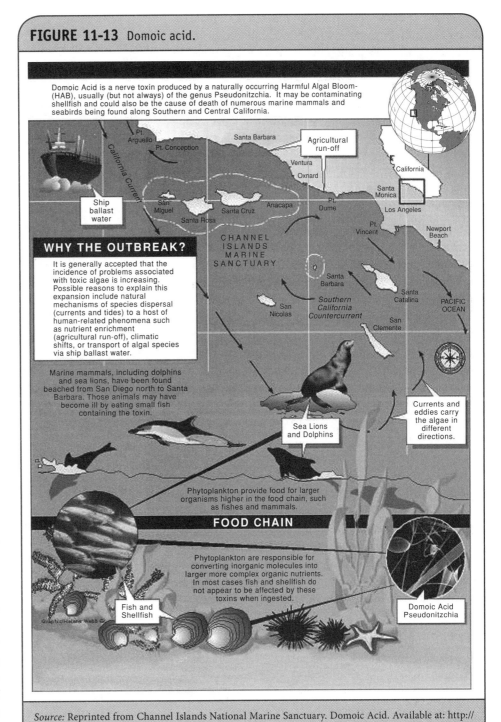

FIGURE 11-13 Domoic acid.

Source: Reprinted from Channel Islands National Marine Sanctuary. Domoic Acid. Available at: http://channelislands.noaa.gov/focus/dom.html. Accessed May 1, 2010.

cases are reported.[53] Marine toxins occur naturally in some types of seafood, which even though contaminated with the toxin may not show any obvious signs such as an off taste or smell. Examples of marine toxins are ciguatoxin, scombroid toxin, paralytic shellfish poison, and puffer fish toxin. Scombroid toxin is elaborated by bacterial deterioration of certain species of fish (e.g., tuna and mackerel). Ciguatoxin and paralytic shellfish poison (PSP) are produced by dinoflagellates (minute sea plants) that become concentrated in certain varieties of fish and shellfish. PSP also is caused by domoic acid toxin produced by other tiny organisms called marine diatoms. (See Figure 11-13.) Puffer fish toxin is present in puffer fish, a delicacy for sushi lovers in Japan. Some forms of poisoning with marine toxins are mild and resolve after a few hours, whereas others (e.g., severe paralytic shellfish poisoning) can be life threatening or fatal.

Mushroom Toxins

Mushroom toxins are produced naturally by several types of mushrooms, referred to commonly as toadstools. The symptoms and effects of mushroom poisoning vary depending upon the amount consumed; some can cause fatal injuries and irreversible organ damage.[54] Persons affected most often are mushroom hunters who misidentify wild mushrooms and persons from foreign countries who mistake US mushroom varieties for wild mushrooms that may be safe in their native country. Most of the mushroom toxins that are linked to human poisoning cannot be deactivated by cooking, canning, freezing, or any other kind of processing; the only sure way to avoid mushroom poisoning is by avoiding consumption of toxic mushrooms.

Heavy Metals

Chapter 6 covered the health effects of heavy metals (e.g., antimony, cadmium, copper, iron, tin, and zinc). When present in high concentrations, heavy metals can cause vomiting that occurs a few minutes to several hours (but in most cases in less than one hour) after ingestion. In addition to metal poisoning caused by high concentrations of heavy metals, there are many possible routes of lower-level exposures to foodborne metals:

- One source of metal poisoning is metals that have leached into foods (especially acidic foods) from metal containers and cooking vessels.
- In California, an instance of lead poisoning occurred when children consumed a variety of lollipops manufactured in Mexico. The candy's wrapper contained extremely high lead concentrations.[55]

- Chicken may contain high levels of arsenic, which is used as an approved food supplement for chickens to control intestinal parasites.[56]
- As noted previously, certain species of fish—shark, swordfish, king mackerel, and tilefish—have levels of mercury that may be high enough to be harmful to developing human fetuses.

Pesticides in Foods

Each year, insects, fungi, and other unwanted pests cause extensive damage to vegetables and fruits, with untold economic losses. Applied to crops to reduce the impact of insects and other hazards, pesticides may leave residues that remain on food crops. These residues should be removed by washing and peeling fruits and vegetables carefully. Dietary sources are one of the principal means of exposure of the population to persistent organic chemicals, which include the family of organochlorine pesticides and polychlorinated biphenyls.[57] As noted in Chapter 7, the health effects of low-level exposures to pesticides are generally unknown or have not been ascertained definitively at this time.

There are several examples of foods that contain low levels of pesticides. In a study of pesticides in baby foods, a public interest group found that 53% of a random sample of jarred fruits and vegetables had traces of at least one pesticide.[58] Nevertheless, the levels found were below federal safety standards for human consumption. However, these levels may not account for the possible special vulnerability of infants to potentially toxic chemicals, coupled with multiple low-level exposures from several different sources, for example, from foods and breast milk.

In comparison with low-level foodborne pesticide exposures, the effects of high-level exposures often are acute. Foodborne pesticides can sicken humans or be potentially toxic if consumed in large amounts. An example is an occurrence of foodborne aldicarb poisoning during early July 1985. Three adults developed symptoms of poisoning following the consumption of a solid green watermelon purchased in Oakland, California.[59] Victims reported the rapid development of symptoms, which included nausea, vomiting, heavy sweating, and reduced heart rate. Around the same time, several persons in Oregon also developed illnesses subsequent to eating striped watermelons. Oregon health officials announced that the pesticide aldicarb had been detected in other watermelons suspected of causing illnesses similar to those already reported in Oregon and California. The California Department of Health Services then issued a statewide embargo on the sale of watermelons and advised residents not to eat them. During the remainder of July, many additional similar illness reports were received. To investigate the cause of the outbreak, officials tested 250 watermelons for aldicarb—only 4% tested positive, possibly due to the lack of sensitivity of the laboratory tests that were used.

This episode was the largest foodborne pesticide illness outbreak ever recorded in North America. California reported 692 probable cases and other states and Canada reported an additional 483 cases. The pesticide aldicarb is regarded as appropriate for use on citrus fruits and potato crops and is not registered for use on melons. This episode demonstrated that aldicarb can cause very severe illnesses if used inappropriately on food crops.

A second example of foodborne pesticide poisoning was a report of endrin poisoning. (Refer to Exhibit 11-5.)

Antimicrobials in Meat

Antimicrobials that are similar or identical to those used by humans are employed for disease prevention and growth enhancement among animals (cattle, swine, poultry, and fish).[60] Four examples of the numerous common antimicrobials that have been approved in the United States for administration to food animals are amoxicillin, penicillin, bacitracin, and erythromycin. In addition, sulfonamide and several other antimicrobials sometimes are administered to farm-raised fish. In a

---

Exhibit 11-5

CASE STUDY:
Pesticide Poisoning with Endrin

In mid-March 1988, three family members in Orange County, California, became dizzy and nauseated within 1 hour of eating taquitos, a snack consisting of a corn tortilla wrapped around a meat filling. Two of the three subsequently had multiple grand mal seizures. The taquitos, a commercial product sold frozen in sealed plastic bags of 48, had been purchased 5 days earlier.

After receiving the reports of illness, the County of Orange Health Care Agency (COHCA) requested that the product be removed from the shelves of the store where the implicated bag was purchased. Several remaining taquitos from the implicated bag were tested by the US Department of Agriculture (USDA), Food Safety and Inspection Service, and found to contain endrin, a pesticide known to cause seizures. Samples of taquitos removed from the store and tested in USDA laboratories were negative for pesticides. The USDA reviewed the operations of the plant where the taquitos were produced, but no evidence of the pesticide was found. However, 90 cases of taquitos were destroyed by the plant owner as a precautionary measure. The USDA concluded that the poisonings were an isolated incident and closed the case April 20, 1988.

Subsequently, in September 1988, COHCA was informed of a 17-year-old boy who, in mid-March, had four seizures 30 minutes after eating taquitos purchased from the same store. After the seizures in March, he had been diagnosed as epileptic and begun on long-term anticonvulsants. At a hearing to determine the 17-year-old's continued eligibility for a driver's license, the hearing officer remarked that he had presided at a similar case (that of the father of the index family) the week before. (In California, seizures and loss of consciousness are reportable conditions for the purpose of determining eligibility for a driver's license.) This new information implicated a second bag of taquitos and indicated that other illnesses may have been misdiagnosed, resulting in serious medical and social consequences. Therefore, the investigation was reopened by the COHCA and the State of California. A state-issued press release and a mailing by the store to over 40,000 customers generated 100 calls to the local health department. As a result of this publicity, [investigators identified] two additional persons who had suffered seizures less than or equal to 12 hours after eating taquitos. All five seizure patients had eaten taquitos purchased from the same discount store within a 5-day period in March. Families other than the index family had no remaining taquitos.

California Department of Food and Agriculture laboratories confirmed the presence of endrin in leftover taquitos from the index family. Endrin was present in the tortillas but not in the meat filling. The store, the manufacturing plant, and the manufacturer's suppliers were thoroughly inspected, but no source of endrin was found.

Because of the limited nature of the outbreak and failure to find evidence of contamination in the plant inspections, the California Department of Health Services suspects deliberate tampering as the cause of the outbreak.

Source: Reprinted from the Centers for Disease Control and Prevention. Endrin poisoning associated with taquito ingestion—California. *MMWR.* 1989;38:345–346.

procedure known as **metaphylaxis**, antimicrobials are given to an entire collection of animals, for example, chickens on a poultry farm or fish raised in pens, for the purpose of curing disease among the sick animals and preventing disease among the remainder. Regarding the use of antimicrobials for growth enhancement of animals (with the exception of farmed fish), antimicrobials increase the efficiency of feeds by reducing the amount of feeds that animals require.

Residues of antimicrobial agents may persist in meat that is destined for human consumption. To reduce the levels of potentially harmful residues in meats, administration of antimicrobials must be discontinued for prescribed periods before feed animals are slaughtered and shipped to market. According to Greenlees,

> Unlike chemical residues, there is an additional concern for the use of antimicrobial animal drugs of an indirect toxicity to the human consumer, characterized by the loss of an effective therapeutic intervention, resulting in adverse health effects. This potential impact on human health has resulted in the concern for microorganisms that are resistant to . . . antimicrobial drugs. . . ."[61(p133)]

At present, because of concerns about potentially undesirable consequences of antimicrobial use, some countries restrict their administration in animal feeds. Improved conditions for raising food animals and the use of vaccines can reduce the need for microbial agents.

Biotechnology and Genetically Modified Foods

Biotechnology and genetically modified (GM) foods hold promise for addressing the need for more food supplies as the world's population increases and, at the same time, available land and water for agricultural uses diminish.[62,63] Examples of GM foods are those that result from genes that have been manipulated (e.g., through recombinant DNA technologies). These technologies may lead to increases in agricultural productivity and food availability for a burgeoning world population. The advantages of GM foods are purported to be the following:

- Develop genetically engineered herbicide-resistant plants that survive application of herbicides used to destroy weeds.
- Increase the amount of arable land by developing plants that are able to grow in poor-quality soils.

- Increase resistance of plants to attacks from insect pests; such resistance would reduce the need for toxic insecticides and thus benefit the environment.
- Improve the nutritional value of food crops.
- Increase the nutritional value of meat, for example, by reducing its fat content.
- Increase the resistance of food animals to disease, thereby reducing costs and protecting the food supply from animal pathogens.

Despite the advantages of GM foods, environmental groups have expressed concerns over their potential negative consequences.[64,65] Some of the concerns raised are the following:

- Use of GM plants may reduce genetic diversity; GM plants used for food crops might be more susceptible to eradication than existing plants in the event of a disaster such as the appearance of a new plant disease.
- GM plants and animals could escape into the environment, supplanting natural species. For example, farm-raised GM salmon might escape their holding pens and compete more successfully for food and reproduction success than wild salmon.
- Concern about the health effects of genetically modified foods (e.g., allergic reactions and carcinogenesis) has led some countries to ban their use.
- Pollen from GM plants could cross-pollinate with non-GM plants, causing loss of biodiversity.
- The number of antibiotic-resistant strains of bacteria might increase.

Although many scientific studies have verified the safety of GM foods, their applications require more research, especially regarding long-term consequences. Some governments, such as the European Parliament, have developed proposals to trace GM foods in the food supply and label items that contain GM products.[66] In the United States, the National Research Council is studying the safety of animal biotechnology as it pertains to food production.[65] The disadvantages of GM foods need to be balanced against their potential advantages. A paper delivered at the National Academy of Sciences stated that

> biotechnology adds value across the system from crop to farmer, customer and consumer. Biotechnology can, and is, enhancing the quality of food in addition to improving the quantity of food. Biotechnology can improve the sustainability of production systems by requiring fewer inputs to control pests and better protect

the quality of water and land mass around us. Biotechnology can add health and vitality to humans. As we look at food production in a more holistic way, biotechnology will be an important component of that holistic system.[67(p5971)]

Food Additives

The term **food additives** is defined as "substances that become part of a food product when added (intentionally or unintentionally) during the processing or production of that food."[68] There are three categories of food additives: intentional, incidental, and malicious:

- *Intentional (direct) additives* are added to foods in order to improve their quality.
- *Incidental (indirect) additives* may be present in foods as a result of unintentional contamination during packaging, storage, and handling. Examples are pesticide residues on fruits, substances from packaging, or antimicrobial agents present in meats; foods may contain parts of insects that were not removed during processing or that have infested a food item.
- *Malicious additives* include substances such as poisons that saboteurs introduce into foods for various

reasons (e.g., poisoning of taquitos from the pesticide endrin).

Examples of types of additives and their purposes are shown in Table 11-6. Additives include emulsifiers, stabilizers, and thickeners; vitamins and minerals; preservatives; and many other substances. Some of the types and functions of additives are explained in the following section.

Preservatives

Preservatives that processors add to foods act as antimicrobial agents and antioxidants. Among the antimicrobial preservatives are nitrates (e.g., sodium nitrate and potassium nitrate), **BHA (butylated hydroxyl anisole)** and **BHT (butylated hydroxytoluene)**, disodium EDTA (ethylenediaminetetraacetic acid), sulfites, proprionates, and parabens. The function of preservatives is to arrest the proliferation of microbes such as bacteria, yeasts, and molds in foods.[69] For example, the preservative sodium nitrite is used on meats for color retention and retardation of the growth of spores that can produce the botulinum toxin. Antioxidants prevent fatty foods from acquiring a rancid taste; they also prevent some foods from turning brown and reduce the loss of vitamins by other foods.

TABLE 11-6 Some of the Types of Food Additives

Type of Additive	Purpose	Examples
Emulsifiers, stabilizers, and thickeners	Impart a consistent texture to products; prevent separation of foods such as salad dressings.	Algin, carrageenan
Anticaking agents	Enable products such as table salt to flow freely.	Calcium silicate
Nutrients	Enrichment (replacement of nutrients lost during processing) and fortification (adding to the nutritional value of foods)	Many types of vitamins, e.g., folic acid, beta-carotene, Vitamin D; many types of minerals, e.g., iron, iodine, calcium.
Preservatives (antimicrobials)	Retard spoiling by microbial agents.	Nitrates, propionates, parabens
Preservatives (antioxidants)	Prevent fats and oils from becoming rancid; prevent cut fresh fruits from turning brown.	BHA, BHT, sulfites (e.g., sodium sulfite)
Leavening agents	Cause bread and baked goods to rise during baking.	Sodium bicarbonate
Flavor enhancers (synthetic and natural)	Enhance flavor of foods.	MSG (monosodium glutamate)
Sweeteners (synthetic and natural)	Add sweetness with or without the extra calories.	Aspartame, sucrose
Color additives (artificial and natural)	Impart color to foods.	FD&C Yellow No. 6, caramel color
Fat replacers	Impart texture and creamy "mouth feel" to foods.	Olestra, cellulose gel

Source: Data from International Food Information Council (IFIC) Foundation and US Food and Drug Administration. *Food Ingredients and Colors.* Washington, DC: International Food Information Council (IFIC) Foundation and US Food and Drug Administration; 2004:2–3.

One concern about the use of nitrates and nitrites is that they may interact with amines (chemicals related to ammonia) to produce substances known as nitrosamines, which have been implicated as suspected carcinogens. To minimize the consumer's exposure to nitrosamines, manufacturers are required to keep sodium nitrate at safe levels that have been set by the US Food and Drug Administration (FDA).

BHA and BHT are used as antioxidants for foods that contain fats and oils; for example, some cereals and other dry foods contain BHT. Sulfites are employed mainly as antioxidants that maintain the color of fruits and vegetables. Because they destroy the vitamin thiamin (vitamin B1), sulfites may not be added to foods such as flour that are used to supply this nutrient. Some individuals are allergic to sulfites and must avoid them in their diets; since 1986, the FDA has banned the use of sulfites in fruits and vegetables that are destined to be consumed raw, e.g., in salad bars. One type of sulfite is sodium sulfite. At present, sodium sulfite "is generally recognized as safe when used with good manufacturing practice, except that it is not used in meats; in food recognized as a source of vitamin B1; on fruits and vegetables intended to be served raw to consumers or sold raw to consumers, or to be presented to consumers as fresh."[69] Proprionates (e.g., sodium proprionate) are used as antimicrobial agents, especially in products that require the use of yeast, because proprionates do not inhibit the action of yeast.[70] In contrast, parabens are antimicrobials that inhibit the actions of unwanted molds and yeast and, consequently, are used to prevent the spoilage of food products by these microbes.

Several concerns about the safety of food additives exist among the general public and health professionals. Some persons have allergic reactions to some additives (e.g., MSG, sulfites, and the artificial sweetener aspartame). Sodium-containing additives (e.g., sodium bicarbonate) may add unwanted sodium to the diets of persons afflicted with hypertension. Finally, other additives may be known or potential carcinogens; for example, nitrosamine compounds are known carcinogens. The artificial sweetener saccharin has been shown to cause cancer in laboratory animals; however, the carcinogenic potency of saccharin for humans is extremely low compared with many other carcinogens. BHA and BHT may be a cause of tumors in laboratory animals. The safety of food additives is monitored by the FDA; this topic is covered in the next section.

REGULATION OF FOOD SAFETY

In the United States, a body of governmental regulations is designed to assure the quality of food products and to protect the public from possible harm resulting from additives and chemicals in food. The FDA is the US agency charged with regulation and enforcement of food safety. The US Department of Agriculture (USDA) regulates the safety of meat and poultry products. Food safety regulations that are in force at present are the result of an incremental process of change: among the significant US food safety regulations that have been legislated or that have evolved over time are the following[71]:

- 1906 Food and Drugs Act
- The Federal Food, Drug, and Cosmetic Act of 1938
- Miller Pesticide Amendments, 1954
- Food Additives Amendment, 1958
- Color Additive Amendments, 1960
- Animal Drug Amendments, 1968
- Food Quality Protection Act (FQPA), 1996

Food, Drug, and Cosmetic Act of 1938

The 1906 Food and Drugs Act prohibited the sale of foods considered "misbranded" or "adulterated."[71] The broadened Federal Food, Drug, and Cosmetic Act, formulated in 1938, introduced several important standards for food, drugs, cosmetics, and medical devices:

> The new law brought cosmetics and medical devices under control, and it required that drugs be labeled with adequate directions for safe use. Moreover, it mandated pre-market approval of all new drugs, such that a manufacturer would have to prove to FDA that a drug were safe before it could be sold. It irrefutably prohibited false therapeutic claims for drugs, although a separate law granted the Federal Trade Commission jurisdiction over drug advertising. The act also corrected abuses in food packaging and quality, and it mandated legally enforceable food standards. Tolerances for certain poisonous substances were addressed. The law formally authorized factory inspections, and it added injunctions to the enforcement tools at the agency's disposal.[72]

The 1938 Act was amended during the period of 1954 to 1968 to take into account the safety of pesticide residues and food additives. A congressional select committee, established in 1952 and chaired by Representative James Delaney of New York, was responsible for initiating many of the amendments designed to regulate pesticides in foods and food additives.

Miller Pesticide Amendments

Adopted in 1954, the Miller Pesticide Amendments to the Food, Drug, and Cosmetic Act of 1938 governed the levels of pesticides that were permitted in foods. Pesticide residues were required to fall within tolerances set by the FDA. The 1938 act and the l954 amendments remain in force, but were modified by additional standards for the regulation of pesticides in foods that were adopted subsequently, as described in the following text.

Food Additives Amendment, 1958

The Food Additives Amendment was implemented in 1958 in recognition of the public's growing concern over chemicals that were being used increasingly in foods. The 1958 amendment, which applies exclusively to the use of food additives as well as chemicals that could come into contact with food (e.g., from food packaging), defined what was meant by the terms *food additive* and *unsafe food additive*. Under the amendment, food manufacturers were required, by means of a premarket review, to demonstrate the safety of food additives to the FDA.[73] As part of the Food Additives Amendment, the Delaney Clause regulated the permissible levels of additives in foods. Specifically, the clause prohibited the use of food additives, including pesticides, that had been determined to cause cancer in human beings or animals.

Many substances that already had been in use over a long period of time and had established safety records were exempted from review. These substances fell under the Generally Recognized as Safe (GRAS) rule; examples of such additives are the many types of salts, flavoring agents, and preservatives that were believed to be safe. Food processors that intended to use other additives not on the GRAS list were required to demonstrate their safety before they could be marketed.

Adopted in 1960, the Color Additive Amendments contained provisions for the premarket approval of colors that were designated for use in foods, drugs, and cosmetics. Finally, the Animal Drug Amendments of 1968 govern the safety and efficacy of drugs and feed additives that are administered to food animals and control the levels of residues of such drugs in meats destined for human consumption.

Food Quality Protection Act (FQPA), 1996

One of the consequences of the Delaney Clause was that it provoked the wrath of food growers and processors by prohibiting the application of any pesticide that might appear in processed foods, should that pesticide carry even a minimal risk of causing cancer. The 1996 FQPA repealed the Delaney Clause and adopted a strict standard for chemicals applied to raw and processed food. The standard was that a substance could not cause a lifetime incidence of more than one cancer case per 1 million exposed persons.[74] According to the EPA,

> The Food Quality Protection Act (FQPA) of 1996 amended the Federal Insecticide, Fungicide, and Rodenticide Act (FIFRA) and the Federal Food, Drug, and Cosmetic Act (FFDCA). These amendments fundamentally changed the way EPA regulates pesticides. The requirements included a new safety standard—reasonable certainty of no harm—that must be applied to all pesticides used on foods.[75]

Overall, FQPA won the favor of environmental groups as well as food processors because it placed into action more effective standards to protect children and to test chemicals for their teratogenic effects.

Agencies That Regulate Food Safety

Figure 11-14 illustrates agencies that regulate food safety at the international level as well as the national, state, and local levels in the United States. For the sake of example, the state of California has been chosen to illustrate the state level. However, the illustration would apply to most of the states in the country. In a similar vein, examples of local jurisdictions chosen are located in Southern California. The choice of these health agencies is arbitrary; similar illustrations could be selected from other local jurisdictions across the United States.

The following are detailed accounts of the functions of each of the agencies shown in Figure 11-14:

- *International:* "The Food and Agriculture Organization of the United Nations (FAO) was founded in 1945 with a mandate to raise levels of nutrition and standards of living, to improve agricultural productivity, and to better the condition of rural populations. Today, FAO is the largest specialized agency in the United Nations system and the lead agency for agriculture, forestry, fisheries and rural development. An intergovernmental organization, FAO has 180 member countries plus one member organization, the European Community. Since its inception, FAO has worked to alleviate poverty and hunger by promoting agricultural development, improved nutrition and the pursuit of food security—defined as the access of all people at all times to the food they need for an active and healthy life."[76]
- *National:* "The Food Safety and Inspection Service (FSIS) is the public health regulatory agency in the

U.S. Department of Agriculture responsible for ensuring that the nation's commercial supply of meat, poultry, and egg products is safe, wholesome, and correctly labeled and packaged."[77]

Figure 11-15 shows poultry that has been condemned by the USDA.

- *National:* The Center for Food Safety and Applied Nutrition (CFSAN) is an arm of the US Food and Drug Administration (FDA). "The Center regulates $417 billion worth of domestic food, $49 billion worth of imported foods, and over $60 billion worth of cosmetics sold across state lines. ... FDA's responsibility in the area of cosmetics covers all domestic and imported products. ... This regulation takes place from the products' point of U.S. entry or processing to their point

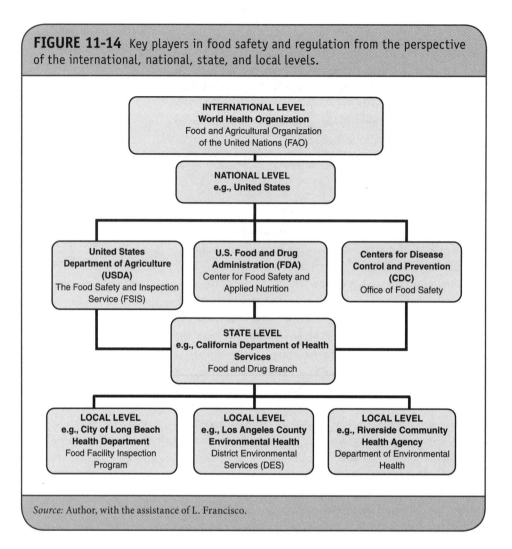

FIGURE 11-14 Key players in food safety and regulation from the perspective of the international, national, state, and local levels.

Source: Author, with the assistance of L. Francisco.

of sale. ... FDA's responsibility in the food area generally covers all domestic and imported food ... [with the following exceptions:]"[78]

- Meat, poultry, and frozen, dried and liquid eggs; these are "under the authority of the U.S. Department of Agriculture (USDA's Food Safety and Inspection Service (FSIS). ...."[78]
- Labeling of alcoholic beverages (above 7% alcohol) and tobacco; these "are regulated by the U.S. Department of the Treasury's Alcohol and Tobacco Tax and Trade Bureau (TTB). ...." [78]
- Establishment of tolerances for pesticide residues in foods and setting of requirements for drinking water; these areas are the responsibility of the US Environmental Protection Agency (EPA).
- *National:* The Centers for Disease Control and Prevention Food Safety Office (FSO) provides leadership in

the control of foodborne illness in the United States. In partnership with local, state, and other federal officials, the agency investigates the sources of foodborne disease outbreaks. The CDC maintains a nationwide system of foodborne disease surveillance (the CDC Foodborne Outbreak Response and Surveillance Unit); it designs and puts in place rapid, electronic systems for reporting foodborne infections, e.g., the Foodborne Diseases Active Surveillance Network (FoodNet). The CDC works with other federal and state agencies to monitor rates of and trends in foodborne disease outbreaks. Another function is to develop state-of-the-art techniques and systems for rapid identification of certain foodborne viruses and DNA fingerprinting of bacteria that may be transmitted by foods; this information helps participating public health officials identify contaminated foods that are implicated in outbreaks.[79]

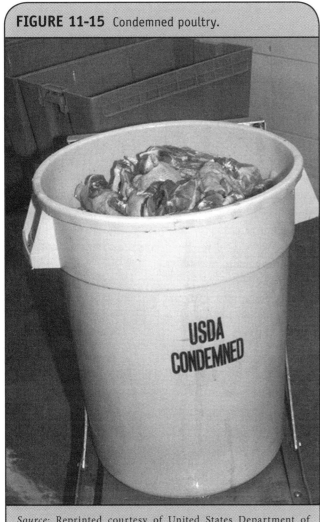

FIGURE 11-15 Condemned poultry.

Source: Reprinted courtesy of United States Department of Agriculture.

- *State:* The mission of the California Department of Health Services, Food and Drug Branch "is to protect and improve the health of all California residents by assuring that foods, drugs, medical devices, cosmetics and certain other consumer products are safe and are not adulterated, misbranded nor falsely advertised; and that drugs and medical devices are effective."[80]
- *Local:* The City of Long Beach Health and Human Services Food Facility Inspection Program oversees the safety of the regulation of food facilities only within the City of Long Beach. "The goal of the food program is to ensure that the food sold and served in the City of Long Beach is safe, wholesome, properly labeled and advertised, and produced under sanitary conditions. ... The Food Inspection Program ... enforces state

and local food safety regulations in over 2,000 food facilities in the city."[81]
- *Local:* The Los Angeles County Department of Health Services, Division of Environmental Health, Bureau of District Environmental Services is an enforcement agency operating as part of the County of Los Angeles, Department of Health Services. The mission of Environmental Health is to protect health, prevent disease, and promote health for all persons in Los Angeles County. "The Bureau of District Environmental Services is comprised of the following two programs: [(1) The Bureau of] District Environmental Services that conducts routine and complaint inspections on retail food establishments, multiple family dwellings, and other miscellaneous facilities as well as residential complaints, and [(2) the] Plan Check Program for retail food facilities."[82]
- *Local:* The mission of the Riverside County Community Health Agency, Department of Environmental Health "is to enhance the quality of life in Riverside County by implementation of effective and efficient environmental health programs to protect the public health, safety and the environment."[83]

FOODBORNE DISEASE PREVENTION

In the United States, two main factors are related to foodborne disease outbreaks: improper temperatures for keeping foods and poor personal hygiene of food handlers.[84] Less developed areas of the world may be deficient in one or both of these elements and in addition not have a reliable water supply. Consider the following two graphic examples of how foodborne illness may erupt in less developed regions of the world. Figure 11-16 shows food preparation techniques found in some parts of the world; in these examples, food is being prepared out in the open, on a street. Such obvious unsanitary conditions for the storing and preparation of food place consumers at risk of illness outbreaks.

Table 11-7 lists risk factors identified by the CDC as being associated with foodborne illnesses, in order of their importance. Note that the percentages total more than 100% because more than one factor at a time can be present as a cause of foodborne illness. Routine inspections of restaurants and food-handling facilities focus on this set of risk factors, some of which are discussed in the following sections.

Safe Cooling and Cold Holding Temperatures

In order to prevent microorganisms from multiplying in foods, they must be kept in the safe temperature range: above

FIGURE 11-16 A: Woman cooking food on the sidewalk in Xian, China. B: A Peruvian street vendor selling a corn-based drink he made at home using a single glass that he fills with a dipper.

A

B

A: *Source:* Reprinted, courtesy of Dr. Edwin P. Ewing, Jr. and the CDC, from Centers for Disease Control and Prevention. Public Health Image Library. ID #755. Available at: http://phil.cdc.gov/Phil/details.asp. Accessed March 24, 2010.

B: *Source:* Reprinted from the CDC Public Image Library. ID #5319. Available at: http://phil.cdc.gov/Phil/details.asp. Accessed March 24, 2010.

140°F for hot foods and below 40°F for foods that are kept in cold storage. The range between 40°F and 140°F is the danger zone, the temperature range in which microbes that can cause foodborne illness produce toxins or multiply. Refer to Figure 11-17.

Preventing Growth of Foodborne Pathogens

Figure 11-18 illustrates four steps to prevent the growth of foodborne pathogens in food. These steps include thorough hand washing, prevention of cross-contamination, cooking at sufficiently high temperatures, and storing cooked and vulnerable foods at proper temperatures in a refrigerator. An example of cross-contamination of foods is the use of a cutting board to cut raw poultry and subsequent use of the same cutting board to cut bread without washing the cutting board before reuse.

The recommended method of safe hand washing is illustrated further in Figure 11-19.

TABLE 11-7 Top Risk Factors for Foodborne Illness

Percentage	Risk Factor
63%	Inadequate cooling and cold holding temperatures
29%	Preparing food ahead of planned service
27%	Inadequate hot holding temperatures
26%	Poor personal hygiene/infected persons
25%	Inadequate reheating
9%	Inadequate cleaning of equipment
7%	Use of leftovers
6%	Cross-contamination
5%	Inadequate cooking or heat processing
4%	Containers adding toxic chemicals
2%	Contaminated raw ingredients
2%	Intentional chemical additives
1%	Incidental chemical additives
1%	Unsafe sources

Percentages refer to foodborne illness outbreaks in which this risk factor is present.

Source: Adapted and reprinted from County of Los Angeles Public Health, Environmental Health. Retail Food Inspection Guide Online. Available at: http://lapublichealth.org/eh/rfig/rfigfiles/cdcrisk.htm. Accessed May 1, 2010.

FIGURE 11-17 Apply the heat chart to determine safe temperature levels for preserving, storing, and cooking foods.

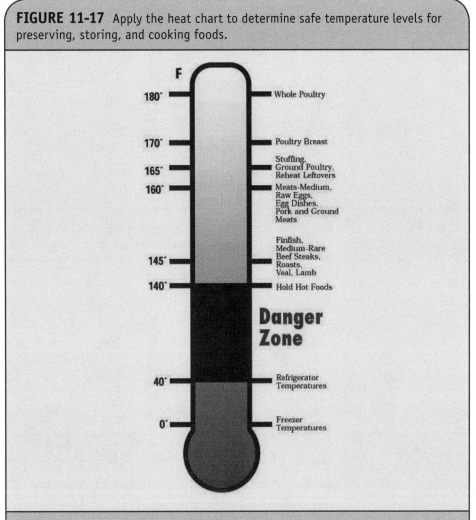

Source: Adapted and reprinted from US Food and Drug Administration, Center for Food Safety and Applied Nutrition. Food safety for moms to be: Educator tools—Apply the heat. Available at: http://www.fda.gov/Food/ResourcesForYou/HealthEducators/ucm109104.htm. Accessed May 1, 2010.

FIGURE 11-18 The Big Four—Clean, Separate, Cook, and Chill—Tools for Educators.

Source: Reprinted from United States Department of Agriculture, Food Safety and Inspection Service. The Food Safety Educator. 2001;6(2). Available at: http://www.fsis.usda.gov/OA/educator/educator6-2a.htm. Accessed March 24, 2010.

FIGURE 11-19 Hand washing techniques.

1. Wet hands with warm water. Lather with soap

2. Lather to your elbows. Scrub hands for 20 seconds.

3. Rinse hands and elbows thoroughly.

4. Dry hands with a single use towel.

5. Use towel to turn off the faucet.

6. Use towel to open the door.

Source: Adapted and reprinted with permission. Prepared by Julie A. Albrecht, Extension Food Specialist, and Susan S. Sumner, Extension Food Microbiologist. Pictures courtesy of Dianne Peters, Food Science and Technology. © 2005 by the University of Nebraska-Lincoln, Cooperative Extension, Institute of Agriculture and Natural Resources. Food safety: Food handling practices. Available at: http://foodsafety.unl.edu/handling/handwashingenglish.pdf. Accessed May 2, 2010.

Irradiation

As noted previously, foodborne illness continues to cause numerous cases of disease and deaths in the United States despite regulations and procedures that are in place to protect the public by monitoring the safety of the food supply. The CDC estimates that reduction in foodborne illness through irradiation of half the meats (ground beef, pork, and poultry; processed luncheon meats) used in the United States could save 352 lives each year as well as prevent 880,000 illness episodes, 8,500 hospitalizations, and 6,660 catastrophic illnesses.[85]

During the process of irradiation, energy from ionizing radiation passes through foods and destroys bacteria and other pathogens; the procedure does not cause food to become radioactive. Exposing foods to radiation does not cause their temperatures to increase as with other methods of food preservation. Hence, irradiation of foods is referred to as cold pasteurization.[86]

The sources of ionizing radiation used in cold pasteurization include gamma radiation from cobalt-60 and cesium-137, electron beam radiation, and X-rays. The latter two sources do not require a radioactive source and can be switched on and off by the operator. A low dose of radiation (< 0.1 kiloGrays) is effective at killing insect pests and parasitic organisms. Medium doses in the range of 1.5 kiloGrays to 4.5 kiloGrays are lethal to most bacteria. High doses up to 45 kiloGrays are needed to kill bacterial spores and some viruses.[87] These doses are needed for immediate eradication of the respective organisms.

Irradiation of food has been certified as a safe method for reducing the risk of foodborne disease.[86] Irradiation also reduces spoilage and increases the shelf life of foods. Use of ionizing radiation for food sterilization has been subjected to evaluation over a period of 50 years. More than 40 countries have approved the irradiation of food, and the procedure has received the endorsements of many health- and food-related organizations.

In the case of many foods, irradiation produces little change in the nutritional value and taste and other sensory qualities of the product. Foods that retain their quality include meat, poultry, seafood, soft fruit and some produce, and grains.[87,88] Leafy vegetables and sprouts wilt following irradiation; meats that have high fat contents may develop slightly unpleasant odors. Cold pasteurization cannot be regarded as a panacea for foodborne illness. Following irradiation, pathogens can be reintroduced into foods during later stages of processing.

FIGURE 11-20 Radura logo, an international symbol used for irradiated food.

Food irradiation has been slow to gain implementation, perhaps because of resistance from the public and possible higher costs.[87,88] Surveys indicate that about half the US population is ready to accept irradiated foods; this percentage may increase once consumers learn of the benefits of irradiation in reducing the risk of foodborne illness. One irradiated product—ground beef—has been available in supermarkets since 2000. Irradiated foods are identified by the Radura logo shown in Figure 11-20.

Hazard Analysis of Critical Control Points

Hazard analysis of critical control points (HACCP) is a system for reducing the risk of foodborne illness.[89] Using HACCP, foods are monitored from the time of harvest to the time of consumption. The methodology was adopted in the 1950s to assure the safety of food used in the US space program. In the 1990s, the FDA established HACCP for the processing of seafood. During the late 1990s, the US Department of Agriculture, which has regulatory oversight of meat and poultry, initiated HACCP for plants that process these products. HACCP was applied to the juice industry beginning in 2002. The seven principles of HACCP are described in the following text box.

Hazard Analysis of Critical Control Points

1. **Perform a Hazard Analysis.** The first principle is about understanding the operation and determining what food safety hazards are likely to occur. [Examples of hazards are microbes, chemicals, and foreign objects.] The manager needs to understand how the people, equipment, methods, and foods all affect each other. The processes and procedures used to prepare the food are also considered. This usually involves defining the operational steps (receiving, storage, preparation, cooking, etc.) that occur as food enters and moves through the operation. Additionally, this step involves determining the control measures that can be used to eliminate, prevent, or reduce food safety hazards. Control measures include such activities as implementation of employee health policies to restrict or exclude ill employees and proper handwashing.

2. **Decide on the Critical Control Points (CCPs).** Once the control measures in principle #1 are determined, it is necessary to identify which of the control measures are absolutely essential to ensuring safe food. An operational step where control can be applied and is essential for ensuring that a food safety hazard is eliminated, prevented or reduced to an acceptable level is a critical control point (CCP).

3. **Determine the Critical Limits.** Each CCP must have boundaries that define safety. Critical limits are the parameters that must be achieved to control a food safety hazard. For example, when cooking pork chops, the *Food Code* sets the critical limit at 145° F for 15 seconds. When critical limits are not met, the food may not be safe. Critical limits are measurable and observable.

4. **Establish Procedures to Monitor CCPs.** Once CCPs and critical limits have been determined, someone needs to keep track of the CCPs as the food flows through the operation. Monitoring involves making direct observations or measurements to see that the CCPs are kept under control by adhering to the established critical limits.

5. **Establish Corrective Actions.** While monitoring CCPs, occasionally the process or procedure will fail to meet the established critical limits. This step establishes a plan for what happens when a critical limit has not been met at a CCP. The operator decides what the actions will be, communicates those actions to the employees, and trains them in making the right decisions. This preventive approach is the heart of HACCP. Problems will arise, but you need to find them and correct them before they cause illness or injury.

6. **Establish Verification Procedures.** This principle is about making sure that the system is scientifically sound to effectively control the hazards. In addition, this step ensures that the system is operating according to what is specified in the plan. Designated individuals like the manager periodically make observations of employees' monitoring activities, calibrate equipment and temperature measuring devices, review records/actions, and discuss procedures with the employees. . . .

7. **Establish a Record Keeping System.** There are certain written records or kinds of documentation that are needed in order to verify that the system is working. These records will normally involve the HACCP plan itself and any monitoring, corrective action, or calibration records produced in the operation of the HACCP system.

Source: Adapted and reprinted from US Food and Drug Administration, Center for Food Safety and Applied Nutrition. *Managing Food Safety: A Manual for the Voluntary Use of HACCP Principles for Operators of Food Service and Retail Establishments.* OMB Control No. 0910-0578. College Park, MD: US Food and Drug Administration, Center for Food Safety and Applied Nutrition; 2006:9–11.

Investigating and Reporting a Foodborne Outbreak

Tracking the cause of a foodborne disease outbreak requires a great deal of detective work and provides many challenges to local public health departments, which often are charged with the responsibility for safety of foods sold in restaurants, grocery stores, and other establishments. The following list provides examples of steps that may be required in the investigation of foodborne illness following a suspected outbreak:

- Identify as many of the cases involved as possible.
- Describe person, time, and place variables (descriptive epidemiologic characteristics) regarding affected and nonaffected persons who were involved in the outbreak. For affected persons, describe their symptoms, including time of onset.
- List the food items served and compare the occurrence of symptoms between those who ate and those who did not eat each particular food listed.

- Create a map of the cases.
- Collect samples of blood, stools, and vomitus for diagnosis of causative agent.
- Collect samples of implicated foods, if possible, and subject to analysis.
- Take corrective actions, as necessary, such as recalling suspected foods.[90]

Employment Roles in Food Safety

Many employment roles, particularly in the government sector, relate to food safety. Restaurant inspectors are responsible for overseeing the safety of foods served in local restaurants. Epidemiologists investigate outbreaks of foodborne illness in their communities. Microbiologists are crucial to the identification of microbes that may be present in foods. The US federal government employs inspectors who are involved with the processing of food animals. The following paragraphs describe the role of food inspectors:

Entry-level food inspectors in private commercial slaughtering plants provide the first line of defense against diseased and adulterated meat and poultry. They are responsible for much of the day-to-day in-plant inspection of animals before and after slaughter.

One career path for a food inspector is to the consumer safety inspector position. Consumer safety inspectors work in one or more privately owned meat, poultry, and egg processing plants. They ensure the plant is operating within its written plans for HACCP, sanitation, and processing.

In addition, they conduct regulatory oversight activities inside the plants in matters relating to other areas of consumer protection, e.g., misbranding.

Another career path for a food inspector is to the import inspector position. Import inspectors are stationed at ports and other points of entry to the United States. They make sure that products imported from other countries are as safe as those produced domestically.[91]

CONCLUSION

This chapter covered food safety, including the causes and prevention of foodborne illness and regulations to protect the safety of the food supply at the international, national, and local levels. Foodborne illness is a major cause of morbidity and mortality in the developing world and also is a growing source of concern for developed countries. Estimates indicate that foodborne illness impacts one-quarter to one-third of the US population each year; also, foodborne illness can be a vexing problem for the closed environments of cruise ships.

Foodborne hazards include biological, chemical, and physical contaminants. Of growing concern for the safety of the food supply are emerging foodborne disease pathogens. Other potential threats to the food supply are residues of pesticides, medicines administered to food animals, genetically modified foods, and additives in foods. In the United States, numerous statutes regulate the quality of the food supply. These statutes are monitored and enforced by regulatory agencies such as the FDA and the USDA as well as by state and local authorities. As a consequence of regulatory and enforcement actions, the food supply of the United States is regarded as one of world's safest.

Study Questions and Exercises

1. Define the following terms:
   a. Foodborne disease
   b. Foodborne outbreak
   c. Passive versus active surveillance systems
   d. Food additive
   e. Radura logo

2. Describe the categories of hazards that may be present in foods and suggest methods for their control or prevention.

3. Name two emerging foodborne disease pathogens. Select one of them and describe an outbreak that involved the pathogen. Describe how foodborne disease outbreaks caused by the pathogen can be prevented.

4. Give examples of pesticides that have caused food-associated poisoning. To what extent can these poisonings be prevented?

5. State the names of two microbial agents of foodborne disease that occur among food animals. Give examples of how these agents may be transmitted by foods and suggest methods for prevention of their occurrence among animals used for food.

6. What foodborne pathogen has been associated with stillbirths? What foods have been suspected of carrying the pathogen? Suggest methods of prevention of foodborne illness from this cause.

7. Name the agent responsible for trichinosis. What foods may be responsible for passing trichinosis to human hosts? To what extent do you believe trichinosis currently poses a hazard to the US food supply? Discuss methods for prevention of trichinosis.

8. What types of microbial agents have been linked to outbreaks of illnesses on cruise ships? What can be done to prevent such outbreaks?

9. Name three acts and/or amendments that regulate food safety in the United States. Describe their purposes and the types of foods and components of foods to which they apply.

10. Give examples of international and national agencies charged with the enforcement of food safety regulations. Contact your state and local health departments and write a brief description of their activities with respect to enforcement of food safety.

11. Discuss the risk factors for foodborne illness. Describe practical methods for the prevention of foodborne illness and indicate how you apply them in your own home or business.

12. What are the procedures that a local health department might use for investigating an outbreak of foodborne illness? (Refer to Exhibit 11-2). What factors could have been responsible for the *S. aureus* outbreak described in the exhibit?

REFERENCES

1. Heymann DL, ed. *Control of Communicable Diseases Manual.* 19th ed. Washington, DC: American Public Health Association; 2008.

2. Rocourt J, Moy G, Vierk K, et al. *The Present State of Foodborne Diseases in OECD Countries.* Geneva, Switzerland: World Health Organization; 2003.

3. Altekruse SF, Cohen ML, Swerdlow DL. Emerging foodborne diseases. *Emerg Infect Dis.* 1997;3:285–293.

4. McMeekin TA, Brown J, Krist K, et al. Quantitative microbiology: a basis for food safety. *Emerg Infect Dis.* 1997;3:541–549.

5. Centers for Disease Control and Prevention. Preliminary FoodNet data on the incidence of infection with pathogens transmitted commonly through food—10 states, 2009. *MMWR.* 2010;59:418–422.

6. Gist GL. Emerging foodborne diseases and NEHA's response. *J Environ Health.* 1999;61:4,61.

7. Centers for Disease Control and Prevention. FoodNet surveillance—what is FoodNet? Available at: http://www.cdc.gov/foodnet/surveillance_pages/whatisfoodnet.htm. Accessed February 22, 2010.

8. Centers for Disease Control and Prevention. FoodNet surveillance—burden of illness pyramid. Available at: http://www.cdc.gov/foodnet/surveillance_pages/burden_pyramid.htm. Accessed February 22, 2010.

9. University of Nebraska Cooperative Extension. Food Safety, HACCP, Physical hazards. Available at: http://foodsafety.unl.edu/haccp/start/physical.html. Accessed April 27, 2010.

10. Morse SS. Factors in the emergence of infectious diseases. *Emerg Infect Dis.* 1995;1:7–15.

11. Woteki CE, Kineman BD. Challenges and approaches to reducing foodborne illness. *Annu Rev Nutr.* 2003;23:315–344.

12. Osterholm MT. Emerging infections—another warning [editorial]. *New Engl J Med.* 2000;342:1280–1281.

13. Centers for Disease Control and Prevention. Multistate outbreak of *Salmonella* serotype Agona infections linked to toasted oats cereal—United States, April–May, 1998. *MMWR.* 1998;47:462–464.

14. Trevejo RT, Courtney JG, Starr M, et al. Epidemiology of salmonellosis in California, 1990–1999: morbidity, mortality, and hospitalization costs. *Am J Epidemiol.* 2003;157:48–57.

15. Centers for Disease Control and Prevention. *Salmonella* surveillance: Annual Summary, 2006. Atlanta, Georgia: US Department of Health and Human Services, CDC; 2008.

16. US Food and Drug Administration, Center for Food Safety and Applied Nutrition. Bad bug book—*Salmonella* spp. Available at: http://www.fda.gov/Food/FoodSafety/FoodborneIllness/FoodborneIllnessFoodbornePathogensNaturalToxins/BadBugBook/ucm069966.htm. Accessed April 27, 2010.

17. Centers for Disease Control and Prevention. Multistate outbreak of *Salmonella* serotype Typhimurium infections associated with drinking unpasteurized milk—Illinois, Indiana, Ohio, and Tennessee, 2002–2003. *MMWR.* 2003;52:613–615.

18. Centers for Disease Control and Prevention. Multistate outbreaks of *Salmonella* serotype Poona infections associated with eating cantaloupe from Mexico—United States and Canada, 2000–2002. *MMWR.* 2002;51:1044–1047.

19. Van Beneden CA, Keene WE, Strang RA, et al. Multinational outbreak of *Salmonella enterica* serotype Newport infections due to contaminated alfalfa sprouts. *JAMA.* 1999;281:158–162.

20. Centers for Disease Control and Prevention. Epidemiologic notes and reports update: milk-borne salmonellosis—Illinois. *MMWR.* 1985;34:215–216.

21. White DG, Zhao S, Sudler R, et al. The isolation of antibiotic-resistant *Salmonella* from retail ground meats. *New Engl J Med.* 2001;345:1147–1154.

22. Centers for Disease Control and Prevention. Outbreak of multidrug-resistant *Salmonella* Newport—United States, January–April 2002. *MMWR.* 2002;51:545–548.

23. US Food and Drug Administration, Center for Food Safety and Applied Nutrition. Bad bug book—*Clostridium botulinum.* Available at: http://www.fda.gov/Food/FoodSafety/FoodborneIllness/FoodborneIllnessFoodbornePathogensNaturalToxins/BadBugBook/ucm070000.htm. Accessed April 26, 2010.

24. Centers for Disease Control and Prevention. Foodborne botulism—Oklahoma, 1994. *MMWR.* 1995;44:200–202.

25. Centers for Disease Control and Prevention. Foodborne botulism from eating home-pickled eggs—Illinois, 1997. *MMWR.* 2000;49:778–780.

26. US Food and Drug Administration, Center for Food Safety and Applied Nutrition. Bad bug book—*Clostridium perfringens.* Available at: http://www.fda.gov/Food/FoodSafety/FoodborneIllness/FoodborneIllnessFoodbornePathogensNaturalToxins/BadBugBook/ucm070483.htm. Accessed April 26, 2010.

27. Centers for Disease Control and Prevention. Clostridium perfringens gastroenteritis associated with corned beef served at St. Patrick's Day meals—Ohio and Virginia, 1993. *MMWR.* 1994;43:137–138, 143–144.

28. US Food and Drug Administration, Center for Food Safety and Applied Nutrition. Bad bug book—*Staphylococcus aureus.* Available at: http://www.fda.gov/Food/FoodSafety/FoodborneIllness/FoodborneIllnessFoodbornePathogensNaturalToxins/BadBugBook/ucm070015.htm. Accessed April 26, 2010.

29. Centers for Disease Control and Prevention. Outbreak of Staphylococcal food poisoning associated with precooked ham—Florida, 1997. *MMWR.* 1997;46:1189–1191.

30. Centers for Disease Control and Prevention. Update: multistate outbreak of *Escherichia coli* O157:H7 infections from hamburgers—western United States, 1992–1993. *MMWR.* 1993;42:258–263.

31. Crump JA, Sulka AC, Langer AJ, et al. An outbreak of *Escherichia coli* O157:H7 infections among visitors to a dairy farm. *New Engl J Med.* 2002;347:555–560.

32. Mead PS, Slutsker L, Dietz V, et al. Food-related illness and death in the United States. *Emerg Infect Dis.* 1999;5:607–625.

33. US Food and Drug Administration, Center for Food Safety and Applied Nutrition. Bad bug book—*Escherichia coli* O157:H7. Available at: http://www.fda.gov/Food/FoodSafety/FoodborneIllness/FoodborneIllnessFoodbornePathogensNaturalToxins/BadBugBook/ucm071284.htm. Accessed April 26, 2010.

34. US Food and Drug Administration, Center for Food Safety and Applied Nutrition. Bad bug book—*Shigella* spp. Available at: http://www.fda.gov/Food/FoodSafety/FoodborneIllness/FoodborneIllnessFoodbornePathogensNaturalToxins/BadBugBook/ucm070563.htm. Accessed April 26, 2010.

35. Altekruse SF, Stern NJ, Fields PI, et al. *Campylobacter jejuni*—an emerging foodborne pathogen. *Emerg Infect Dis.* 1999;5:28–35.

36. Centers for Disease Control and Prevention. Outbreak of *Campylobacter jejuni* infections associated with drinking unpasteurized milk procured through a cow-leasing program—Wisconsin, 2001. *MMWR.* 2002;51:548–549.

37. Beuchat LR. *Listeria monocytogenes*: incidence on vegetables. *Food Control.* 1996;7:223–228.

38. Centers for Disease Control and Prevention. Division of Foodborne, Bacterial and Mycotic Diseases (DFBMD). Disease listing: Listeriosis. Available at: http://www.cdc.gov/nczved/dfbmd/disease_listing/listeriosis_gi.html. Accessed February 22, 2010.

39. Centers for Disease Control and Prevention. Public health dispatch: outbreak of listeriosis—northeastern United States, 2002. *MMWR.* 2002;51:950–951.

40. Centers for Disease Control and Prevention. Parasites and health:

trichinellosis. Available at: http://www.dpd.cdc.gov/dpdx/HTML/Trichinellosis/htm. Accessed April 27, 2010.

41. Centers for Disease Control and Prevention. Parasitic disease information. Fact sheet: trichinellosis. Available at: http://www.cdc.gov/ncidod/dpd/parasites/trichinosis/factsht_trichinosis.htm. Accessed April 27, 2010.

42. Centers for Disease Control and Prevention. Trichinosis—Maine, Alaska. *MMWR*. 1986;35:33–35.

43. Centers for Disease Control and Prevention. DPDx. Parasites and health: taeniasis. Available at: http://www.dpd.cdc.gov/dpdx/html/taeniasis.htm. Accessed April 27, 2010.

44. US Food and Drug Administration, Center for Food Safety and Applied Nutrition. Bad bug book—Hepatitis A virus. Available at: http://www.fda.gov/Food/FoodSafety/FoodborneIllness/FoodborneIllnessFoodbornePathogensNaturalToxins/BadBugBook/ucm071294.htm. Accessed April 26, 2010

45. Hutin YJF, Pool V, Cramer EH, et al. A multistate, foodborne outbreak of hepatitis A. *New Engl J Med*. 1999;340:595–602.

46. Acheson DWK, Fiore AE. Preventing foodborne disease—what clinicians can do. *New Engl J Med*. 2004;350:437–440.

47. Centers for Disease Control and Prevention. Outbreaks of gastroenteritis associated with noroviruses on cruise ships—United States, 2002. *MMWR*. 2002;51:1112–1115.

48. Larkin M. Passengers implicated in gastroenteritis outbreaks on cruise ships. *Lancet*. 2002;360:2052.

49. Charatan F. Viral gastroenteritis sickens hundreds on cruise ships. *BMJ*. 2002;325:1192.

50. Centers for Disease Control and Prevention. Vessel Sanitation Program. Investigation update on the *Carnival Legend*. Investigation update—February 4, 2003. Available at: http://www.cdc.gov/nceh/vsp/surv/outbreak/2003/update_feb4.htm. Accessed February 22, 2010.

51. Cramer EH, Gu DX, Durbin RE, et al. Diarrheal disease on cruise ships, 1990–2000: the impact of environmental health programs. *Am J Prev Med*. 2003;24:227–233.

52. Centers for Disease Control and Prevention. BSE (Bovine spongiform encephalopathy, or mad cow disease). Available at: http://www.cdc.gov/ncidod/dvrd/bse/. Accessed May 4, 2010.

53. Centers for Disease Control and Prevention. Division of Bacterial and Mycotic Diseases. Disease listing: marine toxins. Available at: http://www.cdc.gov/ncidod/dbmd/diseaseinfo/marinetoxins_g.htm. Accessed April 27, 2010.

54. US Food and Drug Administration, Center for Food Safety and Applied Nutrition. Bad bug book—mushroom toxins. Available at: http://www.fda.gov/Food/FoodSafety/FoodborneIllness/FoodborneIllnessFoodbornePathogensNaturalToxins/BadBugBook/ucm070853.htm. Accessed April 26, 2010.

55. U.S. Food and Drug Administration. Supporting document for recommended maximum level for lead in candy likely to be consumed frequently by small children. Available at: http://www.fda.gov/Food/FoodSafety/FoodContaminantsAdulteration/Metals/Lead/ucm172050.htm. Accessed April 26, 2010.

56. Lasky T, Sun W, Kadry A, et al. Mean total arsenic concentrations in chicken 1989–2000 and estimated exposures for consumers of chicken. *Environ Health Perspect*. 2004;112:18–21.

57. Fattore E, Fanelli R, La Vecchia C. Persistent organic pollutants in food: public health implications. *J Epidemiol Community Health*. 2002;56:831–832.

58. Pesticides in baby food. *Environ Health Perspect*. 1995;103:1082–1083.

59. Centers for Disease Control and Prevention. Epidemiologic notes and reports aldicarb food poisoning from contaminated melons—California. *MMWR*. 1986;35:254–258.

60. McEwen SA, Fedorka-Cray PJ. Antimicrobial use and resistance in animals. *Clin Infect Dis*. 2002;34(suppl 3):S93–S106.

61. Greenlees KJ. Animal drug human food safety toxicology and antimicrobial resistance—the square peg. *Int J Toxicol*. 2003;22:131–134.

62. Council on Scientific Affairs, American Medical Association. Biotechnology and the American agricultural industry. *JAMA*. 1991;265:1429–1436.

63. Bouis HE, Chassy BM, Ochanda JO. Genetically modified food crops and their contribution to human nutrition and food quality. *Trends Food Sci Technol*. 2003;14:191–209.

64. Jones L. Science, medicine and the future: genetically modified foods. *BMJ*. 1999;318:581–584.

65. EH Update: NRC reports on concerns about animal biotechnology. *J Environ Health*. 2003;65(6):42.

66. Bosch X. Europe imposes strict GM-food laws. *Lancet*. 2003;362:135.

67. Kishore GM, Shewmaker C. Biotechnology: enhancing human nutrition in developing and developed worlds. *Proc Natl Acad Sci USA*. 1999;96:5968–5972.

68. MedlinePlus. Medical encyclopedia: food additives. Available at: http://www.nlm.nih.gov/medlineplus/ency/article/002435.htm. Accessed April 26, 2010.

69. US Food and Drug Administration. CFR—Code of Federal Regulations Title 21—Food and Drugs. Available at: http://www.accessdata.fda.gov/scripts/cdrh/cfdocs/cfcfr/CFRSearch.cfm?fr=182.3798. Accessed May 7, 2010.

70. Padilla-Zakour O. Chemical food preservatives: proprionates and parabens. New York State Agricultural Experiment Center, Cornell University. *Venture*, Summer 1998. Available at: http://www.nysaes.cornell.edu/necfe/pubs/pdf/Venture/venture3_chemical.html. Accessed April 27, 2010.

71. Merrill RA. Food safety regulation: reforming the Delaney Clause. *Annu Rev Public Health*. 1997;18:313–340.

72. US Food and Drug Administration. FDA History—Part II: The 1938 Food, Drug, and Cosmetic Act. Available at: http://www.fda.gov/AboutFDA/WhatWeDo/History/Origin/ucm054826.htm. Accessed April 27, 2010.

73. US Department of Health and Human Services, Food and Drug Administration. Proposed rules: substances generally recognized as safe. *Federal Register*. 1997;62(74):18937–18964.

74. Lee G. In food safety changes, victories for many. *The Washington Post*. July 28, 1996:A4.

75. US Environmental Protection Agency. About the Region 6 pesticide program. Available at: http://www.epa.gov/region6/6pd/pd-p/index.htm. Accessed April 26, 2010.

76. United Nations Food and Agriculture Organization. World markets for organic fruit and vegetables—Chapter 4: assistance to developing countries in organic agriculture. 2001. Available at: http://www.fao.org/docrep/004/y1669e/y1669e0o.htm. Accessed April 27, 2010.

77. United States Department of Agriculture, Food Safety and Inspection Service. About FSIS. Available at: http://www.fsis.usda.gov/about_fsis/index.asp. Accessed April 26, 2010.

78. US Food and Drug Administration, Center for Food Safety and Applied Nutrition. CFSAN—What we do. Available at: http://www.fda.gov/AboutFDA/CentersOffices/CFSAN/WhatWeDo/default.htm. Accessed April 28, 2010.

79. Centers for Disease Control and Prevention. Food Safety Office Programs and Activities. Available at: http://www.cdc.gov/foodsafety/activities.html. Accessed April 28, 2010.

80. California Department of Public Health, Food and Drug Branch. Available at: http://www.cdph.ca.gov/programs/Pages/FDB.aspx. Accessed April 29, 2010.

81. City of Long Beach, Health and Human Services. Food facility in-

spection program. Available at: http://www.longbeach.gov/health/eh/food/default.asp. Accessed April 26, 2010.

82. County of Los Angeles Department of Public Health. Environmental Health: Bureau of District Environmental Services. Available at: http://www.lapublichealth.org/eh/progs/des/ehdes.htm. Accessed April 26, 2010.

83. Riverside County Community Health Agency. Department of Environmental Health. Available at: http://www.rivcoeh.org/opencms/index.html. Accessed April 26, 2010.

84. Collins JE. Impact of changing consumer lifestyles on the emergence/reemergence of foodborne pathogens. *Emerg Infect Dis*. 1997;3:471–479.

85. Irradiation enhances food safety and quality. [press release] American Council on Science and Health; May 14, 2003. Available at: http://www.acsh.org/news/newsID.200/news_detail.asp. Accessed February 22, 2010.

86. Wood OB, Bruhn CM. Position of the American Dietetic Association: food irradiation. *J Am Diet Assoc*. 2000;100:246–253.

87. Tauxe RV. Food safety and irradiation: protecting the public from foodborne infections. *Emerg Infect Dis*. 2001;7(3 suppl):516–521.

88. Osterholm MT, Potter ME. Irradiation pasteurization of solid foods: taking food safety to the next level. *Emerg Infect Dis*. 1997;3:575–577.

89. University of Rhode Island, Cooperative Extension Food Safety Education. Hazard Analysis of Critical Control Points (HACCP) principles. Available at: http://www.uri.edu/ce/ceec/food/factsheets/haacp.html. Accessed February 22, 2010.

90. Centers for Disease Control and Prevention, Division of Bacterial and Mycotic Diseases. Foodborne illness. How is a foodborne disease outbreak investigated? Available at: http://www.cdc.gov/ncidod/dbmd/diseasinfo/foodborneinfections_g.htm#howoutbreaksdetected. Accessed April 26, 2010.

91. United States Department of Agriculture, Food Safety and Inspection Service. Career opportunities: Food inspector & consumer safety inspector positions. Available at: http://www.fsis.usda.gov/careers/Food_Inspector_&_Consumer_Safety_Inspection_Positions/index.asp. Accessed April 26, 2010.

Solid and Liquid Wastes

INTRODUCTION

This chapter covers two crucial topics for modern society—disposal of solid wastes and treatment and processing of liquid wastes. The first part of this chapter will consider the history of solid waste disposal, challenges caused by the growing volume of waste, and advantages and disadvantages of various methods for waste disposal. This part of the chapter also will review proposed solutions for reduction in solid waste (e.g., source reduction, recycling, and composting). The second part of the chapter will cover the topic of disposal of liquid wastes, including sewage and animal wastes.

The term **waste** is used to describe materials that are perceived to be of negative value.[1] Why should citizens be concerned about waste disposal? One reason is that acute problems can occur if wastes are not disposed of properly. A major concern for waste disposal is the pollution that can result from the process of disposal.[1] The term **hazardous waste** refers to "[b]y-products of society that can pose a substantial or potential hazard to human health or the environment

when improperly managed. [Hazardous waste] [p]ossesses at least one of four characteristics (ignitability, corrosivity, reactivity, or toxicity), or appears on special EPA lists."[2] The term **pollution** "can be defined as the introduction into the natural environment by humans of substances, materials, or energy that cause hazards to human health, harm to living resources and ecological systems, damage to structures and amenities or that interfere with the legitimate uses of the environment."[1(p72)]

Continuing increases in the volume of waste are exacerbating the difficult problem of waste disposal; in some regions of the world, including parts of the United States, space reserved for dump sites is being rapidly depleted. Consequently, during the 21st century much work will need to be done by the global society to cope with its growing output of solid wastes. In addition, a particularly acute problem is the fact that the burgeoning populations of less developed countries are introducing large amounts of liquid wastes directly into waterways and oceans without adequate processing. The presence of such wastes endangers already limited drinking water supplies as well as the viability of aquatic environments.

HISTORICAL BACKGROUND—SOLID WASTE DISPOSAL

The concept of waste management is relatively recent; until the 20th century, the individual was responsible for discarding wastes. Often wastes were discarded carelessly into the environment. The efficient processes that have been realized in the United States and other developed countries were not available early in the 20th century. Since that time, the waste management industry in the United States has evolved to the

FIGURE 12-1 A dumping ground (1866) and street scenes in New York City (1881) demonstrate unsanitary conditions.

Stanley Fox
Dumping ground at the foot of Beach Street, New York City

HAPPY THOUGHT! We return to the simple ways of our grandfathers, and our streets are cleaned once again—more or less.

HYGEIA. "You doubtless think that as all this filth is lying out in the back streets, it is no concern of yours. But you are mistaken. You will find it stealing into your house very soon, if you don't take care."

Street scene in New York

Source: Adapted and reprinted from the US National Library of Medicine, National Institutes of Health, Images from the History of Medicine. Available at: http:/www.nlm.nih.gov. Accessed August 28, 2010.

point where many individuals discard waste without thinking about its ultimate fate. Although some people resent contemporary legislative proposals directed toward abatement of wastes and penalties that are levied against those persons and industries that discharge wastes illegally, almost all people dislike pollution. It is ironic that at the same time, some of the same people who dislike pollution do not recognize that they contribute to the pollution problem through their own consumption practices.[1] For example, foods are wasted and recyclable items are thrown into the trash pile.

New York City, Early 20th Century

The following passage provides a graphic description of the status of solid waste disposal in New York City during the late 19th and early 20th century:

> Until the years following the Civil War, New York City had no municipal health department, no sanitation department, no public water system that could provide pure water to a population that was literally doubling in size every 10 to 15 years. The city was powered, quite literally, by horses—well over 100,000 of them—each depositing between 20 and 25

pounds of manure on the city's streets each day. Dead horses, pigs, goats, and other animals littered the streets and mixed with the overflow of outdoor privies located behind the tenements, shacks, and shanties that housed the city's poor. In 1880, 15,000 horse carcasses were removed from the city's streets; by 1912, over 20,000 horses, cattle, mules, and donkeys were being removed.[3(p14)]

The early methods for waste disposal in New York City were quite primitive and sometimes consisted of dumping garbage into rivers. The sketches and cartoons in Figure 12-1 depict unsanitary conditions in New York City during the mid- to late-19th century.

The Growing Solid Waste Problem

Trash or garbage also is called **municipal solid waste (MSW)**. In 2008, the United States—residents, businesses, and institutions—produced approximately 250 million tons of MSW (before recycling). This amount translates to approximately 4.5 pounds of waste per person per day, which was almost twice the amount for 1960.[4] Refer to Figure 12-2 for trends in MSW generation.

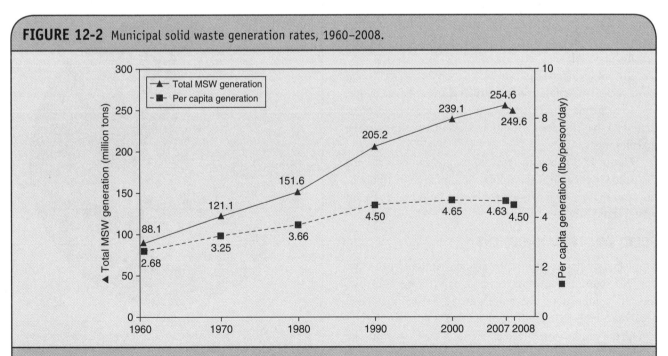

FIGURE 12-2 Municipal solid waste generation rates, 1960–2008.

Source: Adapted and reprinted from US Environmental Protection Agency, Solid Waste and Emergency Response (5306P). Municipal Solid Waste Generation, Recycling, and Disposal in the United States: Facts and Figures for 2008. Washington, DC: US Environmental Protection Agency; 2009, p.1.

Along with the increasing amounts of solid waste that are being produced by US citizens, the expense of disposing of MSW is increasing over time. In areas of the Midwest that at one time had abundant space for waste disposal, landfills are filling up and closing.[5] The shutting down of landfills has caused disposal fees, known as tipping fees, to increase substantially. Average tipping fees per ton in the midwestern United States increased from about $25 in the late 1990s to approximately $30 in 2003. However, at the national level, lack of availability of disposal sites presently does not seem to be a problem.[6]

The problem of waste disposal is not confined to developed countries. The less developed areas of the world also have shown an increase in the amount of solid waste production. Although there are abundant examples, take the case of China. Urban residents of China have experienced a rise in their living standard that has caused a rapid increase in the annual amount of domestic garbage. Now the average city dweller in China produces about 2.5 pounds (about 1.2 kilograms) of garbage per day.[7] This growing waste problem is paralleled in other parts of the developing world.

COMPONENTS OF THE MUNICIPAL SOLID WASTE STREAM

Solid waste includes the subset of materials referred to as municipal solid waste plus other types of solid waste. The components of the municipal solid waste stream include packaging, furniture, clothing, bottles, food waste, papers, batteries, and organic materials such as grass clippings from landscaping.[4] Usually not included as part of MSW are other types of solid waste such as materials from construction sites, sewage sludge, and some forms of industrial wastes that are not hazardous. Refer to Table 12-1 for a list of materials that typically make up solid waste.

Figure 12-3 shows the relative proportion of materials discarded in the municipal solid waste stream. The figure illustrates that paper makes up the largest percentage of solid waste, about 31%.

SOLID WASTE MANAGEMENT

Municipal solid waste disposal is an industrial enterprise that has four main dimensions: recycling, landfilling, composting, and combustion.[8] Refer to Figure 12-4: Note that when MSW decomposes in landfills or is combusted, a by-product can be the production of useful energy. This energy may be produced from methane gas that seeps from disposal sites or by combustion.

The US Environmental Protection Agency (EPA) has developed a hierarchy for the management of MSW.[6] Proce-

---

TABLE 12-1 Some Types of Solid Waste

Municipal solid waste (trash, garbage, refuse)—items that people discard; see Figure 12-3 for a description.

Construction and demolition materials (e.g., concrete, wood, asphalt, and gypsum)

Special wastes (e.g., cement kiln dust, mining waste, oil and gas drilling muds and oil production brines, phosphate rock mining, uranium waste, utility waste from fossil fuel burning)

Medical waste

Discarded material, including solid, liquid, semi-solid, and contained gaseous materials resulting from:
- Industrial and commercial activities
- Mining
- Agricultural activities
- Community activities

Sludge (biosolids) from wastewater treatment and water supply treatment

Source: Adapted from US Environmental Protection Agency. Wastes. Available at: http://www.epa.gov/epawaste. Accessed June 16, 2010.

FIGURE 12-3 Total municipal solid waste generation (by material), 2008—250 million tons (before recycling).

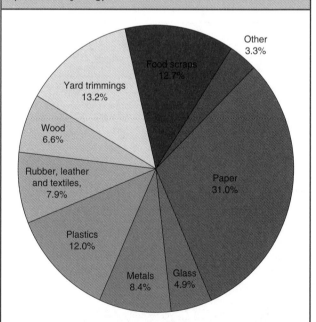

Source: Adapted and reprinted from US Environmental Protection Agency, Solid Waste and Emergency Response (5306P). Municipal Solid Waste Generation, Recycling, and Disposal in the United States: Facts and Figures for 2008. Washington, DC: US Environmental Protection Agency; 2009, p. 4.

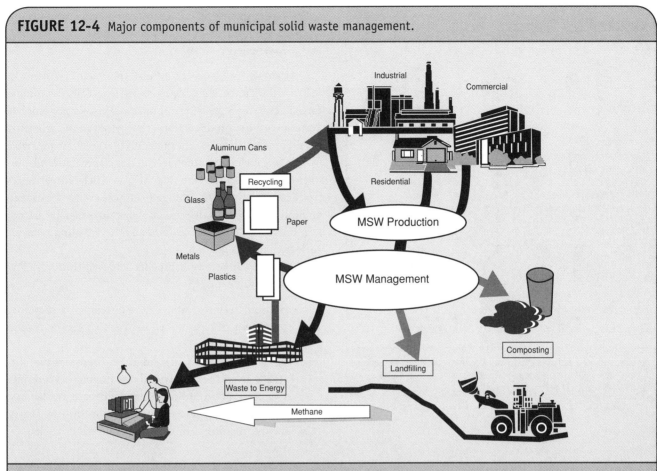

FIGURE 12-4 Major components of municipal solid waste management.

Source: Reprinted from US Department of Energy, Energy Information Administration, Office of Coal, Nuclear, Electric and Alternate Fuels. Available at: http://www.eia.doe.gov/cneaf/solar.renewables/renewable.energy.annual/backgrnd/fig8.htm. Accessed May 2, 2010.

dures at the top of the hierarchy are favored over those at the bottom. The hierarchy is as follows:

- Source reduction (or waste prevention), including reuse of products and onsite, or backyard, composting of yard trimmings.
- Recycling, including offsite, or community, composting.
- Disposal, including waste combustion (preferably with energy recovery) and landfilling.[6(p11)]

Source Reduction

The term **source reduction** refers to "*reducing* the amount of waste created, reusing whenever possible, and then recycling what is left."[6(p11)] Through source reduction, the volume of solid waste that must be deposited in landfills is limited. Two important components of source reduction are *waste reduc-*

tion and *waste recycling*. Waste reduction aims to reduce the amount of waste produced at the source. Waste recycling refers to reuse of materials in the waste.[9] Figure 12-5 shows some of the programs that may be used to achieve source reduction.

The following are examples of source reduction methods that prevent waste from entering disposal channels:

- Financial incentives to homeowners, for example, PAYT, an acronym that refers to "pay-as-you-throw."[5] Municipalities that use the PAYT system require that the amount that residents pay for trash pickup is proportional to the amount of trash that they generate.[10] To illustrate, in a hypothetical PAYT system, residents would purchase stickers for a set price such as $1 each and would affix them to each trash bag disposed. Residents could save money by disposing of fewer bags of trash.[5]

FIGURE 12-5 Programs for recycling wastes.

Reuse Center   Grass cycling   Home Composting

Pay As You Throw   Business Recycling   Business Composting

Drop-Off Recycling Center   Home Yard Trimmings Pick-up   Home Recycling Pick-up (Standard)

Source: Adapted and reprinted from US Environmental Protection Agency. Recycle City, Dumptown Game. Available at: http://www.epa.gov/recyclecity/gameint.htm. Accessed March 25, 2010.

- Improved packaging designs that reduce the amount of materials that must be discarded (e.g., the use of smaller packages for products).
- Design products, such as refillable bottles, that can be reused.
- Design products that have longer service lives so that they will not need to be disposed of so often (e.g., longer-lasting tires for vehicles).

Recycling

The EPA defines **recycling** (reuse) as the process of "Minimizing waste generation by recovering and reprocessing usable products that might otherwise become waste (i.e., recycling of aluminum cans, paper, and bottles, etc.)."[11] The advantages of recycling include the following[12]:

- Reduces emissions of greenhouse gases
- Prevents pollution generated by the use of new materials
- Decreases the amount of materials shipped to landfills, thereby reducing the need for new landfills
- Preserves natural resources

- Opens up new manufacturing employment opportunities and increases US competitiveness
- Saves energy

As shown in Figure 12-6 (left), the rate of recycling of MSW in the United States has increased from 6.4% (5.6 million tons) in 1960 to 33.2% (82.9 million tons) in 2008; automobile batteries are the products that are recycled most frequently (99+% of auto batteries). The materials that are most amenable to recycling include automobile batteries, paper, and landscaping materials. Although they may be placed in landfills, wastes from construction sites, sludge from wastewater treatment, and industrial wastes that are nonhazardous usually are not termed MSW.[13] Figure 12-6 presents the recycling rates for various materials in 2008.

Examples of accomplishments achieved through recycling are the following:

- Missouri (United States) has developed a recycling program that has resulted in diverting 41% of its solid waste stream.[5]
- Japan: The problem of solid waste disposal is very difficult, given the country's dense population, productive economy, and limited landfill space availability. In April 2000, Japanese municipal governments began a recycling program for plastic and paper packaging waste.[9]
- Germany: A very effective program for waste management and recycling of waste is in place. The German city of Freiburg has developed a noteworthy system for waste management.[9]

Composting

Composting is defined as "the aerobic biological decomposition of organic materials [e.g., leaves, grass, and food scraps] to produce a stable humus-like product. . . . Biodegradation is a natural, ongoing biological process that is a common occurrence in both human-made and natural environments."[14(p7–8)] Composting produces a useful material that resembles soil and that can be used in gardening. According to the EPA, composting has the potential for reducing greatly the amount of materials that must be disposed of in landfills, as about one-quarter of household wastes consists of clippings from gardens and food waste.

Some types of materials are acceptable for composting, whereas others are not appropriate. According to the EPA, some food products such as meats may yield poor quality compost or be a magnet for vermin. If you anticipate constructing your own compost bin, refer to Table 12-2 for a list

FIGURE 12-6 Above: Municipal solid waste recycling rates, 1960–2008. Below: Recycling rates of selected products, 2008.*

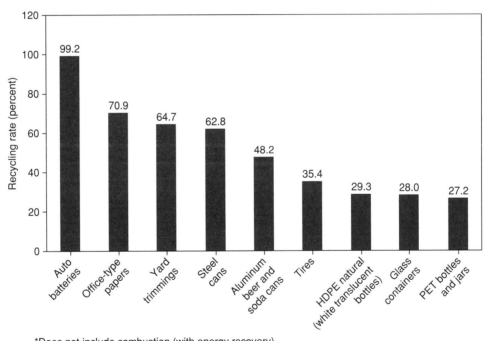

*Does not include combustion (with energy recovery).

Source: Adapted and reprinted from US Environmental Protection Agency, Solid Waste and Emergency Response (5306P). Municipal Solid Waste Generation, Recycling, and Disposal in the United States: Facts and Figures for 2008. Washington, DC: US Environmental Protection Agency; 2009, pp. 2, 3.

TABLE 12-2 Materials to Include and Exclude in Compost

Materials to Include	Materials to Exclude
Animal manure	Black walnut tree leaves or
Cardboard rolls	twigs
Clean paper	Coal or charcoal ash
Coffee grounds and filters	Dairy products
Cotton rags	Diseased or insect-ridden
Dryer and vacuum cleaner	plants
lint	Fats, grease, lard, or oils
Eggshells	Meat or fish bones and scraps
Fireplace ashes	Pet wastes
Fruits and vegetables	Yard trimmings treated with
Grass clippings	chemical pesticides
Hair and fur	
Hay and straw	
Houseplants	
Leaves	
Nut shells	
Sawdust	
Shredded newspaper	
Tea bags	
Wood chips	
Wool rags	
Yard trimmings	

Source: Adapted and reprinted from US Environmental Protection Agency. Composting: Basic information. Available at: http://www.epa.gov/epawaste/conserve/rrr/composting/basic.htm. Accessed March 25, 2010.

(although not all-inclusive) of acceptable and unacceptable materials to include.

Composting breaks down organic materials through the action of physical and chemical processes. If you dig through your own backyard compost pile, you may notice that the temperature of the materials in the compost pile can become quite high. In compost piles that have been maintained properly, optimal temperatures can reach 32°–60°C (90°–140°F) as a result of microbial action.[14] These high temperatures are believed to kill off many harmful components such as pathogenic bacteria, weed seeds, and insect larvae. Nevertheless, a criticism of composting is that it may be insufficient to eliminate pathogenic agents present in the materials that are being composted.[1]

Various types of microorganisms are very important in composting. Other organisms such as invertebrates (e.g., beetles, sowbugs, and earthworms) aid in decomposing the

materials when these living organisms have adequate oxygen and water (provided by well-designed compost bins); however, they play a lesser role in composting than do microorganisms.[14] A specific type of composting, known as vermicomposting (composting by a special kind of earthworm), puts red wigglers to work consuming food scraps and uses their castings as a rich garden fertilizer.

The state of Massachusetts has one of the most successful composting programs in the United States.[15] Yard and food waste are composted, preventing 37,500 tons of waste from entering the disposal process and saving approximately $2 million each year. The state's Department of Environmental Protection Recycling Equipment Grants Program supports the purchase of compost bins. Figure 12-7 shows a citizen at work in a compost program and an example of a compost bin.

The island of Crete, located in the Mediterranean, has developed a noteworthy procedure for composting organic solid wastes.[16] The island has been faced with increasing desertification (gradual conversion of land into desert), exhaustion of landfill capacity for waste disposal, and a chronic lack of organic material for agricultural soils. The island operates programs for composting agricultural organic wastes (e.g., olive leaves, branches, and pressed grape skins), manure, and sewage sludge. The resulting compost will have potential applications for agriculture and landscaping.

Landfills

Materials that cannot be recycled or composted need to be deposited in landfills. A landfill is composed of four major parts: a bottom liner, a system for collecting leachates, a cover, and an appropriate location that minimizes the contamination of groundwater by materials released from the site.[17] The term **leachate** refers to "[w]ater that collects contaminants as it trickles through wastes, pesticides or fertilizers. Leaching may occur in farming areas, feedlots, and landfills, and may result in hazardous substances entering surface water, ground water, or soil."[18] The typical design of a landfill is as follows: The bottom is lined with a dense layer of clay and sealed with thick plastic sheeting to contain leaks of hazardous materials.[19] A flexible membrane liner is designed to hold in toxic chemicals that might contaminate groundwater. A leachate sump collects leachates, which then can be subjected to further treatment. Garbage is piled up in rows that are 10 to 20 feet high; bulldozers and rollers aid in compacting the garbage; at the end of the day, the newly added garbage is covered with soil and other materials. After the garbage is covered, anaerobic bacteria aid in the decomposition of organic materials and produce methane gas. Figure 12-8 shows the profile of a landfill.

FIGURE 12-7 Left: Example of a composting bin. Right: Citizen putting organic materials into a composting bin.

Source: Left: © Harperdrewart/Dreamstime.com. Right: © Gale Verhague/Dreamstime.com.

FIGURE 12-8 Side view of a landfill.

Source: Adapted and reprinted from US Department of Energy, US Energy Information Administration. Energy explained. Available at: http://tonto.eia.doe.gov/energyexplained/images/landfill.gif. Accessed May 4, 2010.

FIGURE 12-9 A municipal solid waste landfill site.

Source: Reprinted with permission from MJ Brackney, The Imagination Factory—Education: Where Is Out? © 1996–2004 Marilyn J. Brackney. Photo credit: Bartholomew County Solid Waste Management District, Columbus, Indiana. Available at: http://www.kid-at-art.com/htdoc/educate.html. Accessed March 25, 2010.

An example of an operating landfill is shown in Figure 12-9. The bulldozer is in the process of crushing the garbage and covering it with soil. This procedure protects the site from seagulls and other scavengers that feed on garbage and can disseminate microbial pathogens into the environment. Newer designs incorporate a method for collecting leachates and disposing of them in an environmentally safe manner. Hazardous wastes such as pesticides and biological materials from hospitals should not be disposed of in MSW waste sites unless those sites are designed to accept such materials, which otherwise need to be processed separately.

Dangers associated with landfills, especially the older designs that were not well-sealed against leakage, include air pollution and groundwater contamination.[20] Considerable amounts of leachate may be generated from landfill sites, even in arid countries, such as Kuwait.[21] Hazardous wastes in landfills may contain toxic heavy metals and old batteries that have been discarded.[22] These materials may contaminate the environment by leaking out. Solvents and cleaning agents are

among the other chemicals that may enter groundwater from leachates. MSW landfills generate methane, volatile organic compounds (VOCs), and other gases.[23] Methane vented from landfills poses a fire hazard and is a greenhouse gas.

Some VOCs are hazardous because of their potential carcinogenic properties. Emissions of VOCs from landfills may cause nearby residents to complain about odors and also may be associated with symptoms of respiratory irritation.[23] In some research, proximity to landfills was related to heightened risk of cancer. Slightly increased risks of cancers (pancreatic, liver, prostate, and non-Hodgkin's lymphomas) were reported among men who lived near an MSW landfill site in Montreal, Canada.[24]

In order to increase the safety of landfills, the EPA adopted federal standards for their construction in 1988.[20] The newer designs that have been implemented reduce leaching of chemicals from landfill sites, minimize air pollution, and limit access by scavengers that could spread disease. Following improved safety standards, the small, previously existing 10,000 landfills were combined into 3,500 larger landfills, which are called **megafills**. These megafills take in from 5,000 to 10,000 tons of trash per day and serve regional needs for waste disposal; some megafills, such as those located in Virginia, serve the disposal needs of several nearby states. The larger landfills tend to be more cost effective than incinerators for disposal of solid waste; consequently, landfills now are used for the disposal of most of the solid waste produced in the United States. Federal standards for the design of landfills are shown in the following text box.

Incineration

Another method for disposal of solid waste is incineration, which can be used to generate energy while at the same time reducing the volume and weight of waste. Incineration for dis-

Federal Landfill Standards

- **Location restrictions**—ensure that landfills are built in suitable geological areas away from faults, wetlands, flood plains, or other restricted areas.
- **Composite liners requirements**—include a flexible membrane (geomembrane) overlaying two feet of compacted clay soil lining the bottom and sides of the landfill, protect groundwater and the underlying soil from leachate releases.
- **Leachate collection and removal systems**—sit on top of the composite liner and remove leachate from the landfill for treatment and disposal.
- **Operating practices**—include compacting and covering waste frequently with several inches of soil to help reduce odor; control litter, insects, and rodents; and protect public health.
- **Groundwater monitoring requirements**—require testing groundwater wells to determine whether waste materials have escaped from the landfill.
- **Closure and postclosure care requirements**—include covering landfills and providing long-term care of closed landfills.
- **Corrective action provisions**—control and clean up landfill releases and achieve groundwater protection standards.
- **Financial assurance**—provides funding for environmental protection during and after landfill closure (i.e., closure and postclosure care).

Source: Adapted and reprinted from US Environmental Protection Agency. Municipal Solid Waste: Landfills. Available at: http://www.epa.gov/osw/nonhaz/municipal/landfill.htm. Accessed March 25, 2010.

posal of MSW takes place in facilities such as the one shown in Figure 12-10. This plant has the capacity to burn about 2,250 tons of MSW per day at temperatures of 2,500 degrees Fahrenheit. No attempt is made to separate the trash into components; at this high temperature glass and aluminum in the trash melt. Metals from the residues of combustion can be recycled into scrap metal; remaining ash is deposited in landfills. The plant has sufficient electric generating capacity for nearly 40,000 homes.[25]

Although the method of incineration of solid wastes can produce valuable energy, some facilities generate hazardous emissions.[1] The substances contained in these emissions may be hazardous to human health and to the environment. Examples of toxic materials that may be emitted from incinerators include polychlorinated biphenyls (PCBs), cadmium, and heavy metals, as well as other potentially carcinogenic substances. These materials may cause air pollution or be deposited on the land.[26] Release of harmful toxins into the environment can be minimized by air pollution control technologies[27]; examples are scrubbers and filters. High temperatures deactivate pathogens and some harmful chemicals.

DISPOSAL OF HAZARDOUS MATERIALS AND WASTES

Hazardous wastes are disposed of legally in the United States by discarding them on the surface of the land, storing them in slurry ponds, dumping them into landfills or into the ocean, and incinerating them.[28] Some waste disposal sites used before the 1970s were designed poorly; untreated wastes were dumped into open pits or deposited onto land. Other wastes were placed in illegal dumping sites via a practice called "midnight dumping." Examples of contaminated lands are urban abandoned properties, old industrial sites, and mines that are no longer in use. Most contaminated land came about from antiquated practices.[29]

Hazardous wastes originate from the following sources (this list is not exhaustive):

- *Hazardous materials used in the home*—Leftover pesticides, cleaning products, automotive products, painting supplies, and other toxic, reactive, flammable, and nonflammable products.[30] Almost every home contains products that incorporate hazardous substances.[31]
- *Medical waste*—In addition to general waste, medical waste may include chemicals, infectious agents, and radioactive materials.[32]
- *Industrial hazardous waste*—Examples include toxic chemicals, solvents, heavy metals from plating operations, and residues from the manufacture of pesticides.
- *Radioactive waste*—Materials from spent nuclear fuel and tailings from uranium processing.
- *Mining wastes and extraction wastes*—Toxic chemicals left over from mining operations include acids and heavy metals.

FIGURE 12-10 Plant for conversion of trash into energy in Baltimore, Maryland.

Source: Reprinted from Energy Information Administration, Energy Kids. Baltimore RESCO waste-to-energy plant. Available at: http://www.tonto.eia.doe.gov/kids/energy.cfm?page=RESCOE_Plant. Accessed May 1, 2010.

Scope of the Hazardous Waste Problem

Worldwide, an enormous quantity of hazardous wastes are produced each year—more that 400 million tons according to some estimates.[33] These toxic substances are being produced in increasing amounts everywhere in the world.[34] For example, India is concerned about the fact that industrial and hazardous wastes are being deposited on the land in an uncontrolled fashion, causing increasing levels of pollution.[35]

The developed world produces most of the toxic wastes. In order to dispose of hazardous materials, industrialized countries have adopted the practice of shipping them to developing countries that welcome cash payments for accepting the shipments. Of concern for the environment is that many developing nations do not have adequate facilities for safe disposal of hazardous wastes, which may endanger the health of the local population and the ecosystem. Several notorious episodes of clandestine shipments of toxic wastes have gained public attention:

> Among these were a number of so-called "toxic cargo" incidents involving ships loaded with hazardous waste that were forced to travel from one international port to another in search of a final disposal site. For example, a vessel named the *Khian Sea* departed from Philadelphia, Pennsylvania, in August 1986 loaded with 14,000 tons of municipal incinerator ash. After dumping 4,000 tons of the ash on a beach in Haiti . . . , the ship plied the waters of five continents for 27 months looking for a country that would accept the remainder of its cargo, most of which is now suspected of having been dumped in the Indian Ocean.[33(pA411)]

In 1989, a treaty titled the Basel Convention on the Control of Transboundary Movements of Hazardous Wastes and Their Disposal came into effect under the sponsorship of the United Nations. The purpose of the treaty is to regulate international transport of hazardous wastes and promote the disposal of such wastes in a safe manner. Of continuing concern is the international trade of hazardous recyclable materials such as lead-acid batteries, which have great commercial value and are being shipped to developing countries. The receiving nations, in many cases, do not possess safe methods for extracting materials from recyclables.

Uncontrolled Hazardous Waste Sites in the United States

Toxic materials contained in uncontrolled hazardous waste sites raise major concerns for public health and the environment in the United States.[36] At least 40,000 of these sites have been reported to federal agencies; as of March 2010, about 1,300 were on the National Priorities List (discussed in Chapter 6). Superfund legislation (described in Chapter 4) mandates the cleanup of hazardous waste sites in the United States. Stakeholders from many sectors of the US population have expressed their concerns about hazardous substances that may be released into the environment from uncontrolled hazardous waste sites. The environmental impacts of releases of toxic materials from hazardous waste sites include potential adverse human health effects, the high costs of cleanup, reductions in property values, and various types of potential ecological damage.[36] Figure 12-11 illustrates a Superfund dump site for hazardous materials. Also shown in the figure are hazardous waste workers dressed in protective clothing.

Environmental Migration of Hazardous Wastes

Toxic chemicals present in hazardous wastes may enter the drinking water supply and, through biomagnification, may enter the food chain. According to one expert,

> Solid wastes deposited in terrestrial environments are subject to leaching by surface and ground waters. Leachates may then be transported to other surface waters and drinking water aquifers through hydrologic transport. Leachates also interact with natural organic matter, clays, and microorganisms in soils and sediments. These interactions may render chemical constituents in leachates more or less mobile, possibly change chemical and physical forms, and alter their biologic activity. Oceanic waste disposal practices result in migration through diffusion and ocean currents. . . . Sediments serve as major sources and sinks of chemical contaminants. Food chain transport in both aquatic and terrestrial environments results in the movement of hazardous chemicals from lower to higher positions in the food web.[28(p295)]

FIGURE 12-11 A: Toxic waste dump, Superfund site. B: Workers in protective clothing to guard against contamination from hazardous waste.

Source: Reprinted from the CDC Public Health Image Library. ID #1193 and ID #1530. Available at: http://phil.cdc.gov/Phil/details.asp. Accessed March 25, 2010.

The foregoing pathways for transport of hazardous chemicals are shown in Figure 12-12.

Love Canal

The Love Canal toxic waste site discussed in this section illustrates some of the concepts presented in Figure 12-12. (Although it is not an ideal example of all the concepts presented in the figure, the Love Canal incident represents a situation in which hazardous wastes entered the water, air, and soil.)

The Love Canal incident is significant to the field of environmental health because it is identified with hazardous chemical exposures and their possible harmful influences on human health.[37] The Love Canal, located near Niagara

FIGURE 12-12 Major physical and biological transport pathways of hazardous chemicals derived from solid waste disposal.

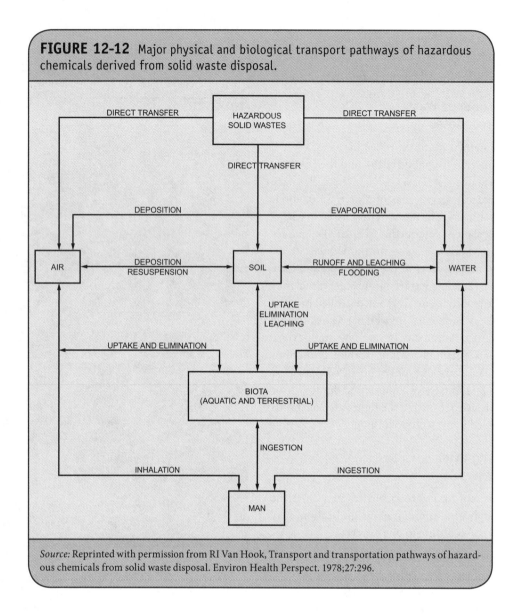

Source: Reprinted with permission from RI Van Hook, Transport and transportation pathways of hazardous chemicals from solid waste disposal. Environ Health Perspect. 1978;27:296.

Falls, New York, was excavated in the 1890s for a proposed hydroelectric power project but never was completed. The Occidental Chemical Corporation, formerly known as Hooker Chemicals and Plastics, used the site beginning in 1942 for the disposal of approximately 20,000 tons of toxic waste sealed in metal drums. The chemical wastes included dioxin, pesticides, and other organic compounds.

When the disposal of toxic chemicals ended 10 years later in 1952, the Love Canal was covered and subsequently deeded to the Niagara Falls Board of Education. The new land that was created then became an area for construction of schools and homes. From the 1960s to the late 1970s, the presence of numerous toxic chemicals was observed near the former

landfill site. Consequently, families who resided on the site were evacuated, and officials declared a national emergency. Residents of the immediate area complained of adverse health outcomes such as miscarriages, birth defects, cancer, and urinary tract diseases.

One of the outcomes of the Love Canal incident was the creation of the Superfund, administered by the EPA. According to Superfund regulations, responsible parties must assume liability for cleanup of environmental hazards that they cause. Both the Occidental Chemical Corporation and the city of Niagara Falls paid more than $20 million to the former residents of the Love Canal site. More than $200 million was paid to New York State and the federal government for cleanup of the

> **TABLE 12-3** Examples of Medical Waste
>
> Blood-soaked bandages
> Culture dishes and other glassware
> Discarded surgical gloves
> Discarded surgical instruments
> Discarded needles used to give shots or draw blood (e.g., medical sharps)
> Cultures, stocks, swabs used to inoculate cultures
> Removed body organs (e.g., tonsils, appendices, limbs)
> Discarded lancets [the little blades the doctor pricks your finger with to get a drop of blood]
>
> ---
>
> *Source:* Reprinted from US Environmental Protection Agency. Wastes: Medical waste. Available at: http://www.epa.gov/osw/nonhaz/industrial/medical/. Accessed May 2, 2010.

site. In the 1990s the site was declared free from toxic waste and the original neighborhood was repopulated.[38–40]

Medical Waste

Medical waste is defined as "any solid waste that is generated in the diagnosis, treatment, or immunization of human beings or animals, in research pertaining thereto, or in the production or testing of biologicals. . . ."[41] The sources of medical wastes include hospitals, doctors' offices, veterinary facilities, and medical laboratories. The United States produces more than 3.5 million tons of medical waste annually.[32] Some examples of medical waste are shown in Table 12-3. The Medical Waste Tracking Act of 1988 provided a system for management of medical wastes. The law was promulgated in response to the public's concerns about potentially hazardous medical wastes such as used syringes and needles that were washing up on the shorelines of several Eastern states.

One of the hazards associated with medical wastes is potential injury by *sharps* (a term that refers to sharp objects such as used needles), which can transmit infectious agents via accidental needle sticks. Otherwise, the levels and amounts of microbial agents in medical wastes are similar to those of household waste.[42] The greatest danger from medical wastes is to those who are occupationally exposed at the point where they are produced; in comparison, the general population has a much lower risk of disease.[43] Consequently, it is permissible to deposit medical waste in sanitary landfills, provided that workers are prevented from coming into contact with the waste during disposal. In addition to disposal in landfills, medical waste may be decontaminated by chemicals, incinerated, irradiated, or subjected to high temperatures (autoclaving).

Safe Disposal of Hazardous Wastes

For a temporary duration, hazardous wastes may be held in storage at waste transfer stations. At the site where they are produced, hazardous wastes are transferred by trucks or rail tank cars to waste storage facilities, which use containers, tanks, or containment buildings. Some communities offer programs for the collection of household hazardous wastes so that they can be disposed of in an environmentally friendly way. These programs help to reduce the amount of hazardous wastes that are dumped down the drain or into landfills that are not designed for the disposal of toxic materials.

Two common technologies for disposal of hazardous waste are land disposal units and injection wells.[44] Land disposal units (landfills, surface storage, waste piles, and land treatment units) are the most frequently employed method for disposal of hazardous wastes. Landfills must be designed with heavy liners and systems for the collection of leachates in order to protect groundwater. A second disposal method is the use of hazardous waste injection wells, into which toxic liquids are injected deep underground at extremely high pressures.

SEWAGE PROCESSING AND DISPOSAL

The remaining part of this chapter covers methods for processing and disposal of sewage. Sewage denotes "[t]he waste and wastewater produced by residential and commercial sources and discharged into sewers."[45] In order to prevent the spread of disease and damage to the environment, municipalities in developed countries pipe sewage to sewage treatment plants, which process sewage by microbial digestion, filtration, aeration, and addition of chemicals."[45]

The methods for sewage disposal evolved over time from the advances of the ancient world to declines in use during the Middle Ages to the innovations of the modern era. The Romans developed technologically advanced sewer systems that in many respects were superior to sewer disposal practices used during the Middle Ages.[46] The Romans constructed a system of underground tunnels for transporting sewage to the Tiber River. A network of aqueducts carried fresh water into Rome.

The Middle Ages were a time of regression for the sanitary disposal of sewage. In medieval cities, the populace casually discarded human waste into the streets, where it coursed through open gutters. Human and animal wastes were not isolated from drinking water supplies, allowing the wastes to seep into drinking water wells. Excrement provided sustenance for rodents and increased the number of ticks and fleas that could spread the plague. Waterborne diseases such as typhoid fever and cholera could be spread easily. The result was that pestilence became rampant in crowded medieval cities, leading to the deaths of hundreds of thousands of people. The connection between human wastes and disease was unknown at the time.

During the 19th century, with the recognition of the connection between sewage-polluted water and cholera, methods for the treatment of sewage began to improve. For example, in London sewers were constructed so that human excrement could be separated from drinking water supplies. In the mid-1800s, New York City installed a system of sewers that drained into nearby rivers. During the 20th century, sewage was processed to remove sludge, which (along with industrial waste) was dumped into the ocean about 100 miles offshore; this practice was banned after 1992.[47]

Modern technology for sewage treatment removes solids, deactivates microbes, and produces wastewater that can be returned safely to waterways or in some cases can be reused or recycled. Sewage treatment involves preliminary processing plus primary, secondary, and tertiary phases; these steps are described in Figure 12-13.

Figure 12-14A–D illustrates primary, secondary, and tertiary sewage processing. The primary stage aims to remove large materials, which can be composted or shipped to landfills. Secondary processing promotes microbial digestion of organic material that remains in the sewage; microorganisms that are present naturally in sewage or that may be added to enhance microbial action aid in the digestion of the liquor during aeration. Figure 12-15 presents a view of microorganisms found in sewage, as seen through a microscope. Following this stage, the sewage sometimes is discharged into waterways.

Tertiary (high-level) processing is directed at removal of remaining solids and microorganisms from the liquid portion of sewage. Various methods exist for high-level processing including filtration through sand and charcoal filters and deactivation of microorganisms (disinfection) by using chlorine or UV radiation. The top of Figure 12-16 demonstrates the progression of sewage from raw effluent to finished product. The bottom of the figure shows the wastewater from sewage after it has been filtered and disinfected.

The finished wastewater may be recycled; for example, the Irvine Ranch Water District in Southern California recycles processed wastewater for watering landscapes and makes it available for flushing toilets in high-rise buildings. Figure 12-17 shows a pond that was created with recycled water.

This use of recycled water from sewage saves millions of gallons of fresh water each year. Most jurisdictions in the United States require that wastewater receive at least secondary treatment. Water that has received only primary treat-

FIGURE 12-13 Diagram of sewage treatment process cycle.

Sewage from domestic, commercial, and municipal properties and certain industries is conveyed by sewer pipes to processing facility.

Preliminary
Screening of large solids

Grit removal by flow attenuation

Primary
Settlement of suspended solids

Secondary
Biological treatment
(bacterial breakdown)
(a) activated sludge process (aerated, agitated liquor)
(b) filter beds (sewage trickled over coarse aggregate coated with bacteria)

Tertiary
Various types of tertiary treatment exist and are applied, in combination, if needed, before piping processed sewage into receiving waters.

Phosphorus and/or nitrate reduction; disinfection by UV or filter membranes

Sewage sludge produced from various stages of the treatment process may be deposited in landfills, incinerated, or disposed of in other ways.

Source: Adapted and reprinted with permission from Department for Environment, Food and Rural Affairs (DEFRA). Sewage treatment in the UK: UK Implementation of the EC Urban Waste Water Treatment Directive. London: Department for Environment, Food and Rural Affairs (DEFRA); 2002:10. © Crown copyright 2002

ment is not recommended for any use and generally needs secondary or tertiary treatment for common purposes such as landscape irrigation. Some municipal water districts augment their supply of potable water by using recycled water that has been subjected to tertiary treatment to recharge aquifers and augment surface waters. Figure 12-18 provides examples of the appropriate uses of recycled water that correspond to the level of treatment of wastewater.

FIGURE 12-14 Primary sewage processing system. A: (upper left) Primary sewage processing tank. B: (upper right) Array of pipes and tanks for secondary sewage processing. C: (lower left) Aeration of sewage during secondary processing. D: (lower right) The inside of an aeration tank that has been emptied for maintenance.

Source: Courtesy of the Irvine Ranch Water District, Irvine, California.

FIGURE 12-15 Microorganisms found in sewage liquor.

Source: Courtesy of the Irvine Ranch Water District, Irvine, California.

FIGURE 12-16 The stages in sewage processing from raw sewage on the left to the finished product on the right (left); the finished product (right).

Source: Courtesy of the Irvine Ranch Water District, Irvine, California.

FIGURE 12-17 Recycled water used to create a pond in an arid region.

Source: Courtesy of the Irvine Ranch Water District, Irvine, California.

FIGURE 12-18 Suggested water recycling treatment and uses.

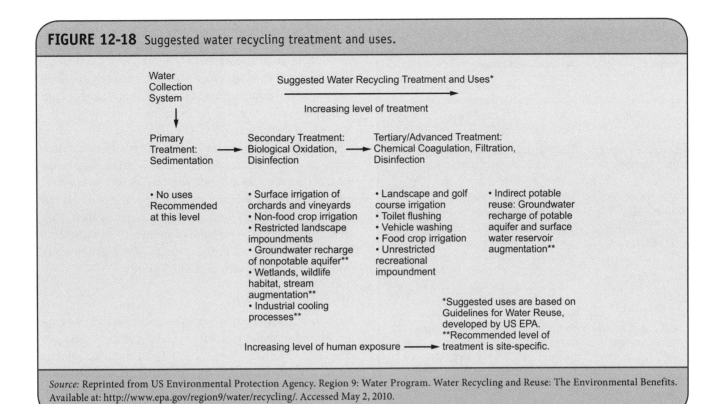

Water Collection System

Suggested Water Recycling Treatment and Uses*

Increasing level of treatment →

Primary Treatment: Sedimentation → Secondary Treatment: Biological Oxidation, Disinfection → Tertiary/Advanced Treatment: Chemical Coagulation, Filtration, Disinfection

• No uses Recommended at this level

• Surface irrigation of orchards and vineyards
• Non-food crop irrigation
• Restricted landscape impoundments
• Groundwater recharge of nonpotable aquifer**
• Wetlands, wildlife habitat, stream augmentation**
• Industrial cooling processes**

• Landscape and golf course irrigation
• Toilet flushing
• Vehicle washing
• Food crop irrigation
• Unrestricted recreational impoundment

• Indirect potable reuse: Groundwater recharge of potable aquifer and surface water reservoir augmentation**

*Suggested uses are based on Guidelines for Water Reuse, developed by US EPA.
**Recommended level of treatment is site-specific.

Increasing level of human exposure →

Source: Reprinted from US Environmental Protection Agency. Region 9: Water Program. Water Recycling and Reuse: The Environmental Benefits. Available at: http://www.epa.gov/region9/water/recycling/. Accessed May 2, 2010.

Other Methods for Sewage Disposal

Composting Toilets

Composting toilets convert human excrement into a soil-like material that must be buried or hauled away for disposal.[48] They require little water to operate and contain and deactivate pathogens in human wastes. The composting of waste occurs as the result of aerobic bacterial action. There are several brands, including the Clivus Multrum (trade name) system shown in Figure 12-19.

Septic System

A **septic system** is a type of underground "well" that receives human sanitary wastes. A septic system includes "a septic tank and a subsurface fluid distribution system."[49] It is "used to dispose of human sanitary waste or effluent from dwellings, businesses, community centers or other places where people congregate."[49] Most septic systems consist of three components,[50] which are described in Table 12-4 and illustrated in Figure 12-20.

Septic systems are a common on-site method for disposal of sewage, especially in rural areas. A home septic system is a passive method for waste (home sewage) treatment that uses both anaerobic and aerobic stages. Anaerobic action treats

FIGURE 12-19 Experimental unit that uses solar energy to aid in composting of human wastes.

SOLAR PROJECT
IN THIS CLIVUS MULTRUM UNIT BACTERIA ACTS ON HUMAN WASTE AND ADDED SAWDUST AND DECOMPOSES IT IN ABOUT THREE YEARS. THE PROCESS IS AIDED BY THE AIR CIRCULATION PROVIDED BY THE FAN RUN BY SOLAR ENERGY. THE COMPOST SIMILAR IN SMELL AND TEXTURE TO FINE TOPSOIL, IS REMOVED AND USED LIKE GARDEN FERTILIZER.

TABLE 12-4 Components of a Home Septic System

Stage	Description of Process
Septic tank (stage one processing)	"waste exits the house via a sewer pipe and enters the septic tank. There, solids settle out and grease and scum float to the top."
Distribution box (next stage)	"liquid effluent flows from the tank through the distribution box to the absorption area."
Absorption field (final stage)	"effluent . . . is distributed to the soil for treatment. If the system is properly designed and maintained, microorganisms on the surface of the soil particles around the absorption area consume the organic pollutants in the effluent before the treated effluent reaches the groundwater."

Source: Data reprinted from US Environmental Protection Agency and Purdue University. Principles and Design of On-Site Waste Disposal with Septic Systems, Principles of Septic Systems. Copyright, 2001 by Purdue Research Foundation. All rights reserved. Available at: http://www.purdue.edu/dp/envirosoft/septics/src/main.htm. Accessed May 5, 2010.

waste material as it sits in the septic tank; solids collect on the bottom of the tank. Effluents from the tank flow to an absorption field, where aerobic microorganisms in the soil aid in sanitizing liquid wastes. Most home septic systems are designed for a 20- to 30-year life, after which they eventually fail because the drain field becomes clogged and the soil loses its ability to assimilate wastes. The life of a septic system can be maximized through proper maintenance (e.g., periodic inspection and pumping out of the septic tank). Also, homeowners should try to minimize the amount of wastewater that is sent into the system (e.g., from dishwashers and washing machines) and limit the use of garbage disposal units. Objects disposed of in a septic system should be limited to biodegradable items; nonbiodegradable materials such as tampons, disposable diapers, solvents, disinfectants, and pesticides are not appropriate for disposal in a septic system. Failed septic systems as well as the presence of numerous septic systems in a densely populated area can contaminate groundwater, causing a potentially serious health hazard.

ANIMAL WASTES

Modern intensive methods of raising livestock crowd large numbers of animals into confined areas in order to maximize efficiency. (Refer to Figure 12-21.) These methods produce substantial quantities of wastes: manure, urine, carcasses of dead animals, and reproductive tissues.[51] For example, the figure shows cattle awaiting slaughter. Often, during this time, huge piles of manure accumulate in the feed lot, where the cattle must be in contact with their own wastes.

Animal wastes are associated with the following components: nutrients, organic materials, microorganisms, residues of animal medicines, and potentially toxic gases. These materials pose a number of environmental hazards including the

FIGURE 12-20 Left: Home septic system. Right: Section view of a septic tank.

Source: Adapted and reprinted with permission from US Environmental Protection Agency and Purdue University. Principles and Design of On-Site Waste Disposal with Septic Systems, Principles of Septic Systems. Copyright, 2001 by Purdue Research Foundation, West Lafayette, Indiana 47907. All rights reserved. Available at: http://www.purdue.edu/dp/envirosoft/septics/src/main.htm. Accessed May 5, 2010.

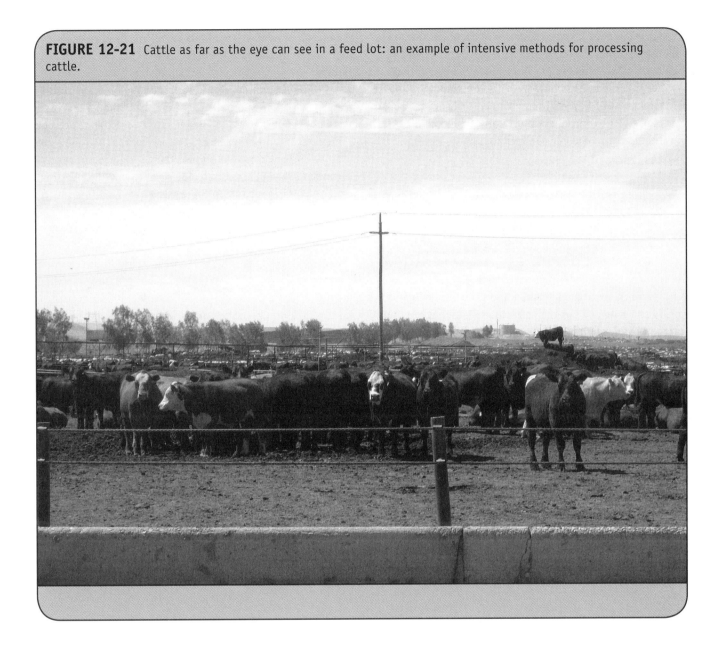

FIGURE 12-21 Cattle as far as the eye can see in a feed lot: an example of intensive methods for processing cattle.

buildup of nutrients on the land, surface contamination, and water pollution due to runoff. Animal manure can be used as a source of fertilizer to improve agricultural productivity; however, application of excessive amounts is an environmentally undesirable practice that can result in the runoff of contaminants that later may infiltrate the water supply.[52]

In addition, workers in contact with livestock and other farm animals are exposed to pathogenic microorganisms contained in feces.[51] Occupational activities involve cleaning of animal holding areas, disposal of wastes, and equipment maintenance. Workers need to handle animals directly during birthing, treatment, and slaughter. During these activi-

ties, workers may be exposed to diseased tissues or inhale or ingest pathogenic materials. Examples of microbes present in manure are *Salmonella*, *E. coli*, protozoa, and zoonotic agents. A Danish study found that wastes from pig farms were contaminated with *Salmonella*; slurry from pig wastes that was disposed of on agricultural soil continued to show contamination with *Salmonella* for up to two weeks after it was deposited on the land.[53]

Antimicrobial agents are given to livestock routinely for therapeutic purposes and for prevention of illness (e.g., spread of disease) and at low doses to promote growth.[51,52] Use of antibiotics and other microbial agents is thought to contribute to the development of resistant strains of bacteria, which may have negative impacts on the health of people in contact with the animals. An estimated 75% of antimicrobial agents that are destined for animals find their way back into the environment via excreta.[51] When the antimicrobials enter the water supply, they may foster the production of antibiotic-resistant organisms that later can become a hazard to human health.

CONCLUSION

This chapter covered two topics related to waste disposal: solid waste and sewage. Before the 20th century, the disposal of waste was handled casually. Often solid waste was dumped onto the land, and liquid waste from human and animal excrement flowed through open sewers without much regard for the environmental consequences of such disposal methods. With increasing industrialization and growing populations worldwide, solid and liquid wastes threaten the environment and require safe methods for their disposal. Of particular concern are hazardous wastes, which can cause dangerous water pollution, contamination of the land, and toxic air pollution.

As a result of intensive methods for raising food animals, excrement from animals represents a growing environmental hazard.

Progress has been made in source reduction and recycling municipal solid waste and industrial waste. Incineration and use of specially designed land disposal units that prevent toxic chemicals from reaching groundwater are two common methods for solid waste disposal. The procedures for sewage disposal include primary, secondary, and tertiary processing. Through high-level processing, wastewater can be made suitable for recycling. Although many industrialized countries have disposal programs in place, developing countries face growing hazards associated with increasing amounts of pollution from sewage and solid waste; developing countries often lack the infrastructure and finances to build waste processing facilities. Through the assistance of international agencies, increased funding and technical know-how could be made available to developing countries in order to help them improve their infrastructures for treatment of wastes.

Study Questions and Exercises

1. Define the following terms in your own words:
   a. Waste
   b. Pollution
   c. Municipal solid waste
   d. Waste recycling
   e. Composting

2. Describe some of the methods of source reduction for solid waste. Visit your local waste management facility; what methods for reduction of solid waste are available in your community?

3. What are the advantages of each of the following methods of waste management?
   a. Landfilling
   b. Composting
   c. Recycling
   d. Incineration

4. Why has recycling become a thriving industry for less developed countries? What hazards can be associated with waste recycling by developing countries?

5. Describe the design of a landfill disposal site. What microbial and physical processes take place in a landfill? How do modern landfills protect the environment from toxic chemicals?

6. What health hazards are associated with uncontrolled and older waste sites in the United States? Describe the processes through which hazardous solid wastes can affect human beings.

7. How do current methods for treating sewage differ from those that were used in the Middle Ages? Historically speaking, what factors spurred the development of today's sanitary sewage systems?

8. Describe the stages for processing sewage. At what stage of processing is it permissible in the United States to dispose of wastewater from sewage into waterways?

9. What health-related considerations relate to the use of recycled water? What level of processing is required in order for wastewater to be recycled? Describe some of the uses for recycled water.

10. Describe alternatives to sewer systems for disposal of human sewage. To what extent could these alternatives replace municipal sewer systems? What are their advantages and disadvantages?

11. Discuss the reasons why the Love Canal incident was significant to the field of environmental health.

REFERENCES

1. Hamer G. Solid waste treatment and disposal: effects on public health and environmental safety. *Biotechnol Adv.* 2003;22:71–79.

2. US Environmental Protection Agency. Terms of environment: glossary: H. Hazardous waste. Available at: http://www.epa.gov/OCEPAterms/hterms.html. Accessed April 28, 2010.

3. Rosner D. Introduction, "hives of sickness and vice." In: Rosner D, ed. *"Hives of Sickness": Public Health and Epidemics in New York City.* New Brunswick, NJ: Rutgers University Press; 1995.

4. US Environmental Protection Agency, Solid Waste and Emergency Response (5306P). *Municipal Solid Waste Generation, Recycling, and Disposal in the United States: Facts and Figures for 2008.* Washington, DC: US Environmental Protection Agency; 2009.

5. Fickes M. Gateway to recycling. *Waste Age.* October 1, 2003. Available at: http://wasteage.com/mag/waste_gateway_recycling/index.html. Accessed May 1, 2010.

6. US Environmental Protection Agency. Office of Solid Waste and Emergency Response. *Municipal Solid Waste in the United States: 2001 Facts and Figures Executive Summary.* Washington, DC: US Environmental Protection Agency; 2003.

7. Jiang Y, Kang M, Liu Z, et al. Urban garbage disposal and management in China. *J Environ Sci.* 2003;15:531–540.

8. Carlin J. Municipal solid waste profile. In: US Department of Energy, Energy Information Administration, Office of Coal, Nuclear, Electric and Alternate Fuels. *Renewable Energy Annual 1996.* Washington, DC: US Department of Energy; 1996.

9. Uela K, Koizumi H. Reducing household waste: Japan learns from Germany. *Environ.* 2001;43:20–32.

10. Canterbury JL. Pay-as-you-throw: a growing MSW management success story. *Resource Recycling.* October 1997;16–22.

11. US Environmental Protection Agency. Terms of environment: Glossary: R. Recycle/Reuse. Available at: http://www.epa.gov/OCEPAterms/rterms.html. Accessed April 29, 2010.

12. US Environmental Protection Agency. Wastes—Resource conservation—Reduce, reuse, recycle: Recycling. Available at: http://www.epa.gov/epawaste/conserve/rrr/recycle.htm. Accessed April 29, 2010.

13. US Environmental Protection Agency, Office of Solid Waste. Municipal solid waste in the United States: 2007 facts and figures. EPA 530-R-08-010. Washington, DC: US Environmental Protection Agency; 2008.

14. US Environmental Protection Agency. Decision Maker's Guide to Solid Waste Management, Volume II. EPA 530-R-95-023. Washington, DC: US Environmental Protection Agency; 1995.

15. US Environmental Protection Agency. Wastes—Information Resources. Massachusetts makes composting a way of life. Available at: http://www.epa.gov/osw/inforesources/news/2003news/11-comp.htm. Accessed May 2, 2010.

16. Manios T. The composting potential of different organic solid wastes: experience from the island of Crete. *Environ Int.* 2004;29:1079–1089.

17. EJNet.org. The basics of landfills. Available at: http://www.ejnet.org/landfills/. Accessed February 24, 2010.

18. US Environmental Protection Agency. Terms of environment: Glossary: L. Leachate. Available at: http://www.epa.gov/OCEPAterms/lterms.html. Accessed April 29, 2010.

19. Utah State University. Intermountain Herbarium. Fun facts about fungi. Waste not, want not: fungi as decomposers. Available at: http://www.herbarium.usu.edu/fungi/funfacts/Decay.htm. Accessed May 5, 2010.

20. Taylor D. Talking trash: the economic and environmental issues of landfills. *Environ Health Perspect.* 1999;107:A404–A409.

21. Al-Yaqout AF, Hamoda MF. Evaluation of landfill leachate in arid climate—a case study. *Environ Int.* 2003;29:593–600.

22. National Institute of Environmental Health Sciences. Hazardous material/waste. Available at: http://www.niehs.nih.gov/health/topics/exposure/haz-waste/. Accessed May 1, 2010.

23. Deloraine A, Zmirou D, Tillier C, et al. Case-control assessment of the short-term health effects of an industrial toxic waste landfill. *Environ Res.* 1995;68:124–132.

24. Goldberg MS, Siemiatyck J, DeWar R, et al. Risks of developing cancer relative to living near a municipal solid waste landfill site in Montreal, Quebec, Canada. *Arch Environ Health.* 1999;54:291–296.

25. Energy Information Administration. Energy Kids: A report from energy ant—my trip to the RESCO trash-to-energy plant in Baltimore, Maryland. Available at: http://www.eia.doe.gov/kids/energy.cfm?page=RESCOE_Plant. Accessed May 1, 2010.

26. Gonzalez CA, Kogevinas M, Gadea E, et al. Biomonitoring study of people living near or working at a municipal solid-waste incinerator before and after two years of operation. *Arch Environ Health.* 2000;55:259–267.

27. US Environmental Protection Agency. Clean Energy: Municipal Solid Waste. Available at: http://www.epa.gov/rdee/energy-and-you/affect/municipal-sw.html. Accessed May 1, 2010.

28. Van Hook RI. Transport and transportation pathways of hazardous chemicals from solid waste disposal. *Environ Health Perspect.* 1978;27:295–308.

29. US Environmental Protection Agency. Chapter 3: Land. In: *EPA's 2008 Report on the Environment.* Washington, DC: National Center for Environmental Assessment. EPA/600/R-07/045F. 2008. Available from the National Technical Information Service, Springfield, VA.

30. US Environmental Protection Agency. Household hazardous waste. Available at: http://www.epa.gov/wastes/conserve/materials/hhw.htm. Accessed May 1, 2010.

31. US Department of Homeland Security, FEMA. Are you ready? Household chemical emergencies. Available at: http://www.fema.gov/areyouready/household_chemical_emergencies.shtm. Accessed May 1, 2010.

32. Lee BK, Ellenbecker MJ, Moure-Ersaso R. Alternatives for treatment and disposal cost reduction of regulated medical wastes. *Waste Manag.* 2004;24:143–151.

33. Schmidt CW. Trading trash: why the US won't sign on to the Basel Convention. *Environ Health Perspect.* 1999;107:A411–A413.

34. Gupta JP, Babu BS. A new Hazardous Waste Index. *J Hazard Mater.* 1999;A67:1–7.

35. Vijay R, Sihorwala TA. Identification and leaching characteristics of sludge generated from metal pickling and electroplating industries by Toxicity Characteristics Leaching Procedure (TCLP). *Environ Monit Assess.* 2003;84:193–202.

36. Johnson BL, DeRosa CT. The toxicologic hazard of Superfund hazardous waste sites. *Rev Environ Health.* 1997;12:235–251.

37. Gibbs LM. Learning from Love Canal: a 20th anniversary retrospective. (1998). The Envirolink Network. Welcome to EnviroArts: Orion Online. Available at: http://arts.envirolink.org/arts_and_activism/LoisGibbs.html. Accessed May 8, 2010.

38. CNN.com. Despite toxic history, residents return to Love Canal. August 7, 1998. Available at: http://www.cnn.com/US/9808/07/love.canal. Accessed May 8, 2010.

39. Questia: Encyclopedia: Love Canal. (from the Columbia Encyclopedia, Sixth Edition Copyright © 2004, Columbia University Press.) Available at: http://www.questia.com/library/encyclopedia/love_canal.jsp. Accessed May 1, 2010.

40. US Environmental Protection Agency. Superfund: EPA removes Love Canal from Superfund list. Available at: http://www.epa.gov/superfund/accomp/news/lovecanal.htm. Accessed April 22, 2010.

41. US Environmental Protection Agency. Wastes: medical waste. Available at: http://www.epa.gov/osw/nonhaz/industrial/medical/. Accessed May 2, 2010.

42. Centers for Disease Control and Prevention. Perspectives in disease

prevention and health promotion summary of the Agency for Toxic Substances and Disease Registry Report to Congress: the public health implications of medical waste. *MMWR*. 1990;39:822–824.

43. US Environmental Protection Agency. Wastes: Medical waste frequent questions. Available at: http://www.epa.gov/wastes/nonhaz/industrial/medical/mwfaqs.htm. Accessed May 2, 2010.

44. US Environmental Protection Agency. Wastes: Land disposal. Available at: http://www.epa.gov/osw/hazard/tsd/td/disposal.htm. Accessed May 2, 2010.

45. US Environmental Protection Agency. Terms of environment: Glossary: S. Available at: http://www.epa.gov/OCEPAterms/sterms.html Accessed May 1, 2010.

46. Northern Arizona University. Onsite Wastewater Demonstration Project: The evolution of sewage treatment. Available at: http://www.cefns.nau.edu/Projects/WDP/resources/History/History.htm. Accessed May 2, 2010.

47. US Environmental Protection Agency. History: Reilly in New York to mark end of sewage sludge dumping. (EPA press release—June 30, 1992) Available at: http://www.epa.gov/history/topics/mprsa/03.htm. Accessed February 24, 2010.

48. US Environmental Protection Agency. Office of Water. Water efficiency technology fact sheet—composting toilets. EPA 832-F-99-066; 1999.

49. US Environmental Protection Agency. Region 5 Water: Glossary of underground injection control terms. Available at: http://www.epa.gov/r5water/uic/glossary.htm. Accessed May 2, 2010.

50. US Environmental Protection Agency and Purdue University. Principles and design of on-site waste disposal with septic systems, principles of septic systems. Copyright, 2001 by Purdue Research Foundation, West Lafayette, Indiana 47907. All rights reserved. Available at: http://www.purdue.edu/dp/envirosoft/septics/src/main.htm. Accessed February 24, 2010.

51. Cole DJ, Hill VR, Humenik FJ, et al. Health, safety, and environmental concerns of farm animal waste. *Occup Med*. 1999;14:423–448.

52. Campagnolo ER, Johnson KR, Karpati A, et al. Antimicrobial residues in animal waste and water resources proximal to large-scale swine and poultry feeding operations. *Sci Total Environ*. 2002;299:89–95.

53. Baloda SB, Christensen L, Trajcevska S. Persistence of a *Salmonella enterica* serovar typhimurium DT12 clone in a piggery and in agricultural soil amended with *Salmonella*-contaminated slurry. *Appl Environ Microbiol*. 2001;67:2859–2862.

Occupational Health

INTRODUCTION

This chapter explores hazardous agents found in the occupational environment, reviews their potential health effects, and identifies procedures for prevention of occupational illnesses and injuries. The field of occupational medicine specializes in detection and prevention of diseases that arise from the work environment.[1] **Occupational disease** is defined as those health outcomes that are "caused or influenced by exposure to general conditions or specific hazards encountered in the work environment."[1(p97)]

You will learn that the occupational environment presents potential health hazards to workers employed in a variety of positions. Among the potential dangers encountered in the workplace are high noise levels, fumes and dusts, toxic chemicals, ionizing and nonionizing radiation, high temperatures, biohazards, and psychological and social hazards including stress. The list of hazards that occur in the workplace is exten-

sive and growing with the introduction of new industrial processes and the expansion of industrialization—an especially acute problem in the developing world. In some instances, exposure to workplace hazards is associated with traumatic injuries and deaths as well as a range of conditions such as hearing loss, respiratory diseases, cancer, and adverse birth outcomes. Nowadays, many individuals telecommute or work at home; the result is an expansion of the work environment to the home setting, with transfer of employment insecurity and job stresses to one's home environment.[1]

Although the scope of occupational hazards and their effects is vast, too little research has been conducted on the health consequences of these hazards. A classic 1972 statement (which remains valid today) on the status of the occupational environment expressed the following poignant sentiment regarding workplace hazards and the health of workers:

> We are dealing here with the tip of a treacherous ecological iceberg. Few exact studies have been made to measure the full dimensions of occupational illness, occupational pollution, [and] occupational exposures. It is, unhappily, mostly guess work. We do know, for instance, how certain occupations lead to a high rate of specific kinds of cancer. But there are only scant and fragmentary epidemiological studies of the health effects of chemical or noise pollution on whole groups of workers. Most of the data consists of broad hints of a far flung, unfathomed problem yet to be accurately measured.[2(p4)]

BACKGROUND AND HISTORY

The history of occupational health contains many notorious examples of how workers' health was impacted by unsafe working conditions. Recognition of occupational risks from mining occurred during Greek and Roman times. Subsequent to the writings of Galen (129–200), through the Dark Ages and the medieval period until the time of Ramazzini (early 1700s), the issue of occupational health was accorded little notice in Europe. However, exceptions during the Renaissance included Agricola's (1494–1555) discussion of the health effects of mining and smelting of gold and silver and the work of Paracelsus (discussed in Chapter 3). From about the 1700s onward, recognition grew with respect to the contribution of occupationally related exposures to adverse health conditions. Many examples of explorations of the impacts of unsafe and hazardous working environments on the health of workers can be cited. One body of writing focused on the effects of miners' exposures to toxic metals and other hazards. Among the persons who made significant contributions to occupational health are those listed in Table 13-1. Note that there was a void in occupational health information during the Dark Ages in Europe; however, during this time scholars in the Middle East and Asia continued to make contributions to the field. A notable Middle Eastern scholar of occupational health was Abu Bakr Muhammad ibn Zakariya al-Razi (about 850–923).

Also known as Rhazes, this Persian scholar used occupational classifications (e.g., goldsmith) in describing medical cases.

Paracelsus (1493–1541) became one of the founders of the field of toxicology, a discipline that is used to examine the toxic effects of chemicals found in environmental venues such as the workplace (see Chapter 3). In 1556, *De Re Metallica*, a book that described the environmental and occupational hazards of mining, was published. The work is attributed to Georgius Agricola, who lived in Germany.

Bernardino Ramazzini, whose likeness is shown in Figure 13-1, has been called the founder of the field of occupational medicine.[3] He is credited with creating elaborate descriptions of the manifestations of occupational diseases among many different types of workers.[1] His descriptions covered a plethora of occupations from miners to cleaners of privies to fabric workers. The father of occupational medicine is also considered to be a pioneer in the field of ergonomics, by pointing out the hazards associated with postures assumed in various occupations. Ramazzini authored *De Morbis Artificum Diatriba (Diseases of Workers)*, published in 1700. His book highlighted the risks posed by hazardous chemicals, dusts, and metals used in the workplace.

Sir Percival Pott tracked the occurrence of scrotal cancer among chimney sweeps in London during the late 1700s. As noted previously in Chapter 2, Pott is regarded as the first person to describe an environmental cause of cancer.

Dr. Alice Hamilton's description of phossy jaw (phosphorus necrosis of the jaw), a condition that occurred among workers who manufactured matches around the late 1900s, was among her contributions to occupational health. The condition, which affected the victims' jawbones, was accompanied by severe pain and abscesses that drained fetid-smelling pus. (Refer to Figure 13-2.) Over time, as the disease process unfolded, the victim gradually became disfigured; surgery, the only means available to save the life of the patient, led to removal of the jaw bone and further disfigurement.

Phossy jaw was caused by exposure to white phosphorus.

TABLE 13-1 Abridged List of Noteworthy Figures in the History of Occupational Health

Name	Dates (Birth–Death)	Contribution
Hippocrates	460–377 BC (estimated)	Discussed hazards of metal working and lead
Pliny the Elder	AD 23–70	Described hazards of dust
Galen	129–200 (estimated)	Described hazards to miners
Rhazes	850–923 (estimated)	Used occupational classifications in medical case descriptions
Paracelsus	1493–1541	Wrote book on occupational diseases
Agricola	1494–1555	Described hazards of mining and producing gold and silver
Bernardino Ramazzini	1633–1714	"Father of occupational medicine"
Sir Percival Pott	1714–1788	Identified scrotal cancer among chimney sweeps
Dr. Alice Hamilton	1869–1970	Publicized dangerous occupational conditions (e.g., phossy jaw)
Irving Selikoff	1915–1992	Identified health effects of asbestos exposure

FIGURE 13-1 Bernardino Ramazzini, founder of occupational medicine.

ISTITUTO NAZIONALE MEDICO FARMACOLOGICO - ROMA

RITRATTI DI MEDICI E NATURALISTI ITALIANI DAL SECOLO XV° AL XVIII°

BERNARDINO RAMAZZINI
(dal busto in marmo esistente nell' Università di Modena)

Source: © National Library of Medicine.

FIGURE 13-2 Patient afflicted with phossy jaw.

Source: Reprinted from New Zealand Department of Labour, Occupational Safety and Health Service. Jaw—Phossy. Available at: http://www.osh.dol.govt.nz/kidz/gore/jphossy.shtml. Accessed April 5, 2010. © Crown copyright [2002].

Affected workers were those who dipped match sticks into white phosphorus paste. Many of the workers were children who labored in vapor-filled, poorly ventilated rooms. The condition, which developed slowly over a period of years, produced debilitation, neurologic disturbances, and lung hemorrhages. Remarkably, phossy jaw was a completely avoidable condition, because red phosphorus worked as well in matches as white phosphorus but was much safer. During the early 20th century, many countries passed laws that prohibited the use of white phosphorus in matches. Exhibit 13-1 provides a graphic description of the condition.

In addition to phossy jaw, described in the foregoing section, other conditions are historically important to the field of occupational health. Some of these work-related diseases are listed in Table 13-2.

Mad Hatter's Disease

The term *mad hatter's disease* stems from Lewis Carroll's 1865 book *Alice in Wonderland*, in which Carroll portrayed the mad hatter as a zany character. The phrase *mad as a hatter* had a grounding in reality. At one time, mercury-containing solutions were applied during the process of converting fur into the felt that was used to manufacture hats. Millinery workers were exposed to mercury fumes in poorly ventilated rooms during the course of their careers. After a period of time, some of the individuals developed "mad hatter's disease," a condition also known as mercurial erethism. This neuropsychiatric syndrome is characterized by symptoms that include irritability, personality change, loss of self-confidence, depression, memory loss, and reduced ability to concentrate. Figure 13-3 shows a hat-maker at work in a poorly ventilated environment in which workers could be exposed to fumes of elemental mercury.

Exhibit 13-1

CASE STUDY:
Phossy Jaw

Physician Alice Hamilton, who crusaded against dangerous industrial working conditions during the late 1800s, wrote the following description of a condition caused by exposure to white phosphorus.

Phossy jaw is a very distressing form of industrial disease. It comes from breathing the fumes of white or yellow phosphorus, which gives off fumes at room temperature, or from putting into the mouth food or gum or fingers smeared with phosphorus. Even drinking from a glass which has stood on the workbench is dangerous. The phosphorus penetrates into a defective tooth and down through the roots to the jawbone, killing the tissue cells which then become the prey of suppurative germs from the mouth, and abscesses form. The jaw swells and the pain is intense, for the suppuration is held in by the tight covering of the bone and cannot escape, except through a surgical operation or through a fistula boring to the surface. Sometimes the abscess forms in the upper jaw and works up into the orbit, causing the loss of an eye. In severe cases one lower jawbone may have to be removed, or an upper jawbone—perhaps both. There are cases on record of men and women who had to live all the rest of their days on liquid food. The scars and contractures left after recovery were terribly disfiguring, and led some women to commit suicide. Here was an industrial disease which could be clearly demonstrated to the most skeptical. Miss Addams told me that when she was in London in the 1880s she went to a mass meeting of protest against phossy jaw and on the platform were a number of pitiful cases, showing their scars and deformities.[4(p116)]

TABLE 13-2 Names of Classic Occupational Diseases Found in Historical Literature

Name of Disease	Definition/Etiology
Miners' asthma	The common name for pneumoconiosis among miners exposed to dusts such as coal dust.
Potters' rot, miners' phthisis	Silicosis, respiratory disease from inhalation of silica dust.
Brass-founders' ague	A type of metal fume fever caused by inhalation of fumes from welding brass. This self-limiting condition is associated with fever and other symptoms that resolve after 24 hours.
Filecutters' paralysis	Paralysis of the hands caused by lead exposure.
Painters' colic	Abdominal pain associated with anemia caused by exposure to white lead in paint.
Bakers' itch	A skin reaction (eczema) caused by contact with the components of baked goods (e.g., sugar).
Mule spinners' cancer, also known as mule spinners' disease	The mule was a textile spinning machine; the disease referred to scrotal cancer that occurred among male cotton textile workers who were exposed to mineral oils over long time periods as they used the mule.
Hatters' shakes; the mad hatter's disease (described in text)	Mercury poisoning among millinery workers.
Caisson disease (decompression sickness)	A disease caused by decompression when workers emerged from caissons, which were used to construct the anchoring piers for the Brooklyn Bridge in New York City and for similar projects. The laborers were exposed to air under very high pressures for extended time periods.
Phossy jaw (described in text)	Phosphorus necrosis of the jaw.

Historically Significant Occupational Accidents

A report published in the *Morbidity and Mortality Weekly Report* observes: "At the beginning of this century [the 20th century], workers in the United States faced remarkably high health and safety risks on the job."[5(p461)] Many workers remained on the job for 16-hour periods during 6- and 7-day workweeks.[6] Two major incidents—the Triangle Shirtwaist Company fire and the Gauley Bridge disaster—illustrated the deplorable conditions that workers often were forced to endure. These poor environmental conditions included contact with hazardous machinery, crowding, lack of ventilation, poor lighting, and infrequent protection against hazards. These two events as well as others led to reforms that resulted eventually in the improvement of working conditions.

Triangle Shirtwaist Company Fire

March 25, 1911, marks the date of New York City's worst factory fire, which occurred at a 10-story structure formerly named the Asch building. The disaster, also one of the worst industrial accidents in American history, claimed the lives of 146 women within the brief time span of 15 minutes. Several hundred women labored on the top three floors used by the

FIGURE 13-3 This photograph shows a man polishing, or "pouncing" a hat in a felt hat-making factory.

Source: Reprinted from the CDC Public Health Image Library. NIOSH Content Provider ID # 6811. Available at: http://phil.cdc.gov/phil/details.asp. Accessed April 5, 2010.

Triangle Shirtwaist Factory. Doors were locked to prevent the women from leaving their sewing machines; fire escapes were nonfunctional. As a result, when a fire erupted about 4:30 in the afternoon, many of the women (especially on the ninth floor) perished from the fire when they were unable to escape or were killed when they jumped from windows or attempted to slide down elevator cables.[7,8]

Gauley Bridge Disaster

Beginning about 1931, workers began a tunneling project near the small town of Gauley Bridge, located in West Virginia. During tunneling operations, workers were exposed to high levels of silica dust from which they did not have adequate protection. Estimates indicated that as many as 1,500 workers contracted the lung disease silicosis and 1,000 died from this cause.[9] (More information on silicosis is provided later in this chapter.)

SIGNIFICANCE OF THE OCCUPATIONAL ENVIRONMENT FOR HEALTH

Currently, fatal and nonfatal occupational illnesses and injuries exact a significant social and economic toll in the United States. The National Institute for Occupational Safety and Health (NIOSH) reported that on a typical day during the 1990s, 11,000 employees endured disabling injuries; occupationally related diseases caused the deaths of 130 individuals.[10] The direct costs of all occupational injuries and illnesses in 2002 were about $45.8 billion and the indirect costs as much as $229 billion.

During 2001, approximately 5.2 million nonfatal work-related illnesses and injuries were reported in private industry.[11] This number includes both illnesses and injuries that required time off from work and those that did not. Of this total, the vast majority (93.6%) were injuries. (Refer to Figure 13-4.) The remaining 6.4% (333,800) were illnesses, a category that includes repeated trauma, disorders due to physical agents, poisonings, respiratory conditions due to toxic agents, dust diseases of the lungs, and skin diseases or disorders. Figure 13-5 demonstrates time trends in reported illnesses from 1972 to 2001. The numbers peaked between 1992 and 1996 and subsequently declined. During 2002, the number of newly reported nonfatal injuries and illnesses declined to slightly more than 4.7 million cases.

Since 2002, the number of occupational injuries and illnesses has continued to decline. According to the Bureau of Labor Statistics, 3.7 million cases of nonfatal occupational injuries and illnesses were reported by private industry employers in 2008; slightly more than half of these cases were classified as serious nonfatal occupational injuries,[12] which

FIGURE 13-4 Injuries and illnesses in private industry, 2001.

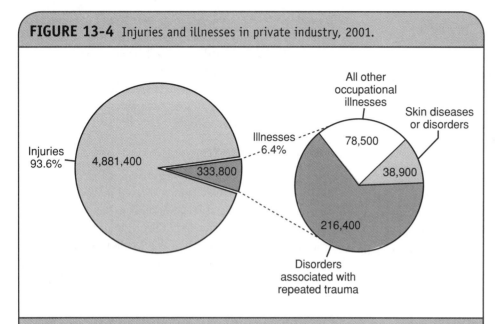

Source: Sestito JP, Lunsford RA, Hamilton AC, Rosa RR, eds. Worker Health Chartbook 2004. NIOSH Publication Number 2004-146. Cincinnati, OH: Department of Health and Human Services, Centers for Disease Control and Prevention, National Institute for Occupational Safety and Health; 2004:19.

FIGURE 13-5 Number of illness cases in private industry by type of illness, 1972–2001.

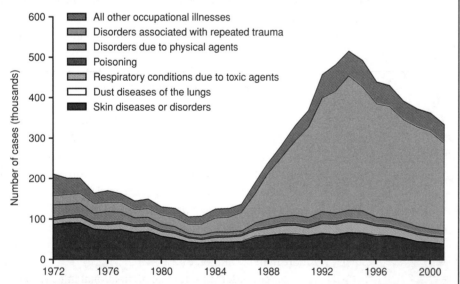

Source: Sestito JP, Lunsford RA, Hamilton AC, Rosa RR, eds. Worker Health Chartbook 2004. NIOSH Publication Number 2004-146. Cincinnati, OH: Department of Health and Human Services, Centers for Disease Control and Prevention, National Institute for Occupational Safety and Health; 2004:19.

are defined as those that require recovery away from work and extend in duration beyond the day of occurrence.[11] Figure 13-6 presents the relative distribution of occupational injuries and illnesses by nature, 2008. The leading causes of such conditions were sprains and strains (total number = 416,620; 38.6% of all cases of injury and illness); cuts, lacerations, and punctures (9.3%); and bruises and contusions (8.7%). In 2008, a total of 71.2% of injuries took place in the service-providing sector, with the remainder (28.8%) happening in goods-producing industries.[12]

OVERVIEW OF AGENTS OF OCCUPATIONAL DISEASE

A large number of agents and a diversity of unhealthful workplace settings are associated with occupational disease. (Refer to Table 13-3.) To some extent, many of the agents shown in the table have been covered in previous chapters. Nevertheless, a review and discussion of the relevance of these disease-causing factors to the work environment is in order.

As indicated by Table 13-3, agent factors associated with occupational diseases and injuries include noise, dusts, toxic heavy metals and their fumes, carbon monoxide, chemicals, ionizing radiation, microbial agents, lifting heavy weights, repetitive motion, accidents, and work-related stress. The following paragraphs describe some of these agent factors and their health effects.

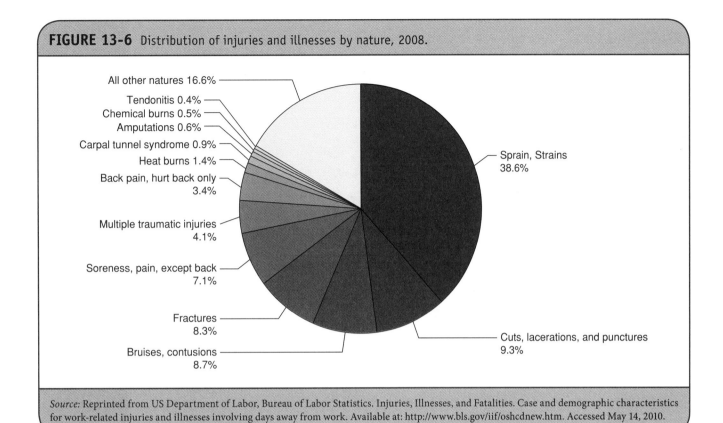

FIGURE 13-6 Distribution of injuries and illnesses by nature, 2008.

All other natures 16.6%
Tendonitis 0.4%
Chemical burns 0.5%
Amputations 0.6%
Carpal tunnel syndrome 0.9%
Heat burns 1.4%
Back pain, hurt back only 3.4%
Multiple traumatic injuries 4.1%
Soreness, pain, except back 7.1%
Fractures 8.3%
Bruises, contusions 8.7%
Sprain, Strains 38.6%
Cuts, lacerations, and punctures 9.3%

Source: Reprinted from US Department of Labor, Bureau of Labor Statistics. Injuries, Illnesses, and Fatalities. Case and demographic characteristics for work-related injuries and illnesses involving days away from work. Available at: http://www.bls.gov/iif/oshcdnew.htm. Accessed May 14, 2010.

Noise

The term *ototoxic* refers to agents that can produce hearing loss. Ototoxic agents include very loud sounds and several classes of drugs and chemicals used in the work environment; there also may be synergistic effects among ototoxic agents (e.g., noise and workplace chemicals). Noise-induced hearing loss is cumulative; generally speaking, exposure to high noise levels for extended time periods is associated with hearing loss and other hearing disorders. Some research has linked noise with psychological disturbances and mental disorders.

What is meant by **noise**? Sound and noise are similar from the perspective of physics and are defined as follows:

- Sound[13]
  - Produced by vibrating bodies
  - A form of mechanical energy
  - Carried in the air as longitudinal waves
  - Impinges upon the auditory system and produces physiological responses
- Noise[14]

- A type of sound that is unwanted
- Can be made up of pure tones, a narrow band of frequencies, and sound impulses

Noise can be subjectively annoying, can disrupt performance, and has the capacity to produce adverse health effects. One consequence of high noise levels in the work environment is a sharp reduction in hearing acuity among workers in certain occupations, such as construction.

Dusts

Dusts found in many occupational environments are linked to lung diseases. For instance, black lung disease (also known as coal miners' pneumoconiosis or coal workers' pneumoconiosis) is an occupational hazard of the coal mining industry (although the threat from this condition is abating in the United States due to improved procedures and higher safety standards). Cotton and textile dusts are a cause of brown lung disease. In addition to pneumoconiosis, exposure to dusts may induce emphysema, lung cancer, and other pulmonary conditions.

TABLE 13-3 Categories of Occupationally Associated Diseases or Injuries, Agent Factors, and Associated Work Settings

Disease or Injury	Agent Factors	Work Settings
Hearing loss	Noise	Transport, manufacturing, construction
Lung diseases: asthma, chronic obstructive pulmonary disease, pneumoconiosis	Dusts, e.g., coal dust, cotton and textile dusts	Mining, textile manufacturing, construction
Cancer and lead poisoning	Toxic heavy metals (e.g., lead) and their fumes	Metal working, plumbing, ceramics manufacture
Carbon monoxide poisoning	Carbon monoxide	Mining, smelting, indoor use of gasoline-powered engines
Allergic and irritant dermatitis	Chemicals	Manufacturing, numerous industries
Fertility and pregnancy abnormalities	Chemicals, ionizing radiation	Manufacturing, hospitals
Infectious diseases	Microbial agents, e.g., bacteria and viruses	Health care, public utilities, agriculture
Low-back disorders	Lifting heavy weights	Manufacturing, health care
Musculoskeletal disorders of the upper extremities	Repetitive motion	Manufacturing, office work
Traumatic injuries	Workplace accidents	All occupations potentially at risk
Adverse mental health outcomes	Work-related stress	All occupations potentially at risk

Toxic Heavy Metals and Their Fumes

Some metals used in the work environment have potentially toxic or injurious properties, as noted previously in Chapter 6. The toxic heavy metals (arsenic, lead, mercury, cadmium, chromium, and nickel) are potential hazards to human health. During the processing and milling of heavy metals, employees are at risk of breathing fumes and dusts that contain toxic levels of these metals. Consider the widespread occupational exposures to lead: Workers who have potential for such exposures are plumbers, radiator repair workers, painters, ceramic workers, and metal workers. Another group of lead-exposed individuals are those who patronize or work in firing ranges; such workers include coaches and law enforcement personnel who regularly practice shooting guns. (Refer to the following text box.)

Carbon Monoxide

Carbon monoxide (CO), which is odorless and can pose an undetected threat, is one of the hazardous toxic gases found in the work environment. CO causes death by depriving the body of oxygen; CO combines more readily than oxygen with the hemoglobin in the blood, thus accounting for CO's hazardous

nature. The product formed by the combination of CO and hemoglobin is known as carboxyhemoglobin (COHb). The oxygen-carrying capacity of blood decreases in proportion to the amount of COHb that is present. In comparison to healthy individuals, workers who have preexisting diseases that affect the circulation and oxygen-carrying capacity of the blood are at increased risk of the effects of CO poisoning. Persons who should avoid CO exposure are those who have conditions such as lung disease, heart disease, and anemia. Cigarette smoking is known to increase blood COHb levels.

Among the many sources of CO in the occupational environment are small gasoline-powered engines (e.g., those used in lawn mowers, pressure washers, and generators). Care should be taken to provide adequate ventilation when using these devices. Other sources of CO are kilns, furnaces, forges, space heaters, and fires and explosions. Some mines can have high levels of CO.

Chemicals

Literally thousands of chemical substances are used in the modern workplace. For example, the list of substances associated with the manufacture of plastics and paints includes

Lead Exposure from Indoor Firing Ranges among Students on Shooting Teams—Alaska, 2002–2004

Firing ranges have been recognized as potential sources of lead exposure since the 1970s. Lead-containing dust is produced by 1) the combustion of lead-containing primers, 2) the friction of bullets against the gun barrel, and 3) fragmentation as bullets strike the backstop. Lead dust inhaled into the lungs is highly bioavailable, with an absorption rate near 100%. The Occupational Safety and Health Administration (OSHA) has established acceptable standards for airborne lead exposure in the workplace, including indoor firing ranges, since 1979. Guidelines for proper design and operation include use of a separate ventilation system for firing lanes, written protocol for range maintenance, use of wet mopping or HEPA vacuuming instead of dry sweeping to remove dust and debris, and use of copper-jacketed bullets.

CDC recognizes blood lead levels (BLLs) of $\geq$ 25 µg/dL in adults and $\geq$ 10 µg/dL in children aged " 6 years as levels of concern; no similar level has been set for older children and adolescents. During 2002–2004, the Alaska Environmental Public Health Program (EPHP) conducted lead-exposure assessments of school-based indoor shooting teams in the state, after a BLL of 44 µg/dL was reported in a man aged 62 years who coached a high school shooting team in central Alaska. This report summarizes the results of the EPHP investigation of potential lead exposure in 66 members of shooting teams, aged 7–19 years, who used five indoor firing ranges. The findings suggest that improper design, operation, and maintenance of ranges were the likely cause of elevated BLLs among team members at four of the five firing ranges. Public health officials should identify indoor firing ranges that have not implemented lead-safety measures and offer consultation to reduce the risk for lead exposure among shooters, coaches, and employees.

The shooting-team coach was asymptomatic for lead exposure; in January 2002, he sought BLL testing from his health-care provider after reading about potential lead exposure at firing ranges. The BLL test result of 44 µg/dL was reported to EPHP in accordance with the Alaska lead surveillance system, which requires laboratories to report all BLLs $\geq$ 10 µg/dL. An epidemiologic investigation by EPHP revealed that the man was the chief range officer and shooting-team coach for firing range A, which was used primarily by adolescents. In February 2002, EPHP tested BLLs for all seven members of the shooting team, who were aged 15–17 years. The mean BLL was 24.3 µg/dL (range: 21.0–31.0 µg/dL). BLLs for 14 nonshooting family members were significantly (p < 0.05) lower (mean: 3.5 µg/dL; range: 1.0–7.0 µg/dL). EPHP advised parents of the team members that their children should discontinue use of the firing range.

Source: Adapted and reprinted from the Centers for Disease Control and Prevention. Lead exposure from indoor firing ranges among students on shooting teams—Alaska, 2002–2004. *MMWR.* 2005;54:577, 579.

epoxy resins, acrylates, and formaldehyde. Other widely used industrial chemicals are colorants, dyes, disinfectants, pharmaceuticals, preservatives, and solvents.[15] Chemical exposures have been associated with dermatoses, liver disease, and many other conditions. As noted previously, agricultural workers are exposed routinely to potentially toxic pesticides.

Ionizing Radiation

Sources of ionizing radiation exist in many occupational settings. One example is found in healthcare facilities, such as nursing homes, specialized clinics, dentistry suites, and hospitals. Commonly, healthcare personnel might encounter ionizing radiation from sources such as radionuclides and X-ray machines. Other occupational venues that involve the use of ionizing radiation include research facilities, nuclear

generating plants, and plants for the production of nuclear weapons. Chapter 8 discussed hazards associated with ionizing radiation.

Microbial Agents

Microbial agents (sometimes referred to as biologic agents) of disease are a source of health risks for workers in many occupational categories, for example, hospital employees, workers exposed to sewage, and agricultural workers. Persons on the front line of patient contact—physicians and nurses—interact directly with patients who may be affected by communicable diseases. Microbial agents originate from a number of sources including human and animal blood and bodily fluids, feces from humans and animals (e.g., manure, droppings from rodents), persons who are carrying infectious diseases, infected primates and other animals, and disease-carrying insects. For example, of particular concern are the following agents and associated diseases:

- Bloodborne pathogens, examples:
  - Hepatitis B virus (HBV)
  - Hepatitis C virus (HCV)
  - Human immunodeficiency virus (HIV)
- Bacteria
  - Tuberculosis
  - Anthrax
- Viruses
  - Influenza
  - Other communicable respiratory diseases

Work-Related Stresses

Beyond the category of physical and chemical hazards are the psychological and somatic effects of work-related stresses. Chronic stress has been implicated in a range of somatic conditions (e.g., coronary heart disease) and mental disorders including depression. The term *going postal* refers to employees of the post office and other companies who react to stressful conditions of their environment, particularly the work environment, by committing violent acts.

SPECIFIC OCCUPATIONALLY ASSOCIATED DISEASES AND CONDITIONS

Referring back to Table 13-3, you will observe examples of the conditions that have been associated with occupational hazards. In particular, NIOSH developed the National Occupational Research Agenda (NORA) that targets 21 research priorities. These priorities include dermatologic conditions, lung diseases, fertility and pregnancy abnormalities, hearing loss, infectious diseases, low-back disorders, musculoskeletal disorders of the upper extremities, and traumatic injuries as areas for special focus.[16] In addition, included below are adverse mental health outcomes associated with the hazard of work-related stress.

Allergic and Irritant Dermatitis (Contact Dermatitis)

Because of direct exposure to the occupational environment, the skin is one of the most common sites of contact with chemicals used in the work setting.[16,17] Consequently, the skin is vulnerable to numerous injuries and dermatologic conditions; the full extent of job-related dermatoses is unknown, because many skin diseases that result from occupational sources are not reported. Workers at highest risk of occupational skin diseases are employed in manufacturing, construction, food

FIGURE 13-7 Occupational contact dermatitis.

Source: Reprinted from MM Key, AF Henschel, J Butler, et al., eds. *Occupational Diseases: A Guide to Their Recognition.* (Rev. ed.) Washington, DC: National Institute for Occupational Safety and Health; 1977:78.

production, and activities such as metal plating and engine service.[18] Referring back to Figure 13-4, observe that in 2001 there were 38,900 reports of occupationally related skin diseases or disorders in private industry, approximately 12% of occupational illnesses (excluding injuries). Figure 13-7 shows a case of dermatitis, which has affected the subject's forearms, wrists, and hands.

Occupationally Associated Respiratory Diseases

A number of significant respiratory diseases are linked to occupational exposures. Examples of these conditions, listed in

TABLE 13-4 Occupationally Associated Respiratory Diseases

Name of Lung Disease	Symptoms or Condition	Exposure
Asbestosis	Progressive scarring of lung tissue	Asbestos fibers
Coal workers' pneumoconiosis	Breathing difficulties	Coal dust
Silicosis	Presence of scar tissue in lungs	Crystalline silica from various sources
Byssinosis (brown lung disease)	Obstruction of small airways; impaired lung function	Dusts from hemp, flax, and cotton
Malignant mesothelioma	Uncommon cancer of chest lining	Asbestos
Hypersensitivity pneumonitis	Inflammation of air sacs of lungs; loss of normal breathing function	Organic dusts, fungus spores, bird droppings
Asthma	Symptoms of asthma (e.g., wheezing, difficulty breathing)	Allergens in workplace (e.g., pollen, animal dander)
Chronic obstructive pulmonary disease	Chronic cough, loss of lung function	Air pollution and contamination
Respiratory tuberculosis	Symptoms of tuberculosis (e.g., night sweats, persistent cough)	Tuberculosis bacillus
Occupationally associated lung cancer	Cancer of the lung, trachea, and bronchus	Workplace carcinogens (e.g., beryllium, radon)
Disorders due to smoking in the workplace	Lung cancer, chronic bronchitis, cough	Side-stream tobacco smoke

Table 13-4, include asbestosis, coal workers' pneumoconiosis, silicosis, byssinosis, mesothelioma, lung cancer, and other noteworthy diseases that affect the respiratory system. Many of the work-related respiratory diseases are chronic conditions that have long latency periods. Some of the respiratory diseases are indirect or underlying, and not a direct cause of mortality; hence the frequency of their contributions as causes of morbidity and mortality is likely to be underestimated. Hazards arise not only from visible dust particles, but also from unseen dust particles. A discussion of some of the major conditions follows.

Chronic Obstructive Pulmonary Disease (COPD) and Asthma

- As reported in statistics for the leading causes of death, COPD is called "Chronic lower respiratory diseases (CLRD)" and includes chronic and unspecified bronchitis, emphysema, asthma, and other chronic lower respiratory diseases.[19] In 2006, the category of CLRD (COPD) was the fourth leading cause of mortality in the United States.[19] COPD causes significant loss of work time, economic losses, morbidity, and, ultimately, increases in the risk of mortality. Here are some additional facts regarding diseases in this classification[16]:

- About 30% of cases of COPD and asthma can be linked to occupational exposures.
- Asthma has become the most frequently diagnosed occupational respiratory disease in the United States.
- Occupational exposures may exacerbate preexisting asthma.
- COPD is related to workplace exposure to dusts.

Pneumoconiosis

The term pneumoconiosis is defined as "'the accumulation of dust in the lungs and the tissue reactions to its presence. For the purpose of this definition, 'dust' is meant to be an aerosol composed of solid inanimate particles.'"[20] Pneumoconiosis can result in fibrosis of the lungs (development of fibrous tissues) and lung nodules. The following list provides examples of substances that when inhaled may cause pneumoconiosis:

- Asbestos (associated with asbestosis and a lung condition known as mesothelioma, defined below)
- Cotton dust (byssinosis)
- Silica-containing dusts (silicosis)
- Coal dust (black lung disease, coal workers' pneumoconiosis)

FIGURE 13-8 Number of deaths of US residents aged 15 or older with pneumoconiosis recorded as an underlying or contributing cause on the death certificate, 1968–1999.

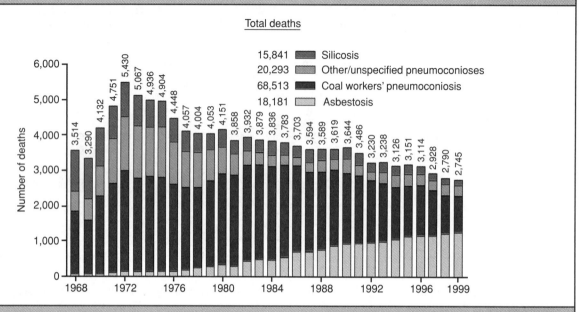

Source: Sestito JP, Lunsford RA, Hamilton AC, Rosa RR, eds. Worker Health Chartbook 2004. NIOSH Publication Number 2004-146. Cincinnati, OH: Department of Health and Human Services, Centers for Disease Control and Prevention, National Institute for Occupational Safety and Health; 2004.

Figure 13-8 reports trends in mortality from pneumoconioses. After 1972, the number of deaths from this cause declined, shrinking to 2,745 cases in 1999. Formerly, coal workers' pneumoconiosis was a leading cause of lung-associated mortality; recently, mortality from asbestosis has shown an increasing trend.

Asbestosis

Asbestosis refers to a type of pulmonary fibrosis that is associated with exposure to asbestos, the name assigned to six different fibrous minerals found in nature. Asbestosis results from inhalation of large amounts of asbestos fibers over long time periods. The condition occurs mainly among workers exposed to asbestos and is uncommon among the larger population. Asbestosis is related to declines in pulmonary function and increased risk of lung cancer, especially among smokers. Asbestos-associated mesothelioma is a rare form of cancer that invades the chest lining. From 1968 to 1999, over 18,000 deaths were caused by asbestosis. (Refer to Figure 13-8.)

The epidemiologist Irving Selikoff identified hazards of asbestos exposure during the 1950s. Although their use has declined greatly, asbestos-containing products were in-

corporated for many years into materials for fireproofing, insulation, and motor vehicle brakes. Asbestos has many useful attributes such as fire resistance and insulating ability. In 1973, the EPA banned the spraying of materials that contained asbestos on buildings; in 1989, the agency issued a regulation that would prohibit most other uses of asbestos. The EPA's 1989 regulation was overturned in 1991 by a court action that continued to permit many uses of asbestos.[21] Currently asbestos is banned from six categories of products including certain types of construction materials, certain paper goods, and all new applications of asbestos. The majority of car manufacturers have adopted substitutes for asbestos-containing brake linings.

Coal Workers' Pneumoconiosis (Black Lung Disease)

Coal workers' pneumoconiosis (CWP) is a potentially fatal lung disease that is associated with breathing coal dust, which then becomes deposited in the lungs as shown in Figure 13-9. Over time, the lungs of persons who are afflicted with CWP lose their elasticity, causing respiration to become increasingly difficult.

FIGURE 13-9 Section of a lung showing coal workers' pneumoconiosis. The dark areas are caused by coal deposits.

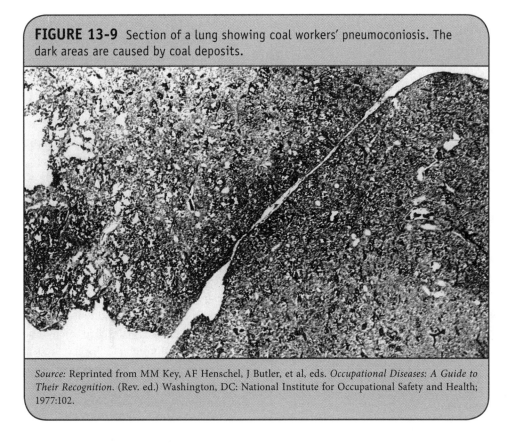

Source: Reprinted from MM Key, AF Henschel, J Butler, et al, eds. *Occupational Diseases: A Guide to Their Recognition.* (Rev. ed.) Washington, DC: National Institute for Occupational Safety and Health; 1977:102.

In the United States, the federal government regulates dust levels in coal mines. Following the enactment of the Federal Coal Mine and Safety Act of 1969, average dust levels declined sharply in coal mines. The 1969 law provided black lung disability benefits to coal miners who had incurred disabilities caused by mine-related dust exposure. Figure 13-10 shows a poster that proclaims the availability of such benefits.

Silicosis

The lung disease *silicosis* is a condition caused by inhaling respirable crystalline silica dust. Silicosis, a disabling condition that is fatal in many instances, presents in three major forms: *chronic silicosis* (associated with long-term exposures to silica at low levels—10–20 years); *accelerated silicosis* (a rapidly progressing form that is associated with exposure to large amounts of silica during short time periods—5–10 years); and *acute silicosis* (caused by very heavy exposures to silica during short time periods—up to 5 years).[22]

Workers encounter crystalline silica during activities such as sandblasting, cutting tiles and masonry, and grinding cement. The dangers of silica dust are not limited to particles of visible size, because very fine, invisible silica particles also may be drawn into the lungs. Chronic silicosis takes many years to develop: Early in the course of the disease, few symptoms may be present or, if observable, may consist of coughing and shortness of breath. Long after initial exposure to silica (e.g., 10 or more years), nodules may develop on the lobes of the lungs. More severe cases, designated as complicated silicosis, may result in pulmonary fibrosis and loss of lung function. Persons afflicted with silicosis are at increased risk of tuberculosis. Figure 13-11 shows a worker who is not protected from silica dust. The inset illustrates a close-up of silica dust.

Fertility and Pregnancy Abnormalities

Fertility and pregnancy abnormalities include dysfunctions that affect fetuses and infants; examples are birth defects, prematurity, low birth weight, spontaneous abortions, and developmental disabilities. There are many opportunities for workers to be exposed to workplace hazards that could be associated with these abnormalities. A special exposure group includes women of childbearing age and pregnant women. Here are some observations regarding workplace hazards and fertility and pregnancy abnormalities[16]:

- A total of 4 million chemicals in use commercially have not been tested for their reproductive effects.

FIGURE 13-10 This 1970 poster announced the availability of black lung benefits for disabled coal miners.

black lung benefits

coal miners
who are disabled by coal dust disease

and widows
of coal miners who had this disease

may now receive black lung cash benefits under the new Federal Coal Mine Health and Safety Act.

If you think you may be entitled to these monthly benefits and have not already applied, do it now at any social security office.

U.S. DEPARTMENT OF HEALTH, EDUCATION, AND WELFARE
Social Security Administration

Source: Reprinted from US Social Security Administration. Social Security history: black lung benefits. Available at: http://www.ssa.gov/history/blung.html. Accessed April 5, 2010.

- Most of the 1,000 chemicals used in the work environment that have been demonstrated to cause adverse reproductive effects among animals have not been tested with humans.
- Some hazards to human reproduction are known—lead, solvents, and ionizing radiation.

The etiologies of most birth defects and developmental disabilities have not been ascertained. With the exception of some known teratogens, the role of occupational exposures in these outcomes is largely unknown and unexplored.

Hearing Loss Caused by Noise

Hearing loss caused by noise in the work environment occurs very commonly and takes a major toll. Here are some facts regarding hearing loss in the workplace[23]:

- The second most-commonly self-reported occupational injury or illness is noise-induced hearing loss.

- As many as 10 million workers in the United States suffer from noise-induced hearing loss.
- Almost one half of carpenters and plumbers are afflicted by noise-induced hearing loss.

Noise, a term that stems from the Latin word "nausea," is a feature of modern life that at best is an annoyance and at worst can affect our health adversely, both physically and mentally. According to a professor of otolaryngology, "Noise is the most ubiquitous global pollutant, which permeates all aspects of life throughout the inhabited world."[24(p3)] Although one of the primary direct consequences of excessive noise is hearing loss, other health consequences may include cardiovascular effects (e.g., exacerbation of high blood pressure), increases in stress levels, and sleep deprivation.[25] Noise has been recognized as harmful for more than 2,500 years: As early as 600 BC, the Sybarites of Greece banned metal work that involved noise-producing hammering within city limits.[14]

Noise is a pervasive environmental problem, whether it arises from motor vehicles, home landscape maintenance, construction projects, jet aircraft flying overhead, hovering helicopters, or even an inconsiderate person playing a boom box too loudly. Those of us (the majority in any urban area) who live near a major highway (e.g., an interstate highway in the United States, the *autobahn* in Germany, the *autostrada* in Italy, or any other highway in the world) are aware of the roar of trucks and other motor vehicles. Homeowners who are unfortunate enough to live under the flight path of an airport must endure the ear-splitting sounds produced by jets taking off, landing, and flying overhead. City dwellers who rely on public transportation—as in New York City—are subjected to the head-splitting screech of subway trains. When you walk around in most cities, you are impacted involuntarily by the deafening sounds emitted by emergency vehicle sirens and honking horns. In the suburbs, especially on weekends, one cannot fail to notice the racket produced by power lawnmowers, leaf blowers, trimmers, and similar machines. It is difficult to escape the din of modern society; even in remote national parks, noise from motor vehicles, snowmobiles, and aircraft intrudes.

As many as 30 million persons in the United States (11% of the population), and a similar percentage of Europeans, face the risk of hearing loss due to excessive noise. Estimates suggest that about 12% of the population of the developing world is confronted with potential hearing loss due to high noise levels. The residents of megacities in Asia must cope with the incessant cacophony from motor vehicle engines, blowing of horns, and crowded shopping areas.

FIGURE 13-11 The worker shown is sawing bricks while unprotected from breathing silica dust.

Close up of fine silica dust.

Source: Reprinted from the CDC, National Institute for Occupational Safety and Health (NIOSH). Silicosis: Learn the Facts. DHHS (NIOSH) Publication No. 2004-108. Washington, DC: NIOSH; 2004:6.

Even when noise levels are not sufficient to damage hearing, they may interfere with everyday life and impact the quality of our lives adversely. Some reactions to noise are annoyance, sleep disturbance, and reduction in cognitive performance. Think of the difficulty of trying to conduct classes in an environment such as a university located in a large, noisy city or under the flight path of an airport. Noise in the work environment may interfere with workers' alertness and communication and induce stress over time. Some experts believe that prolonged exposure to noise may result in psychological reactions that have adverse consequences for people's immune system status and physical well-being.[26]

Physiology of Hearing

The human ear translates the energy from sound waves into neurological impulses that are heard as sound through the actions of the ear canal, eardrum, bones of the middle ear,

cochlea, and cochlear nerve. (Refer to Figure 13-12, which illustrates the major parts of the ear.) After sounds enter and pass through the ear canal, they create vibrations in the tympanic membrane (eardrum). These vibrations cause the ossicles—bones in the middle ear (hammer, anvil, and stirrup)—to move. The function of the bones in the middle ear is to amplify sounds that move the oval window of the cochlea. In turn, this movement causes fluid in the cochlea to move and to stimulate hairs, which then stimulate cells that send neurological impulses along the cochlear nerve to the brain. These impulses are perceived as sound.

The Nature of Sound and Hearing

Sound is produced by oscillating waves of various frequencies. The term *Hertz (Hz)* denotes the number of cycles per second associated with the oscillation of a given sound wave, with low Hz numbers characterizing low tones and high Hz numbers

FIGURE 13-12 The outer, middle, and inner ear.

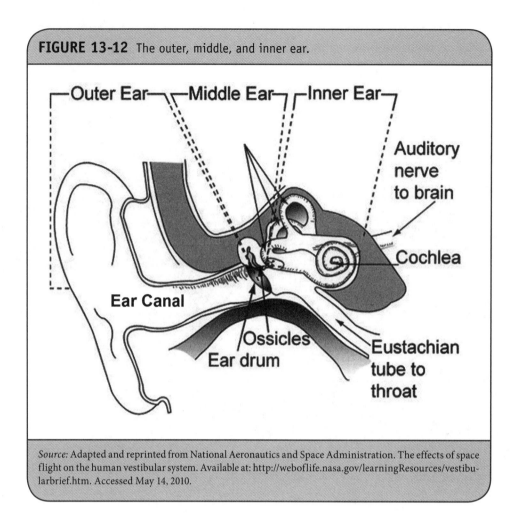

Source: Adapted and reprinted from National Aeronautics and Space Administration. The effects of space flight on the human vestibular system. Available at: http://weboflife.nasa.gov/learningResources/vestibularbrief.htm. Accessed May 14, 2010.

characterizing high tones. The approximate range of human hearing is from a low of 20 Hz to 20,000 Hz on the upper end of the frequency scale. The usual sounds we hear in everyday life range from about 60 Hz to about 6,000 Hz.

Audiologists measure hearing level (HL) with an audiometer, an instrument that generates test tones of known intensities. In a type of hearing test known as air conduction testing, hearing is measured by using pure tones generated by an audiometer; the hearing threshold refers to the lowest level of a tone to which a subject responds correctly 50% of the time. A patient's hearing level is defined as the difference between the threshold level that the tested person can hear and the average level that the general population can hear.

The sound pressure level (SPL) is a measure of the intensity of sound. The SPL is reported on a logarithmic scale that uses **decibels (dBs)**, the standard measure of the strength of a sound. While the issue of sound measurement is complex, the dB scale refers to 10 times the log of a ratio to the base 10.

To illustrate, the logs of 10, 100, and 1,000 to the base 10 are 1, 2, and 3, respectively. Thus, 10 dB is 10 times the log of 10; a level of 30 dB is 10 times the log of 1,000; and a level of 60 dB is 10 times the log of 1,000,000—and so forth, for various points on the scale. Thus, an increase of 10 dB (e.g., from 20 dB to 30 dB) represents a 10-fold increase in sound intensity and not a linear jump of 10 units. Human beings can perceive differences between sound intensities from the lowest levels to the highest levels, which vary by a factor of more than 1 trillion. A logarithmic scale is advantageous for characterizing the large variability in the range of sounds that the human ear can perceive.

The dB scale is useful for describing SPLs of common sounds, HLs, and the sound levels that are associated with hearing loss:

- The threshold of hearing is 0 dB/HL.
- Sounds at 85 dB/SPL can produce slight hearing loss.

FIGURE 13-13 Typical range of common sounds.

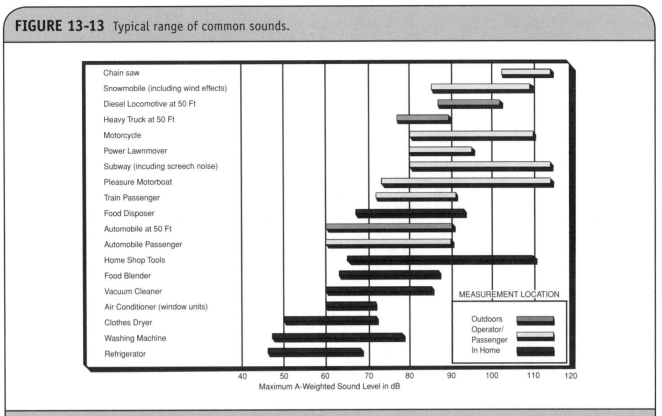

Source: Reprinted from US Environmental Protection Agency. Protective Noise Levels: Condensed Version of EPA Levels Document. EPA 550/9-79-100. Washington, DC: US EPA, Office of Noise Abatement & Control; November 1978:5.

- Brief exposure to sounds at 100 dB/SPL can cause severe, permanent hearing loss.

Figure 13-13 lists the approximate SPLs in dB of common sounds: for example, refrigerator (45–68 dB), subway (80–115 dB), and chain saw (105–115 dB). The SPLs of some other sounds not shown in the chart are breathing (10 dB), quiet sounds in an office (50–60 dB), average traffic noise (80 dB), shotgun firing (130 dB), close proximity to a jet engine (140 dB), and threshold for pain (about 125 dB).[27]

Noise in the Workplace

Noise is a significant feature of most work environments, ranging from "quiet" offices to active construction sites. Two examples of employment categories affected greatly by noise are construction and health care.

Construction industry. Sources of noise in the construction industry include bulldozers, heavy trucks, and loading machines. Other noisy equipment includes jackhammers, nail guns, and drills. As a result, construction workers of almost all types are exposed to high noise levels.[28] Figure 13-14 shows the sound levels associated with tools used by carpenters. For example, a chain saw produces sounds that reach the 110 dB level; other power tools used in carpentry may exceed this level.

As a consequence of exposure to high noise levels, many older carpenters have diminished hearing acuity. In addition, carpenters who are 25 years old have the hearing acuity of persons who are 50 years old and who have had no noise exposure. (Refer to Figure 13-15.)

Healthcare industry. Noise levels in hospital operating rooms are reported to reach 118 dB; sources include high-speed bone-cutting drills and suctioning devices.[29] Operating room physicians, nurses, and other personnel are exposed to high noise levels from these sources. In dental offices, dentists and hygienists are exposed to excessive noise from air compressors, ultrasonic instrument cleaners, high-speed dental drills, and scalers.[30]

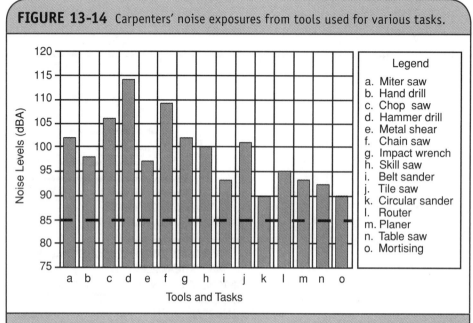

FIGURE 13-14 Carpenters' noise exposures from tools used for various tasks.

Legend
a. Miter saw
b. Hand drill
c. Chop saw
d. Hammer drill
e. Metal shear
f. Chain saw
g. Impact wrench
h. Skill saw
i. Belt sander
j. Tile saw
k. Circular sander
l. Router
m. Planer
n. Table saw
o. Mortising

Source: Reprinted from the CDC, National Institute for Occupational Safety and Health (NIOSH). Noise and Hearing Loss Prevention. Available at: http://www.cdc.gov/niosh/topics/noise/pubs/toolnoiselevel. html. Accessed April 6, 2010.

FIGURE 13-15 The average 25-year-old carpenter has the ears of a 50-year-old person who has not been exposed to noise.

Source: Reprinted from the CDC, National Institute for Occupational Safety and Health (NIOSH). Noise and Hearing Loss Prevention. Available at: http://www.cdc.gov/niosh/topics/noise/pubs/50yearold.html. Accessed April 6, 2010.

Permissible noise levels in the workplace.   The NIOSH recommended exposure limit (REL) for noise exposure in the workplace during an eight-hour shift is 85 dBA (using a type of weighting on a sound meter called "A-weighting" and meaning that exposure is an eight-hour time-weighted average).[31] Employers are required to post warning signs in work areas where noise levels exceed 85 dBA. For higher noise levels, exposure times must be limited, as shown in Figure 13-16.

Infectious Diseases

The transmission of infectious diseases can occur in various occupations with many different modes of transmission.[16] Here are a few examples:

- Healthcare workers are at increased risk of exposure to the hepatitis virus (e.g., hepatitis B and C) and the human immunodeficiency virus (HIV), particularly through accidental needle sticks. Other sources of exposure include biohazards resulting from direct patient contact as well as contact with blood and blood products.
- Public utility workers may be exposed to the hazards of disease carried in raw sewage.
- Agricultural workers are at increased risk of exposure to zoonotic diseases through contact with animals and disease agents contained in the soil.
- Social service workers and corrections personnel may be exposed to tuberculosis.

FIGURE 13-16 Permissible noise levels in the US workplace.

Source: Reprinted from the CDC, National Institute for Occupational Safety and Health (NIOSH). Noise and Hearing Loss Prevention. Available at: http://www.cdc.gov/niosh/topics/noise/pubs/lookatnoise. html. Accessed April 6, 2010.

- Clinical laboratory specialists may be exposed to infectious agents from specimens including bloodborne pathogens, viruses, and bacterial agents (e.g., *Y. pestis* and *S. typhi*, among others).
- Mortuary workers are exposed to a range of microbial agents as human bodies are embalmed or exhumed from burial sites.
- Adult film industry workers are at risk from a range of bloodborne and sexually transmitted infections.

Musculoskeletal Disorders

The term **musculoskeletal disorder (MSD)** refers to "an injury or disorder of the muscles, nerves, tendons, joints, cartilage, or spinal disks."[12(p6)] Musculoskeletal disorders of the upper extremities include tendonitis (rotator cuff tendonitis), sprains, neck pain, and carpal tunnel syndrome. These conditions occur widely in the work environment and cost the US economy more that $2 billion annually in expenditures for workers' compensation.[16] A total of 317,440 cases of musculoskeletal disorders were reported in 2008. Of this total, about 74% were caused by sprains, strains, and tears. Refer to Figure 13-17.

Carpal Tunnel Syndrome (CTS)

Carpal tunnel syndrome is a condition that presents with numbness, pain, or tingling of the fingers, wrist, and back of the hand. These anatomic areas are innervated by the median nerve, which passes through the carpal tunnel of the wrist and may become compressed or squeezed.[32,33]

Of work-related injuries and illnesses reported during 2003, 5.1% were due to CTS, which is the most frequently reported upper-extremity musculoskeletal disorder. The condition necessitates long periods of recuperation and absence from work. CTS is related to repetitive work activities with the hand and wrist; one of the work domains that has been described as having a high frequency of CTS is the meat packing industry. The use of computer keyboards for extended time periods also has been identified as a risk factor for CTS.

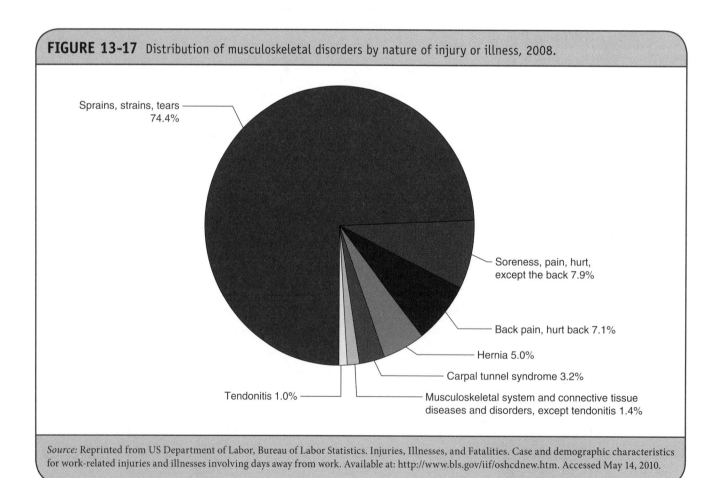

FIGURE 13-17 Distribution of musculoskeletal disorders by nature of injury or illness, 2008.

Sprains, strains, tears 74.4%

Soreness, pain, hurt, except the back 7.9%

Back pain, hurt back 7.1%

Hernia 5.0%

Carpal tunnel syndrome 3.2%

Musculoskeletal system and connective tissue diseases and disorders, except tendonitis 1.4%

Tendonitis 1.0%

Source: Reprinted from US Department of Labor, Bureau of Labor Statistics. Injuries, Illnesses, and Fatalities. Case and demographic characteristics for work-related injuries and illnesses involving days away from work. Available at: http://www.bls.gov/iif/oshcdnew.htm. Accessed May 14, 2010.

Low-Back Disorders

Low-back disorders are an extremely common and important musculoskeletal problem associated with the work environment.[16] In 2003, a total of 5.4% of the 435,180 cases of MSD that resulted in days away from work were caused by back pain or a hurt back. Back injuries accounted for about 23% of all the occupational injuries and illnesses that required time away from work in 2003.[12] One of the occupations with a high risk of back injuries is the nursing profession, in which back injuries may occur when nurses or aides are required to lift patients. Approximately 38% of nurses are reported to have sustained back injuries.[34] Such injuries may be caused by lifting over barriers or lifting from an awkward position. Other workers with a high frequency of back problems include laborers, carpenters, and drivers.

Work-Related Injuries and Fatalities

Work-related injuries and fatalities have continued to be an issue of major consequence for society worldwide, in terms of both human suffering and economic costs. In the United States, workplace injuries exact billions of dollars each year in medical expenses, foregone wages, reduced productivity, and other costs.[16]

What is meant by an injury? Injuries are defined as the result of energy applied to the human body in such a manner that the energy exceeds the body's physiological tolerance. Refer to Chapter 14 for more information on this definition and the topic of injuries in general. The present section focuses primarily on fatal occupational injuries.

Work-related traumatic injuries are serious injuries from causes such as vehicle collisions, workplace violence, and falls. In 2007, approximately 15 workers died every day in the United States from traumatic injuries.[35] Consequently, because of the large toll that they take, fatal injuries in the workplace are a very significant public health concern. The National Institute for Occupational Safety and Health (NIOSH) states:

> Over 93,000 workers were fatally injured while working in the United States from 1980 through 1995. Each day an average of 16 people died—simply by doing their jobs. These deaths result from exposure to many different hazards on the job. Leading causes of traumatic occupational fatalities include motor vehicles, homicides, machines, falls, electrocutions, and falling objects. . . . Workers are at risk of fatal injury in many different ways. Workers who operate motor vehicles or machines risk injury due to over-

turns or collisions. Taxicab drivers risk being killed during robbery attempts while construction workers risk fatal falls while working from heights. Electrical linemen risk electrocution while repairing power lines and loggers risk being struck by a falling tree during tree harvesting operations. These scenarios highlight some of the risks that are a daily presence in many of the industries and occupations in the United States. These jobs are frequently noted as being the jobs with the highest fatal injury rates. However, the potential for work-related injury exists in any job where injury risks are present and not controlled.[36(pxi)]

Sources of information on occupational fatalities include NIOSH and the Bureau of Labor Statistics (BLS) in the US Department of Labor. NIOSH gathers information on fatal occupational injuries among workers aged 16 years and older.[36] This information is derived from cases of work-related injury reported on death certificates from 52 vital statistics–reporting units that encompass the 50 US states, New York City, and the District of Columbia. The National Traumatic Occupational Fatalities (NTOF) Surveillance System was developed by NIOSH in the 1980s to conduct a census of death certificate–based information in order to perform descriptive and analytic epidemiologic analyses of causes of job-related mortality.[11] A second source of occupational fatality information is the BLS Census of Fatal Occupational Injuries (CFOI), which collects information from various sources, including death certificates, police reports, and worker compensation reports.

The BLS reported a total of 5,214 fatal occupational injuries in 2008. (Refer to Figure 13-18.) Most fatalities (63%) concerned transportation incidents and highway deaths; about one-fifth (18%) involved contact with objects and equipment. In 2007, the fatality rates among younger (aged 15–24) workers were lower than those among older (aged 25 and older) workers. The respective rates were 3.6 per 100,000 and 4.4 per 100,000 full-time equivalent workers.[37]

In 2008, several industrial categories accounted for the largest number of deaths—construction; transportation and warehousing; and agriculture, forestry, fishing, and hunting. (Refer to Figure 13-19.) A total of 975 fatal injuries occurred in the construction industry alone. With respect to fatality rates, the category of agriculture, forestry, fishing, and hunting had the highest rate (30.4 per 100,000). Other industries with high fatality rates were mining and the category of transportation and warehousing.

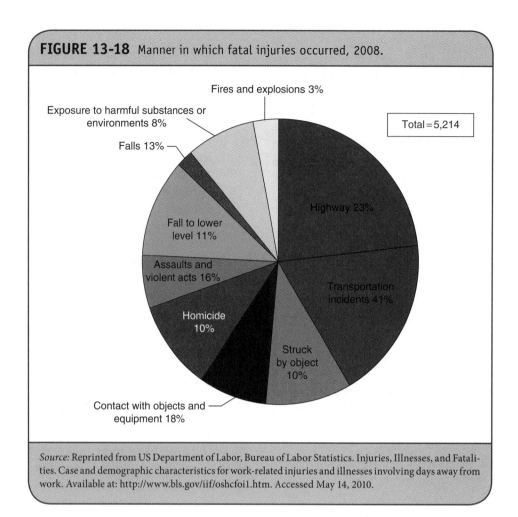

FIGURE 13-18 Manner in which fatal injuries occurred, 2008.

Fires and explosions 3%

Exposure to harmful substances or environments 8%

Falls 13%

Fall to lower level 11%

Assaults and violent acts 16%

Homicide 10%

Contact with objects and equipment 18%

Struck by object 10%

Transportation incidents 41%

Highway 23%

Total = 5,214

Source: Reprinted from US Department of Labor, Bureau of Labor Statistics. Injuries, Illnesses, and Fatalities. Case and demographic characteristics for work-related injuries and illnesses involving days away from work. Available at: http://www.bls.gov/iif/oshcfoi1.htm. Accessed May 14, 2010.

The number of fatal work-related injuries reported in 2008 was the smallest number since the CFOI began in 1992.[38] In part this finding may have been attributable to economic influences such as substantial reductions in employment in the construction industry. Declines in fatalities were reported for transportation, falls, and homicides, although workplace suicides increased.

Job Stress and Associated Conditions

Job stress can affect the health of workers adversely and results in significant time away from work. The term **job stress** is "defined as the harmful physical and emotional responses that occur when the requirements of the job do not match the capabilities, resources, or needs of the worker. Job stress can lead to poor health and even injury."[39(p6)] The BLS reported 5,659 cases of anxiety, stress, and neurotic disorders that involved absence from work in 2001.[11] As shown in Figure 13-20, the rates of anxiety, stress, and neurotic disorders declined from 0.8 per 10,000 full-time

workers to 0.6 per 10,000 workers (about 25%) between 1992 and 2001.

Figure 13-21 demonstrates that the highest percentage of anxiety, stress, and neurotic disorder cases involved the job classification of technical, sales, and administrative support (39.9%), followed by the category of managerial and professional specialty (23.6%).

Job-related stressors may provoke extreme reactions, such as those embodied in the concept of *going postal*. Employees may feel that they have been treated unfairly by their employers and commit a violent act against their supervisors and coworkers. *Critical incident stress* refers to intense reactions that arise from witnessing violent behavior or from dealing with traumatic incidents such as those experienced by paramedics or personnel who are first responders to disasters. Critical incident stress management (CISM) is a method of helping persons cope with the aftermath of the experience of a traumatic event. One form of CISM involves debriefing the individual.[40]

FIGURE 13-19 Number and rate of fatal occupational injuries by industry sector, 2008.

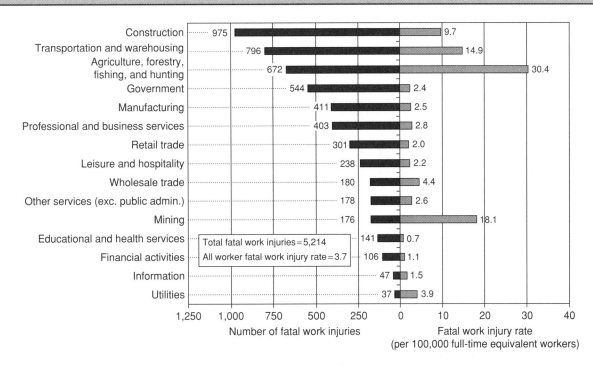

Source: Reprinted from US Department of Labor, Bureau of Labor Statistics. Injuries, Illnesses, and Fatalities. Case and demographic characteristics for work-related injuries and illnesses involving days away from work. Available at: http://www.bls.gov/iif/oshcfoi1.htm. Accessed May 14, 2010.

FIGURE 13-20 Annual rates of anxiety, stress, and neurotic disorder cases involving days away from work in private industry, 1992–2001.

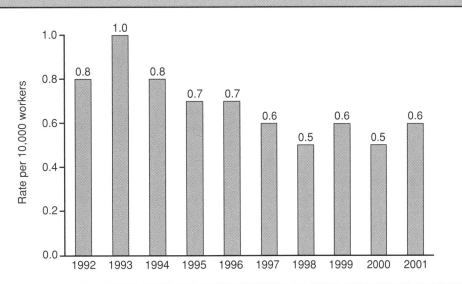

Source: Sestito JP, Lunsford RA, Hamilton AC, Rosa RR, eds. *Worker Health Chartbook 2004*, Chapter 2: Fatal and Nonfatal Injuries, and Selected Illnesses and Conditions. NIOSH Publication Number 2004-146. Cincinnati, OH: Department of Health and Human Services, Centers for Disease Control and Prevention, National Institute for Occupational Safety and Health; 2004:35.

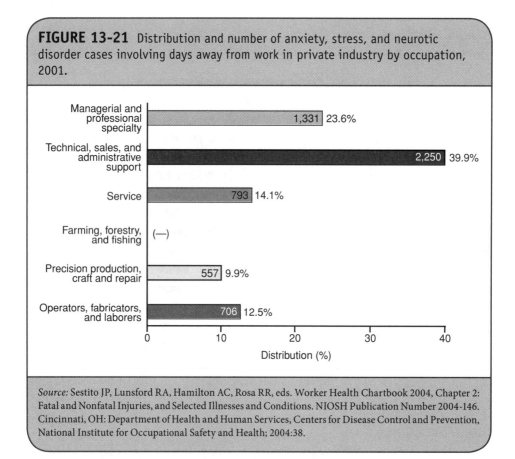

FIGURE 13-21 Distribution and number of anxiety, stress, and neurotic disorder cases involving days away from work in private industry by occupation, 2001.

Source: Sestito JP, Lunsford RA, Hamilton AC, Rosa RR, eds. Worker Health Chartbook 2004, Chapter 2: Fatal and Nonfatal Injuries, and Selected Illnesses and Conditions. NIOSH Publication Number 2004-146. Cincinnati, OH: Department of Health and Human Services, Centers for Disease Control and Prevention, National Institute for Occupational Safety and Health; 2004:38.

Sources of job stress include:

- Work overload—long hours, high-pressure deadlines
- Job dissatisfaction
- Job insecurity due to fear of layoff, changes in the nature of work, global competition, and deregulation of labor
- Workers' lack of control over their environment and conditions of employment; e.g., employment insecurity and shift work are associated with work-related stress.[41]
- Assembly line work that involves repetitive tasks
- Dealing with members of the public who may be abusive
- Inadequate compensation and lack of benefits such as health insurance

Job stress has been researched extensively as a possible contributor to both impaired mental health status and poor physical health status. In one example that addressed mental health, a large, one-year, prospective study of employed men and women in Belgium found that the cumulative experience of stress was associated with indicators of poor mental health.[42]

One aspect of job stress is job strain, which arises from employment that combines low control over the decision-making process with high psychological demands. The association between job strain and the risk of morbidity and mortality from coronary heart disease (CHD) is a focus of research on the physical health consequences of stress. The findings with respect to this hypothesized association have been controversial and span a vast body of research literature. Here are two of many examples: A prospective cohort study conducted among employees in the metal industry in Finland followed workers who were free from cardiovascular diseases at baseline. At follow-up approximately two and a half decades later, employees who had high job strain experienced more than a twofold increase in risk of cardiovascular mortality.[43] In contrast, a prospective study conducted among subjects from the Framingham Offspring Study did not find that job strain was a significant risk factor for CHD or CHD mortality in men and women.[44]

PREVENTION OF OCCUPATIONAL DISEASE

The best method for control of occupational hazards is primary prevention, which includes the following[45]:

- Engineering controls
- Modification of work practices
- Administrative controls

Examples of engineering controls are physical modifications of the work environment to reduce hazards, such as use of quieter machinery, installation of protective guards, and improvement of building ventilation to remove dusts and vapors. Examples of modification of work practices include use of safety education and training programs in order to change work procedures so that they are safer than the usual methods. Examples of administrative controls are organization of work shifts and rotation of employees to minimize exposure to hazards. Several other methods for protecting workers from occupational hazards are use of personal protective equipment, public health surveillance, and establishment and enforcement of exposure limits.

Personal Protective Equipment

A procedure for reducing exposure to workplace hazards, and the one that is the last line of defense, is the use of personal protective equipment. The US Occupational Safety and Health Administration (OSHA) defines **personal protective equipment (PPE)** as apparatuses "designed to protect employees from serious workplace injuries or illnesses resulting from contact with chemical, radiological, physical, electrical, mechanical, or other workplace hazards. Besides face shields, safety glasses, hard hats, and safety shoes, PPE includes a variety of devices and garments such as goggles, coveralls, gloves, vests, earplugs, and respirators."[45]

Devices to Protect against Airborne Hazards

The two basic types of PPE for protecting workers against airborne hazards are contaminant removers and clean air suppliers. Contaminant removers filter airborne particles or remove airborne chemicals and gases. Clean air suppliers are either at-

tached to a line that brings in clean air from a remote source or are self-contained breathing apparatuses that issue clean air from tanks.[46] Figure 13-22 illustrates some of the types of PPE for protection against airborne hazards.

Devices to Protect Hearing

Examples of devices used to protect hearing are ear plugs and ear muffs, as shown in Figure 13-23.

FIGURE 13-22 Respirators for protection against gases and chemicals.

Source: Reprinted from US Department of Labor, Occupational Safety and Health Administration, Woodworking eTool, Finishing/Chemicals, Personal Protective Equipment. Available at: http://www.osha.gov/SLTC/etools/woodworking/finishchems_ppe.html. Accessed April 6, 2010.

FIGURE 13-23 Hearing protection devices. Earplugs (left) and ear muffs (right).

Protective Eyeware

Protective eyeware includes goggles, face shields, safety glasses, and respirators that cover the full face. Eyeware protects against solid objects such as flying chips, metal fragments, and other small objects that could injure the eye. Another purpose of eyeware is to form a barrier against fluids and gases (e.g., liquids that contain chemical or biological hazards, hot water, and steam). Unless welders wear protective goggles, they are at risk of retinal burns caused by ultraviolet radiation. Figure 13-24 demonstrates a worker who is wearing a protective shield.

Public Health Surveillance

Public health surveillance is defined as "the ongoing systematic collection, analysis, and interpretation of health data essential to the planning, implementation, and evaluation of public health practices, closely integrated with the timely dissemination of these data to those who need to know."[47(p2)] Surveillance systems include the collection of information about occupational injuries and illnesses and maintenance of databases on exposures (exposure databases) to occupational hazards such as noise, industrial chemicals, and ionizing radiation. Exposure surveillance systems and databases can be instrumental in advancing the health and safety of the workplace.[48] These systems can provide the foundation for epidemiologic studies of adverse health outcomes in the workplace.

Several US federal agencies collaborate in surveillance programs; these agencies include NIOSH, the National Center for Health Statistics (NCHS), BLS, OSHA, and the Mine Safety and Health Administration (MSHA).[47] Examples of surveillance programs operated by NIOSH are:

- National Surveillance System of Pneumoconiosis Mortality (NSSPM)
- National Traumatic Occupational Fatalities (NTOF) Surveillance System
- State-based Sentinel Event Notification System for Occupational Risks (SENSOR)

A noteworthy example of state-level surveillance of occupational diseases and injuries is the Occupational Health Surveillance and Evaluation Program (OHSEP) operated by the State of California's Department of Health Services.[49] OHSEP examines the occurrence of conditions such as work-related respiratory disease, pesticide-related illnesses, and carpal tunnel syndrome through data obtained from reporting systems. The Doctor's First Report of Occupational Injury or Illness is one of the reporting forms used by OHSEP. (Refer to Figure 13-25.)

Exposure Limits

In most situations, workplace exposures to hazardous agents are higher than the exposures of the general public. In order to protect workers from these higher exposure levels to hazardous agents, organizations and government agencies have established guidelines and regulations for limitation of exposures. These standards make

FIGURE 13-24 Worker who is wearing protective goggles and a face shield.

Source: Reprinted from US Department of Labor, Occupational Safety and Health Administration. Shipyard Employment eTool, Ship Repair, PPE Selection, Eye and Face Protection. Available at: http://www.osha.gov/SLTC/etools/shipyard/standard/ppe/general_ppe/eye_face.html. Accessed April 6, 2010.

FIGURE 13-25 Doctor's first report of occupational injury or illness.

STATE OF
CALIFORNIA **DOCTOR'S FIRST REPORT OF OCCUPATIONAL INJURY OR ILLNESS**

Within 5 days of your initial examination, for every occupational injury or illness, send two copies of this report to the **employer's workers' compensation insurance carrier** or the **self-insured employer.** Failure to file a timely doctor's report may result in assessment of a civil penalty. **In the case of diagnosed or suspected pesticide poisoning,** send a copy of this report to Division of Labor Statistics and Research, P.O. Box 420603, San Francisco, CA 94142-0603, and notify your local health officer by telephone within 24 hours.

	PLEASE DO NOT USE THIS COLUMN
1. **INSURER NAME AND ADDRESS**	
2. **EMPLOYER NAME**	Case No.
3. Address No. and Street City Zip	Industry
4. Nature of business (e.g. food manufacturing, building construction, retailer of women's clothes)	County

5. **PATIENT NAME** (first name, middle initial, last name)	6. Sex ☐ Male ☐ Female	7. Date of Mo. Day Yr. Birth	Age
8. Address: No. and Street City Zip		9. Telephone number ( )	Hazard
10. Occupation (Specific job title)		11. Social Security Number __ __	Disease
12. Injured at: No. and Street City County			Hospitalization
13. Date and hour of injury or onset of illness Mo. Day Yr. Hour _____ a.m. _____ p.m.		14. Date last worked Mo. Day Yr.	Occupation
15. Date and hour of first examination or treatment Mo. Day Yr. Hour _____ a.m. _____ p.m.		16. Have you (or your office) previously treated patient? ☐Yes ☐ No	Return Date/Code

Patient please complete this portion, if able to do so. Otherwise, doctor please complete immediately. Inability or failure of a patient to complete this portion shall not affect his/her rights to workers' compensation under the California Labor Code.
17. **DESCRIBE HOW THE ACCIDENT OR EXPOSURE HAPPENED** (Give specific object, machinery or chemical. Use reverse side if more space is required.)

18. **SUBJECTIVE COMPLAINTS** (Describe fully. Use reverse side if more space is required.)

19. **OBJECTIVE FINDINGS** (Use reverse side if more space is required)
    A. Physical examination

    B. X-ray and laboratory results (State if none or pending.)

20. **DIAGNOSIS** (if occupational illness specify etiologic agent and duration of exposure.) Chemical or toxic compounds involved? ☐ Yes ☐ No
    ICD-9 Code __ __ __ . __ __

21. Are you findings and diagnosis consistent with patient's account of injury or onset of illness? . ☐Yes ☐No   If "no", please explain.

22. Is there any other current condition that will impede or delay patient's recovery? ☐Yes ☐No   If "yes", please explain.

23. **TREATMENT RENDERED** (Use reverse side if more space is required.)

24. If further treatment required, specify treatment plan/estimated duration.

25. If hospitalized as inpatient, give hospital name and location   Date admitted   Mo. Day Yr.   Estimated stay

26. **WORK STATUS** - is patient able to perform usual work? ☐ Yes ☐ No
    If "no", date when patient can return to: Regular work _____ / _____ / _____
    Modified work _____ / _____ / _____   Specify restrictions _____

Doctor's Signature _____   CA License Number _____
Doctor Name and Degree (please type) _____   IRS Number _____
Address _____   Telephone Number ( ) _____

FORM 5021 (REV. 4)
1992   Any person who makes or causes to be made any knowingly false or fraudulent material statement or material representation for the purpose of obtaining or denying workers' compensation benefits or payments is guilty of a felony.

Source: Reprinted from California Department of Industrial Relations, Division of Labor Statistics and Research. Available at: http://www.dir.ca.gov/dlsr/dlsrform5021.pdf. Accessed May 6, 2010.

use of the terms ***threshold limit values (TLVs), biological exposure indices (BEIs), permissible exposure limits (PELs),*** and ***maximum allowable concentrations (MACs)***. The definitions of the foregoing terms are as follows:

- *Threshold limit value (TLV)*—"Refers to airborne concentrations of substances and represents conditions under which it is believed that nearly all workers may be unaffected."[50] Guidelines for TLVs are published annually by the American Conference of Governmental Industrial Hygienists (ACGIH) for use by industrial hygienists to guide them in making decisions about safe levels of exposure to chemicals and other agents found in the occupational environment.[51]
- *Biological exposure indices (BEIs)*—"A measure of the amount of chemical absorbed into the body."[50] The ACGIH also publishes BEIs annually.
- *Permissible exposure limits (PELs)*—"An OSHA standard . . . [that] is subject specific and has the supporting documentation for promulgation and enforcement of occupational health regulations. [PELs denote] [a]n allowable exposure level in the workplace air [that is] averaged over an eight-hour shift."[50] This type of average is called a time-weighted average (TWA). PELs refer to airborne concentrations of substances, although they may refer also to dermatologic exposures.[52]
- *Maximum allowable concentrations (MAC)*—" define permissible levels of exposure to chemicals."[50]

CONCLUSION

The scope of the occupational environment is diverse and poses hazards to workers who are employed in many different types of employment settings. The field of occupational health has a lengthy history, beginning with the first humans who engaged in occupations such as mining and smelting metals. During the Industrial Revolution, the 19th century, and the early 20th century, workers often were required to work long hours under extremely hazardous conditions. Work-related diseases such as black lung disease and silicosis affected a large proportion of miners. With the introduction of labor laws and industrial reforms, the contribution of the occupational environment to adverse health conditions among workers has diminished. Nevertheless, occupational illnesses and injuries are a substantial cause of morbidity and mortality in the United States. Primary prevention programs—those directed at eliminating adverse health outcomes before they occur—should be a goal of occupational physicians and nurses, policymakers, employers, and industrial hygienists. Through the use of surveillance systems for monitoring occupational illnesses, introduction of environmental controls, and supplying of personal protective equipment, employers can achieve the realistic goal of minimizing the occurrence of adverse health outcomes that are associated with work.

Study Questions and Exercises

1. Define the following terms:
   a. Pneumoconiosis
   b. Byssinosis
   c. Mesothelioma
   d. Black lung disease
   e. Ototoxic
   f. Decibel (dB)
   g. Trauma
   h. Mule spinners' cancer

2. List five persons who were significant to the history of occupational health and state their contributions.

3. The following list describes occupations that involve exposures to hazardous substances (e.g., metals or chemicals). Indicate the hazards associated with each occupation. Which of these occupations, if any, no longer exist?
   a. Chimney sweep
   b. Welder
   c. Farm worker
   d. Miner
   e. Attendant at a firing range
   f. Pottery maker

4. What are two of the most common occupational illnesses (as opposed to injuries found in private industry)? What are the causal factors for these conditions?

5. The following is a list of agents of occupationally associated diseases and injuries. Describe the work settings in which they may be encountered and the types of adverse health outcomes they produce:

a. Microbial agents
b. Toxic chemicals and metals
c. Repetitive motion
d. Noise
e. Work-related stress

6. In recent years, what has been the leading cause of fatal occupational injuries? What are the top three causes of fatal occupational injuries? Which five industry sectors tend to have the highest rates of fatal occupational injuries (as of 2008)?

7. For the construction industry, a total of 975 fatal injuries were reported in 2008, whereas the number for agriculture, forestry, fishing, and hunting was 672. The rate of fatal injuries was higher for the category that included agriculture, forestry, fishing, and hunting than for the category of construction. Explain how the rate could be lower for construction than for agriculture, forestry, fishing, and hunting.

8. In your own words, describe methods for preventing occupational fatalities.

9. What are the five leading causes of nonfatal occupational injuries? What can be done to prevent such injuries?

10. The number of occupational illnesses has declined since 1994. What factors have led to this decline? What steps can be taken to reduce occupational hazards and thereby improve the health of workers?

11. Even though workers in professional occupations usually are not exposed directly to hazardous agents, they are prone to occupationally associated illnesses.
    a. What types of hazards predominate in professional occupations?
    b. What illnesses are associated with these hazards?
    c. What interventions would you propose to mitigate these hazards?

REFERENCES

1. Gochfeld M. Chronologic history of occupational medicine. *J Occup Environ Med.* 2005;47:96–114.

2. Wallick F. *The American Worker: An Endangered Species.* New York, NY: Ballantine Books; 1972.

3. Franco G. Ramazzini and workers' health. *Lancet.* 1999;354:858–861.

4. Hamilton A. *Exploring the Dangerous Trades: The Autobiography of Alice Hamilton, M.D.* Boston, MA: Little, Brown and Company; 1943.

5. Centers for Disease Control and Prevention. Improvements in workplace safety—United States, 1900–1999. *MMWR.* 1999;48:461–469.

6. Rosner D, Markowitz G. Labor Day and the war on workers. *Am J Public Health.* 1999;89:1319–1321.

7. US National Park Service. Triangle Shirtwaist factory building. Available at: http://www.nps.gov/history/nr/travel/pwwmh/ny30.htm. Accessed February 24, 2010.

8. University of Missouri–Kansas City School of Law. The Triangle Shirtwaist Factory Fire Trial, by Doug Linder (2002). Available at: http://www.law.umkc.edu/faculty/projects/ftrials/triangle/trianglefire.html. Accessed May 14, 2010.

9. Kuschner WG. Introduction to the symposium. *Postgraduate Medicine.* 2003;113(4). Available at: http://www.postgradmed.com/index.php?art=pgm_04_2003?article=1397. Accessed May 6, 2010.

10. US Department of Health and Human Services, Public Health Service. *Healthy People 2010.* Progress review: occupational safety and health. February 18, 2004. Available at: http://www.healthypeople.gov/data/2010prog/focus20/OccSafetyHealth.pdf. Accessed May 10, 2010.

11. Sestito JP, Lunsford RA, Hamilton AC, Rosa RR, eds. *Worker Health Chartbook 2004.* NIOSH Publication Number 2004-146. Cincinnati, OH: Department of Health and Human Services, Centers for Disease Control and Prevention, National Institute for Occupational Safety and Health; 2004.

12. US Department of Labor, Bureau of Labor Statistics. *News Release: Workplace Injuries and Illnesses—2008.* Washington, DC: US Department of Labor, Bureau of Labor Statistics; October 29, 2009.

13. Berglund B, Lindvall T, eds. *Community Noise.* Archives of the Center for Sensory Research. 1995;2(1):1–195.

14. Kam PCA, Kam AC, Thompson JF. Noise pollution in the anaesthetic and intensive care environment. *Anaesthesia.* 1994;49:982–986.

15. European Agency for Safety and Health at Work. Factsheet 40—Skin sensitisers. Available at: http://osha.europa.eu/en/publications/factsheets/40/view. Accessed May 10, 2010.

16. Centers for Disease Control and Prevention, National Institute for Occupational Safety and Health. National Occupational Research Agenda. NORA priority research areas. Available at: http://www.cdc.gov/niosh/docs/96-115/diseas.html. Accessed April 21, 2010.

17. Centers for Disease Control and Prevention. Current trends leading work-related diseases and injuries. *MMWR.* 1986;35:561–563.

18. Peate WF. Occupational skin disease. *Am Fam Physician.* 2002;66:1025–1032, 1039–1040.

19. Heron MP, Hoyert DL, Murphy SL, Xu JQ, Kochanek KD, Tejada-Vera B. Deaths: Final data for 2006. National vital statistics reports; vol 57 no 14. Hyattsville, MD: National Center for Health Statistics; 2009.

20. Stellman JM, ed. *Encyclopaedia of Occupational Health and Safety.* 4th ed. Geneva, Switzerland: International Labour Organization; 1998.

21. US Environmental Protection Agency. Asbestos: asbestos ban and phase out. Available at: http://www.epa.gov/asbestos/pubs/ban.html. Accessed February 24, 2010.

22. SilicosisFYI.com. Are you a victim of silica exposure? Available at: http://www.silicosisfyi.com. Accessed April 19, 2010.

23. National Institute on Deafness and Other Communication Disorders (NIDCD). Wise Ears!* At work! Available at: http://www.nidcd.nih.gov/health/wise/wiseears_atwork.asp. Accessed April 19, 2010.

24. Alberti PW. Noise, the most ubiquitous pollutant. *Noise & Health.* 1998;1:3–5.

25. Noise Pollution Clearinghouse (NPC). About noise, noise pollution, and the Clearinghouse. Available at: http://www.nonoise.org/aboutno.htm. Accessed February 24, 2010.

26. Prasher D. Issue of environmental noise and annoyance [editorial]. *Noise & Health.* 1999;3:1.

27. National Institute on Deafness and Other Communication Disorders (NIDCD). Common sounds. Available at: http://www.nidcd.nih.gov/health/education/teachers/common_sounds.asp. Accessed April 24, 2010.

28. Schneider S, Johanning E, Bélard J-L, et al. Noise, vibration, and heat and cold. *Occup Med.* 1995;10:363–383.

29. Ray CD, Levinson R. Noise pollution in the operating room: a hazard to surgeons, personnel, and patients. *J Spinal Disord.* 1992;5:485–488.

30. Merrell HB, Claggett K. Noise pollution and hearing loss in the dental office. *Dent Assist J.* 1992;61(3):6–9.

31. Centers for Disease Control and Prevention, National Institute for Occupational Safety and Health. *Criteria for a Recommended Standard: Occupational Noise Exposure, Revised Criteria 1998.* DHHS (NIOSH) Publication No. 98-126. Cincinnati, Ohio: US Department of Health and Human Services; 1998.

32. Isolani L, Bonfiglioli R, Raffi GB. Different case definitions to describe the prevalence of occupational carpal tunnel syndrome in meat industry workers. *Int Arch Occup Environ Health.* 2002;75:229–234.

33. National Oceanic and Atmospheric Administration, Southeast Fisheries Science Center. Computer ergonomics self help guide. Available at: http://www.sefsc.noaa.gov/HTMLdocs/ComputerErgonomics.htm. Accessed May 11, 2010.

34. Stetler CB, Burns M, Sander-Buscemi K, et al. Use of evidence for prevention of work-related musculoskeletal injuries. *Orthop Nurs.* 2003;22(1):32–41.

35. Centers for Disease Control and Prevention, National Institute for Occupational Safety and Health. Traumatic occupational injuries. Available at: http://www.cdc.gov/niosh/injury/default.html. Accessed April 19, 2010.

36. Marsh SM, Layne LA. *Fatal Injuries to Civilian Workers in the United States, 1980–1995 (National and State Profiles).* DHHS (NIOSH) Publication No. 2001-129S. CDC, National Institute for Occupational Safety and Health; 2001.

37. Centers for Disease Control and Prevention. Occupational injuries and deaths among younger workers—United States, 1998–2007. *MMWR.* 2010;59:449–455.

38. US Department of Labor, Bureau of Labor Statistics. Economic news release: Census of fatal occupational injuries summary, 2008. Available at: http://www.bls.gov/news.release/cfoi.nr0.htm. Accessed April 24, 2010.

39. Centers for Disease Control and Prevention, National Institute for Occupational Safety and Health. *Stress . . . at Work.* DHHS (NIOSH) Publication No. 99-101. Cincinnati, OH: National Institute for Occupational Safety and Health; 1999.

40. MedicineNet.com. Definition of critical incident stress management. Available at: http://www.medterms.com/script/main/art.asp?articlekey=26281. Accessed April 24, 2010.

41. Elovaino M, Kuusio H, Aalto AM, et al. Insecurity and shiftwork as characteristics of negative work environment: psychosocial and behavioural mediators. *J Adv Nurs.* 2010;66:1080–1091.

42. Godin I, Kittel F, Coppieters Y, et al. A prospective study of cumulative job stress in relation to mental health. *BMC Public Health.* 2005;5:67.

43. Kivimaki M, Leino-Arjas P, Luukkonen R, et al. Work stress and risk of cardiovascular mortality: prospective cohort study of industrial employees. *BMJ.* 2002;325:857.

44. Eaker ED, Sullivan LM, Kelly-Hayes M, et al. Does job strain increase the risk for coronary heart disease or death in men and women? The Framingham Offspring Study. *Am J Epidemiol.* 2004;159:950–958.

45. US Department of Labor, Occupational Safety and Health Administration. OSHA fact sheet: personal protective equipment. Washington, DC: Occupational Safety and Health Administration; 2002.

46. Centers for Disease Control and Prevention, National Institute for Occupational Safety and Health, National Personal Protective Technology Laboratory. Respirators. Available at: http://www.cdc.gov/niosh/npptl/topics/respirators. Accessed April 19, 2010.

47. Centers for Disease Control and Prevention, National Institute for Occupational Safety and Health. *Tracking Occupational Injuries, Illnesses, and Hazards: The NIOSH Surveillance Strategic Plan.* DHHS (NIOSH) Publication No. 2001-118. Cincinnati, Ohio: NIOSH; 2001.

48. LaMontagne AD, Herrick RF, Van Dyke MV, et al. Exposure databases and exposure surveillance: promise and practice. *AIHA J.* 2002;63:205–212.

49. California Department of Public Health, Occupational Health Branch. Occupational Health Surveillance and Evaluation Program (OHSEP). Available at: http://www.cdph.ca.gov/programs/ohsep/Pages/default.aspx. Accessed May 11, 2010.

50. Extension Toxicology Network (EXTOXNET). Toxicology information brief: standards. Available at: http://pmep.cce.cornell.edu/profiles/extoxnet/TIB/standards.html. Accessed April 19, 2010.

51. American Conference of Governmental Industrial Hygienists (ACGIH). Statement of position regarding the TLVs and BEIs. Available at: http://www.acgih.org/TLV/PosStmt.htm. Accessed April 19, 2010.

52. US Department of Labor, Occupational Safety and Health Administration. Permissible exposure limits (PELs). Available at: http://www.osha.gov/SLTC/pel/index.html. Accessed February 24, 2010.

Injuries with a Focus on Unintentional Injuries and Deaths

INTRODUCTION

From the worldwide perspective, injuries of all types account for an estimated 5 million deaths annually[1]; unintentional injuries cause more than 3.5 million deaths, 6 percent of all deaths, and two-thirds of all injury deaths during a typical year.[2] With respect to the United States, unintentional injuries are the fifth leading cause of mortality in the population as a whole and the leading cause of death for the population aged 1 to 44 years.[3] These dramatic contributions to mortality (as well as to morbidity) worldwide and domestically often are preventable and can be linked with environmental influences. Accordingly, because of their association with environmental factors, injuries are a noteworthy topic for an environmental health textbook. Chapter 14 delimits the scope of injuries (both intentional and unintentional), describes how environmental factors contribute to such injuries, and suggests methods for prevention of injuries. The field of injury studies covers a vast domain, e.g., car crashes, falls, poisonings,

shootings, recreational injuries, and industrial injuries. The present chapter will focus primarily on unintentional injuries and consider in detail three major areas: motor vehicle injuries and transport-related injuries, life stages and unintentional injuries, and methods of injury prevention. The chapter will also describe methodologies used in injury research, identify some of the most important types of injuries, and discuss the economic impact of injuries.

HOW INJURIES ARE CLASSIFIED

Specialists in the field of injury research have devoted considerable attention to methods for describing and classifying injuries. Development of a standardized framework for classification of injuries facilitates making comparisons internationally and domestically within the United States. For example, the rates for various types of injuries can be compared more easily from one year to the next as well as across states and regions. Accurate and reliable information helps policy makers develop injury prevention and intervention programs.

One of the methods for classifying injuries uses the *International Classification of Diseases* (ICD) Injury Matrices, which organize injury data into helpful groupings in order to make international and national comparisons.[4] The ICD classifies injuries according to two dimensions: *external cause* (e.g., car crash) and *nature of the injury or diagnosis* (e.g., fracture). Within each of these two dimensions are two axes, which are collapsed into a single code. For example, the first dimension, external cause, is presented as a single code that combines the mechanism of injury (e.g., firearm) and intent of injury (e.g., intentional). The second dimension is the nature of the injury, also a single code for a two-factor variable that aggregates the nature of the injury itself (e.g., open wound) with the region of the body affected (e.g., chest).[4,5]

The term **injury** refers to "the physical damage [to the person] that results when a human body is suddenly or briefly subjected to intolerable levels of energy. It can be a bodily lesion resulting from acute exposure to energy in amounts that exceed the threshold of physiological tolerance, or it can be an impairment of function resulting from a lack of one or more vital elements (i.e.[,] air, water, warmth), as in drowning, strangulation or freezing. The time between exposure to the energy and the appearance of an injury is short."[6(p5)] Examples of energy that can cause injuries are mechanical force, radiant energy from light or shock waves, extremes of temperature, electrical energy, and chemical energy. Injuries that do not result in death—nonfatal injuries—are defined as "bodily harm resulting from severe exposure to an external force or substance (mechanical, thermal, electrical, chemical, or radiant) or a submersion. This bodily harm can be unintentional or violence-related."[7]

The **cause (mechanism) of injury** denotes "the way in which the person sustained the injury; how the person was injured; or the process by which the injury occurred. . . . The underlying cause is what starts the chain of events that leads to an injury. The direct cause is what produces the actual physical harm. The underlying and direct causes can be the same or different. For example, if a person cuts his or her finger with a knife, the cut is both the underlying and direct cause. However, if a child falls and hits his head on a coffee table, the fall is the underlying cause (the action that starts the injury event), and the contact with the table is the direct cause (the action that causes the actual physical harm)."[7] Examples of definitions for causes of nonfatal injuries used by WISQARS™ Nonfatal are shown in the text box.[7] (Also see Table 14-1.)

Another aspect of injuries is the **intent of injury**, which refers to "[w]hether an injury was caused by an act carried out on purpose by oneself or by another person(s), with the goal of injuring or killing."[7] Three terms for classifying the intent of injuries are unintentional, intentional, and undetermined. Intentional injuries include those that result from self-harm (e.g., suicide), legal intervention (e.g., action of the police), interpersonal actions (e.g., assault), and acts of war. An **unintentional injury** is an "[i]njury or poisoning that is not inflicted by deliberate means (i.e., not on purpose). This category includes those injuries and poisonings described as unintended or "accidental," regardless of whether the injury was inflicted by oneself or by another person."[7]

An unintentional injury is the consequence of an unanticipated event that results in harm or death. The use of the

Examples of Causes of Nonfatal Injuries

Cut/pierce/stab: Injury resulting from an incision, slash, perforation, or puncture by a pointed or sharp instrument, weapon, or object. This category does not include injury from being struck by or against a blunt object (such as the side of a night stand) or bite wounds; these injuries fall in the category "struck by/against."

Inhalation/ingestion/suffocation: Inhalation, aspiration, or ingestion of food or other object that blocks the airway or causes suffocation; intentional or accidental mechanical suffocation due to hanging, strangulation, lack of air in a closed place, plastic bag or falling earth. This category does not include injury resulting from a foreign body that does not block the airway.

Natural/environmental: Injury resulting from exposure to adverse natural and environmental conditions (such as severe heat, severe cold, lightning, sunstroke, large storms, and natural disasters) as well as lack of food or water.

Poisoning: Ingestion, inhalation, absorption through the skin, or injection of so much of a drug, toxin (biologic or non-biologic), or other chemical that a harmful effect results, such as drug overdoses. This category does not include harmful effects from normal therapeutic drugs (i.e., unexpected adverse effects to a drug administered correctly to treat a condition) or bacterial illnesses.

Struck by/against or crushed: Injury resulting from being struck by (hit) or crushed by a human, animal, or inanimate object or force other than a vehicle or machinery; injury caused by striking (hitting) against a human, animal, or inanimate object or force other than a vehicle or machinery.

Transportation-related causes: Injury involving modes of transportation, such as cars, motorcycles, bicycles, and trains. This category is divided into four subcategories according to the person injured: motor vehicle occupant, motorcyclist, pedal cyclist, pedestrian, and other transport. This category also involves another factor—whether the injury occurred in traffic (on a public road or highway).

Pedal cyclist: Injury to a pedal cycle rider from a collision, loss of control, crash, or some other event involving a moving vehicle or pedestrian. This category includes riders of unicycles, bicycles, tricycles, and mountain bikes. This category does not include injuries unrelated to transport (moving), such as repairing a bicycle.

Source: Adapted and reprinted from the Centers for Disease Control and Prevention, Injury Center. Definitions for WISQARS Nonfatal. Available at: http://www.cdc.gov/Ncipc/wisqars/nonfatal/definitions.htm. Accessed May 21, 2010.

term unintentional injury is preferred to accident; the latter implies a random event that cannot be prevented. Most unintentional injuries are highly preventable; for example, laws that require seat belts and air bags in cars have contributed to a decline in motor vehicle driver and passenger deaths. Other preventive measures include safety messages directed to the public via media campaigns, prohibition of consumption of alcoholic beverages in public parks, school-based safety programs for school children, and licensing of firearms.

In practice—for example, in some government reports—the terms unintentional injury and accident often are used interchangeably, perhaps because of the public's familiarity with the latter term and its use in common parlance. An **accident** is defined as "An unanticipated event—commonly leading to INJURY or other harm—in traffic, the workplace, or a domestic or recreational setting. The primary event in a sequence that leads ultimately to injury if that event is genuinely not predictable. Epidemiological studies have demonstrated that the risk of accidents is often predictable and that accidents are preventable. This word is preferably avoided in many types of scientific works."[8] The World Health Organization states, "There is clear, scientific evidence that injury-related deaths can be avoided and the effect of injury mitigated. . . . [R]esearch, development of data collection systems, the introduction of specific prevention measures such as improvements in the local environment, legislation, public education, product safety, and improvements in the level and quality of emergency care [have led to the reduction of injury deaths among children]."[1]

Because the word *accident* is not in favor as a scientific term, the National Center for Health Statistics has added the term "unintentional injuries" in parentheses next to the category of accidents, the fifth leading cause of death in the United States.[5] The National Highway Traffic Safety Administration (NHTSA) favors the use of the term car *crash* to *accident*.

Injury epidemiology is a branch of epidemiology that studies the distribution and determinants of injuries in the population. The results of epidemiologic investigations are applied to the prevention and control of injuries. For example, descriptive epidemiologic studies aid in the development of analytic research into the risk factors for and causes of injuries. From this information, policies and procedures to prevent injuries are facilitated. Currently, such research programs may be coupled with ongoing injury surveillance programs and databases that store information about the occurrence of injuries.

Chapter 2 covered the use of natural experiments, one of the study designs employed in analytic epidemiology. When new laws to increase safety are adopted (e.g., improvement of automobile safety through the mandatory use of passenger safety belts), they are similar to natural experiments, which can be evaluated by the use of epidemiologic methods.

Sources of Injury Data

As noted previously, high quality (reliable and valid) data are necessary for developing descriptive and analytic research on the occurrence of and risk factors for unintentional injuries. See Table 14-1 for examples of data sources; as shown in the table, one method for collecting information about injuries is the use of **surveillance systems**. Public health surveillance refers to the systematic and continuous gathering of information about the occurrence of diseases and other health phenomena. As part of the surveillance process, personnel analyze and interpret the data they have collected and distribute the data and associated findings to planners, health workers, and members of the community. Injury surveillance systems specialize in collecting information about injuries, for example, occupational injuries, motor vehicle injuries, risk behaviors, traumatic brain injuries, and injuries to consumers.

In addition to listing information regarding surveillance data, Table 14-1 gives other examples of data sources that may be accessed for information about injuries. The National Hospital Discharge Survey compiles information about patients who receive hospital care for injuries. The National Vital Statistics System collects and reports data on injuries listed on death certificates. The *National Vital Statistics Reports* published by the CDC is an example of a report that displays information on the frequency and distribution of intentional and unintentional injuries. Many of the data sources shown in the table can be accessed via the Internet.

THE SIGNIFICANCE OF INJURIES

Injuries are a significant phenomenon worldwide because everyone is at risk. As noted, approximately 5 million people succumb to fatal injuries worldwide each year.[1] (This total includes both intentional and unintentional injuries.) The death toll from injuries is projected to increase substantially by the year 2020.[9] Beyond the direct harm to people, injuries burden the healthcare system and rehabilitation facilities. The adverse effects caused by injuries include the immediate impact not only upon the affected individual but also upon that person's family members and social support system. Nonfatal injuries can lead to permanent disability and drastically affect one's independence—not to mention the pain and suffering that may be experienced by the injured person.[10] Injuries may create stress and severe emotional responses among family members and exact a substantial economic cost.

TABLE 14-1 Data Sources and Types of Information Available on Injuries

Data Source	Sponsor	Population Coverage	Information Available
Behavioral Risk Factor Surveillance System	The CDC	All of United States (persons aged 18 years old and older)	Risk behaviors for leading causes of injury and death; injury-related data, e.g., occurrence of falls, use of seat belts.
Central nervous system surveillance: traumatic brain injury (TBI)	The CDC	Participating US states	Extent of injury among persons who experience TBIs. Risk factors for TBI.
National Electronic Injury Surveillance System—All Injury Program	US Consumer Product Safety Commission	US hospitals	Originally for injuries associated with consumer products. Now includes all nonfatal injuries treated in hospital emergency departments.
National Hospital Discharge Survey	The CDC—National Center for Health Statistics	US national sample of about 500 hospitals	Injuries among persons who survive and are discharged from inpatient hospital care.
National Vital Statistics System	The CDC—National Center for Health Statistics	All of United States	Deaths causes by injuries and violence.
Web-based Injury Statistics Query and Reporting System (WISQARS)	The CDC	All of United States	Injury morbidity and mortality data. Fatal and nonfatal unintentional and violent injuries. Permits online user queries via interactive database.

Source: Data from National Center for Injury Prevention and Control. *CDC Injury Fact Book.* Atlanta, GA: Centers for Disease Control and Prevention; 2006:16.

Noteworthy is the fact that injuries manifest characteristic social and demographic distributions, disproportionately affecting the poor in all countries of the world.[6] A total of 90% of unintentional injury deaths transpire in low- and middle-income countries.[2] Some environmental conditions found in many less developed countries increase the likelihood of unintentional injuries; these aspects of the environment include poorly maintained sidewalks, lack of paved streets, unavailability of pedestrian zones in cities, public transportation facilities in disrepair, and unsafe working conditions in factories.

At the international level, persons between the ages of 5 and 44 years are at special risk of injuries of all types; among this age group injury-related causes account for 6 of the 10 leading causes of death. About half of injury-related mortality occurs in the group aged 15 to 44 years; mortality from injuries among men is double that among women.[9] Injuries account for approximately one-third of deaths among children aged 1 to 14 years in Europe, although death rates differ greatly between Eastern and Western European countries.[11] For ex-

ample, the main contributors to injury deaths among children in the former Soviet Union countries of Eastern Europe are drowning, poisoning, fires, and falls. Traffic-related injuries are the leading cause of injury-related mortality among children and young people in the northwestern part of Europe.

In the United States, all forms of injuries accounted for 179,065 deaths during 2006. (Refer to Figure 14-1.) These were distributed according to the five general categories shown on the left of Figure 14-1. These categories, defined according to International Classification of Diseases (ICD) codes, are unintentional injuries, suicide, homicide, undetermined, and legal intervention/war (shown as legal intervention in the figure). The three leading causes of death from injuries were unintentional injuries, suicide, and homicide. Fatalities from unintentional injuries are discussed later in the chapter. Note that these aggregate categories can be subdivided into finer subcategories and rearranged into other classifications. For example, the general category of suicide can also fall under specific mechanisms and intent of death (e.g., firearm suicide, suicide by drowning, and suicide by poisoning).

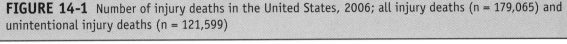

FIGURE 14-1 Number of injury deaths in the United States, 2006; all injury deaths (n = 179,065) and unintentional injury deaths (n = 121,599)

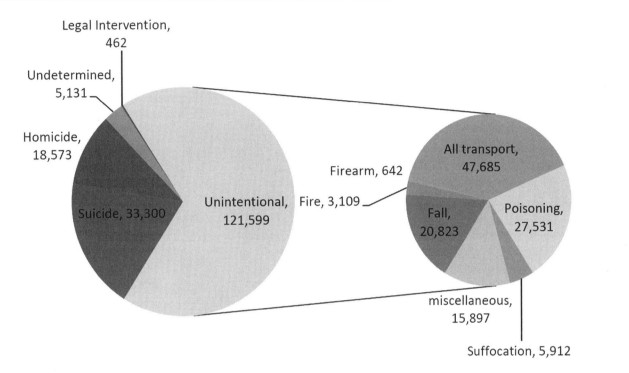

Source: Data from Heron M, Hoyert DL, Murphy SL, et al. Deaths: Final data for 2006. National vital statistics reports; vol 57 no 14. Hyattsville, MD: National Center for Health Statistics; 2009, p. 89.

Time trends in age-adjusted death rates for the three leading causes of injury death are presented in Figure 14-2. According to the CDC,

> During 1979–2004, the three leading causes of injury death in the United States were motor-vehicle traffic, firearm, and poisoning (including drug overdose). In 2004, for the first time since 1968, when such data first became available, the number of reported poisoning deaths (30,308) and the age-adjusted poisoning death rate (10.3 per 100,000 population) exceeded the number of firearm deaths (29,569) and the firearm death rate (10.0), respectively. During 1999–2004, the poisoning death rate increased 45%, whereas the firearm death rate declined 3%; during the same period, no change occurred in the rate

(14.7) for motor-vehicle traffic deaths [number = 43,432]."[12(p1363)]

The three leading causes of injury deaths shown in Figure 14-2 encompass the following subcategories:

- Motor vehicle traffic deaths include fatalities to occupants of motor vehicles, motorcyclists, pedal cyclists, pedestrians, other, and unspecified (2006 data: number = 43,664; rate = 14.4 per 100,000).
- Firearm deaths include unintentional firearm deaths, suicide, homicide, undetermined, and legal intervention/war (2006 data: number = 30,896; rate = 10.2 per 100,000).
- Poisoning deaths include unintentional poisoning deaths, suicide, homicide, undetermined, and legal intervention/war (2006 data: number = 30,309; rate = 10.3 per 100,000).

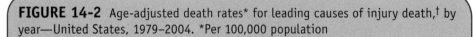

FIGURE 14-2 Age-adjusted death rates* for leading causes of injury death,† by year—United States, 1979–2004. *Per 100,000 population

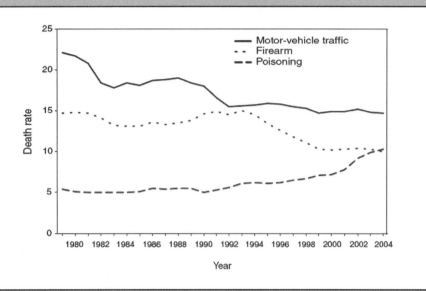

†Coded according to the International Classification of Diseases Ninth Revision during 1979–1998 and according to the Tenth Revision during 1999–2004.

Source: Reprinted from Centers for Disease Control and Prevention. QuickStats: Age-Adjusted Death Rates* for Leading Causes of Injury Death,† by Year—United States, 1979-2004. *MMWR.* 2006;55:1363.

UNINTENTIONAL INJURIES

The term *unintentional injury* was defined in an earlier section. Five of the categories of unintentional injuries are

- Injuries to children—e.g., children who live in substandard housing units are at increased risk of injuries, as are youngsters who play in unsupervised playgrounds.
- Motor vehicle injuries—Associated factors are human errors coupled with poorly designed highways. Although progress has been made in recent years, unsafe vehicles continue to contribute to the toll of injuries on public roadways; consider the case of an engineering defect that is alleged to have caused one brand of motor vehicle to accelerate out of control.
- Firearm injuries—Failure to educate the public about safe methods for storage and handling of weapons contributes to the number of unintentional firearm deaths.
- Falls—Inadequately illuminated stairways and slippery surfaces contribute to falls, a major cause of morbidity among the elderly.

- Workplace injuries—The work setting, a venue for the use of dangerous machinery and exposure to toxic chemicals, is a domain for numerous injuries to employees. This topic was covered previously in Chapter 13.

In the United States, unintentional injuries are the fifth leading cause of mortality. During 2006, a total of almost 121,599 deaths from unintentional injuries (5% of the total deaths) were recorded.[3] Figure 14-1 indicates that of the 121,599 deaths due to unintentional injuries, the three leading causes of death were transport-related fatalities, poisonings, and falls. The category of transport injuries included motor vehicle traffic injuries (e.g., vehicle occupants, motorcyclists, and pedestrians), other land transport injuries, and injuries that occurred on water and in the air and space. The crude and adjusted death rates for unintentional injuries were 40.6 and 39.8 per 100,000, respectively. During 2006, a total of 27.7 million visits were made to hospital emergency departments for unintentional injuries.[13] The three most frequent types of visits were for falls (8.6 million), motor vehicle traffic events (4.0 million), and "struck against or struck accidentally by objects or persons" (2.9 million). Figure 14-3 displays the percentage distribution of visits to emergency departments for unintentional injuries.

The top ten causes of unintentional injuries among age groups from under age 1 to age 65 and older are presented in Figure 14-4. You can see that unintentional motor vehicle traffic injuries dominate as the leading cause of injury deaths in all age groups combined and in 6 of the 10 age groups shown in the chart. Among infants (younger than 12 months old), suffocation is the leading cause of unintentional injury, followed by homicide (unspecified) and motor vehicle traffic injuries. With respect to children and young adults (persons aged 1 year to 24 years) and adults aged 25 to 34 years, motor vehicle traffic injuries lead the causes of injury death; also,

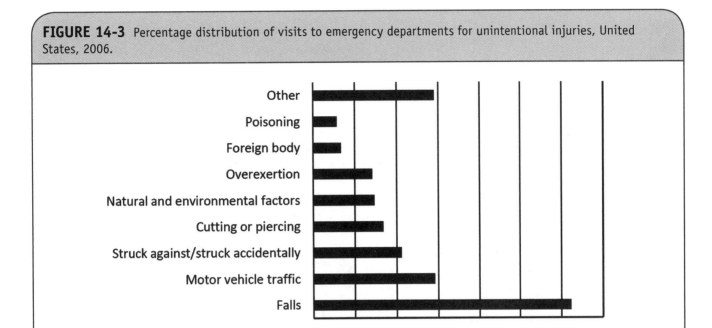

FIGURE 14-3 Percentage distribution of visits to emergency departments for unintentional injuries, United States, 2006.

Source: Data from Pitts SR, Niska RW, Xu J, et al. National Hospital Ambulatory Medical Care Survey: 2006 emergency department summary. National health statistics reports; no 7. Hyattsville, MD: National Center for Health Statistics; 2008, p. 28.

unintentional drowning, homicide/firearm, and fires and burns are frequent causes of mortality from injuries. In age groups 35 to 44 and 45 to 54, unintentional poisonings are at the top of the list of causes of injury deaths. In the 55 to 64 age group, motor vehicle traffic incidents are the most common cause of injury deaths. Unintentional falls are the leading cause of injury death among persons 65 years of age and older. Refer to the figure for information about other major causes of injury death.

Economic Impacts of Unintentional Injuries

The economic impacts of unintentional injuries include direct medical costs for treatment and indirect costs such as those due to:

- Lost productivity at work and home
- Charges for rehabilitative therapies (for physical and mental health)
- Coverage of caregiver expenses
- Personal injury lawsuits and other forms of litigation
- Other nonmedical expenses such as purchase of wheelchair ramps.[10]

Estimates of medical expenditures for treatment of injuries were $117 billion in 2000. (Refer to Table 14-2.) These expenditures are comparable to those for treatment of the effects of such major public health problems as diabetes and smoking.[10] Table 14-2 demonstrates that the costs were highest among the 45–64 age group and that women in this age group had the highest costs of any age group when men and women were classified separately. However, overall, men had slightly higher expenditures than women.

The remainder of this chapter will cover several of the major types of injuries that are among the most burdensome for society in terms of economic costs as well as the extent of morbidity and mortality that they produce. Among the topics that we will explore are:

- Motor vehicle injuries and other types of transport injuries. Related topics are pedestrian injuries, child passenger safety, teenage and older adult drivers, risk factors for injuries, and methods for prevention of such injuries.
- Unintentional injuries among children and young adults. Examples are recreational and sports-related injuries.

FIGURE 14-4 Ten leading causes of injury death by age group highlighting unintentional injury deaths, United States—2006.

Rank	<1	1–4	5–9	10–14	15–24	25–34	35–44	45–54	55–64	65+	Total
1	Unintentional suffocation 843	Unintentional MV traffic 471	Unintentional MV traffic 515	Unintentional MV traffic 703	Unintentional MV traffic 10,739	Unintentional MV traffic 7,162	Unintentional poisoning 7,542	Unintentional poisoning 8,234	Unintentional MV traffic 4,317	Unintentional fall 16,650	Unintentional MV traffic 43,664
2	Homicide unspecified 179	Unintentional drowning 458	Unintentional drowning 142	Homicide firearm 175	Homicide firearm 4,827	Unintentional poisoning 5,267	Unintentional MV traffic 6,470	Unintentional MV traffic 6,396	Suicide firearm 2,562	Unintentional MV traffic 6,738	Unintentional poisoning 27,531
3	Unintentional MV traffic 139	Unintentional fire/burn 202	Unintentional fire/burn 118	Suicide suffocation 137	Unintentional poisoning 2,936	Homicide firearm 3,767	Suicide firearm 2,821	Suicide firearm 3,481	Unintentional poisoning 2,415	Unintentional unspecified 4,989	Unintentional fall 20,823
4	Homicide other spec., classifiable 75	Homicide unspecified 166	Homicide firearm 62	Unintentional drowning 114	Suicide firearm 1,978	Suicide firearm 2,150	Homicide firearm 1,987	Suicide poisoning 1,841	Unintentional fall 1,592	Suicide firearm 3,828	Suicide firearm 16,883
5	Unintentional drowning 51	Unintentional suffocation 137	Unintentional other land transport 50	Unintentional other land transport 66	Suicide suffocation 1,509	Suicide suffocation 1,597	Suicide suffocation 1,694	Suicide suffocation 1,399	Suicide poisoning 1,028	Unintentional suffocation 3,211	Homicide firearm 12,791
6	Undetermined suffocation 42	Unintentional pedestrian, other 113	Unintentional suffocation 50	Unintentional fire/burn 64	Unintentional drowning 616	Suicide poisoning 800	Suicide poisoning 1,517	Unintentional fall 1,290	Suicide suffocation 598	Adverse effects 1,605	Suicide suffocation 7,491
7	Homicide suffocation 34	Homicide other spec., classifiable 51	Homicide unspecified 24	Suicide firearm 62	Homicide cut/pierce 473	Undetermined poisoning 625	Undetermined poisoning 991	Homicide firearm 1,185	Homicide firearm 468	Unintentional fire/burn 1,130	Unintentional unspecified 6,345
8	Unintentional fire/burn 28	Homicide firearm 42	Unintentional other transport 22	Unintentional suffocation 58	Undetermined poisoning 389	Homicide cut/pierce 476	Unintentional fall 628	Undetermined poisoning 1,049	Unintentional fire/burn 467	Unintentional poisoning 1,025	Suicide poisoning 6,109
9	Three* tied 23	Unintentional fall 38	Unintentional pedestrian, other 22	Suicide firearm 62	Suicide poisoning 342	Unintentional drowning 436	Unintentional drowning 466	Unintentional drowning 491	Unintentional suffocation 463	Suicide poisoning 570	Unintentional suffocation 5,912
10	Three* tied 23	Unintentional natural/ environment 37	Two** tied 18	Unintentional other transport 30	Unintentional other land transport 280	Unintentional fall 318	Homicide cut/pierce 424	Unintentional fire/burn 491	Unintentional unspecified 393	Unintentional natural/ environment 555	Unintentional drowning 3,579

Age Groups

*Three causes are: Adverse effects, undetermined unspecified and unintentional falls
**Two causes are: Unintentional firearm and unintentional poisoning

Source: Reprinted from the Centers for Disease Control and Prevention. Ten Leading Causes of Death and Injury (Charts), Causes of Injury Death: Highlighting Unintentional Injury. Available at: http://www.cdc.gov/injury/Images/LC-Charts/10lc%20-Unintentional%20Injury%202006-7_6_09).jpg. Accessed May 20, 2010.

TABLE 14-2 Percentage and Number[a] of Persons Reporting Treatment for an Injury and Percentage and Amount of Medical Expenditures Attributable to Injuries, by Selected Characteristics—United States, 2000

Characteristic[b]	Persons reporting treatment for an injury (%)	Persons reporting treatment for an injury No.[c]	Medical expenditures attributable to injuries %	Medical expenditures attributable to injuries MEPS[d]	Injury-attributable expenditures ($) NHA[e]	Injury-attributable expenditures ($) Per capita, NHA
Total	(16.3)	44.7	10.3	64.7	117.2	427
Sex						
Male	(17.3)	23.1	12.5	33.2	59.8	448
Female	(15.4)	21.6	9.2	31.8	57.4	409
Age group (yrs)						
<10	(11.9)	4.8	7.8	3.1	5.7	141
10–19	(17.9)	7.2	16.6	7.4	13.4	333
20–29	(15.8)	5.7	6.8	2.7	5.0	137
30–44	(17.8)	11.3	12.2	14.6	26.5	417
45–64	(16.7)	10.2	10.6	20.9	37.9	621
>65	(16.7)	5.5	8.7	16.0	29.0	881
Sex by age group						
Male						
<10	(13.7)	2.8	9.4	1.6	3.0	145
10–19	(20.7)	4.3	26.3	5.1	9.2	445
20–29	(18.0)	3.2	7.9	1.0	1.7	98
30–44	(20.0)	6.2	15.3	7.5	13.6	438
45–64	(15.5)	4.6	7.9	7.6	13.7	463
>65	(14.2)	2.0	11.8	9.6	17.4	1,233
Female						
<10	(9.9)	1.9	6.7	1.3	2.3	118
10–19	(15.0)	3.0	11.9	3.0	5.4	272
20–29	(13.6)	2.5	4.8	1.4	2.5	139
30–44	(15.7)	5.1	9.4	6.7	12.1	373
45–64	(17.9)	5.7	12.5	12.9	23.3	732
>65	(18.5)	3.5	6.7	7.1	12.9	680

[a]In millions.

[b]On the basis of Medical Expenditure Panel Survey (MEPS) estimates.

[c]Results were weighted to be nationally representative.

[d]In billions. MEPS estimate of US medical expenditures in 2000 is restricted to the civilian, noninstitutionalized population.

[e]In billions. National Health Accounts (NHA) estimates include the US-based military and institutionalized populations and are calculated by multiplying the NHA estimate of US medical expenditures in 2000 by the percentage of medical expenditures attributable to injuries estimated by MEPS.

Source: Adapted from National Center for Injury Prevention and Control. *CDC Injury Fact Book*. Atlanta, GA: Centers for Disease Control and Prevention; 2006:3.

- Common injuries such as falls among elderly persons
- A framework for injury prevention

MOTOR VEHICLE INJURIES

In the United States, motor vehicle crashes were the leading cause of unintentional deaths in 2006 and accounted for 43,664 fatalities, the largest number (11,015) of which occurred among persons aged 15 to 24 years. When one encounters the scene of a car crash, often the event is frightening and evokes intense emotions. (Refer to Figure 14-5.) Unfortunately, motor vehicle crashes are an all too common event on America's highways. Since the early 2000s, the occurrence of such fatalities has not declined over time. Motor vehicle fatalities and injuries vary according to the demographic characteristics of the victims, geographic region, and risk factors associated with crashes. Data suggest that young male drivers are the group most likely to be involved in fatal crashes.

During the years 1999–2005, the number of motor vehicle–related deaths totaled 311,356.[14] From the late 1960s to 1992, death rates showed a 43% decline, and then did not de-

FIGURE 14-5 Emergency treatment at the scene of a car crash.

Source: Reprinted from National Highway Traffic Safety Administration. NHTSA Image Library, Img 138 H. Available at: http://www.nhtsa.dot.gov/nhtsa/ImageLibrary/display.cfm. Accessed May 20, 2010.

cline thereafter, despite the continuing introduction of safety measures and laws to prevent motor vehicle injuries. (Refer to Figure 14-2.) The annual death rates from 1999 to 2005 did not vary substantially; the rates ranged from 15.2 per 100,000 to 15.7 per 100,000.[14]

Time trends in death rates for motor vehicle fatalities vary by sex and age of victim. The annual death rate for motor vehicle fatalities during 1999 to 2005 for males (21.7 per 100,000) was more than double the rate for females (9.4 per 100,000). During this same period, persons aged 15 to 24 years and 75 years and older had the highest rates, 26.8 per 100,000 and 25.9 per 100,000, respectively.[14] Figure 14-6 presents data on time trends in motor vehicle fatalities by age group; during the time period shown, the total number of licensed drivers increased by about 13%.[15] The age group 16 to 20 years of age had the highest death rate from motor vehicle fatalities during the decade 1998–2008; however, the number of fatalities among drivers in this age group declined by 20%.[16] The rate of traffic fatalities among persons aged 65 years of age and older also reflected a declining trend; and, among persons aged 75 years and older, the average annual death rate from motor vehicle–related causes declined by 14% between 1999 and 2005.[14] Figure 14-7 demonstrates that the excess of male over female motor vehicle fatalities persisted across age groups (e.g., age group 16 to 20 years through age group 65 years and older).

Motor vehicle death rates vary by geographic region of the country, reaching the highest level in the South and the lowest in the Northeast. The respective rates by region were South (19.5 per 100,000), Midwest (14.7 per 100,000), West (14.2 per 100,000), and Northeast (9.8 per 100,000).[14] The rates for this cause also vary by race and ethnicity. American Indians/Alaska Natives had the highest rate (27.2 per 100,000) among four racial classifications. (Refer to Figure 14-8.)

Other Types of Transport-Related Injuries

Another type of transport-related injury is associated with the use of all-terrain vehicles (ATVs). A motorized ATV has low-pressure tires that enable it to travel off road. According to data for the 1990s, West Virginia had death rates from ATV crashes that were about eight times higher than the national average.[17] The state enacted several laws to reduce ATV fatalities; examples were reducing the distance that is permitted to travel on paved roads, reducing the speed of the vehicle, and requiring helmet use. Nevertheless, between 1999 and 2006, fatal ATV crashes increased by about 14% per year. (Refer to Figure 14-9.) During this period, 250 people died from ATV crashes in West Virginia. Factors related to ATV fatalities were lower socioeconomic status, being single or divorced, and having lower levels of education.

FIGURE 14-6 Motor vehicle traffic fatality rates by age group, 1998–2008.

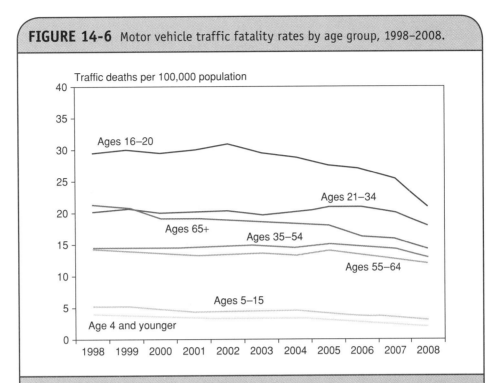

Source: Reprinted from NHTSA. Traffic Safety Facts: 2008 Data. Available at: http://www-nrd.nhtsa.dot. gov/Pubs/811161.PDF. Accessed March 24, 2010.

FIGURE 14-7 Driver involvement rates in fatal crashes by age and sex, 2008.

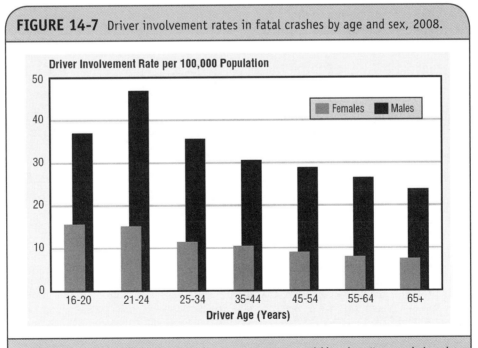

Source: Reprinted from NHTSA. Traffic Safety Facts: 2008 Data. Available at: http://www-nrd.nhtsa.dot. gov/Pubs/811161.PDF. Accessed March 24, 2010.

FIGURE 14-8 Number of motor vehicle-related deaths by race, United States, 1999–2005.

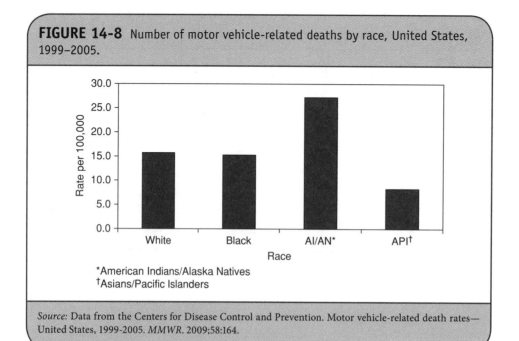

*American Indians/Alaska Natives
†Asians/Pacific Islanders

Source: Data from the Centers for Disease Control and Prevention. Motor vehicle-related death rates—United States, 1999-2005. *MMWR.* 2009;58:164.

FIGURE 14-9 Death rate* attributed to fatal all-terrain vehicle crashes, by age group† and crash classification§— West Virginia¶, 1999—2006.

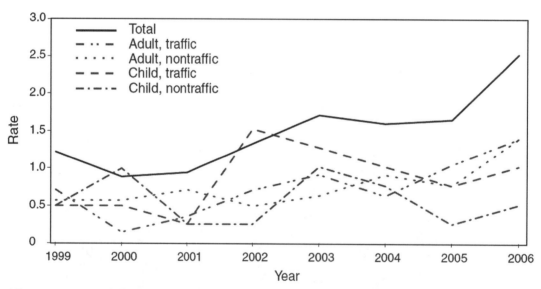

* Per 100,000 population.
† Adult is defined as a person aged ≥18 years; child is defined as a person aged <18 years.
§ Based on *International Classification of Deaths, 10th Revision.* Traffic crash defined as occurring on a public highway; nontraffic crash occurs entirely in any place other than a public highway.
¶ Includes only decedents who were West Virginia residents involved in crashes that occurred in West Virginia (N = 215).

Source: Reprinted from the Centers for Disease Control and Prevention. All-terrain vehicle fatalities—West Virginia, 1999-2006. *MMWR.* 2008;57:314.

Pedestrians and Motor Vehicles

During 2006, 5,021 transport-related deaths to pedestrians were reported. A large proportion of the deaths occurred among child pedestrians. In comparison with injuries to automobile passengers who are involved in crashes, injured pedestrians have a much higher likelihood of death.[18] Environmental factors are strongly implicated in pedestrian injuries. In illustration, roads in many US communities are devoid of sidewalks and shoulders, forcing pedestrians to walk close to vehicles. Convenient and safe pedestrian crossings may not be available: In the interest of promoting the flow of traffic, authorities may place crosswalks far apart, creating the temptation to jaywalk. Pedestrian fatalities can be prevented through the thoughtful design of roads and sidewalks. Other measures for enhancing pedestrian safety include:

- Increasing the awareness of the public, pedestrians, and drivers regarding pedestrian safety
- Developing safe-walking programs for children
- Modifying city streets to maximize pedestrian safety and encourage walking as a form of exercise
- Creating warning signs for motorists as well as speed-bumps in areas frequented by children and other pedestrians

Older Adult Drivers

In 2007, the number of older drivers (aged 65 years and older) had increased by almost one-fifth over the previous decade to 31 million licensed drivers—about 15% of all licensed drivers.[15] The injury toll for older drivers was more than 183,000 persons in 2008.[19] Methods for the prevention of motor vehicle crashes among this age group include (1) maintaining a regimen of regular exercise to increase strength and flexibility; (2) reviewing personal use of medications that may impair driving; (3) obtaining annual vision checks; (4) creating a safe environment within the car's interior by eliminating distractions, e.g., turning down the radio and not using a cell phone; and (5) completing a driver's training course for senior drivers. Other facts related to older drivers are shown in the text box.

Teen Drivers

Figure 14-6 demonstrates that during 1998 to 2008, persons aged 16 to 20 years had the highest rate of motor vehicle traffic fatalities. Approximately 3,500 teenagers (ages 15 to 19) died from crashes in 2008. As many as 100 times more teenagers were treated in hospital emergency rooms for this cause. Some risk factors for motor vehicle crashes in this age group are inexperience in driving a vehicle, failure to use seat

Older Adult Drivers: Who Is Most at Risk?

- Motor vehicle crash deaths per capita among males and females begin to increase markedly starting at ages 70–74. . . .
- Per mile traveled, fatal crash rates increase starting at age 75 and increase notably after age 80. This is largely due to increased susceptibility to injury, particularly chest injuries, and medical complications among older drivers rather than an increased tendency to get into crashes. . . .
- Age-related declines in vision and cognitive functioning (ability to reason and remember), as well as physical changes, may affect some older adults' driving abilities. . . .
- Across all age groups, males had substantially higher death rates than females. . . .

Source: Adapted and reprinted from the Centers for Disease Control and Prevention. Older adult drivers: fact sheet. Available at: http://www.cdc.gov/MotorVehicleSafety/Older_Adult_Drivers/adult-drivers_factsheet.html. Accessed April 10, 2010.

belts, driving without adult supervision while other teens are passengers, and drinking and driving. Reduction of motor vehicle fatalities can be accomplished through increased use of educational programs for teenage drivers and their parents. Graduated drivers licensing programs have proved to be highly effective in reducing crashes among drivers who are 16 years old.[20]

Summary of Risk Factors for Motor Vehicle Injuries

Several risk factors associated with car crashes were noted previously. These include:

- Drinking and driving: alcohol-impaired driving was implicated in almost one-third (about 12,000) of all fatalities caused by car crashes in 2008.[21] Most at risk were young persons, motorcyclists, and those who had prior drunk driving convictions. In addition to alcohol consumption, impaired driving can be caused by use of prescription medications and substance abuse.
- Failure to "buckle-up."

In recent years, many US states have instituted laws that mandate the use of automobile safety belts. Figure 14-10 provides data on the prevalence of always using a seat belt. Primary laws (referring to primary enforcement of safety-belt laws) permit law enforcement personnel to stop drivers and passengers who are not wearing belts and issue citation for noncompliance.[22] Secondary laws allow police officers to issue a citations for noncompliance only when motorists have been stopped for some other violation. Evidence suggests that primary laws are more effective than secondary laws for encouraging motorists to wear safety belts and reducing fatalities caused by automobiles. (See Figure 14-10) Seat belt use tends to increase during both daytime and nighttime driving hours among jurisdictions that transition from secondary seat belt laws to primary laws.[23]

Child Safety Seats

Child safety seats, essential for protecting infants and young children during a car crash or sudden stop, should be placed in the rear seat of a passenger vehicle and never in the front seat because of the risk of injury from air bags. When transporting infants who are younger than one year old and weigh less than 20 pounds, the seats should face toward the rear of the vehicle. Figure 14-11 shows an infant who has been secured correctly in the seat.

FIGURE 14-10 Prevalence of always using a safety belt among persons aged ≥ 18 years, by area—Behavioral Risk Factor Surveillance System, United States, 2002

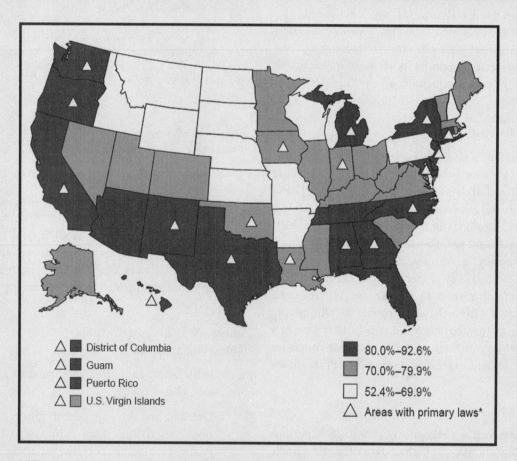

△ ■ District of Columbia	■ 80.0%–92.6%
△ ■ Guam	■ 70.0%–79.9%
△ ■ Puerto Rico	□ 52.4%–69.9%
△ ■ U.S. Virgin Islands	△ Areas with primary laws*

*Allow police to stop a motorist and issue a citation solely for being unbelted.

Source: Reprinted from the CDC. Impact of primary laws on adult use of safety belts—United States, 2002. *MMWR.* 2004;53:260.

FIGURE 14-11 Infant positioned correctly in a rear-facing infant-only car seat.

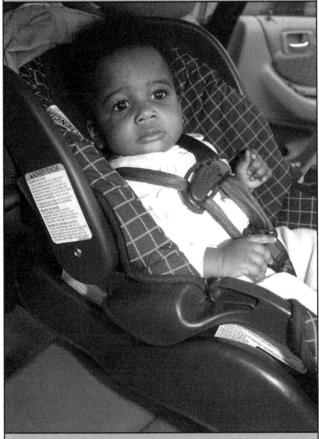

Source: Reprinted from the CDC Public Health Image Library. ID# 8426. CDC/American Academy of Pediatrics Content Providers. Available at: http://phil.cdc.gov/phil/details.asp. Accessed May 18, 2010.

UNINTENTIONAL INJURIES AMONG CHILDREN

In the United States, unintentional injuries are the top source of morbidity and mortality among children.[24] Despite the fact that the statistics regarding injuries disclose this alarming fact, injuries among children tend to be an under-recognized public health issue. During the years 2000–2005, the death rate for unintentional injuries among children was 15.0 per 100,000. Figure 14-12 reveals that males aged 15 to 19 years had the highest mortality rate of the groups shown. The respective overall mortality rates among males and females were 19.3 per 100,000 and 10.4 per 100,000. The rates for males exceeded those for females across all age groups.

For all forms of injury (intentional and unintentional), substantial disparities exist among childhood injury death

rates by race across age groups. The CDC reported that "The disparity between rates among blacks and whites was greatest in infancy, when the rate for blacks was 2.5 times that for whites. Rates among AI/AN (American Indian/Alaska Native) children were consistently two times those of white children for nearly every age from 0 to 19 years. Overall, for Hispanic children, injury death rates were comparable with or just below those for white children; in contrast, rates for A/PI (Asian/Pacific Islander) children were significantly lower than those for white children." [25(p4)] Refer to Figure 14-13 for information on trends in unintentional injury death rates between 1982 and 2002; the figure demonstrates that these disparities among racial and ethnic groups have tended to persist over time.

Key Facts about Unintentional Injury Deaths among Children, United States—2000–2006

- On average, 12,175 children 0 to 19 years of age died each year in the US from an unintentional injury.
- Males had higher injury death rates than females.
- Injuries due to transportation were the leading cause of death for children.
- The leading causes of injury death differed by age group.
- Risk for injury death varied by race. Injury death rates were highest for American Indian and Alaska Natives and were lowest for Asian or Pacific Islanders. Overall death rates for whites and African Americans were approximately the same.
- Injury death rates varied by state depending upon the cause of death.
- For injury causes with an overall low burden, death rates greatly varied by age.

Source: Adapted and reprinted from NN Borse, J Gilchrist, AM Dellinger, et al. *CDC Childhood Injury Report: Patterns of Unintentional Injuries among 0–19 Year Olds in the United States, 2000–2006.* Atlanta, GA: Centers for Disease Control and Prevention, National Center for Injury Prevention and Control; 2008:3–4.

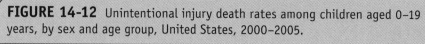

FIGURE 14-12 Unintentional injury death rates among children aged 0–19 years, by sex and age group, United States, 2000–2005.

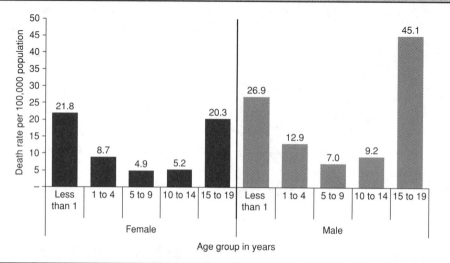

Source: Reprinted from Borse NN, Gilchrist J, Dellinger AM, et al. CDC Childhood Injury Report: Patterns of Unintentional Injuries among 0–19 Year Olds in the United States, 2000-2006. Atlanta, GA: Centers for Disease Control and Prevention, National Center for Injury Prevention and Control; 2008, p. 26.

FIGURE 14-13 Trends in unintentional injury death rates* among children aged 0–19 years, by race/ethnicity[†] and year—United States, 1982–2002.

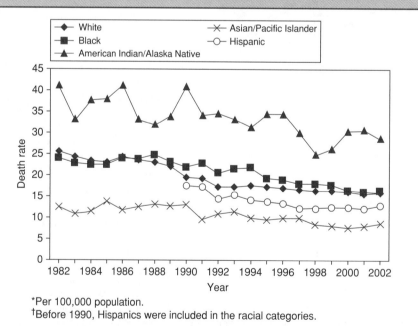

*Per 100,000 population.
[†]Before 1990, Hispanics were included in the racial categories.

Source: Reprinted from Bernard SJ, Paulozzi LJ, Wallace LJD. Fatal injuries among children by race and ethnicity—United States, 1999-2002. In: CDC Surveillance Summaries, May 18, 2007. Centers for Disease Control and Prevention. *MMWR.* 2007;56(No. SS-5):16

The most frequent cause of unintentional injury death during 2000 through 2005 was transportation related: 9.8 per 100,000. (See Figure 14-14.) Transportation-related causes include fatalities that occur among occupants of a motor vehicle, pedal cyclists, pedestrians, and users of other forms of transportation. Other major causes of deaths from unintentional injuries include drowning, falls, fires or burns, poisoning, and suffocation. The CDC notes that there are 11 major causes of injuries among children; these include child maltreatment (abuse and neglect), child passenger safety, fireworks-related injuries, playground injuries, poisonings, residential fire-related injuries, suicide, traumatic brain injury, water safety, young drivers, and youth violence.[26] See the text box titled "Key Facts about Unintentional Injury Deaths among Children, United States—2000–2006" for additional information.

The rate of injury death for all types of injuries among children aged 0 to 9 years by race/ethnicity in the United States (1999–2002) is shown in Figure 14-15. The highest death rates from injuries among children occur during the first five years of life and then stabilize by age nine. These data suggest the need for targeted interventions for reducing the toll of unintentional injuries among children, particularly during the early years of life. For example, such interventions should take into account the fact that infants and very young children are curious about their environment and like to explore, thus increasing their risk for poisoning and drowning. Older children are susceptible to bicycle and playground injuries because of immature cognitive development and limited physical coordination.

Playground Injuries

Playground injuries are a significant cause of nonfatal injuries and traumatic brain injuries among children. Annually in the United States, between 2001 and 2005, a total of 7,398 playground injuries resulted in hospitalizations and about 4.7 percent were traumatic brain injuries (TBIs). Refer to Table 14-3 for more information. Environmental factors such as safe design of playground equipment and surfaces reduce the possibility of injuries. The surfaces shown in Figure 14-16 are made of either soft sand or thick, padded rubber; these surfaces protect children in the event of falls. Playground sets should not have sharp edges and should be constructed securely so that they will not collapse. Playground equipment designed for home use may be flimsy and made of wood that can splinter or that contains toxic preservatives. Some older playground installations used lead-based paint, which children could ingest.

Sports- and Recreation-Related Injuries

In the United States, almost 40 million children and adolescents take part in organized sports; about 170 million adults engage in physical activity not connected with work. Participation in these activities incurs the risk of TBI, which can cause long-lasting adverse health effects such as behavioral changes and memory loss. A TBI is a type of brain injury that may occur from an external force such as a blow to the head. Many individuals present to hospital emergency departments for

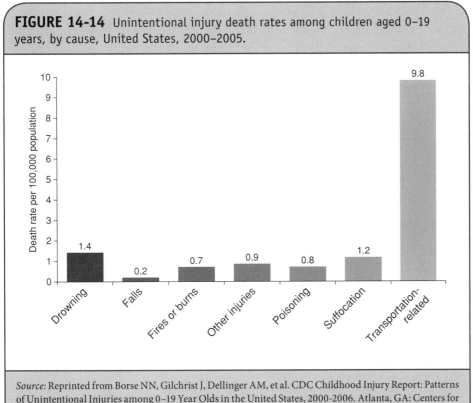

FIGURE 14-14 Unintentional injury death rates among children aged 0–19 years, by cause, United States, 2000–2005.

Source: Reprinted from Borse NN, Gilchrist J, Dellinger AM, et al. CDC Childhood Injury Report: Patterns of Unintentional Injuries among 0–19 Year Olds in the United States, 2000-2006. Atlanta, GA: Centers for Disease Control and Prevention, National Center for Injury Prevention and Control; 2008, p. 27.

FIGURE 14-15 Rate* of injury death among children aged 0–9 years, by race/ethnicity†—United States, 1999–2002

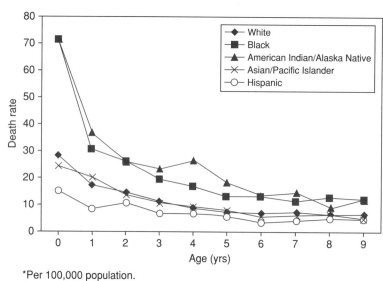

*Per 100,000 population.
†Hispanics are not included in any of the racial categories.

Source: Reprinted from Bernard SJ, Paulozzi LJ, Wallace LJD. Fatal injuries among children by race and ethnicity—United States, 1999-2002. In: CDC Surveillance Summaries, May 18, 2007. Centers for Disease Control and Prevention. *MMWR.* 2007;56(No. SS-5):14.

FIGURE 14-16 Example of an outdoor playground set with safe surfaces.

treatment of sports- and recreation-related injuries; a significant proportion of these injuries require hospitalization. About 18% of hospitalizations for sports-related injuries are for TBIs.

As the CDC reported,

> During 2001–2005, an estimated 207,830 patients with [sports and recreation] SR-related TBIs were treated in US hospital EDs [emergency departments] each year, accounting for 5.1% of all SR-related ED visits. . . . Overall, males accounted for approximately 70.5% of SR-related TBI ED visits. The highest rates of SR-related TBI ED visits for both males and females occurred among those aged 10–14 years, followed by those aged 15–19 years (Figure [14-17]). Activities associated with the greatest number of TBI-related ED visits included bicycling, football, playground activities, basketball, and riding all-terrain vehicles (ATVs). Activities for which TBI accounted for greater than 7.5% of ED visits for that activity included horseback riding (11.7%), ice skating (10.4%), riding ATVs (8.4%), tobogganing/sledding (8.3%), and bicycling (7.7%).[27(p733)]

Table 14-3 summarizes data on the estimated annual number of hospitalizations for nonfatal injuries and nonfatal TBIs in the United States related to sports and recreational activities among all ages and ages 5 through 18 years during 2001 through 2005. Among persons aged 5 through 18 years, the five activities most frequently associated with hospitalizations for all injuries related to sports and recreational activities were bicycling, driving ATVs, riding mopeds/minibikes/dirt bikes, football, baseball/softball, and use of playgrounds. Among the same age group, activities that had the highest proportions (20% or more) of hospitalizations for TBIs as a proportion of all hospitalizations for that activity were golfing, bicycling, driving ATVs, riding scooters, and playing baseball/softball.

Participation in collegiate sports, e.g., volleyball, can be a cause of injuries. The National Collegiate Athletic Association collected injury surveillance data for participation in women's volleyball from 1988–1989 through 2003–2004. Results indicated 2,216 injuries reported from 50,000 games and 4,725 injuries from 90,000 practices. The majority of reported injuries affected the lower extremities; ankle injuries were the most frequently reported type of injury.[28]

Prevention of Unintentional Injuries among Children

Among the major types of children's unintentional injuries are those related to motor vehicles (e.g., injuries to child passengers and young drivers), burns (e.g., from residential fires and improper handling of fireworks), playground mishaps, poisonings, and drowning. Environmental factors bear an important relationship to unintentional injuries among children, for example, at home and in recreational areas.[29] The impact of these influences is particularly acute for children who come from low-income and minority families. Environmental factors that contribute to unintentional injuries include:

- Aging, substandard housing facilities that increase risk of falls and other injuries
- Unavailability of safe playgrounds in combination with a lack of parental supervision while children are playing
- Failure to install home protective devices such as smoke alarms, locks on storage cabinets, and electrical outlet covers

Among the measures for preventing injuries are installing fences around pools in order to prevent children's unsupervised access, improving the design of playground equipment and surfaces, implementing municipal building codes that require smoke alarms and fire safety standards for construction, securing water heaters to prevent them from toppling over, packaging pharmaceuticals in child-safe containers, and mandating the use of car safety seats by small children.

INJURIES AMONG THE ELDERLY

Many forms of injuries (including those caused by violence) threaten the health and well-being of older adults—persons 65 years of age and older.[30] Individuals in this age group have an increased risk of numerous types of injuries that may cause deaths or disability. In comparison with all other age groups, persons over the age of 64 years have the highest risk of fatal injuries and injuries that lead to a hospital stay.[31] Among individuals who have attained the age of 75 years or older, the rate of such injuries is three times the rate for the general population. Moreover, with the continuing growth of the elderly population in the United States in the future, the total number of serious injuries among the elderly is projected to increase as are the costs for hospitalizations and trauma care. During the first decade of the 21st century, morbidity and mortality from several types of fatal and nonfatal injuries have shown an increasing trend among the 65 years and older age group. For example, mortality from falls, motorcycle

TABLE 14-3 Estimated Annual Number of Hospitalizations[a] for All Nonfatal Injuries and Nonfatal Traumatic Brain Injuries (TBIs) Related to Sports and Recreation Activities, for All Ages and for Ages 5–18 Years, by Selected Activity—National Electronic Injury Surveillance System—All Injury Program, United States, 2001–2005

| | All ages | | | | | | Ages 5–18 yrs | | | | | |
| | All injuries | | TBIs | | | | All injuries | | TBIs | | | |
Activity	No.[b]	(95% CI[c])	No.	(95% CI)	% of all injury hospitalizations[d]	% resulting in hospitalization[e]	No.	(95% CI)	No.	(95% CI)	% of all injury hospitalizations	% resulting in hospitalization
Bicycle	25,062	(17,858–32,267)	6,296	(3,636–8,957)	25.1	15.6	11,396	(8,958–13,835)	3,026	(1,993–4,059)	26.6	12.9
All-terrain vehicle	16,503	(10,195–22,810)	3,383	(1,649–5,117)	20.5	30.2	6,413	(3,897–8,929)	1,622	(698–2,545)	25.3	31.1
Moped/minibike/dirt bike[f]	6,095	(3,848–8,341)	1,039	(442–1,636)	17.0	21.9	2,653	(1,683–3,623)	517	(233–801)	19.5	20.5
Football	6,809	(5,588–8,030)	891	(633–1,148)	13.1	3.9	5,639	(4,590–6,688)	775	(521–1,029)	13.7	3.8
Baseball/softball	3,759	(2,895–4,623)	811	(491–1,130)	21.6	5.6	1,926	(1,481–2,371)	419	(198–640)	21.8	4.5
Playground	9,669	(7,714–11,624)	529	(332–727)	5.5	3.3	7,398	(5,727–9,069)	349	(200–497)	4.7	3.3
Basketball	4,816	(4,057–5,575)	465	(274–656)	9.7	3.2	2,674	(2,110–3,238)	365	(218–513)	13.6	3.2
Skateboard	3,068	(1,700–4,437)	432	(216–647)	14.1	8.2	2,304	(1,389–3,219)	350	(170–529)	15.2	7.9
Scooter	2,011	(1,586–2,437)	372	(191–552)	18.5	10.5	1,429	(1,090–1,769)	329	(154–504)	23.0	11.8
Golf[g]	1,586	(1,016–2,156)	366	(159–573)	23.1	13.6	504	(299–708)	178	(87–269)	35.3	15.8

Swimming/diving	3,915	(2,380–5,449)	352	(155–549)	9.0	6.0	1,304	(820–1,789)	198	(81–315)	15.2	5.1
Skating[h]	2,946	(2,148–3,745)	263	(126–399)	8.9	4.8	1,571	(1,114–2,029)	153	(63–243)	9.7	4.0
Soccer	2,653	(1,625–3,681)	198	(84–312)	7.5	2.1	1,602	(999–2,206)	161	(66–256)	10.0	2.1
Other specified[i]	37,790	(27,470–48,110)	5,916	(3,264–8,567)	15.7	11.5	13,557	(10,359–16,755)	2,351	(1,340–3,361)	17.3	8.2
Total	126,683	(97,146–156,220)	21,311	(13,258–29,364)	16.8	10.3	60,372	(49,416–71,329)	10,790	(7,461–14,120)	17.9	8.0

[a]Includes those for patients hospitalized and those for patients transferred to another facility for additional care.

[b]Estimates might not sum to totals because of rounding.

[c]Confidence interval.

[d]Percentage of all hospitalizations attributed to TBI = (number of TBI hospitalizations for activity/number of all hospitalizations for activity) × 100.

[e]Percentage of TBIs resulting in hospitalization = (number of TBI hospitalizations for activity/number of TBI-related emergency department visits for activity) × 100.

[f]Includes other two-wheeled, powered off-road vehicles and dune buggies.

[g]Includes injuries related to golf carts.

[h]Includes ice, in-line, and roller skating.

[i]Includes trampoline, toboggan/sled, go-cart, gymnastics, bowling, hockey, racquet sports, volleyball, miscellaneous ball games, track/field, combative, exercise, amusement attractions, water skiing, surfing, personal watercraft, snow skiing, snowmobile, snowboarding, camping, fishing, archery, darts, table tennis, nonpowder/BB guns, and billiards.

Source: Adapted from the Centers for Disease Control and Prevention. Nonfatal traumatic brain injuries from sports and recreation activities—United States, 2001–2005. MMWR. 2007;56:735.

FIGURE 14-17 Estimated annual rate* of nonfatal sports- and recreation-related traumatic brain injuries treated in emergency departments, by age group and sex—National Electronic Injury Surveillance System-All Injury Program, United States, 2001–2005.[†]

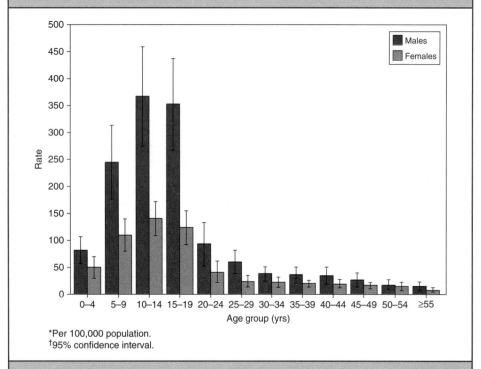

*Per 100,000 population.
[†]95% confidence interval.

Source: Reprinted from the Centers for Disease Control and Prevention. Nonfatal traumatic brain injuries from sports and recreation activities—United States, 2001-2005. *MMWR.* 2007;56:735.

TABLE 14-4 Types of injury and violence that pose the greatest threat to older adults in the United States

Elder abuse and maltreatment
   With the aging process some elderly persons become more dependent on others and, as a result, more vulnerable to abuse.

Falls among older adults (refer to text.)

Injuries among older adult drivers

Residential fire-related injuries

Sexual abuse among older adults

Suicide among older adults

Traumatic brain injury (especially among persons 75 years of age and older)

Source: Data from the Centers for Disease Control and Prevention. Injury Center: Injuries among older adults. Available at: http://www.cdc.gov/NCIPC/olderadults.htm. Accessed May 19, 2010.

crashes, machinery, poisoning, and drowning increased.[32]

As shown in Figure 14-4, the leading causes of injury death among older people include falls (described in the following section), motor vehicle injuries, firearm deaths, fires and burns, and poisoning. Table 14-4 provides a list of frequent causes of injuries among older persons. For some elderly individuals, a concomitant of the aging process is the loss of independence, which is the consequence of affliction with debilitating chronic diseases and other conditions. Consequently, some elderly persons are vulnerable to injury from maltreatment by care givers and other forms of abuse, as shown in the table.

Injuries and Fatalities that Result from Falling

According to the CDC, falls are the leading cause of fatal and nonfatal injuries for persons aged 65 years and older.[33] Interviews from the 2006 Behavioral Risk Factor Surveillance System (BRFSS) indicated that 16,650 persons in this age group succumbed to falls during 2006. Of the 16,650 individuals, 15.9% fell during the three months that preceded the interview, and 31.3% were injured at least one time. Older respondents were more likely to report falling than younger individuals; for example, the percentage of falling among persons 65 to 69 years of age was 13.4% and increased to 15.7% and 20.8%, respectively, among individuals aged 75 to 79 years and 80 years and older.

Data from the BRFSS revealed that race and ethnicity, health status, and sex were related to falling. With respect to race and ethnicity, the highest prevalence of falling occurred among American Indian/Alaska natives; the highest prevalence of injuries among those who fell occurred among Hispanic persons. Regarding health status, persons who had poor health status were more than three times as likely to report falling as those who had excellent health status. Concerning sex, the prevalence of falling was similar for men and women, although women had a greater percentage of fall-related injuries than men.

Falls among persons aged 65 and older were associated with 15,802 deaths in 2005.[33] As shown in Figure 14-18, the rates of fatal falls were higher among men than among women. The rates of fall-related death tended to increase between 1987 and 1996. Hip fractures are one of the consequences of falling and often are linked to death soon afterward. The rate of hospitalization for hip fractures was more than twice as high among women as among men between 1987 and 1996. (See Figure 14-19.)

Prevention of Falls

Among the elderly, factors associated with falls are dizziness, impaired balance, and reduced visual acuity. Also, many elderly persons may be afflicted with symptoms associated with chronic illnesses and the sequelae of strokes. Community-based assessments of risk factors for falling linked with coordinated interventions are one possible method for the prevention of falls. An example was a clinical trial that consisted of visits to the homes of independent-living elderly persons who had fallen; during these visits researchers assessed risk factors and household hazards that might lead to falling; referrals were made for appropriate interventions in the community as well as exercise programs that provided strength and balance training.[34] Another program investigated risk factors associated with falling among elderly women who had experienced strokes and who lived at home.[35] Among the most important risk factors for falling in this group were problems with balance while dressing. The findings suggested that interventions are needed to improve balance among female stroke victims when they are engaging in complex activities of daily living such as dressing; clinicians also should take into account the special risks and needs of stroke patients with respect to falling.

SCHEMA FOR INJURY PREVENTION

This chapter has demonstrated that injuries, both intentional and unintentional, rank among the leading causes of morbidity and mortality worldwide and in the United States. As a result, injuries are a significant public health problem that warrants preventive interventions at the population level. Prevention of injuries requires a systematic approach such as that depicted in Figure 14-20. The CDC identifies four components for the development of a strategy for the prevention of unintentional injuries.[10]

Problem definition refers to gathering data and analyzing datasets for patterns and trends. In this phase, injury specialists define subgroups of the population that have the highest prevalence of specific types of injuries. Descriptive epidemiologic studies form one of the keystones of problem identification. To illustrate, many types of injuries differ according to demographic variables and show disparities according to race and socioeconomic level. One example discussed previously is the higher rate of motor vehicle fatalities among men in comparison with women. Another example is the increased risk of falling among older persons in comparison with younger persons.

Risk factors are variables that increase the probability of the occurrence of an injury. Personal behavior and environmental components contribute to the risk of unintentional injuries. Examples of behavioral risk factors for motor vehicle fatalities are alcohol consumption, failure to wear seat belts, and driving while distracted. Examples of environmental risk

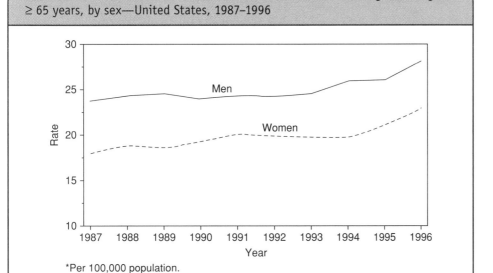

FIGURE 14-18 Rate* of unintentional fall-related death among adults aged ≥ 65 years, by sex—United States, 1987–1996

*Per 100,000 population.

Source: Reprinted from Stevens JA, Hasbrouck L, Durant TM. Surveillance for injuries and violence among older adults. In: CDC Surveillance Summaries, December 17, 1999. *MMWR.* 1999; 48(No. SS-8):34.

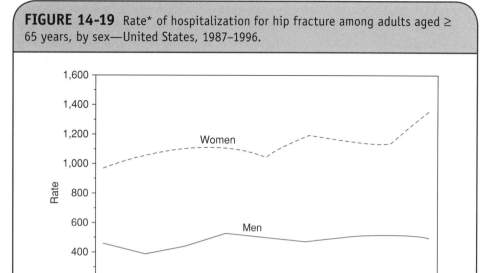

FIGURE 14-19 Rate* of hospitalization for hip fracture among adults aged ≥ 65 years, by sex—United States, 1987–1996.

*Per 100,000 population.

Source: Reprinted from Stevens JA, Hasbrouck L, Durant TM. Surveillance for injuries and violence among older adults. In: CDC Surveillance Summaries, December 17, 1999. *MMWR.* 1999; 48(No. SS-8):35

Protective factors are those that reduce the probability of an injury. Child safety seats and air bags protect the occupants of automobiles from severe or fatal injuries during a collision. Examples of protective factors for older drivers include the fact that in comparison with other drivers they are more likely to wear seat belts, drive when the weather and others conditions are safest, and avoid the use of alcohol when driving.[19]

Prevention strategies are methods to prevent the occurrence of future injuries. These strategies flow from empirical information that has been gathered and should be consistent with identified risk and protective factors. For example, prevention strategies could be directed at identifying risk factors for falls among the elderly and modifying the environment in order to reduce the incidence

factors pertain to both the home setting and the physical environment outside the home. At home, unsafe environmental conditions increase the risk of adverse outcomes such as falling, poisoning, and injuries to children; outside the home, environmental conditions are implicated in many types of injuries, including harm to pedestrians, playground mishaps, and sports-related injuries.

of falling. Other prevention strategies may address motor vehicle injuries (e.g., use of seat belts and child safety seats, assignment of designated drivers), injuries from fires and burns (e.g., installation of smoke alarms, wearing nonflammable clothing), drowning (barriers around swimming pools), and injuries from firearms (storage of weapons and ammunition in locked vaults).[36]

Widespread adoption means that successful prevention strategies are disseminated widely in order to encourage their adoption on a broad scale. Implementation of safety laws (such as mandated use of seat belts) is one means of increasing the probability that prevention strategies will be successful.

CONCLUSION

An under-recognized problem that affects public health signifi-

FIGURE 14-20 The public health approach to injury prevention.

Define the problem → Identify risk and protective factors → Develop and test prevention strategies → Assure widespread adoption

Source: Reprinted from National Center for Injury Prevention and Control. CDC Injury Fact Book. Atlanta, GA: Centers for Disease Control and Prevention; 2006, p.4.

cantly, injuries cause approximately 5 million deaths globally each year; more than two-thirds of these fatalities are from unintentional injuries. The fifth leading cause of mortality in the United States, unintentional injuries accounted for about 121,000 deaths in 2006. In addition to their contribution to morbidity and mortality, injuries can have devastating social and economic consequences; these include impacts upon the individual, family members, and society in terms of lost productivity, direct costs of health care, and related economic burdens.

The term *unintentional injury* is preferred to *accident*, which suggests that such events are random and cannot be prevented; in fact much progress has been achieved through the systematic examination of the distribution and causes of injuries. Injuries have differential distributions according to age, sex, race, and other variables. For example, males from all age groups are much more likely than females to die from injuries. Among the total US population, the top three categories of deaths from unintentional injuries are motor vehicle fatalities, firearm-related deaths, and poisonings. Falls are the leading cause of fatal injuries among persons aged 65 years and older. The public health approach to injury prevention involves four components that have implications for identification of environmental risk factors and development of intervention strategies, which are then disseminated widely.

Study Questions and Exercises

1. Define the following terms:
   a. Injury
   b. Causes of injuries
   c. Intent of injury
   d. Intentional injury
   e. Unintentional injury
   f. Injury epidemiology

2. Differentiate between the terms *unintentional injury* and *accident*. Why is the use of *unintentional injury* preferred?

3. Why do you need to be concerned about injuries? Discuss the significance of unintentional injuries for morbidity and mortality globally and in the United States. How do unintentional injuries rank in comparison with other causes of mortality? Describe the potential economic, social, and emotional costs of unintentional injuries.

4. Describe how the causes of unintentional injury death differ according to age group. Using your own ideas, discuss possibilities for prevention.

5. Describe variation in motor vehicle–related fatalities by demographic characteristics such as age, sex, and race. How can such fatalities be prevented among high-risk groups such as young male drivers?

6. Why do you think that death rates from motor vehicle injuries have not declined very much in recent years, despite the continuing introduction of safety measures and new laws to prevent motor vehicle injuries?

7. Why is the rate of fatalities so high among ATV drivers? What can be done to reduce the number of ATV-associated injuries?

8. Describe what is meant by disparities in the occurrence of unintentional injuries. Give some examples from the global and domestic (US) perspectives. How do you account for these disparities? Be sure to link them to environmental factors in your response.

9. What are the five most common sports and recreation activities associated with nonfatal injuries among all ages in the United States? How does the frequency of all injuries from sports and recreation activities compare with the frequency of traumatic brain injuries caused by sports and recreation activities? Using your own ideas, suggest methods for the prevention of the traumatic brain injuries linked with sports and recreation activities.

10. Describe the patterns and causes of unintentional injuries among children and the elderly. What can be done to protect vulnerable populations such as children and the elderly from unintentional injuries?

11. Invite a trauma specialist to your classroom and ask this individual to discuss the types of injuries seen in the hospital trauma center.

12. Arrange a debate in your classroom to discuss the causes and consequences of unintentional injuries. Assume that little can be done to prevent such events because they are random occurrences. Ask one group of students to present the *pro* side of this assumption and another group to present the *con* side of the assumption.

13. Conduct a walk-through of your home and identify potential injury hazards. Record these in a list and discuss them in class. Suggest how to eliminate these hazards.

REFERENCES

1. World Health Organization. How can injuries be prevented? Available at: http://www.who.int/features/qa/36/en/print.html. Accessed May 21, 2010.

2. Disease Control Priorities Project. Burden and causes of unintentional injuries. Available at: http://www.dcp2.org/pubs/DCP/39/Section/5525. Accessed February 1, 2010.

3. Heron M, Hoyert DL, Murphy SL, et al. Deaths: Final data for 2006. National vital statistics reports; vol 57 no 14. Hyattsville, MD: National Center for Health Statistics, 2009.

4. Centers for Disease Control and Prevention. Injury data and resources: ICD injury matrices. Available at: http://www.cdc.gov/nchs/injury/injury_matrices.htm. Accessed May 21, 2010.

5. Bergen G, Chen LH, Warner M, et al. *Injury in the United States: 2007 Chartbook*. Hyattsville, MD: National Center for Health Statistics; 2008.

6. Holder Y, Peden M, Krug E, et al. (Eds). *Injury Surveillance Guidelines*. Geneva, Switzerland: World Health Organization; 2001.

7. Centers for Disease Control and Prevention, Injury Center. Definitions for WISQARS Nonfatal. Available at: http://www.cdc.gov/Ncipc/wisqars/nonfatal/definitions.htm. Accessed May 21, 2010.

8. Porta M, ed. *A Dictionary of Epidemiology*. 5th ed. New York, NY: Oxford University Press, 2008.

9. Peden M, McGee K, Sharma G. *The Injury Chart Book: A Graphical Overview of the Global Burden of Injuries*. Geneva, Switzerland: World Health Organization; 2002.

10. National Center for Injury Prevention and Control. *CDC Injury Fact Book*. Atlanta, GA: Centers for Disease Control and Prevention; 2006.

11. WHO/Europe. Children at Risk! Main health effects of exposure to environmental risk factors. Fact sheet EURO/05/03. Available at: http://www.euro.who.int/document/mediacentre/fs0503e.pdf. Accessed March 28, 2010.

12. Centers for Disease Control and Prevention. QuickStats: age-adjusted death rates for leading causes of injury death, by year—United States, 1979–2004. *MMWR*. 2006;55:1363.

13. Pitts SR, Niska RW, Xu J, et al. National Hospital Ambulatory Medical Care Survey: 2006 emergency department summary. National health statistics reports; no 7. Hyattsville, MD: National Center for Health Statistics; 2008.

14. Centers for Disease Control and Prevention. Motor vehicle-related death rates—United States, 1999–2005. *MMWR*. 2009;58:161–165.

15. NHTSA. Traffic Safety Facts: 2008 data. Older population. Available at: http://www-nrd.nhtsa.dot.gov/Pubs/811161.PDF. Accessed March 24, 2010.

16. NHTSA. Traffic Safety Facts: 2008 Data. Young drivers. Available at: http://www-nrd.nhtsa.dot.gov/pubs/811169.pdf. Accessed May 23, 2010.

17. Centers for Disease Control and Prevention. All-terrain vehicle fatalities—West Virginia, 1999–2006. *MMWR*. 2008;57:312–315.

18. Shieber RA, Vegega ME, eds. Executive summary: reducing childhood pedestrian injuries. *Injury Prevention*. 2002;8(suppl I):i3–i8.

19. Centers for Disease Control and Prevention. Older Adult Drivers: fact sheet. Available at: http://www.cdc.gov/MotorVehicleSafety/Older_Adult_Drivers/adult-drivers_factsheet.html. Accessed April 10, 2010.

20. Centers for Disease Control and Prevention. Teen Drivers: fact sheet. Available at: http://www.cdc.gov/MotorVehicleSafety/Teen_Drivers/teend-drivers_factsheet.html. Accessed April 10, 2010.

21. Centers for Disease Control and Prevention. Impaired Driving. Available at: http://www.cdc.gov/MotorVehicleSafety/Impaired_Driving/impaired-drv_factsheet.html. Accessed April 10, 2010.

22. Centers for Disease Control and Prevention. Impact of primary laws on adult use of safety belts—United States, 2002. *MMWR*. 2004;53:257–260.

23. Masten S. Traffic safety facts: research note. The effects of changing to primary enforcement on daytime and nighttime seat belt use. Washington, DC: National Highway Transportation Safety Administration; 2007. DOT HS 810 743.

24. Borse NN, Gilchrist J, Dellinger AM, et al. *CDC Childhood Injury Report: Patterns of Unintentional Injuries among 0–19 Year Olds in the United States, 2000–2006*. Atlanta, GA: Centers for Disease Control and Prevention, National Center for Injury Prevention and Control; 2008.

25. Bernard SJ, Paulozzi LJ, Wallace LJD. Fatal injuries among children by race and ethnicity—United States, 1999–2002. In: *CDC Surveillance Summaries*, May 18, 2007. Centers for Disease Control and Prevention. *MMWR*. 2007;56(No. SS-5):1–16.

26. Centers for Disease Control and Prevention. Injury Center: Injuries among children and adolescents. Available at: http://www.cdc.gov/NCIPC/factsheets/children.htm. Accessed: May 21, 2010.

27. Centers for Disease Control and Prevention. Nonfatal traumatic brain injuries from sports and recreation activities—United States, 2001–2005. *MMWR*. 2007;56:733–737.

28. Agel J, Palmieri-Smith RM, Dick R, et al. Descriptive epidemiology of collegiate women's volleyball injuries: National Collegiate Athletic Association Injury Surveillance System, 1988–1989 through 2003–2004. *Journal of Athletic Training*. 2007;42:295–302.

29. Grad J, Kunseler E. Policies to reduce unintentional injuries from falls, drowning, poisoning, fires and choking in children and adolescents. Copenhagen, Denmark: World Health Organization–Regional Office for Europe; 2007.

30. Centers for Disease Control and Prevention. Injury Center: Injuries among older adults. Available at: http://www.cdc.gov/NCIPC/olderadults.htm. Accessed May 19, 2010.

31. MacKenzie EJ. Epidemiology of injuries: current trends and future challenges. *Epidemiologic Reviews*. 2000;22:112–119.

32. Hu G, Baker SP. Recent increases in fatal and non-fatal injury among people aged 65 years and over in the USA. *Inj Prev*. 2010;16:26–30.

33. Centers for Disease Control and Prevention. Self-reported falls and fall-related injuries among persons aged ≥65 years—United States, 2006. *MMWR*. 2008;57:225–229.

34. Elley CR, Robertson MC, Kerse NM, et al. Falls Assessment Clinical Trial (FACT): design, interventions, recruitment strategies and participant characteristics. *BMC Public Health*. 2007;7:185.

35. Lamb SE, Ferrucci L, Volapto S, et al. Risk factors for falling in home-dwelling older women with stroke: the Women's Health and Aging Study. *Stroke*. 2003;34:494–501.

36. WHO. Facts about injuries: preventing global injuries. Available at: http://www.who.int/violence_injury_prevention/resources/publications/en/injury_factsheet.pdf. Accessed May 21, 2010.

Glossary

accident	An unanticipated event commonly leading to injury or other harm; this term is not appropriate for use in scientific discourse.
acid rain	The precipitation of acidic compounds formed when components of air pollution (e.g., SO_2 and NO_x) interact with other components in the air such as water, oxygen, and oxidants.
additive	The combination of two chemicals produces an effect that is equal to their individual effects added together.
aerosol particles	Particulate matter, including dust, soot, and other finely divided solid and liquid materials, which are suspended in and move with the air.
agenda setting	Setting priorities, deciding at what time to deal with an environmental problem, and determining who will deal with the problem.
agent	A factor, such as a microorganism, chemical substance, or form of radiation, whose presence, excessive presence, or (in deficiency diseases) relative absence is essential for the occurrence of a disease.
air pollution	Air pollution refers to the presence, in various degrees, of substances not found in perfectly clean air.
Air Quality Index (AQI)	An index for reporting daily air quality, which tells the public how clean or polluted the air is.
alpha particle	A subatomic particle made up of the nucleus of a helium atom that is ejected from a radioactive atom.
analytic epidemiology	Examines causal (etiologic) hypotheses regarding the association between an exposure and health condition(s).
antagonism	Occurs when two chemicals administered together interfere with each other's actions or one interferes with the action of the other.
aquifer	A layer or section of earth or rock that contains freshwater, known as groundwater.

Note: Some definitions are quoted from other sources; refer to text for citations.

arboviral diseases	A group of viral diseases that are acquired most frequently when blood-feeding arthropod vectors—including ticks, sand flies, biting midges, and mosquitoes—infect a human host.
aromatic compound	An organic molecule that contains a benzene ring; for example, benzene and toluene.
asthma	A chronic respiratory illness characterized by difficulty breathing and tightness of the chest in response to muscle contractions that constrict the trachea, lungs, and other parts of the airway.
beta particle	An electron that is emitted from the nucleus of a radioactive atom.
bias	Deviation of results or inferences from the truth, or processes leading to such deviation. Any trend in the collection, analysis, interpretation, publication, or review of data that can lead to conclusions that are systematically different from the truth.
bioaccumulation	Occurs when trace amounts of substances (such as heavy metals) become more concentrated and potentially more harmful as they move up the food chain; sometimes called biomagnification.
biodiversity	Generally refers to the different types and variability of animal and plant species and the ecosystems in which they live.
biomagnification	See bioaccumulation.
bovine spongiform encephalopathy (BSE)	A neurological disease in cattle hypothesized to be caused by prions; also known as mad cow disease.
breast cancer 1, early onset (BRCA1)	First breast cancer gene identified.
building-related illness (BRI)	An identified diagnosable illness attributed directly to airborne building contaminants.
built environment	Urban areas and structures (e.g., roads, parks, and buildings) constructed by human beings, as opposed to undeveloped, rural areas.
burden of disease	The total significance of disease for society beyond the immediate cost of treatment; measured in years of life lost to ill health as the difference between total life expectancy and disability-adjusted life expectancy.
butylated hydroxyl anisole (BHA)	Antioxidant used for foods that contain fats and oils.
butylated hydroxytoluene (BHT)	Antioxidant used for foods that contain fats and oils.
carbon dioxide (CO_2)	A by-product of combustion of fossil fuels, carbon dioxide is a greenhouse gas.
carbon monoxide (CO)	A colorless, odorless, poisonous gas, produced by incomplete burning of carbon-based fuels, including gasoline, oil, and wood.
carboxyhemoglobin	A combination of carbon monoxide and hemoglobin, which at high levels limits the oxygen-carrying capacity of blood.
carcinogen	A chemical (or substance) that causes or is suspected of causing cancer, a disease associated with unregulated proliferation of cells in the body.
carrying capacity	The population that an area will support without undergoing environmental deterioration.
case–control study	A study in which subjects who participate are defined on the basis of the presence (cases) or absence (controls) of outcome of interest. Association between exposure and outcome is measured by the odds ratio (OR).

case series study	Study in which information about individual patients who share a disease in common is gathered over time.
cause (mechanism) of injury	The way in which a person sustains an injury.
chemical allergy	An immunologically mediated adverse reaction to a chemical resulting from previous sensitization to that chemical or to a structurally similar one.
chronic obstructive pulmonary disease (COPD)	A group of conditions subsumed under the category of "chronic lower respiratory diseases"; includes chronic and unspecified bronchitis, emphysema, asthma, and other chronic lower respiratory diseases.
coalitive interaction	Several agents that individually have no known toxic effects interact to produce a toxic effect.
cohort study	A type of study in which subjects are classified according to their exposure to a factor of interest and then are observed over time to document the occurrence of new cases (incidence) of disease or other health events. Relative risk (RR) is the measure of association.
common units	A system of measurement of radiation; still used often in the United States, it has been superseded by the SI system.
composting	The controlled decomposition (breaking down through the action of physical and chemical processes) of organic materials, such as leaves, grass, and food scraps, by microorganisms.
composting toilets	Units that convert human excrement into a soil-like material that should be buried or hauled away for disposal.
confounding	A situation in which a measure of the effect of an exposure on risk is distorted because of the association of the exposure with other factor(s) that influence(s) the outcome under study. The other factor or factors were not controlled for in the study design.
Creutzfeldt-Jakob disease, new variant (vCJD)	Type of dementia in humans hypothesized to be caused by prions.
criteria air pollutants	A group of very common air pollutants regulated by the EPA, including ozone, nitrogen dioxide, carbon monoxide, sulfur dioxide, particulate matter, and lead.
cross-sectional study	A study that examines the relationship between diseases (or other health-related characteristics) and other variables of interest as they exist in a defined population at one particular time.
Curie (Ci)	A common unit of measure used to describe the amount of radioactivity in a sample of material.
decibel (dB)	A logarithmic scale designed to measure sound pressure levels.
demographic transition	Alterations over time in a population's fertility rate, mortality rate, and composition.
descriptive epidemiology	The depiction of the occurrence of disease in populations according to classification by person (e.g., sex, age, race), place, and time variables.
dioxin(s)	Dioxin usually refers to the chemical TCDD (2,3,7,8-tetrachlorodibenzo-p-dioxin), but dioxins refer to a family of dioxin-like compounds that are unintentional by-products of certain industrial, nonindustrial, and natural processes, usually involving combustion.
disability-adjusted life expectancy	The number of years of healthy life expected in a particular population.
dose	The amount of a substance administered at one time.

dose–response relationship	The relationship of observed outcomes (responses) in a population to varying levels of a protective or harmful agent such as a form of medication or an environmental contaminant.
ecologic study	A study in which the units of analysis are populations or groups of people, rather than individuals; also called ecological study.
ecological model	Proposes that the determinants of health (environmental, biological, and behavioral) interact and are interlinked over the life course of individuals.
ecosystem	A dynamic complex of plant, animal, and microorganism communities and the nonliving environment interacting as a functional unit.
emerging zoonoses	Zoonotic diseases that are caused by either apparently new agents or by known agents that occur in locales or species that previously did not appear to be affected by these known agents.
environment	The complex of physical, chemical, and biotic factors (such as climate, soil, and living things) that acts upon an organism or an ecological community and ultimately determines its form and survival.
environmental epidemiology	The study of diseases and health conditions that occur in the population and are linked to environmental factors.
environmental health	Comprises those aspects of human health, including quality of life, that are determined by physical, chemical, biological, social, and psychosocial factors in the environment. It also refers to the theory and practice of assessing, correcting, controlling, and preventing those factors in the environment that potentially can affect adversely the health of present and future generations.
environmental impact assessment (EIA)	A process for reviewing the potential impact of anthropogenic (human-related) activities (e.g., a proposed construction project) with respect to their general environmental consequences.
environmental justice	The equal treatment of all people in society irrespective of their racial background, country of origin, and socioeconomic status, especially concerning environmental laws and policies.
environmental objectives	Statements of policy intended to be assessed using information from a monitoring program.
environmental policy	A statement by an organization (public or private) of its intentions and principles in relation to its overall environmental performance.
environmental risk transition	Changes in environmental risks that happen as a consequence of economic development in the less developed regions of the world.
environmental sustainability	The concept that resources should not be depleted faster than they can be regenerated; the concept also specifies that there should be no permanent change to the natural environment.
environmental tobacco smoke (ETS)	Secondhand smoke; also known as sidestream smoke.
environmental toxicology	The study of how ecological systems—their structure, dynamics, and function—are affected by pollutants.
epidemiologic transition	A shift in the pattern of morbidity and mortality from causes related primarily to infectious and communicable diseases to causes associated with chronic, degenerative diseases.
epidemiologic triangle	Fundamental model of disease causality that includes three major categories of factors: agent, host, and environment.
epidemiology	The study of the distribution and determinants of health and diseases, morbidity, injuries, disability, and mortality in populations.

essential metals	Metals (e.g., copper, zinc, manganese, and iron) necessary for human nutrition in trace amounts, but that can be toxic if ingested in excessive amounts.
exposure	Proximity and/or contact with a source of a disease agent in such a manner that effective transmission of the agent or harmful effects of the agent may occur.
extraterrestrial radiation	Primary cosmic rays, which originate from outer space (e.g., the earth's galaxy and the sun) and interact with the earth's atmosphere to produce secondary cosmic rays.
extremely low frequency radiation (ELF)	A form of nonionizing radiation in the range of 50 to 60 hertz that originates from electric power poles, wiring in the walls of buildings, and some electrical appliances.
finished water	Water leaving a treatment plant and ready to be used by consumers after being collected, treated, and, usually, filtered.
fluorosis	A dental condition in which teeth have been discolored by fluoride.
food additives	Substances that become part of a food product when added (intentionally or unintentionally) during the processing or production of that food.
food insecurity	A situation in which supplies of wholesome foods are uncertain or may have limited availability.
foodborne diseases	Illnesses acquired by consumption of contaminated food; they are frequently and inaccurately referred to as food poisoning.
foodborne infections	Foodborne diseases induced by infectious agents such as some bacteria (e.g., *Salmonella*) that cause foodborne illness directly.
foodborne intoxications	Foodborne diseases incited by agents that do not cause infections directly but produce spores or toxins as they multiply in food; these toxins then can affect the nervous system (neurotoxins) or the digestive system.
foodborne outbreak	The occurrence among two or more people of cases of a similar illness, which an investigation has linked to consumption of a common meal or food items. In the instance of botulism, one case constitutes an outbreak.
freshwater lake	A lake usually located at a high latitude containing freshwater as opposed to saltwater.
gamma rays	Consisting of photons, these high-energy rays are part of the electromagnetic spectrum and are the most highly penetrating type of radiation.
glaciers and icecaps	Frozen freshwater located in high elevations and near the earth's poles.
global warming	An increase in the near-surface temperature of the earth, in part due to increased emissions of greenhouse gases and deforestation.
greenhouse gases	Gases that arise from natural sources and anthropogenic activities such as the burning of fossil fuels and that may accumulate in the atmosphere. They are referred to as greenhouse gases because in sufficient concentrations in the atmosphere, they may have the effect of trapping heat and causing the earth's temperature to rise.
groundwater	Any water that is stored naturally deep underground in aquifers or that flows through rock or soil, supplying springs and wells; this water is less susceptible to contamination than surface water.
hazard	The inherent capability of an agent or a situation to have an adverse effect; a factor or exposure that may adversely affect health.
hazard analysis of critical control points (HACCP)	A system for reducing the risk of foodborne illness in which foods are monitored from the time of harvest to the time of consumption.

hazardous waste	By-products of society that can pose a substantial or potential hazard to human health or the environment when improperly managed. It possesses at least one of four characteristics (ignitability, corrosivity, reactivity, or toxicity), or appears on special EPA lists.
health impact assessment (HIA)	A method for describing and estimating the effects that a proposed project or policy may have on the health of a population.
healthy worker effect	The observation that employed populations tend to have lower mortality rates than the general population.
heavy metal	A metal that has a high atomic weight with a specific gravity that exceeds the specific gravity of water by five or more times. Examples include arsenic, lead, and mercury.
hormesis	The belief that some nonnutritional toxic substances also may impart beneficial or stimulatory effects at low doses, but at higher doses they produce adverse effects.
host	A person or other living animal, including birds and arthropods, that affords subsistence or lodgment to an infectious agent under natural conditions.
hydrocarbon	A substance that consists of only carbon and hydrogen atoms. Benzene is an example.
hydrological cycle	The natural cycle by which water evaporates from oceans and other water bodies, accumulates as water vapor in clouds, and returns to oceans and other water bodies as precipitation.
incidence	The occurrence of new disease or mortality within a defined period of observation (e.g., a week, month, year, or other time period) in a specified population.
incidence rate	A rate formed by dividing the number of new cases of disease or mortality that occur during a time period by the number of individuals in the population at risk.
injury	Physical damage to a body that results when it is suddenly or briefly subjected to intolerable levels of energy.
injury epidemiology	A branch of epidemiology that studies the distribution and determinants of injuries in the population.
insecticide	A pesticide compound specifically used to kill or prevent the growth of insects.
intent of injury	Whether an injury was caused by an act carried out on purpose or by accident.
intervention study	An investigation involving intentional change in some aspect of the status of the subjects. An example of such a change is the introduction of a preventive or therapeutic regimen.
ionizing radiation	Radiation that has enough energy to remove tightly bound electrons from atoms, thus creating ions.
isotopes	Atoms of a chemical element that have the same atomic number (which denotes the number of protons in an atom), but have different masses.
itai-itai disease	A condition attributed to ingestion of cadmium and characterized by excruciating pain across the entire body.
job stress	The harmful physical and emotional responses that occur when the requirements of the job do not match the capabilities, resources, or needs of the worker.
latency	The time period between initial exposure to a factor and a measurable response.
leachate	A liquid produced as water percolates through wastes, collecting contaminants.
lethal dose 50 (LD_{50})	The dosage (mg/kg body weight) that causes death in 50% of exposed animals.
life expectancy	The expectation of the number of years of life at birth.
medical waste	Any solid waste that is generated in the diagnosis, treatment, or immunization of human beings or animals, in research pertaining thereto, or in the production or testing of biologicals.

megacities	Urbanized areas that have 10 million or more inhabitants.
megafills	Landfills that take in 5,000–10,000 tons of trash per day and serve regional needs for waste disposal.
melanosis	A dermatologic condition that can cause the darkening of the skin of the entire body (diffuse melanosis) or spotted pigmentation of the skin or tissues inside the mouth (spotted melanosis); associated with chronic low-level arsenic exposure.
metaphylaxis	A procedure in which antimicrobials are given to an entire collection of animals, for example, chickens on a poultry farm or fish raised in pens, for the purpose of curing disease among the sick animals and preventing disease among the remainder.
methyl isocyanate (MIC)	An intermediate chemical used for the manufacture of carbamate pesticides.
microwave radiation	A form of nonionizing radiation produced by radar; a major use is to heat foods. Microwave radiation is associated with ocular effects (lens opacities such as cataracts and clouding of the lenses of the eyes) at high levels.
Minamata disease	A neurologic condition associated with ingestion of mercury; characterized by numbness of the extremities, deafness, poor vision, and drowsiness.
municipal solid waste (MSW)	Trash or garbage; includes packaging, furniture, clothing, bottles, food waste, papers, batteries, and organic materials such as grass clippings from landscaping.
musculoskeletal disorder (MSD)	An injury or disorder of the muscles, nerves, tendons, joints, cartilage, or spinal discs.
National Priorities List (NPL)	The EPA's list of the most serious uncontrolled or abandoned hazardous waste sites identified for possible long-term remedial action under Superfund legislation.
natural experiments	Naturally occurring circumstances in which subsets of the population have different levels of exposure to a supposed causal factor, in a situation resembling an actual experiment where human subjects would be randomly allocated to groups.
nitrogen oxides (NO_x)	Gases made up of a single molecule of nitrogen combined with varying numbers of molecules of oxygen; produced from burning fuels, which react with volatile organic compounds to form smog and with water to form acid rain.
noise	A type of sound that is unwanted; can be made up of pure tones, a narrow band of frequencies, and sound impulses.
nonionizing radiation	Radiation that has enough energy to move atoms in a molecule around or cause them to vibrate, but not enough to remove electrons. Examples are sound waves, visible light, and microwaves.
nonrenewable water	Water in aquifers and other natural reservoirs that is not recharged by the hydrological cycle or is recharged so slowly that significant withdrawal for human use causes depletion.
nuclide	A nucleus with a specific number of protons and neutrons and a specific energy state; nuclides include radioactive and nonradioactive atoms.
occupational disease	Those health outcomes that are caused or influenced by exposure to general conditions or specific hazards encountered in the work environment.
odds ratio (OR)	The measure of association between exposure and outcome used in case–control studies. The OR refers to the ratio of the odds in favor of exposure among the disease group (the cases) to the odds in favor of exposure among the no-disease group (the controls).

organic chemical	Generally speaking, a substance that contains carbon atoms, although this definition is not always true, as in the case of the gas carbon dioxide (CO_2). (CO_2 contains carbon atoms but is not an organic chemical.) Organic chemicals are found in all living organisms, although many also can be synthesized.
organochlorines	A wide range of chemicals that contain carbon, chlorine, and, sometimes, several other elements; these chemicals include many herbicides, insecticides, and fungicides as well as industrial chemicals such as polychlorinated biphenyls (PCBs).
organophosphate (OP) pesticides	Pesticides that act on the nervous systems of insects and higher organisms by disrupting the transmission of nerve impulses.
ozone (O_3)	A gas that consists of three oxygen atoms bonded together into a molecule; it is a main component of ground-level, photochemical smog.
particulate matter (PM)	Refers generically to a mixture of airborne particles that can vary in size; it is one of the constituents of air pollution.
passive smoking	The involuntary breathing of cigarette smoke by nonsmokers in an environment where there are cigarette smokers present; also known as exposure to sidestream cigarette smoke or environmental tobacco smoke (ETS).
persistent organic pollutants (POPs)	Carbon-containing chemical compounds that, to varying degrees, resist photochemical, biological, and chemical degradation.
personal protective equipment (PPE)	Apparatuses designed to protect employees from serious workplace injuries or illnesses resulting from contact with chemical, radiological, physical, electrical, mechanical, or other workplace hazards.
pesticide	Any substance or mixture of substances intended for preventing, destroying, repelling, or mitigating pests. Also, any substance or mixture intended for use as a plant regulator, defoliant, or desiccant.
pests	Unwanted organisms such as insects, rodents, and weeds.
photoallergy	A type of dermatitis that is activated by sunlight, which sensitizes the skin to allergens.
phototoxicity	A severe reaction to sunlight that occurs sometimes in conjunction with drugs (e.g., antibiotics and diuretics) that a person may be taking.
phthalates	A class of plasticizer that is used to increase the flexibility of plastics; also used as additives in cosmetics, aspirin, and insecticides.
plasticizer	A substance that is added during the manufacture of a plastic to make it more pliable and softer.
pneumoconiosis	The accumulation of dust in the lungs and the tissue reactions to its presence. For the purpose of this definition, "dust" is meant to be an aerosol composed of solid inanimate particles.
point prevalence	All cases of a disease that exist at a particular point in time relative to a specific population from which the cases are derived.
poison	Any agent capable of producing a deleterious response in a biological system.
policy cycle	The distinct phases involved in the policy-making process; comprises five stages: (1) problem definition, formulation, and reformulation; (2) agenda setting; (3) policy establishment (i.e., adoption and legislation); (4) policy implementation; and (5) policy assessment.
polluter-pays principle	States that the polluter should bear the expenses of carrying out pollution prevention and control measures.

pollution	The introduction into the natural environment by humans of substances, materials, or energy that cause hazards to human health, harm to living resources and ecological systems, and damage to structures and amenities, or that interfere with the legitimate uses of the environment.
polychlorinated biphenyls (PCBs)	Classified as dioxin-like chemicals, these substances comprise an extensive class of organochlorines.
polycyclic aromatic hydrocarbons (PAHs)	A group of over 100 different chemicals that are formed during the incomplete burning of coal, oil and gas, garbage, or other organic substances such as tobacco or charbroiled meat.
population at risk	Those members of the population who are capable of developing the disease or condition being studied.
population dynamics	The ever-changing interrelationships among the set of variables that influence the demographic makeup of populations as well as the variables that influence the growth and decline of population sizes.
potentiation	One chemical that is not toxic causes another chemical to become more toxic.
precautionary principle	States that preventive, anticipatory measures should be taken when an activity raises threats of harm to the environment, wildlife, or human health, even if some cause-and-effect relationships are not fully established.
preservatives	Additives to foods that act as antimicrobial agents and antioxidants, retard spoiling by microbial agents, prevent fats and oils from becoming rancid, and prevent cut fresh fruits from turning brown.
prevalence	The number of existing cases of a disease, health condition, or deaths in a population at some designated time.
prevention strategies	Methods to prevent the occurrence of future injuries.
problem definition	The process of gathering data and analyzing datasets for patterns and trends in order to prevent injuries.
protective factors	Variables that reduce the probability of an injury.
public health surveillance	The ongoing systematic collection, analysis, and interpretation of health data essential to the planning, implementation, and evaluation of public health practices, closely integrated with the timely dissemination of these data to those who need to know.
radiation	Energy traveling through space. Some types of radiation associated with radioactivity are alpha and beta particles and gamma and X-rays. Radiation also includes neutrons, which are uncharged.
radio frequency (RF) radiation	Occurs when an electric charge alternates (oscillates back and forth) very rapidly in a radio antenna to produce radio waves, which move at the speed of light.
radioactivity	The spontaneous emission of radiation from the nucleus of an unstable atom. As a result of this emission, the radioactive atom is converted, or decays, into an atom of a different element that might or might not be radioactive.
radioisotope	A natural or artificially produced isotope that is radioactive.
radiological dispersal device (RDD)	Combines a conventional explosive, such as dynamite, with radioactive material; commonly known as a dirty bomb.
radionuclide	An atom that has an unstable nucleus; when a radionuclide decays, it can emit X- or gamma rays and/or subatomic particles.
recycling	The process of minimizing waste generation by recovering and reprocessing usable products that might otherwise become waste (e.g., recycling of aluminum cans, paper, and bottles).

relative risk (RR)	The ratio of the incidence rate of a disease or health outcome in an exposed group to the incidence rate of the disease or condition in a nonexposed group; the measure of association between exposure and outcome used in cohort studies.
rem (roentgen equivalent in man)	A measure of radiation dose related to biological effect (i.e., the equivalent dose or effective dose). A rem is a measure of dose deposited in body tissue, averaged over the mass of the tissue of interest. One rem is approximately the dose from any radiation corresponding to one roentgen of gamma radiation.
renewable water	Freshwater that is continuously replenished by the hydrological cycle for withdrawal within reasonable time limits; includes water in rivers, lakes, or reservoirs that fill from precipitation or runoff.
risk	The likelihood of experiencing an adverse effect.
risk assessment	The process of determining risks to health attributable to environmental or other hazards; involves (1) hazard assessment, (2) dose–response assessment, (3) exposure assessment, and (4) risk characterization.
risk management	The adoption of steps to eliminate identified risks or lower them to acceptable levels (often as determined by a government agency that has taken into account input from the public).
runoff	Water originating as precipitation on land that then runs off the land into rivers, streams, and lakes, eventually reaching the oceans, inland seas, or aquifers, unless it evaporates first.
septic system	A "well" that is used to emplace sanitary waste below the surface and typically comprises a tank and subsurface fluid distribution system or disposal system.
sewage	The wastewater generated by people in homes and businesses.
SI (System International) units	International System of Units, which has been implemented more recently than the common units system for measurement of radiation.
sick building syndrome (SBS)	A situation in which building occupants experience acute health and comfort effects that appear to be linked to time spent in a building, but no specific illness or cause can be identified.
sister chromatid exchange (SCE)	A reciprocal exchange of DNA between a pair of DNA molecules.
smog	A mixture of pollutants, principally ground-level ozone, produced by chemical reactions in the air among certain chemicals (e.g., volatile organic chemicals).
smog complex	Symptoms associated with smog, including eye irritation, irritation of the respiratory tract, chest pains, cough, shortness of breath, nausea, and headache.
social environment	Influences upon the individual that arise from societal and cultural factors.
solvent	A liquid substance capable of dissolving other substances.
source reduction	Reduction of the amount of waste created, reusing waste whenever possible, and then recycling what is left.
source water	The untreated and unfiltered water in rivers, streams, lakes, and aquifers from which water utilities draw water to be treated, filtered, and tested to produce drinking water.
spectrum of toxic dose	The toxicity or hazards that are related to exposure to a particular chemical.
sulfur dioxide (SO_2)	Gas produced by burning sulfur contaminants in fuel (such as coal).
Superfund	A federal fund provided through the Comprehensive Environmental Response, Compensation, and Liability Act (CERCLA) to clean up uncontrolled or abandoned hazardous-waste sites, as well as accidents, spills, and other emergency releases of pollutants and contaminants into the environment.

surface water	Water from lakes, streams, rivers, and surface springs.
surveillance system	The systematic gathering of information about the occurrence of diseases, injuries, and other health phenomena.
synergism	As applied to toxicology, indicates that the combined effect of exposures to two or more chemicals is greater than the sum of their individual effects.
temperature inversion	An atmospheric condition during which a layer of warm air stalls above a layer of cool air that is closer to the surface of the earth.
threshold	As applied to toxicology, the lowest dose of a chemical at which a particular response may occur.
threshold limit value (TLV)	Refers to airborne concentrations of substances and represents conditions under which it is believed that nearly all workers may be unaffected.
total fertility rate (TFR)	A hypothetical estimate of completed fertility; indicates how many births a woman would have by the end of her reproductive life.
toxic agent	A material or factor that can be harmful to biological systems.
toxic substance	A material that has toxic properties.
toxicants	Toxic substances that are man-made or result from human (anthropogenic) activity.
toxicity	The degree to which something is poisonous; denotes the amount of a substance that can produce a deleterious effect.
toxicologist	Scientist who investigates in living organisms the adverse effects of chemicals (including their cellular, biochemical, and molecular mechanisms of action) and assesses the probability of the occurrence of such effects.
toxicology	The study of the adverse effects of chemicals on living organisms.
toxin	Usually refers to a toxic substance made by living organisms including reptiles, insects, plants, and microorganisms.
trace metals	See definition for essential metals.
trichloroethylene (TCE)	A grease-dissolving solvent that evaporates readily; added to some cleaning agents, paint removers, and adhesives.
ultraviolet radiation (UVR)	A form of nonionizing radiation in the optical range. Sources of UVR include the sun, welders' arcs, lamps used for tanning beds, and some flood lamps used in photography.
unintentional injury	An injury or poisoning that is not inflicted on purpose. This category includes those injuries and poisonings described as unintended or "accidental," regardless of whether the injury was inflicted by oneself or by another person.
vector	An insect or any living carrier that transports an infectious agent from an infected individual or its wastes to a susceptible individual or its food or immediate surroundings.
vector-borne infection	A type of infection transmitted by a vector; the several classes of vector-borne infections are determined by the interaction among the infectious agent, the human host, and the vector.
volatile organic compounds (VOCs)	Organic compounds (often in paints and solvents) that easily become vapors or gases. Along with carbon, they contain one or more elements such as hydrogen, oxygen, fluorine, chlorine, bromine, sulfur, and nitrogen.
waste	In the context of solid or liquid waste disposal, any material perceived to be of negative value.
water reservoir	An artificial lake, produced by constructing physical barriers across flowing rivers, which allows the water to pool.
water scarcity	An annual supply of renewable freshwater less than 1,000 cubic meters per person.

water stress	An annual supply of renewable freshwater between 1,000 and 1,700 cubic meters per person.
water withdrawal	Removal of freshwater for human use from any natural source or reservoir, such as a lake, river, or aquifer.
waterborne diseases	Conditions that are transmitted through the ingestion of contaminated water, which acts as the passive carrier of the infectious agent.
wetlands	Swamps, bogs, marshes, mires, lagoons, and floodplains.
widespread adoption	Dissemination of prevention strategies on a broad scale.
xenobiotics	Chemical substances that are foreign to the biological system; they include naturally occurring compounds, drugs, environmental agents, carcinogens, and insecticides.
x-rays	Penetrating electromagnetic radiation whose wavelengths are shorter than those of visible light.
zoonosis	An infection or infectious disease transmissible under natural conditions from vertebrate animals to humans.

Index

Exhibits, figures, and tables are indicated by exh, f, and t following the page numbers.